Critical Care And Hospitalist Medicine

Made Ridiculously Simple

Michael Donahoe, M.D.
Professor of Medicine
Division of Pulmonary, Allergy, and Critical Care Medicine
University of Pittsburgh School of Medicine and UPMC

Mark T. Gladwin, M.D.
Chair of the Department of Medicine
Director, Pittsburgh Heart, Lung, Blood and Vascular Medicine Institute
Division of Pulmonary, Allergy, and Critical Care Medicine,
University of Pittsburgh School of Medicine and UPMC

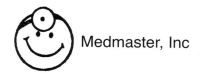

Medmaster, Inc

Critical Care and Hospitalist Medicine Made Ridiculously Simple aims at current approaches to intensive care problems. However, since guidelines may change, please confirm with the latest literature and pharmacologic manufacturer recommendations for evaluation and treatment.

ISBN 13: 978-1-935660-34-7

Made in the United States of America
Published by
MedMaster, Inc.
P.O. Box 640028
Miami, FL 33164

Contents

Introduction

In the olden days, the hospital was a place for many different types of patients with a broad range of disease severity. Many patients were not very sick, waiting for access to the CT machine, waiting for a particular elective procedure, or monitoring many days after an acute illness. Times have changed dramatically. *In today's world, the hospital is one big intensive care unit.* Patients are rapidly moved to home care, a medical home environment or a skilled care facility, leaving behind only the unstable patients, particularly in large referral centers. In this new world, if you see patients in the hospital, you will need to have critical care medicine skills and knowledge.

This book has been conceived with this new world in mind, with the idea that the contents will form a strong base of logically organized knowledge of critical care medicine that will be useful for the intensivist, hospitalist, internist, specialist, and community physician charged with the care of the sick hospitalized patient.

Similar to **Microbiology Made Ridiculously Simple**, the information is organized in a logical conceptual manner, using plain English for rapid assimilation of information, and focusing on critical facts and approaches required to keep the critically ill patient alive and thriving. This book is designed to provide both introductory information as well as a complete base of knowledge that will be useful for all levels of the trainee from medical student, to resident, to fellow, to practicing hospitalist and intensivist. We fully expect this book to provide a solid foundation to enhance the practice of critical care and hospitalist medicine.

Both of us have practiced and taught critical care medicine and hospital-based medicine for decades and bring this experience, and a healthy sense of humor, to this new book. We hope that it will help you save lives and develop confidence, comfort, and expertise in the "combat" environment of the modern hospital.

Mark T. Gladwin, MD

Michael Donahoe, MD

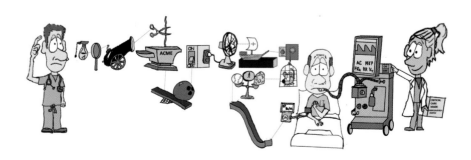

Contributors

The Illustrator

Physician by day, cartoonist by night, Jonathan Gotfried is an attending gastroenterologist in Philadelphia, PA, where he lives with his wife and three children. He started drawing cartoons as a memory aid during anatomy lab in medical school and continues to use his illustrations when teaching medical students, residents, and fellows.

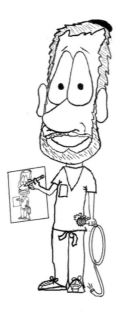

The Consultant for Point of Care Ultrasound (POCUS)

Dr. Phil Lamberty is the Director of the MICU at Presbyterian University Hospital. He has a lifelong commitment to the education and training of medical students, housestaff, and fellows. His particular focus is point of care ultrasound, and he is recognized for his expertise and enthusiasm in the application of this diagnostic tool in the critically ill patient population.

1

The Art of the Patient Presentation

1.1 Welcome to Acute Hospital Medicine

Let's start by giving you a patient with eight different medical problems, 10-20 data inputs per problem, ten minutes to synthesize and present the information to a large crowd, about 30-45 seconds to make a handful of critical decisions, and then.... Let's move on to the next patient. *Whew! How do you get this all organized?* Despite the intensity of the process, a hospital rotation is a critical time in your training experience because you will learn to organize and present patient information quickly and efficiently. The experience will train you to approach organ system problems logically, make efficient and hard decisions, and study the pathophysiology and anatomy of human disease.

Patient rounds function as a time for health professionals to come together to develop an integrated patient care plan, improve the quality of patient care, share information, address patient problems, plan and evaluate treatment, and provide learning opportunities for staff. Patient rounds have been called "storytelling events" because they inject (narrative) structure into the working day and educational and supervisory relationships. Think of yourself as a "storyteller" with facts.

The teaching effectiveness of rounds is critically dependent on compact, organized patient presentations from the house officer. As a physician in any discipline, the ability to briefly present a patient's history, problems, and plan of action is highly valued. This skill is ever more important in our current era of medical shifts and frequent "hand-offs" of information. Much like a pilot running a checklist prior to takeoff, this information transfer improves care and saves lives. From a more selfish point of view, your ability to present information will be one of the most common ways you are evaluated and judged by your peers and professors. Repeated presentations to different physicians are a good tool to refine those skills. Your initial presentations will be slow and disorganized. But with persistence, your efficiency will improve over your training period. The patients are complex with multi-organ system problems, and the ability to synthesize this at times overwhelming amount of information is initially intimidating. Here are a few suggestions to help you organize your presentations.

1.2 How To Summarize Your Patient

As a storyteller. You don't need to include every specific element of your story unless the information is critical to the story. Learn to summarize patients quickly, and then move to the critical elements of the day, using a more structured format. A typical "equation" for this summary is:

Age + Gender + key past medical history + presenting with chief complaint of X + a short 3-5 point list of major signs, symptoms and lab abnormalities

For example:

"Mr. Jones is a 65-year-old male with a past medical history of coronary artery disease, adult-onset diabetes, and coronary

artery bypass with an aortic valve replacement in 2010, who presents with a chief complaint of severe dyspnea, and arrives in the ICU status post-intubation in the emergency department with diffuse rales, peripheral edema, diffuse pulmonary infiltrates on chest radiograph, and an increased creatinine level of 3.5."

As the diagnoses during the ICU or hospital stay become clear, the items on the list can be replaced by more concrete diagnoses:

"with a new diagnosis of congestive heart failure with an ejection fraction of 35%, a new anterior wall motion abnormality, and cardiorenal syndrome."

As you will see, the presentation becomes a language of its own, replete with abbreviations denoting the more common medical diagnoses and disease signs and symptoms.

1.3 Structure Those Random Thoughts

In the ICU setting, clinicians prefer a system-based or organ-based approach to presentation. Alternatively, some physicians use a problem-based approach. The method is less important than working consistently. You must develop the skill to organize complex information, and a consistent approach will help this happen and will help you to avoid missing critical patient details. With each organ-system or problem-based discussion, begin to group relevant pieces of the physical exam, laboratory data, and patient data. This will not only help your presentation, but will also help you organize your decision-making for the care of your patient.

One easy way to remember this is to start from the top of the head and move down: head (neurologic), chest (respiratory and cardiovascular), infectious disease (hits the center of the body!), abdomen (renal, GI and endocrine), and skin (integument) (**Figure 1-1**). Always finish off with prophylaxis and family communication. If you really want to make friends, at the end of every presentation turn to your team and ask: "Any other input from nursing, respiratory therapy, or from the pharmacy?" An outline to get you started is shown in **(Figure 1-2)**.

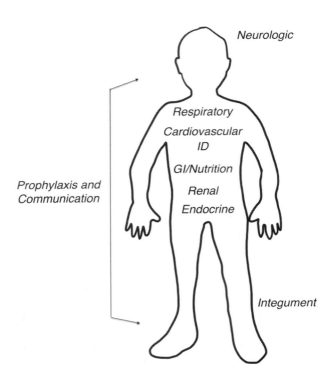

Figure 1-1 A structure for a system based patient presentation.

System	Problem-Based	Items to Include
Neurologic	Delirium	Signs of consciousness (eye-opening, motor responses, vocal responses), lateralizing signs, sedative and relaxant medication and dosing, intracranial pressure (ICP), external ventricular drain, CT scan, EEG
Respiratory	Acute Respiratory Failure	Type of airway, patency, tracheobronchial secretions, cough, ventilator settings, ABG, weaning progress and plans
Cardiovascular	Septic Shock	Vital signs, vasoactive medications and dose. Fluid input and output (balance) from all sites
Infectious Disease	Streptococcal Bacteremia	Culture results and sensitivities, antibiotics with day and duration, antibiotic drug levels
GI/Nutrition	Malnutrition	Feeding method, tolerance, bowel function
Renal/ Electrolyte	Acute Renal Insufficiency	Urine output, creatinine, indications for hemodialysis, measures of renal function and electrolytes
Endocrine	Diabetes Mellitus	Glucose levels and management
Integument	Decubitus Ulcer	Wound care
Prophylaxis and Maintenance	Prophylaxis and Maintenance	Deep vein thrombosis (DVT) and GI prophylaxis. Tubes, lines, catheters with duration and ability to remove
Communication	Communication	Family meetings

Figure 1-2 Organization for patient history presentation.

1.4 Think Data—Diagnosis—Direction

Whether using a problem-based or system-based approach, each item should be approached using the 3 *D's* of *Data, Diagnosis,* and *Direction* (**Figure 1-3**). With each problem or organ system summary you move in steps:

- Summarize the *DATA* relative to that specific problem.
- Conclude about your working *DIAGNOSIS.*
- Provide your *DIRECTION* for patient care on that day.

There are critical pieces of data for each system that are required to make decisions. For example, the blood gas values are not helpful unless you know the ventilator settings (respiratory rate, TV, PEEP and FiO_2), and the blood pressure is not helpful if you do not know what type and dose of vasopressor a patient is getting. Your attending may become annoyed by a presentation that includes: "the vital signs are stable with MAP of 73 and HR of 67." One patient is on no vasopressors and is having a good urine output while another patient is on an infusion of 0.5 mcg/kg/min norepinephrine and has no urine output. Very different patient with the same vital signs!

It is OK to make a mistake in your conclusions and to have your attending or team modify your proposed plan. But these are your patients, and you should assume responsibility for their care. Your analysis of the problem and plan may not be correct, but the repeated exercise

will quickly improve your assessment skills with time. Close the loop with each system with a diagnosis and plan for the day.

You will also find that when you first see an ICU patient, the information is overwhelming: Drugs hanging on pumps, ventilator at the bedside with hundreds of values, hemodynamic monitoring, lots of lines and tubes, and thousands of lab values. By approaching your evaluation of the patient by system, and one by one organizing your data, establishing your diagnosis and generating a direction of care, you will find the complexity will melt away!

You will learn a new language with lots of "shorthand" used during ICU presentations. **Figure 1-4** will help you define some of these abbreviations.

1.5 A Sample Presentation

Here is an example of a patient presentation to help you. *We wrote it so it must be right!!*

Our patient has Staphylococcus endocarditis and ARDS. We will start with a brief introduction about who the patient is:

Mr. Jones is a 47 yo male intravenous drug abuser, who presents with Staph aureus aortic valve endocarditis, septic shock, and evolving ARDS.

Summarize important events overnight:

Events overnight included a trip to the CT scanner and an episode of atrial fibrillation requiring a change of vasopressors from norepinephrine to neosynephrine and addition of amiodarone. He converted after the interventions.

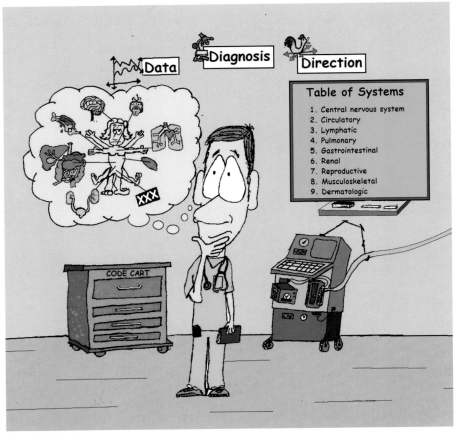

Figure 1-3 *Organize your random thoughts around Data-Diagnosis-Direction.*

Summarize your three D's (Data, Diagnosis, and Direction) by system:

I will review his physical examination, laboratory results, therapies and plan by system.

From a neurological standpoint Mr. Jones is currently sedated on 100 micrograms of fentanyl and 2 mg of midazolam, with a Riker scale of 3. His pupils are equally round and reactive to light, and he moves all extremities to deep pressure.

His head CT is normal, and a lumbar puncture was normal. We are currently stopping sedation daily to assess his level of consciousness but are not ready to stop sedation secondary to his severe ARDS and high pressure and PEEP requirements. No further action is necessary today.

From a respiratory standpoint, the patient is intubated and sedated secondary to his sepsis. Mr. Jones' lung examination reveals coarse rhonchi anteriorly with no wheezes. He has clear thin white and minimal secretions and is synchronizing well with the ventilator. His oxygen saturation is 92% on the current ventilator settings of FiO2 of 0.70, PEEP of 15, respiratory rate of 30, and tidal volume of 420 ml. His settings are unchanged since yesterday. His blood gas is 7.35, $PaCO_2$ of 50 and PaO_2 of 63. His chest radiograph today reveals diffuse alveolar opacities in all lung fields, which are stable compared with yesterday's film with no effusions and normal cardiac size, and the tubes are in good positions. My impression is that he has ARDS with no evidence of seeding of his Staph aureus to the lung. We continue to manage him with our ARDS protocol of 6 cc of tidal volume per kg of ideal body weight. He is not ready to wean now based on his high oxygen and PEEP requirements. Our goal today is to wean his oxygen as tolerated and maintain his sedation.

From a cardiac standpoint, he has Staph aureus bacteremia, which I will discuss under the infectious disease system. His vital signs reveal a heart rate of 74 in normal sinus rhythm on an amiodarone drip and a MAP of 67 on 0.5 mcg/kg/min mcg per minute of neosynephrine. We have been unable to wean the neosynephrine overnight. His last trans-esophageal echocardiogram revealed no evidence of abscess in the aortic valve but he has a 0.25 cm vegetation on the valve. The valve is still functional with no aortic insufficiency. CT surgery is on board as are the Infectious disease consultants. With preserved MAP and good urine output we can continue to manage him medically with antibiotics. Our plan for the day is to stop the amiodarone and wean the neosynephrine as tolerated for a MAP greater than 65 mm Hg.

From an infectious disease standpoint, the patient has methicillin sensitive Staph aureus and is currently on day number three of intravenous nafcillin. His blood cultures were all positive for Staph aureus, so we have discontinued his cefepime and vancomycin. He has no current evidence of embolic disease to the extremities or lungs and we are monitoring with daily physical examination. We will repeat his blood cultures today to make sure they are now negative and continue to appreciate input from our infectious disease consultants.

And this should continue for each system: ***Data, Diagnosis, and Direction...***

Note you must make judgments about what data to cover in what system. You can more clearly communicate if you tell people your plan: "He has Staph aureus bacteremia, which I will discuss under the infectious disease system."

When you first present a complex ICU patient, it is helpful to write your data, diagnosis and direction down for each system. As you gain experience, you will be more efficient.

Here Is What They Say	Here Is What They Mean
ATN	Acute tubular necrosis
ARDS	Adult respiratory distress syndrome
Day #	Usually refers to the number of days a patient has received a medication
Effusions	Pleural effusions
FiO_2	Fraction of inspired oxygen
GCS	Glascow coma score
HR	Heart rate
I/O	Refers to fluid balance (intake and output)
Lines	Central and peripheral venous catheters
MAP	Mean arterial pressure
PEEP	Positive end-expiratory pressure
Pressors	Vasopressors
RR	Respiratory rate
Temp	Temperature
Tubes	Endotracheal tube and/or nasogastric tube
Tubed	Patient was intubated

Figure 1-4 *Common "medical speak" and definitions.*

2

Acute Care Chest Radiology

The goal of this chapter is to introduce you to the necessary nuts and bolts of reading a chest X-ray and lung CT scan during hospital rounds. Our goal is to teach you the top ten most essential X-ray problems you will see. The portable digitalized chest radiograph you will get is one of the most basic of studies. Because the X-ray beam shoots from the front of the chest to the plate on the back, this study will magnify the anterior mediastinum and make the heart look bigger than it should. It will also make the definition of structures a little fuzzy. Worse yet, the typical sick hospital patient chest X-ray kind of looks like a sandstorm in Afghanistan, and only gets worse in the sicker patient. What is the point of this film? There are three main things you want from this film:

1. *Diagnosis.* The X-ray helps make a basic diagnosis: Is this heart failure, ARDS, pneumonia, pneumothorax, effusion, etc.?
2. *Progression.* Are we getting worse or better? Are infiltrates progressing? Is the pneumothorax resolving?
3. *Tubes and Disasters.* The safe location of the spaghetti salad of endotracheal tubes, central lines, feeding tubes and surgical drains has to be examined. Also, the X-ray helps you keep an eye out for disasters. The portable film may be your first look at a new pneumothorax, subcutaneous air, tube migration, increasing effusion or infiltrates, and a collapsed lobe or lung.

As you learn to read a chest X-ray on rounds, you can run through these three elements so as not to miss anything: Diagnosis? Progression? Tubes and disasters?

2.1 Basics of Reading Portable Chest Radiographs

2.1.1 Is the Radiograph Worth Reading?

First things first: Is the CXR any good? Does the film capture the entire thorax and include the costophrenic angle? Is the film under-exposed or underpenetrated? Both problems will give you a whiter film, and both might make lung infiltrates look worse. This is not a problem with CT scans, which have their own problems!

- *Under-exposed.* Look at the armpit area of soft tissues. If you are comparing yesterday's and today's film, you want the soft tissues to look about the same. If the soft tissues are very white, this can suggest that the film was under-exposed.
- *Under-penetrated.* Look at the spine behind the heart. If you can see the vertebra, the radiograph is well penetrated. You should make sure the penetration is similar in today's and yesterday's film. If you can only see vertebra, you have fried right through the heart and might not be able to see infiltrates, line position, etc.

- *CT scan motion artifacts.* If a patient is breathing rapidly or moves in the CT scanner, the image can look blurry. This movement can make it difficult to define heart or vessel borders and may give the appearance of more infiltrates in the lung parenchyma than there should be.

Figure 2-1 shows two portable chest radiographs in the same patient over 24 hours. The right panel is underexposed compared to the left panel, giving the appearance of worsening pulmonary infiltrates. The patient was clinically unchanged.

Figure 2-2 is an underpenetrated portable chest radiograph. Note the spine detail is poorly visualized

A CT scan "slice" can integrate images over a range of thicknesses, for example from 1 cm to as thin as 0.5 mm. A thicker cut will provide a more blurred image as the cut will integrate proximal structures, from the air in alveoli to blood in the vasculature. A thin or high-resolution cut will provide the clearest image of alveolar septae, nodules, air bronchograms, emphysematous changes, and other smaller details. **Figure 2-3** shows motion artifact in the lower lung zones on the representative CT image.

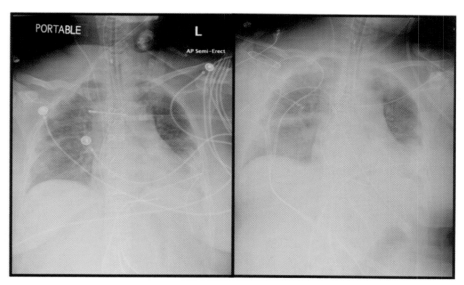

Figure 2-1 Underexposed image (right panel) compared to baseline (left panel).

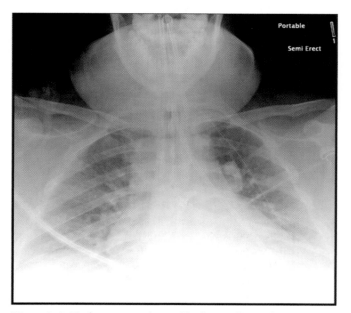

Figure 2-2 Underpenetrated portable chest radiograph.

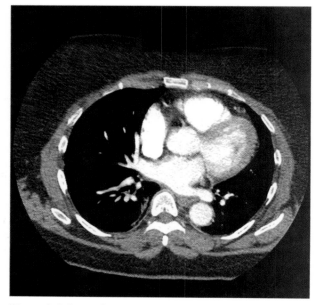

Figure 2-3 Lower lung zone motion artifact.

2.1.2 Ignore the Most Interesting Findings

The first thing that you will be tempted to look at in the CCU is the heart, and the first thing in the MICU is the lung. Stop yourself, take a deep breath, and first look at the soft tissue and bones. Remember that the best way to read a chest X-ray is to move from the outside inward. The soft tissue can reveal asymmetry to suggest tissue swelling or a hematoma. An essential thing to look for is subcutaneous air, which dissects along the rib cage or can make the skin look like it has black waves or is streaky (**Figure 2-4).**

Look for lines of air around the heart or aortic root (pneumomediastinum) or under the diaphragm. Free abdominal air is suggested by a radiolucency under the hemidiaphragm (**Figure 2-5**). If in a tuberculosis or fungal endemic area, look for calcified supraclavicular lymph nodes (so-called Kings Evil or Scrofula).

Examine the bones for missing ribs, fractures to suggest a traumatic lung contusion, a rib that is missing to suggest old surgery or an osteoclastic malignant process eating away at the bone (multiple myeloma). Now you can start moving in.

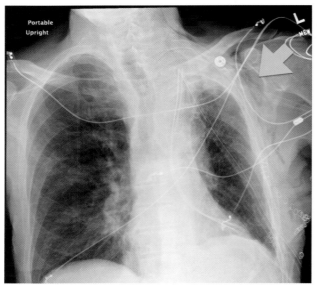

Figure 2-4 Subcutaneous air outside the left upper chest (yellow arrow).

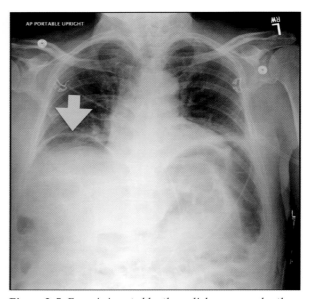

Figure 2-5 Free air is noted by the radiolucency under the right hemidiaphragm (yellow arrow).

2.1.3 Get to the Heart of the Matter

The heart is magnified in an AP (anteroposterior) or portable film, so a large heart can fool you. In general, the heart should be less than half the width of the thorax as defined by the distance between lateral ribs. **Figure 2-6** outlines the heart silhouette and the structures. Starting at the top right (patient's left) is the aortic arch, which can be enlarged with an aortic dissection, then the aortopulmonary window, which can be full of lymph nodes from cancer or sarcoidosis. Then the pulmonary artery, which is enlarged in pulmonary hypertension, hilar lymph nodes, then the left ventricular border, which can be enlarged in heart failure. Starting at the upper left (patient's right) is the superior vena cava running into the azygous vein just above the right

mainstem bronchus. The azygous vein can be enlarged in heart failure or fluid overload. Moving downward is the right atrial wall.

Note that you cannot see the right ventricle on an AP film. The right ventricle is only evident on a lateral view where the anterior shadow under the sternum is caused by the right ventricle, and if normal in size, should only occupy about 2/3 of the space below the sternum (**Figure 2-7**). The left atrium can barely be seen on an AP film, if at all. Its size can be estimated by its pushing against the right and left mainstem bronchi to push them up to make the carina more of an obtuse angle.

One should also take a good look at the trachea. It is a clear empty structure running down to the carina, where it separates into the left and right main stem bronchi.

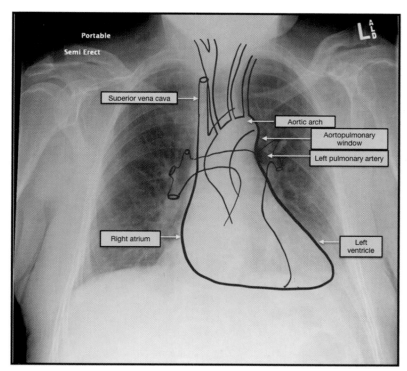

Figure 2-6 *Portable chest radiograph with key structures defined.*

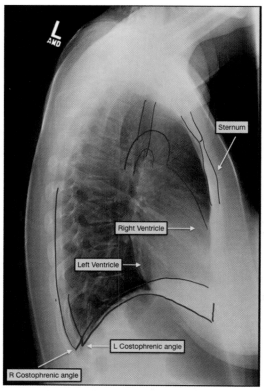

Figure 2-7 *Lateral radiograph with key structures defined.*

A right paratracheal "stripe" is visible along the right side of the trachea on a frontal chest X-ray and represents the combination of the right tracheal wall, the adjacent pleural surfaces, and any additional mediastinal fat between them. The stripe should be less than 4 mm, and if thickened, suggests that there are enlarged paratracheal nodes, which are common in sarcoidosis.

2.1.4 The Pleural Space and Costophrenic Angles

Next look at the pleural space. You should see sharp angles where the visceral pleura under the ribs meets the diaphragm, at a location called the costophrenic angle. If this is whitened out, it suggests the presence of a pleural effusion (**Figure 2-8**).

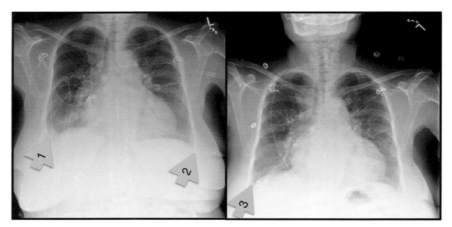

Figure 2-8 *In the left image, the right costophrenic angle is blunted (1) and the left costophrenic angle is normal (2). Following diuresis the right image from the same patient post diuresis now shows a normal right costophrenic angle (3).*

If the costophrenic angle is hyperlucent or black and runs deep into the lateral abdomen, this can suggest a *deep-sulcus sign*, seen in a supine patient with a pneumothorax, where the air moves up above the lower thorax (**Figure 2-9**).

Follow the lines of the diaphragm to look for a sliver of air under the diaphragm (free air in the abdomen)

or a plaque of white calcification (suggestive of asbestosis). If you see bilateral loss of the costophrenic angles and a large heart, this might add weight to a diagnosis of congestive heart failure. If only one side has the loss of the costophrenic angle, you might think of a localized process such as a parapneumonic effusion.

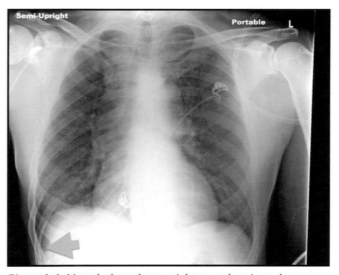

Figure 2-9 *Note the hyperlucent right costophrenic angle consistent with a deep sulcus sign.*

2.1.5 Finally, the Lungs!

Now you can look at the lung itself for *infiltrates*. Usually the lung is black with superimposed silhouettes of the ribs and pulmonary vasculature. You might see areas of patchy or streaky opacities (whiteness) and areas where the opacities blur the normal borders of structures like the left ventricle or right atrium or hilar vasculature. The loss of easily defined heart borders suggests there is an infiltrate that is making the density of the lung equal to the density of the adjoining structures, providing a hint that there is an infiltrate and where the infiltrate is located. Infiltrates just indicate that the density has increased. Infiltrates can be caused by three things:

1. *Alveolar consolidation.* BLOOD, WATER, PUS... This means that the air sacks or alveoli are filled with stuff: blood from pulmonary hemorrhage, inflammatory material (neutrophils, fibrin, bacteria, etc.) or fluid (edema fluid, etc.).
2. *Collapse or atelectasis.* This means the lung has collapsed, making it appear solid. You can have a whole lobe or lung collapse or just segments of the lung.
3. *Pleural fluid.* Enough pleural fluid can make any lung white, which makes you think of infiltrates.

But the opacification is actually outside the lung in the pleural cavity!

How to tell these apart is a critical part of reading an X-ray and will be covered as we talk about the main X-ray problems you will have to know.

2.2 Our Top Ten X-Ray Bad Guys

We picked ten significant things you must be able to diagnose on a CXR. Mastering the *TOP TEN* will set you on your way to clinical excellence. We will start from least essential/least common to the most essential/most common, so if you are in a rush, you should start at the end

2.2.1 #10 Mediastinal and Hilar Masses

The mediastinum can look very big, bulky, and full if there is a mass on one side or both. If on both sides, this suggests sarcoidosis or lymphoma, while if asymmetric, one would worry about a localized cancer, such as lung cancer. **Figure 2-10** and **Figure 2-11** show bilateral hilar adenopathy as seen in sarcoidosis.

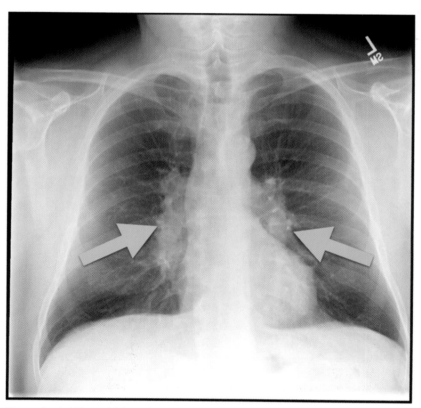

Figure 2-10 *Bilateral hilar adenopathy (arrows).*

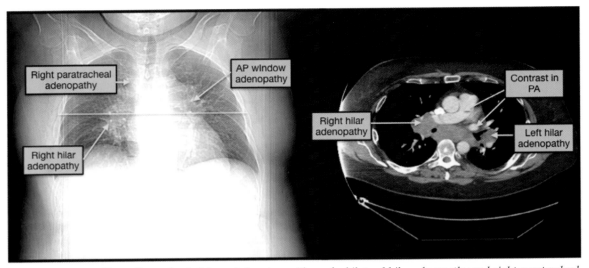

Figure 2-11 *Plain film radiography (left image) showing evidence for bilateral hilar adenopathy and right paratracheal adenopathy. A corresponding CT cross-sectional image at the level of the white line on the plain film radiograph is presented in the right image.*

2.2.2 #9 Pericardial Effusion and Tamponade

A large heart on the plain film radiograph usually indicates a cardiomyopathy with heart failure but look out for a pericardial effusion with possible cardiac tamponade. This could be seen in patients presenting to the ICU with hypotension.

Figure 2-12 shows a 71 yo male presenting with nausea, dyspnea, and worsening renal function.

2.2.3 #8 Pulmonary Hypertension and Pulmonary Emboli

As more patients survive longer with advanced lung diseases like COPD and lung fibrosis, we are seeing more patients with pulmonary hypertension. Pulmonary hypertension is difficult to diagnose on an AP film, but you should look at the left and right main pulmonary arteries. A big hump on the left main pulmonary artery (the hump after the aortic pulmonary window on the left side of the cardiac silhouette) is a giveaway. The right pulmonary artery is seen next to the right main stem bronchus, and the thickness should be less than 1 cm. Pulmonary hypertension is much more apparent on the CT scan when you are looking at the mediastinal vessels. Intravenous contrast will help you identify the aortic root and next to it the main pulmonary artery. While not a very specific finding, if the main pulmonary artery is bigger than the aortic root, this suggests pulmonary hypertension **(Figure 2-13)**.

Pulmonary emboli are seen with CT scan protocols that provide images using a rapid CT scanner during a fast infusion of intravenous contrast. A computer

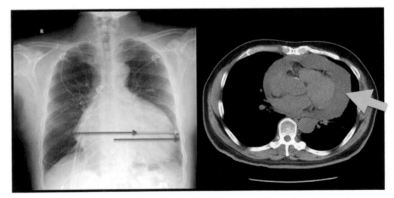

Figure 2-12 *The plain film radiograph (left image) shows an enlarged cardiac silhouette. Note the cardiac dimension (blue plus yellow arrow) is greater in width than ½ the thorax (blue arrow only). The CT scan in this patient (right image) shows a moderate pericardial effusion (large arrow).*

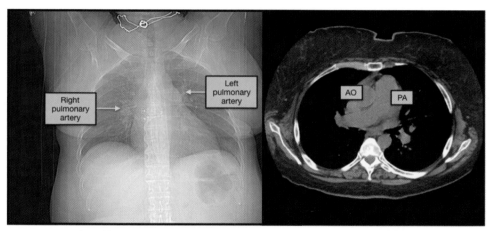

Figure 2-13 Plain film radiograph (left image) of a patient with moderate pulmonary hypertension showing right and left enlarged pulmonary arteries. The CT scan in the same patient (right image) illustrates enlargement of the main pulmonary artery (PA) in comparison to the aorta (AO).

program times the images during the injection of contrast so that more of the contrast is in the pulmonary arteries. Clots appear as space voids (holes) in the contrast. To identify these "defects," you follow the vessel up and down and make sure that a space void falls within the vessel, is seen on multiple cuts/slices, and ideally has contrast above and below the space void. Note the two images in **Figure 2-14,** which look at the contrast "holes" in the right pulmonary artery viewed in two different planes (see arrows).

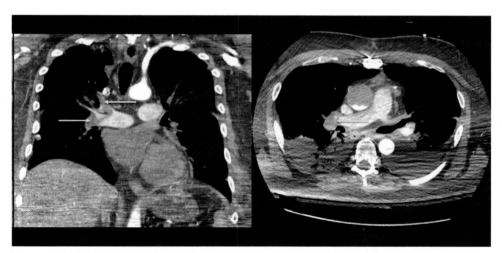

Figure 2-14 The left image demonstrates a sagital CT image with a constrast filling defect in the right pulmonary artery (arrow). A cross-sectional view in the right image shows the same filling defect.

2.2.4 #7 Tube Mishaps

Every time you finish endotracheal intubation, obtain a CXR to make sure the endotracheal tube is in the correct place. A complication occurs when the tube is advanced too far and goes into the right mainstem bronchus **(Figure 2-15)**. This will result in over-aeration of the right lung and collapse of the left lung. If the tube is too far down and past the right upper lobe, this can also cause right upper lobe (RUL) collapse as the RUL takeoff is higher up in the right mainstem bronchus. Other essential tube placements should also be confirmed with each CXR.

Additional "tube" problems are feeding tubes in the esophagus, central lines up the internal jugular vein or out in the arm brachial vein, or, more rarely, lines can go down the chest into the mammary vein **(Figures 2-16 and 2-17)**. A chest tube can be misplaced along the outer rib cage and not even be in the chest.

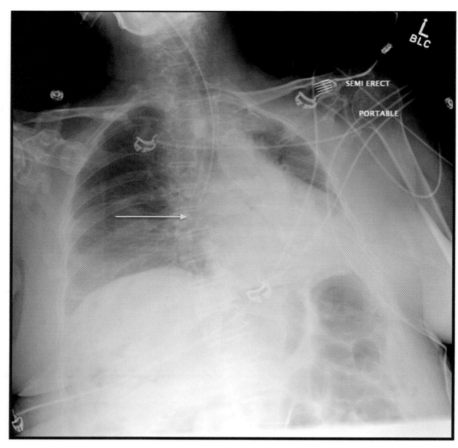

Figure 2-15 *Portable chest radiograph shows right mainstem intubation (arrow) with partial collapse of the left lung and over aeration of the right lung.*

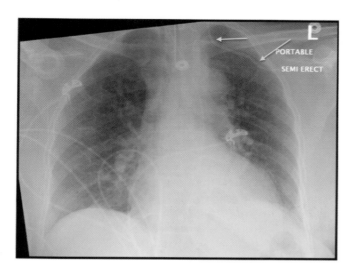

Figure 2-16 *A left subclavian catheter (arrow) has been inadvertently directed up the left internal jugular vein and must be repositioned.*

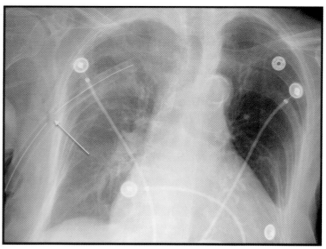

Figure 2-17 *A right sided chest tube (arrow) shows the proximal air port outside the pleural activity.*

2.2.5 #6 Pneumothorax and Barotrauma

Now we are getting to even more life-threatening and common problems. With mechanical ventilation, patients can develop barotrauma and volutrauma, which can both result in a pneumothorax. Air looks blacker and can appear along the mediastinum (mediastinal air), can dissect into the neck and chest subcutaneous tissue (subcutaneous air, which appears wispy or streaky black), and can get into the pleura as a pneumothorax **(Figure 2-18)**.

You must look carefully for a small pneumothorax in all mechanically ventilated patients after placing central lines in the subclavian or internal jugular veins. Look between the ribs for a small line of the pleura **(Figure 2-19, left image)**. A large pneumothorax can cause a tension pneumothorax when the air in the pleural space is large and trapped so that it pushes the lungs and heart over, compressing the vena cava and atrium. A tension pneumothorax reduces venous blood return to the heart and limits cardiac output (hypotension and shock!). Look for the sneaky deep sulcus sign in a recumbent patient, which may be an early sign of a pneumothorax **(Figure 2-19, right image)**. Picking up a deep sulcus sign will impress your attending and save a patient!

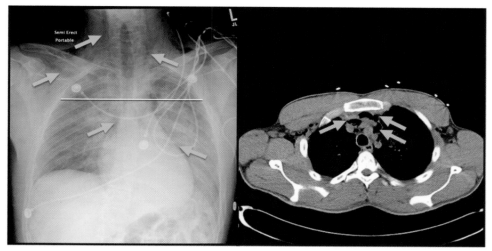

Figure 2-18 *The left image portable chest xray shows evidence for mediastinal and subcutaneous air (arrows) with no proof of a pneumothorax. A CT image (right) from this same patient shows the distribution of the air located primarily in the anterior mediastinum.*

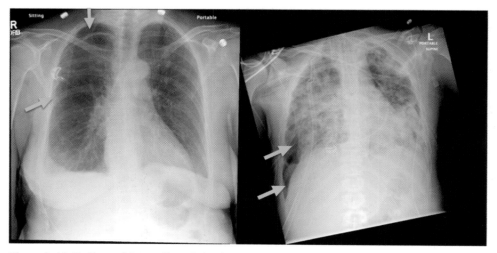

Figure 2-19 *Radiographic manifestations of a pneumothorax. The left image shows a small pneumothorax adjacent to the right rib margin with an apical pleural line (arrows). The right image shows a deep sulcus sign (arrows).*

2.2.6 #5 Effusions, Empyema, and Hemothorax

Fluid in the pleural space can form a clear fluid meniscus, but often shows as a graded opacification as one moves from top to bottom in a portable ICU radiograph. The costo-phrenic angle is blunted.

When an asymmetric effusion is present, it needs to be tapped to sample the fluid to both determine a cause for the effusion and drain a large effusion. A pleural effusion can form because of an imbalance in oncotic and hydrostatic forces. This imbalance in forces results in a transudate since the fluid has low total protein and is not inflamed. The Light's Criteria are the traditional method for defining an exudate vs. a transudate. If the pleural fluid characteristics fulfill any of the exudate criteria in **Figure 2-20**, the fluid is considered an exudate. As outlined in **Figure 2-21**, examples of a transudate include low albumin conditions, such as cirrhosis and protein starvation or malabsorption. Conditions with high hydrostatic pressure, such as congestive heart failure,

can also produce a transudative effusion. An exudative effusion results from inflammation around the pleura with an increase in pleural permeability. Disorders that cause pleural inflammation and exudative effusion include a parapneumonic effusion, a malignant effusion, and lung infarction from a pulmonary embolus.

A few things can cause both an exudative or a transudative effusion. A pulmonary embolus if bad enough causes a lung infarction, and the dying tissue gets leaky and inflamed and causes an exudative effusion, while a pulmonary embolus can also cause right heart failure, which results in decreased drainage of the pleural space to the right heart and causes a hydrostatic transudative effusion. Excessive diuresis of patients with a transudative effusion from congestive heart failure can result in concentration of the effusion until it is a little exudative.

Criteria	Transudate	Exudate
Pleural fluid protein/serum protein ratio	≤ 0.5	> 0.5
Pleural fluid LDH/serum LDH	≤ 0.6	> 0.6
Pleural fluid LDH	< 2/3 upper limit of laboratory normal	> 2/3 upper limit of laboratory normal

Figure 2-20 *Criteria to distinguish a transudative and exudative pleural effusion.*

Transudative Effusions	Exudative Effusions	Either—But Most Commonly Exudative
Congestive heart failure	Parapneumonic effusion	Amyloidosis
Hepatic hydrothorax	Subdiaphragmatic abscess	Chylothorax
Nephrotic syndrome	Esophageal perforation	Constrictive pericarditis
Hypoalbuminemia	Malignancy	Hypothyroidism
Urinothorax	Connective tissue disease	Malignancy
Cerebrospinal fluid leak into the pleural space	Pancreatitis	Pulmonary embolism
Peritoneal dialysis	Meig's syndrome	Sarcoidosis
	Malignant ascites	Superior vena cava obstruction
	Yellow nail syndrome	Trapped lung
	Lymphangioleiomyomatosis	
	Pancreatitis	
	Benign asbestos effusion	
	Uremic pleurisy	
	Postcardiac injury syndrome	

Figure 2-21 *Etiologies of a pleural effusion by classification.*

Parapneumonic effusions lie on the same side as the lung infiltrate. A complicated parapneumonic effusion refers to one that is infected with bacteria (positive Gram stain or culture on the diagnostic tap) or has frank pus in it (empyema) or has so many white cells in it that it causes the pH to be very low (pH < 7.2) in the pleural fluid sample. A parapneumonic effusion may also be loculated (encapsulated in fibrous material). These complicated effusions lie on the same side as the pneumonia and if loculated will not layer when taking an X-ray in different positions (lateral decubitus angle for example). While most pneumonias result in the development of a simple parapneumonic exudative effusion, a complicated pleural effusion may need complete drainage with a chest tube **(Figure 2-22)**.

2.2.7 *#4 Atelectasis and Lobar Collapse*

Atelectasis is a partial or complete collapse of a lung. So, you have an increase in lung opacification because the alveoli and interstitial tissues are all smashed together. The key to the diagnosis of atelectasis is that you must have a shadow (collapsed lung) with evidence of volume loss. You must remember the radiographic signs of volume loss. *There is only one DIRECT SIGN OF VOLUME LOSS, and there are FOUR INDIRECT SIGNS OF VOLUME LOSS*:

Direct sign of volume loss. The lungs are separated into lobes by major fissures. If you can see a major fissure that has moved to make the lobe smaller, this indicates you have volume loss. The trick is that you can only see one of the major fissures on an anterior-posterior (AP) or posterior-anterior (PA) film (films looking at the front of the patient): this is the right middle lobe fissure. If this moves up, the right upper lobe is atelectatic or collapsed, and if it moves down, the right middle lobe or right lower lobes may be collapsed **(Figure 2-23)**. On the lateral CXR you can see the right and left major fissures, and on a CT scan you can see them all.

Figure 2-24 illustrates a right upper lobe collapse. Note the movement of the minor fissure towards the upper mediastinum (arrow #1). Just because you are happy you found the right upper lobe collapse, do not miss the high endotracheal tube (arrow #2) or the vascular catheter coiled in the right subclavian vein. vessel (small arrow).

Indirect signs of volume loss suggest a portion of the lung collapsed. These signs include: 1) elevation of a hemidiaphragm, 2) movement to one side of the mediastinum and heart, 3) narrowing of the rib spaces on one side of the chest, and 4) a relative lucency of the lung next to the atelectatic or collapsed lobe, suggesting it is being pulled to the collapsed side and opened **(Figure 2-25)**.

Patients on mechanical ventilation in the supine position have the heart pushing down on the left lower lobe, which often collapses. This can cause the heart to shift left, the left hemidiaphragm to rise, and the left upper lobe to look more lucent.

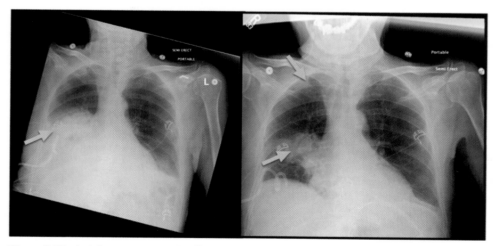

Figure 2-22 *A right parapneumonic effusion (left image) is shown (arrow). In the right image, a drainage catheter partially drained the effusion, but a residual collection remains loculated in the region of the right minor fissure (right image, bottom arrow). The drainage of the effusion has also been associated with incomplete lung re-expansion, which gives the appearance of a small pneumothorax in the lung apex (right image, top arrow).*

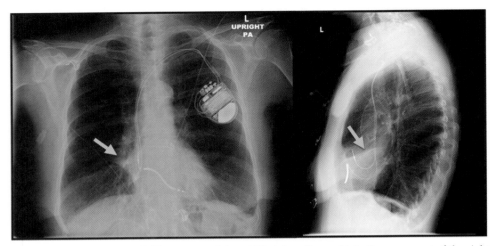

Figure 2-23 *The radiograph illustrates a right middle lobe collapse. Note the movement of the right minor fissure on both the posterior-anterior (PA) (left image) and lateral radiograph (right image). The edge of the fissure is highlighted (arrow).*

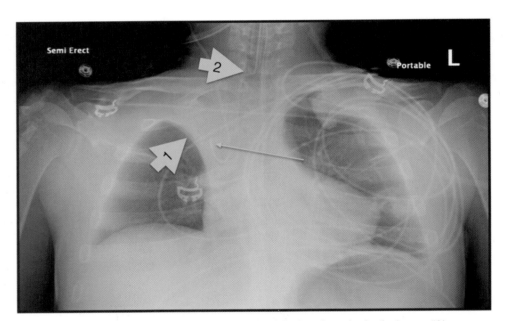

Figure 2-24 *Right upper lobe collapse (arrow #1) with high endotracheal tube (arrow #2) and coiled catheter in subclavian vein (small arrow).*

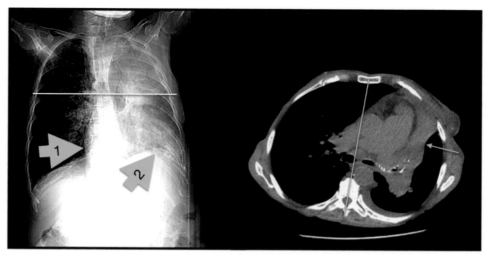

Figure 2-25 *Indirect signs of volume loss with the collapse of the left upper lobe. On the left image, note arrow #1) the shift of the heart and mediastinum to the left chest and arrow #2) the elevation of the left hemidiaphragm to compensate for the volume loss. The right CT image corresponds to the level of the white line on the plain film. Note the movement of the major fissure seen on the CT (arrow) and the shift of the mediastinum and left lower lobe to fill the volume loss created by the collapse of the left upper lobe.*

2.2.8 #3 Congestive Heart Failure

You will often hear your radiologists, attending or fellow, say, "This looks like CHF," but you rarely hear them tell you why they think this. *How do you determine if this fuzzy mess is CHF?!?* A few elements help to make this diagnosis:

- *Hilar prominence and fuzziness.* The hilum usually has crisp blood vessels, meaning every vessel coming from it has a smooth outer vessel wall. With CHF these are fuzzy, looking like someone took an eraser to the edges and rubbed and blurred them. The hilum is also large (a big, blurred, juicy hilum) **(Figure 2-26)**.
- *Acinar shadows.* The acinus is the smallest unit of the alveoli with a feeding terminal respiratory bronchiole. This unit is 1-4 mm and fills with edema fluid giving tiny 1-4 mm blurred dots. As the acini are filled, they form fuzzy opacities. With a good resolution chest radiograph, one can often see these acinar shadows, which look like a stippled pattern made by a paintbrush dabbed in white paint and tapped on black **(Figure 2-27).**
- *Bat wing pulmonary edema and vascular cephalization.* As CHF gets worse, the acinar shadows and hilar prominence coalesce to form hazy opacities that are greater in the center of the hilum than at the pleural edge, giving a butterfly or bat wing appearance **(Figure 2-28)**. If the film is obtained with the patient sitting up, the vasculature can be appearing engorged moving up to the upper lobes, rather than tapering from thick to thin as would be expected. This is called cephalization, meaning thickening of vasculature moving cephalad toward the head.

Other tricks:

- *Septal lines and Kerley B lines.* Fluid will fill the broncho-vascular bundles as the lymphatics engorge and leak. This creates blurry lines coming from the hilum and also septal lines, which are horizontal lines running from the pleural edge inward (these septal lines are also called Kerley A lines). Kerley B lines represent interlobular septa represented by horizontal lines running at the lung periphery to the pleura, usually less than 1 cm in length, and parallel to one another at right angles to the pleura **(Figure 2-29)**.
- *Bronchial wall thickening.* In the upper hilum, especially on the patient's left side, one can find small airways cut on the end that look like a fine ring. With CHF these thicken and can be a nice way to appreciate changes.
- *And of course, a big heart and bilateral effusions.* Don't forget that you want to look for the bad company your disease keeps. Bad guys hang out with bad guys. In other words, CHF is more likely if a big heart and pleural effusions accompany the other radiographic abnormalities of CHF.

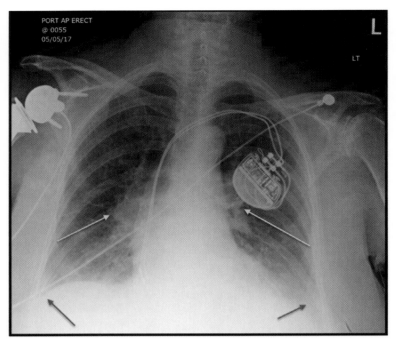

Figure 2-26 *Portable radiograph shows bilateral hilar prominence (yellow arrows) with fuzziness. Note the blunting of both costophrenic angles (red arrows) and the increase in interstitial lung markings. These findings are all consistent with pulmonary edema from congestive heart failure.*

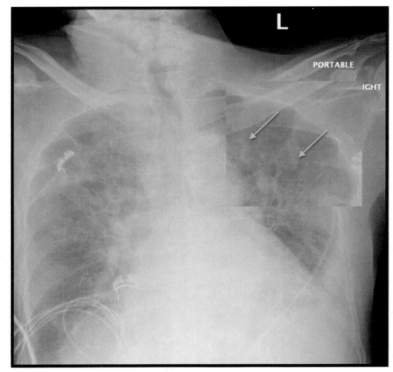

Figure 2-27 *illustrates a patient with pulmonary edema. Note vascular redistribution in the upper lung zones. Acinar shadows are evident in the magnified view of the left upper lobe (arrows).*

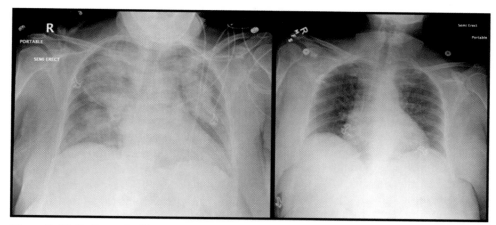

Figure 2-28 *Radiographs illustrate bat wing, butterfly pulmonary edema before (left image) and following 8 days of diuresis (right image).*

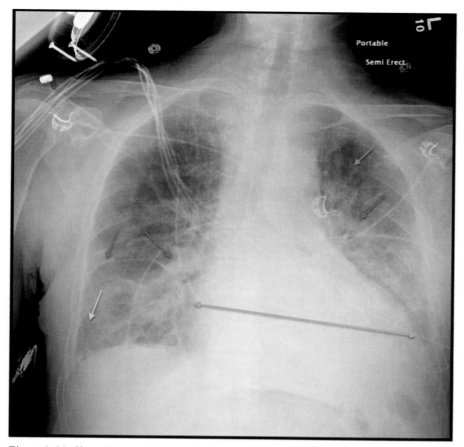

Figure 2-29 *Shows bilateral hilar prominence (red arrows), cardiac enlargement (orange arrow), fluid in the minor fissure (green arrow), Kerley B lines (yellow arrow), and vascular redistribution (blue arrows) – all signs of hydrostatic pulmonary edema.*

2.2.9 #2 Pneumonia

Pneumonia is an infiltrate, usually without volume loss, and may have an associated unilateral effusion. The key to diagnosing pneumonia on the ventilator is the associated clinical signs and symptoms of inflammation and infection such as a new fever, leukocytosis, and increasing quality and quantity of sputum production, often with worsening oxygenation. A pneumonia on CXR will show a hazy to dense infiltrate, often filling specific segments or lobes of the lung. A major indication that one has a pneumonia is that the airways are open and run like dark tubes into the dense white infiltrate. These are called air bronchograms. Because pneumonias consist of alveoli filled with fluid, fibrin, white blood cells and other solid material, the infiltrate has a similar density to that of the tissue structures around it. A pneumonia is suspected with the loss of a distinct border with an adjoining structure (**Figure 2-30**). For example, a basilar infiltrate or pneumonia causes the loss of a clean diaphragm border at the lung base (**Figure 2-31 and 2-32**). Left lower lobe pneumonia is evident by a loss of the diaphragm behind the heart. Right middle lobe pneumonia is suggested by a loss of the right atrial wall line. CT scans are easier to read, and the location can be determined by the airway that leads to the infiltrate. This approach requires knowledge of the airway anatomy, which is beyond the focus of this brief review.

And now! The number one (on our list) radiographic diagnosis in the modern ICU is…

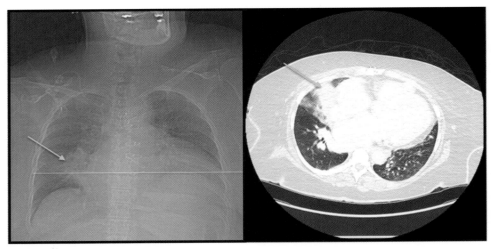

Figure 2-30 *Radiographic findings of a right middle lobe pneumonia (arrow) on CXR showing loss of the right atrial wall border with a corresponding CT image (at level of white line) with infiltrate adjacent to heart border.*

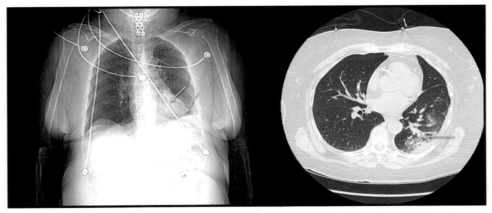

Figure 2-31 *Radiographic signs of a left lower lobe pneumonia. Note rather subtle findings of an elevated left hemidiaphragm with an infiltrate apparent behind the heart. The CT image shows a clear left lower lobe pneumonia with a small adjacent pleural effusion (arrow).*

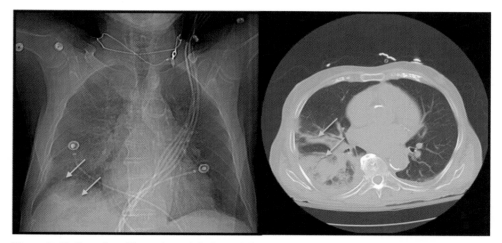

Figure 2-32 *Reveals evidence for a right lower lobe pneumonia on the plain film radiograph (left image). Note the elevated hemidiaphragm and the infiltrate behind the diaphragm on the plain film radiograph (arrows). The chest CT (right image) illustrates the dense right lower lobe consolidation with the presence of air bronchograms (arrows).*

2.2.10 #1 Adult Respiratory Distress Syndrome

ARDS is non-cardiogenic pulmonary edema. In many ways, ARDS looks like CHF but in a patient with normal cardiac function **(Figure 2-33)**. A difference between congestive heart failure with cardiogenic pulmonary edema and ARDS is the anatomical distribution. ARDS tends to be more heterogeneous and patchy, does not have the classic bat wing appearance of cardiogenic pulmonary edema, and should not have evidence of hydrostatic pulmonary edema (cephalization, effusions, cardiac enlargement). A patient can have ARDS with fluid overload, making these distinctions difficult in some patients. On CT scan, ARDS classically shows patchy alveolar consolidation that is often worse in gravity-dependent areas **(Figure 2-34)**. Remember that ARDS can arise from many sources of primary lung injury or systemic disease so that a CXR can start with pneumonia and then progress to ARDS.

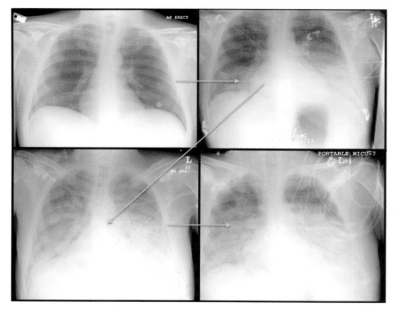

Figure 2-33 *A series of radiographs that illustrate the progression (follow arrows) in a patient presenting with fevers, chills, productive cough. Over 24 hours she rapidly progressed to bilateral airspace infiltrates with normal cardiac function consistent with ARDS.*

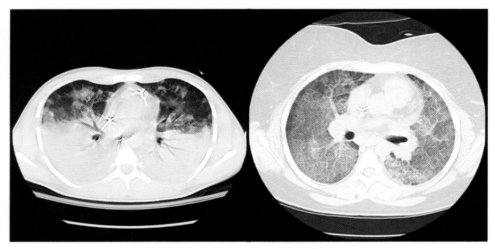

Figure 2-34 *CT images show the appearance of ARDS. The left image is the more common densely consolidated dependent lung infiltrate pattern. The right image is the less common diffuse symmetric infiltrate pattern. Both of these images fit the radiographic definition of ARDS but may represent two very different clinical phenotypes of ARDS.*

Your skills at reading the chest X-ray and CT scan will increase over time with practice and case-by-case instruction. We will provide additional examples related to diseases throughout this book to help you refine your skills and knowledge. Just remember your approach: You are looking to make a *Diagnosis,* establish *Progression,* check on *Tubes and Disasters.* You will do this by starting on the outside and moving in and you will be facing a common top ten list of public enemies *(BAD GUYS)!*

Suggested Reading

- Fraser RS et al. Fraser and Pare's Diagnosis of Diseases of the Chest: 4-Volume Set / Edition 4 1999.

3

Point of Care Ultrasound (POCUS)

Contributed By Phillip Lamberty, MD

You may find that your intensive care unit, emergency department, or floor unit provides an ultrasound (US) machine for central venous catheter placement. If you look closer at the device, you may notice some more probes and buttons, and you may have witnessed a user placing these probes not just on a patient's neck, but on other parts—chest, back, abdomen, even lumbar spine, and eyes. You may have even lifted your butt from your work station and asked the ultrasound operator, "Hmmm, so whatcha doin?" She may have responded, "Since your patient with pneumonia is in shock, I thought I should learn *NOW* if the patient has adequate LV and RV function. I will rule out a pericardial effusion, and make sure the patient has no gross mitral regurgitation. Since you asked, I can tell right *NOW* if your empiric fluid boluses are giving the patient pulmonary edema... I'll also make sure she doesn't have a pleural effusion to aspirate and does not have a proximal deep vein thrombosis." You respond, "I thought I just ordered an ECHO, morning chest X-ray, and lower extremity venous ultrasound studies. They should be ready in the next 24-36 hours. I'll present the data on rounds this week."

So, you get it? Point of care ultrasound (POCUS) gives the bedside practitioner information IMMEDIATELY that can assist with diagnosis, procedural guidance, and management. It complements a thorough history and exam. We're not talking extensive studies here.

We don't have the time to spend an hour in the room doing triphasic US studies of both lower extremities. In this chapter, we will review some common scenarios where POC ultrasound can aid and assist management.

3.1 The Three Goals of POCUS

3.1.1 Procedural Guidance

If you are sticking a needle in a vessel or body cavity, ultrasound usually can make the entire procedure safer and quicker. For example, use it for venous and arterial cannulation. It has been shown in numerous studies to facilitate and reduce complications for internal jugular, subclavian and femoral vein cannulation. It has also been shown to speed up arterial cannulation and require fewer sticks. Thoracentesis and paracentesis are much safer and successful when using real-time US.

3.1.2 Diagnosis

Thoracic ultrasound techniques can 1) identify or narrow down the causes of dyspnea or respiratory failure; 2) identify pneumothorax and a site for chest tube placement; 3) identify an infection source, such as ascites, pleural fluid, and lung consolidation; 4) identify causes of renal dysfunction, such as volume depletion by inferior vena cava collapse analysis, left ventricular dysfunction, hydronephrosis, and obstructed bladder; 5) identify proximal deep vein thrombosis with accuracy; and 6) identify raised intracranial pressure.

3.1.3 Shock Management

Using basic critical care echo techniques, US can identify gross cardiac dysfunction and volume status to tailor resuscitation and vasopressor doses. Bedside US allows frequent re-assessment as a patient's shock state evolves. Caution—you may use a lot of ultrasound gel. Have your unit Director buy a big box of the stuff.

3.2 POCUS Lingo

How does one *LEARN* POC ultrasound? Great question. If your training program does not offer a pathway to competence, then you will have to be creative and persistent. Find an ultrasound mentor—this could be a cardiologist with extensive echo expertise or an echo technician who can show you how to obtain standard views and troubleshoot your technique. After asking around, you may find out that lots of people are scanning away—your emergency medicine colleagues, anesthesiologists, and pulmonary and critical care specialists. Take a courses offered by emergency medicine and critical care societies conducted by experts that often provides live models and instruction on acquisition and interpretation. Read papers and watch lectures and podcasts. Visit some of the many websites out there—ultrasound is dynamic and you need to look at many video clips.

Scan, scan, scan. Not just sick people, but well people. You want to gauge what is normal.

Now that you are getting hungry for POCUS knowledge, let's review the basics.

Ultrasound waves are very high-frequency waves that humans cannot hear. The centerpiece of your US machine is the transducer probe. The transducer probe both creates the sounds waves and receives the echos. Electrical energy vibrates tiny crystals within the transducer probe that produces the sound waves (called a piezoelectric effect). The reverse piezoelectric effect occurs when sound or pressure waves return to hit the crystals,

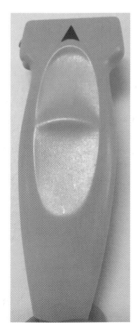

Figure 3-1 Vascular probe

causing them to emit electrical current. Most ultrasound systems use a pulse echo mode, which has the crystals spend part time generating ultrasound waves and part time receiving ultrasound waves. Diagnostic ultrasound transmits waves in a frequency range of 1 to 15 MHz far above the range of normal human hearing. A higher frequency ultrasound probe translates to decreased tissue penetration but higher resolution. A lower frequency ultrasound probe enables deeper tissue penetration but a lower resolution.

There are two probes most POC ultrasonographers master. Linear transducers are often called "vascular" or high frequency probes **(Figure 3-1)**. The higher frequency probe (~10 MHz) resolves superficial structures well, including blood vessels and the pleural surface. A different probe with a lower frequency (2-4 MHz) is used to resolve deeper structures such as solid organs. This probe is called the phased array probe **(Figure 3-2)** and is used to image the heart or abdomen.

The waves, when applied to a patient (with some gel in between) travel through tissue and variably bounce back to the probe, depending on the tissue properties. Through data processing the ultrasound processor unit will transform the reflected wave data into an image.

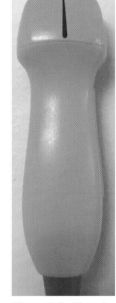

Figure 3-2 Phased array probe

There are lots of dials and buttons on your machine that are devoted to enhancing your image. Novices should adjust their scanning depth to place the object of interest in the center of the screen (example: the internal jugular vein) and adjust the gain to resolve all neighboring structures as clearly as possible. Oh yeah. What's up with that dot at the top of the screen? Most US systems want you to know what is left and right without picking up the probe and touching the probe with your finger. Most probes have a knob or plastic protrusion on the side of the probe that matches the "dot" on the screen. Make sure the dot on the screen is on the same side as the protrusion on the probe **(Figure 3-3)**. If the protrusion is left on your probe and the dot is left of screen, your screen will appropriately demonstrate right and left.

A few key additional POCUS terms apply to images:

- *Anechoic—Black as night* (maybe gray if your gain is set too high). Anechoic imaging is caused by fluid not reflecting or scattering the US as seen with pleural fluid, ascites, and blood.

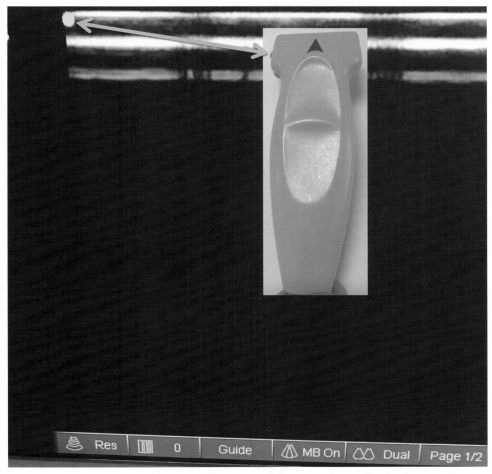

Figure 3-3 POCUS screen shows green dot in upper left corner. Line up the plastic protrusion with the dot to help with right to left orientation.

- *Hypoechoic – Gray.* This is caused by reflecting some waves and letting most pass through. This is the typical image of fat/muscle.
- *Hyperechoic – Bright and white.* The tissue reflects waves well and produces a bright image. This is typical for bone, tough tissue like the diaphragm, muscle, heart valves, teeth, and blood vessel walls.

3.3 Our Top Ten POCUS Findings in the ICU

3.3.1 Vessel Location for Catheter Placement

An ideal vein for cannulation is compressible with no thrombosis, big enough to accept the catheter, and with a target trajectory that will avoid cannulation of a neighboring artery. The vein will be thin-walled with an irregular shape, in contrast to the rounder neighboring artery with a thicker wall and with more discernible pulsations **(Figure 3-4).** If the artery is in front of or behind the vein, there is an increased risk of arterial cannulation. Push the probe up and down; the vein will compress, while the artery will remain round and pulsatile. Image the wire in the vein prior to advancing the dilator to prevent arterial cannulation.

Figure 3-5 illustrates an internal jugular vein position with the carotid artery under the vein. In this view, the clinician would risk arterial puncture if the needle passed through the posterior wall of the internal jugular vein.

3.3.2 Pneumothorax

Wouldn't it be great to know if your patient has a pneumothorax immediately without waiting for a portable X-ray? That US machine can do just that. Just place your probe between the ribs and look for lung sliding. Lung sliding is a normal thing to see and is

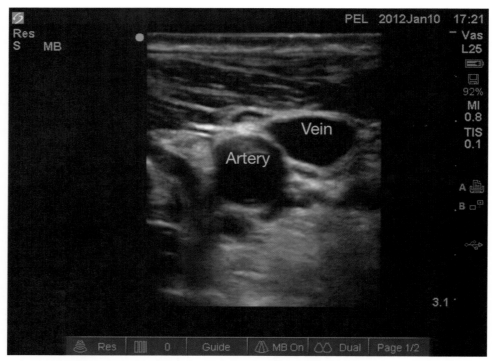

Figure 3-4 *Illustrates contrast of artery and vein in a cross-sectional image*

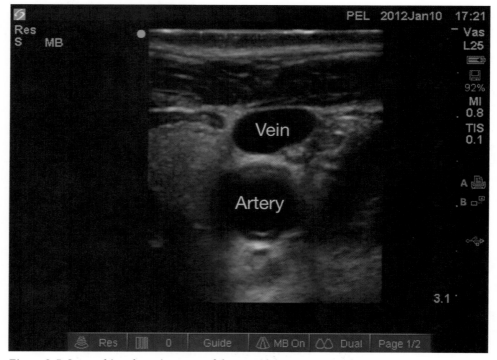

Figure 3-5 *Internal jugular vein on top of the carotid artery.*

the effect of the parietal and visceral pleura moving against each other during exhalation and inhalation. Remember again—air scatters US waves. Thus, air from a pneumothorax will block resolution of visceral (lung) pleura so you will not see the visceral pleura moving and will create a "quiet" and "still" pleura.

While the presence of lung sliding rules out a pneumothorax at the examined location, the lack of lung sliding does not confirm a pneumothorax. Right mainstem intubation (quiet left lung pleura), hyperinflation, consolidation, and low tidal volume ventilation can all be associated with absent lung sliding. So, if you suspect pneumothorax, systematically scan all rib space regions, starting with non-dependent areas first (where air collects—anterior and cephalad).

Look for B-lines that move with respiration. The presence of B lines rules out a pneumothorax at the region of the probe. If you detect *NO* sliding, move the probe until you see sliding. The transition point where you go from lung sliding to no sliding is called the *lung point sign* and is highly suggestive of pneumothorax.

Scan for lung sliding before and after CVC placement and thoracentesis and in your examination of your patient in shock and respiratory distress. Direct your chest tube where you have outlined the pneumothorax.

3.3.3 Pleural Fluid

Using your phased array probe, you can identify the hypoechoic diaphragm, the spleen or liver beneath the diaphragm, and an anechoic space above the diaphragm, which means there is fluid there **(Figure 3-6)**. By visualizing atelectatic lung moving in and out of this anechoic space, one feels much more confident this space is pleural fluid. Always discern adjacent structures before inserting needles. There may be "smoke" or loculations that suggest the fluid is not a simple transudative liquid. The appearance may have you place a larger tube or refer to a thoracic surgeon.

3.3.4 Lung Patterns

As air is an enemy to sound waves, the lung should not be amenable to ultrasound. But you can learn a great deal about the lung with POCUS if you know what you are looking to see. The vascular probe (higher frequency) is great for the lung periphery.

To examine the lung, we need to peek between ribs, because calcified ribs fully reflect US waves (hyperechoic) and cause shadows behind them. One can get information at the rib space, acknowledging that things change at other rib spaces. Only by surveying many rib spaces can we learn what is truly happening in the hemithorax. Unfortunately, or fortunately, air scatters US waves, producing gray snow. Therefore, we cannot resolve well the normally aerated lung.

The initial hyperechogenic line > 0.5 cm deep to the probe is the interface between the soft tissue of the chest wall and the aerated lung or the "pleural" line. Air in the lung stops the progression of the ultrasound

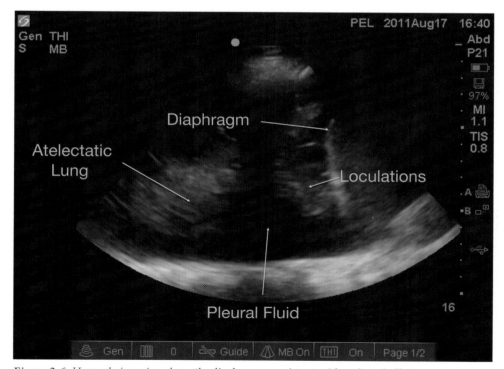

Figure 3-6 *Hypoechoic region above the diaphragm consistent with a pleural effusion*

beam so air artifacts are created that arise from the pleural line. Two different types of artifacts may appear on your screen:

- A-lines **(Figure 3-7)**. *When you see A-lines, everything is A-OK!* Normally aerated lung produces a typical artifact pattern consisting of horizontal lines that run parallel to the pleura and are called A-lines. If you see this pattern, you feel confident that the region of the thorax where you placed the probe is well aerated. Remember, we cannot "see" air-filled lung, but we can usually identify the pleural surface.
- B-lines **(Figure 3-8)**. *Your patient is B-UMMING!!!* Engorgement or thickening of interlobular septa in the peripheral lung will produce a B-line artifact pattern as fluid increases in the lung. A few scattered B lines can be physiologic in more dependent lung regions. However, more than 3 per field in a rib interspace is considered abnormal. Note that B-lines look like a beam of light going from the intercostal space down. *You can remember this by thinking of, "B-eam me up Scottie, I got to get to the sick bay for my pulmonary edema!"*

These B-lines are also called *lung rockets*, a type of *"comet tail"* artifact (These ultrasound guys are very creative!). B lines are believed to represent artifacts generated by the interaction of fluid and air bubbles, but the exact mechanism that produces the artifact is not known. B lines can be present in a focal lung region due to inflammation caused by pneumonia, infarction, or contusion. The more diffuse B line pattern suggests pulmonary edema (cardiac and non-cardiac), pulmonary fibrosis, and ARDS. In pulmonary edema, B-lines can often precede a positive CXR. The Presence of A-lines anteriorly without B-lines suggests that there is no pulmonary edema.

In conditions where the air is not present in the lung, the ultrasound appearance takes on that of a more solid organ or tissue (hepatization) **(Figure 3-9)**. Air bronchograms may be present as hyperechoic artifacts within the lung. Lung sliding may be absent in regions of consolidation.

3.3.5 Left Ventricle and Right Ventricle Dysfunction

The basic critical care echocardiography exam is focused and does not attempt to rule out all cardiac pathology. Often the operator is trying to answer the question, "Are the LV and RV contracting normally." Using global visual assessment ("eyeball technique"), one can determine if the LV has depressed function. The differential for myocardial depression is not small. Your patient may have preexisting heart disease or may be experiencing myocardial depression from sepsis. Sequential exams may suggest the depression is only temporary or improved by giving an inotrope.

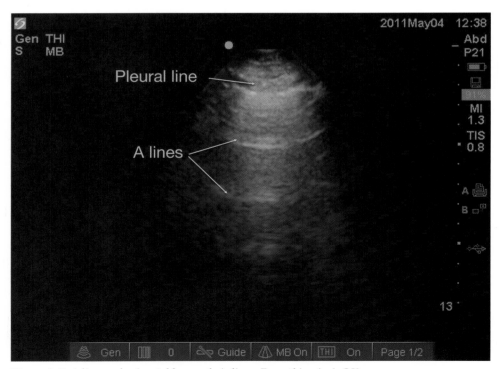

Figure 3-7 *A lines as horizontal hyperechoic lines. Everything is A-OK.*

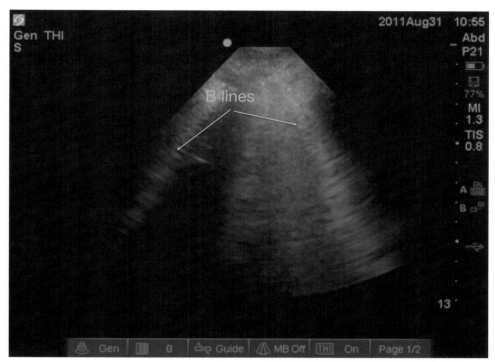

Figure 3-8 *B lines, also called lung rockets or comet tails, are characteristic of the alveolar-interstitial syndrome. B-eam me up Scottie, I got to get to the sick bay for my pulmonary edema.*

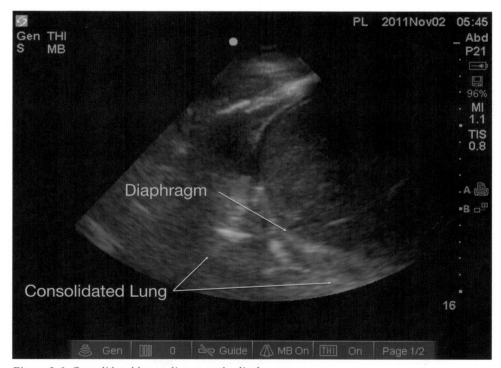

Figure 3-9 *Consolidated lung adjacent to the diaphragm.*

Learning the fundamental views for cardiac imaging can get you started. There is an extensive literature on measurements to assess left and right ventricular function, which is beyond the scope of this introductory chapter.

The parasternal long axis view (PLAX) is shown in **Figure 3-10** and is obtained by placing the transducer between the 3rd and 4th ribs just to the patient's left of the sternum. The indicator points to the patient's right shoulder. The ideal image should include the left atrium (LA), the mitral valve (MV), the left ventricle (LV), the aortic valve (AV), and the aortic root (AR). The descending aorta (DA) is adjacent and deep to the left atrium. The apex of the ventricle will often be outside the image. Only the anterior wall of the right ventricle (RV) is seen.

The parasternal short axis view (PSAX) is achieved by rotating the transducer 90 degrees clockwise from the PLAX view so that the transducer is pointing to the patient's left shoulder **(Figure 3-11)**. The image captured will be at the level of the midventricle or papillary muscles. Tilting the tail of the transducer toward the patient's right shoulder will point the transducer toward the apex. Progressively tilting the transducer tail from 10 on the watch dial to 4 on the watch dial will change the image from

- *PSAX midventricle.* Left ventricle with papillary muscles at 3 and 7 o'clock

- *PSAX base.* Left ventricle with mitral valve leaflets
- *PSAX apex.* Left ventricle with no papillary muscles or mitral valve leaflets

You obtain the apical four chamber view (A4C) **(Figure 3-12)** at the point of maximum cardiac impulse, preferably with the patient in the left lateral decubitus position. The transducer is placed between the ribs at the location of the apical impulse and gently lifted upwards as if you are lifting the pectoralis muscle. The indicator is pointed straight at the patient's left or 3 o'clock position.

3.3.6 Valvular Vegetation

Your patient with shock and dyspnea may have endocarditis. A quick bedside exam may reveal a large valvular vegetation before blood cultures turn positive or a formal echo can be obtained and interpreted **(Figure 3-13)**. Color Doppler examination may reveal severe regurgitation. Lack of valvular vegetations does not rule out endocarditis. A transesophageal echo remains the gold standard for achieving this diagnosis.

3.3.7 Inferior Vena Cava (IVC) Size

The inferior vena cava is a very compliant vessel, and its caliber shrinks with volume depletion. Spontaneous

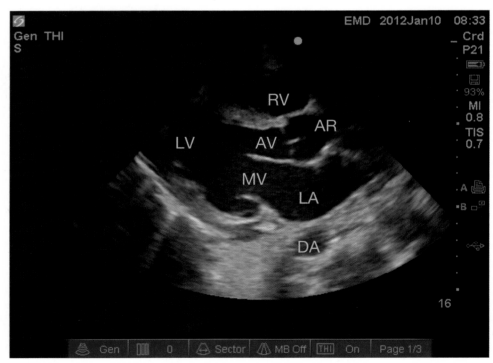

Figure 3-10 *Parasternal long axis view of the heart with components illustrated including the left atrium (LA), the mitral valve (MV), the left ventricle (LV), the aortic valve (AV), the aortic root (AR), the descending aorta (DA), and the right ventricle (RV).*

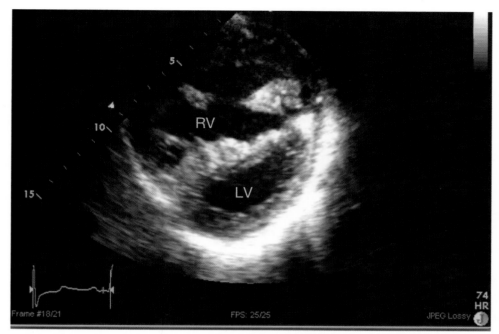

Figure 3-11 *A PSAX apex view of the left ventricle. Usually the left ventricle (LV) appears round and symmetric, but in this image the adjacent right ventricle (RV) is dilated and compressing the LV. The images confirm a right ventricle pressure overload.*

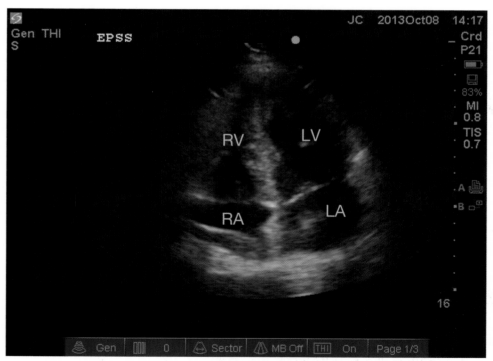

Figure 3-12 An apical 4 chamber view of the heart illustrates the right atrium (RA), right ventricle (RV), left atrium (LA), and left ventricle (LV).

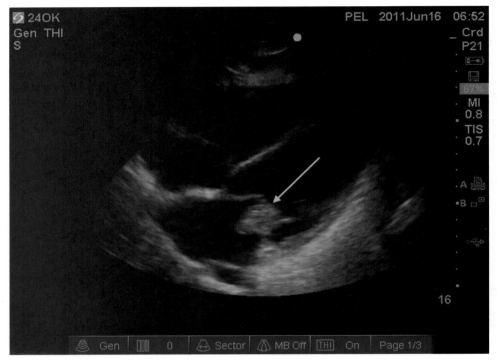

Figure 3-13 A PLAX view with a large vegetation on the mitral valve (arrow).

respiration may collapse a dry IVC during the inspiratory phase, while positive pressure ventilation may expand the IVC during the inspiratory phase. This respiratory variation in the IVC size has been used extensively by investigators to predict "fluid responsiveness" in the ICU patient.

Visualize the IVC from the subcostal view. The patient is imaged supine, preferably with the hips and knees partially flexed to relax the abdominal muscles. Place the probe a few centimeters below the xiphoid. An overhand grip is preferred to hold the probe, which is flattened by rotating the tail down. The indicator is pointed to the patient's left (3 o'clock). From the subcostal view, one can center the RA in the screen and rotate the probe to obtain the IVC in longitudinal view entering the RA. Two to three centimeters caudal to this juncture, one can freeze the image and use the caliper function to measure the IVC diameter at end inspiration and expiration. We will talk more about the significance of these measurements in Chapter 7 on *Hemodynamic Monitoring*

Figure 3-14 illustrates the IVC entering the right atrium. Visualizing the IVC at the entrance to the right atrium helps distinguish this vessel from the aorta. Often the hepatic vein might be visualized as it joins the IVC.

Bedside POCUS cardiac imaging in your patient with shock or respiratory distress can assist with determining the etiology and define the scope of the patient's critical illness. Again, we are not interested in a formal and thorough echo study interrogating each valve and

myocardial segment. The operator is trying to answer specific questions regarding the etiology of shock or respiratory distress. Using four standard views, the basic critical care echocardiographer is trying to determine the following:

1. Presence of a pericardial effusion
2. Presence of LV or RV dilation or dysfunction
3. LV/RV abnormal contraction patterns
4. Severe valvular regurgitation with color Doppler
5. IVC size and respiratory variation to detect fluid responsiveness

Achievement of competence with POCUS will take study, practice, and interaction with expert operators. Make a play date with a friendly cardiologist or other US skilled colleague, and you will learn the skills for this rapid assessment.

A few more uses for POCUS ....

3.3.8 Distended Bladder

Your critically ill patient may have anuria. Your nurse has flushed the Foley, and your exam skills do not detect any abdominal abnormalities. A quick scan of the anterior pelvis may reveal a very distended bladder from a poorly functioning bladder catheter **(Figure 3-15)**. Move the probe to find the Foley balloon. Now you know if you have to reinsert another Foley catheter.

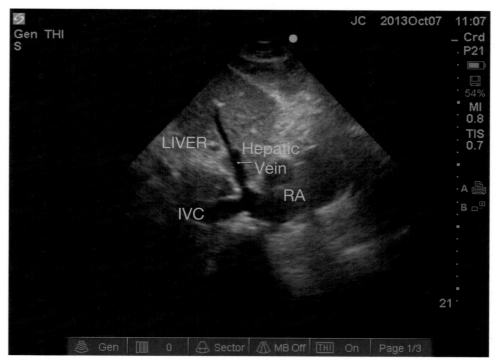

Figure 3-14 *The inferior vena cava (IVC) entering the right atrium (RA). Visualizing the IVC at the entrance to the right atrium helps distinguish this vessel from the aorta. Often the hepatic vein might be visualized as it joins the IVC.*

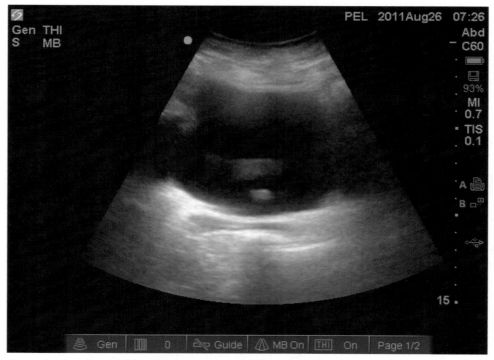

Figure 3-15 *A distended bladder from an occluded Foley catheter.*

3.3.9 Peritoneal Fluid

A scan of the abdomen with your phased array probe in your critically ill patient may reveal an anechoic fluid collection in the abdomen. In the focused assessment with sonography for trauma exam (FAST), your healthy patient should have NO fluid in the abdomen. If you find an anechoic collection or stripe, you assume the patient is having traumatic bleeding. In the FAST exam, one scans the most dependent portions of the abdomen in the supine patient to identify ANY fluid. You should focus on the hepatic and hepato-renal space, spleno-renal space, pelvis, and pericardium. A negative test assumes you acquired excellent images of those areas and found no anechoic collections. In your non-trauma patient (for instance, your critically ill cirrhotic patient), identification of ascites can direct paracentesis and sampling **(Figure 3-16)**. US guidance may reveal a safe needle path to ascites free of bowel or adhesions. Large volume ascites drainage or placement of a catheter may relieve pressure and abdominal compartment syndrome.

3.3.10 Deep Venous Thrombosis (DVT)

Your linear array probe can identify a vessel for cannulation, but before scanning you may notice something just isn't right with that vessel. Something echogenic is in that venous lumen **(Figure 3-17 and Figure 3-18)**. The vein is not compressible any longer. The walls don't kiss with a light pressure from the ultrasound probe. That would be a thrombus. Even if you are not looking to place a venous catheter, one can use that probe to diagnose a DVT. Studies have shown that nominally trained physicians can detect proximal lower extremity DVT using just compression, with excellent accuracy compared to a formal triphasic study performed by ultrasonographers. Order your confirmatory study, but a POCUS study may lead to immediate therapy instead of waiting hours or days.

3.4 POCUS Focus

As your skill advances, the shock patient deserves a more comprehensive exam. The RUSH (rapid ultrasound for shock and hypotension) exam (RUSH the Hocus-POCUS!) is designed to provide a rapid but comprehensive assessment for medical etiologies associated with cardiac arrest.[1] The RUSH exam is simplified as three components: the pump, the tank, and the pipes. The position of the probe for each portion of the exam is illustrated by **Figure 3-19**, which corresponds to the numbers in the text description of the exam.

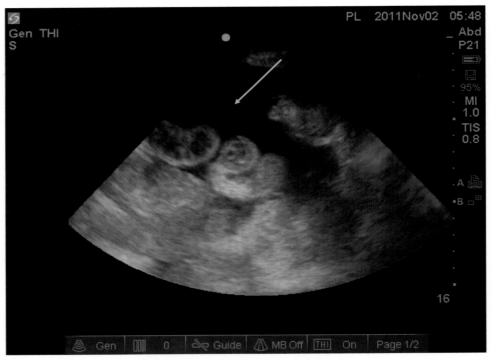

Figure 3-16 *Ascites fluid (arrow) found between loops of small bowel.*

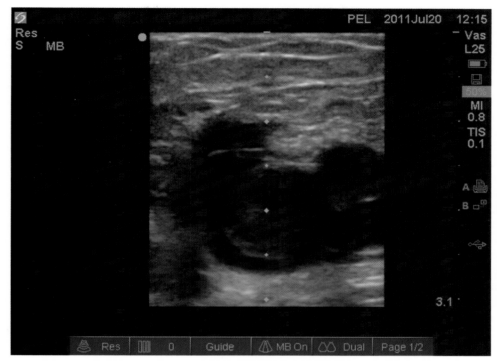

Figure 3-17 *A deep venous thrombosis in a cross-sectional view.*

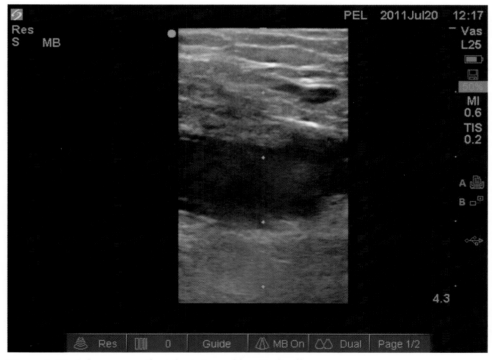

Figure 3-18 *A deep venous thrombosis imaged longitudinally*

The components of the RUSH exam are outlined below:

- The PUMP
  - *Cardiac exam.* The cardiac portion of the exam uses 1) the parasternal long axis cardiac view and 2) the apical four-chamber view. The exam is intended to look for three specific findings: pericardial effusion, left ventricular contractility, and right ventricular dilation.
- The TANK
  - *Inferior vena cava.* The four- chamber subxiphoid view (3) is used to identify the convergence of the inferior vena cava with the right atrium. The dimensions of the inferior vena cava are evaluated approximately 2 cm from the junction of the vessel with the right atrium. If the inferior vena cava is not visualized, the internal jugular vein can be used as an alternative assessment. The relative vessel size and respiratory dynamics provide an estimate of volume status. An inferior vena cava dimension ≥ 2.1 cm with less than 50% collapse during inspiration suggests a central venous pressure that is elevated.
  - *Chest and abdominal fluid.* In trauma patients, you are looking for blood in the chest or within the peritoneum. In medical patients, fluid in the lung, pleural space, or peritoneal cavity will more commonly suggest "tank overload." The probe is placed in the mid-axillary line at about the 8th to 11th interspace on the right (4). With the patient in the supine position (or even better in Trendelenburg), the most dependent region in the upper peritoneum is Morison's pouch – the region between the liver and the kidney. A similar exam on the left examines the area between the spleen and kidney (5). Slide the probe cephalad in each location to obtain a view of the diaphragm and look for pleural fluid. A pelvic view is also obtained since the pelvis is the most dependent part of the peritoneal space (6). Place the probe in the midline just cephalad to the pubic bone with the marker-dot pointed cephalad to obtain a longitudinal view.
  - *The lungs.* Lung ultrasound can identify pulmonary edema as another marker of excess fluid in the tank. Scan the lungs in the anterolateral chest between the second and fifth rib interspaces (7 and 8). Detection of pulmonary edema with ultrasound relies on seeing a special type of lung ultrasound artifact, termed *ultrasound B-lines* or *"lung rockets."* The lung exam can also be used to assess for pneumothorax, looking for lung

sliding. The lack of pleural sliding may indicate a pneumothorax, a mainstem intubation, or inadequate ventilation.

- The PIPES
  - *Aorta.* You should pay attention to the abdominal aorta in the region below the renal arteries (7). The maximal diameter of the aorta from the outer wall to outer wall is used as an indicator with a ruptured aneurysm. The parasternal long axis view of the heart also provides evidence for a proximal aortic dissection.
  - *Venous circulation.* A compression evaluation of the lower extremity venous system including the common femoral vein, proximal femoral vein, and the popliteal vein (8 and 9)

POCUS requires advanced training and significant practice to gain confidence in your imaging. Although many different shock protocols exist, the protocols have common components that often reorder the sequence of the examination. Mastering the skill set to allow confident image acquisition will be your main challenge.

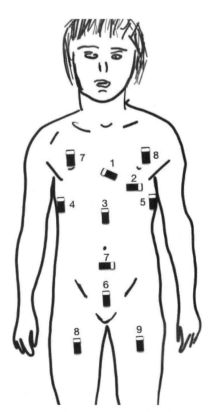

Figure 3-19 *The ultrasound probe positions for the components of the RUSH exam as outlined in the text.*

4

Sepsis and Resuscitation

4.1 Sepsis Defined

If you are a hospitalist, intensivist, surgeon or just about any category of physician who works in a hospital setting, you are going to spend a fair amount of time diagnosing and treating patients with sepsis. So, let's start with this most common of hospital problems. Early treatment and recognition saves a life!

The inflammatory response and tissue injury produced by infection is called sepsis. In sepsis, organ systems remote from the initial infection suffer from the more generalized effects of vasodilation, capillary permeability, and local inflammation. The term *systemic inflammatory response syndrome* (SIRS) was introduced in 2001 to describe the host inflammatory response to infection and injury.[2] The criteria for SIRS required that two of four specific components be present:

- Temperature > 38°C (100.4°F) or < 36°C (95°F)
- Heart rate > 90 beats per minute
- Respiratory rate > 20 breaths/min or $PaCO_2$ < 32 mm Hg
- WBC >12,000 cells/mm^3, <4000 cells/mm^3, or >10% immature (band) forms

The range of host responses to an infection were outlined based upon the presence or absence of SIRS:

- *Bacteremia* – bacterial infection in the blood without SIRS
- *Sepsis* – infection (suspected or probable) with SIRS criteria (~10% mortality)

- *Severe Sepsis*—sepsis with hypoperfusion and/or organ dysfunction (~17-20% mortality)
- *Septic Shock* – sepsis-induced hypotension that persists after volume resuscitation (~40-55% mortality)

The use of SIRS criteria in sepsis definitions is problematic. SIRS criteria lack sensitivity for defining sepsis, as many patients with infection and organ dysfunction do not meet two of the SIRS criteria. SIRS criteria also lack specificity, as the majority of ICU patients without infection often meet SIRS criteria on any given day.

To address the limitations of SIRS criteria in defining sepsis, a 2016 consensus conference report updated the terminology for sepsis (termed Sepsis-3).[3] The Sepsis-3 definition no longer uses SIRS criteria and has only two categories to consider: *sepsis (without shock)* and *sepsis with shock* .

- *Sepsis* – defined as life-threatening organ dysfunction due to a dysregulated host response to infection. The clinical criteria for organ dysfunction include one of two measures
  - A 2-point or greater increase in the Sequential Organ Failure Assessment (SOFA) score **(Figure 4-1)** or
  - A risk for prolonged ICU stay or hospital mortality identified at the bedside, using a modified organ failure score called the qSOFA

SOFA Score Point Value	0	1	2	3	4
PaO$_2$/FiO$_2$ mm Hg	≥400	<400	<300	<200	<100
Platelets × 10^3/uL	>150	<150	<100	<50	<20
Bilirubin mg/dL	<1.2	1.2-1.9	2.0-5.9	6.0-11.9	>12
Mean arterial pressure (MAP) mm Hg	≥70	<70	Dopamine < 5 ug/kg/min or dobutamine (any dose)	Dopamine > 5 ug/kg/min or epi/norepi ≤ 0.1 ug/kg/min	Dopamine > 15 ug/kg/min or epi/norepi > 0.1 ug/kg/min
Glascow Coma Score points	15	13-14	10-12	6-9	<6

Figure 4-1 *Sequential Organ Failure Assessment (SOFA) score point value based on the 5 measured variables.*

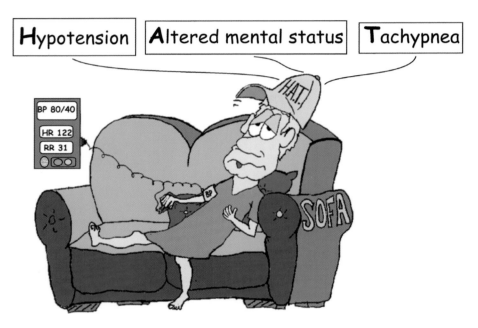

Figure 4-2 *HAT variables to remember for qSOFA scoring.*

qSOFA stands for *quick Sepsis Organ Failure Assessment.* The qSOFA is calculated based upon the presence or absence of three parameters with 1 point per variable if present.

- **H**ypotension: systolic blood pressure < 100 mm Hg
- **A**ltered mental status: any Glascow Coma Score < 15
- **T**achypnea: respiratory rate ≥ 22

Note the variables in the qSOFA score can be remembered with the mnemonic *HAT* **(Figure 4-2)**.

A qSOFA score ≥ 2 (meaning two of the three variables are present) in a patient outside the ICU identifies a high-risk infected patient with a 3- to 14-fold increase in hospital mortality compared to a qSOFA < 2.[3]

Summary: INFECTION + ORGAN DYSFUNCTION (HAT) = SEPSIS

- *Septic shock* is defined as a subset of sepsis in which underlying circulatory and cellular / metabolic abnormalities are profound. The Sepsis-3 clinical criteria for septic shock include:
  - Persistent hypotension requiring vasopressors to maintain the mean arterial pressure (MAP) greater than 65 mm Hg
  - Lactate greater than 2 mmol/L

Summary: INFECTION + ORGAN DYSFUNCTION (HAT) + SHOCK = SEPTIC SHOCK

Should you use SOFA or qSOFA to determine if your patient has sepsis?

SOFA Score on Admission	Hospital Mortality
0 to 5	< 11%
6 to 7	22%
8 to 9	33%
10 to 11	50%
>11	> 90%

Figure 4-3 The relationship between the admission SOFA score and ICU mortality from one series.[4]

When you are busy resuscitating your patient, you are not going to sit down beside your septic patient and calculate the SOFA score. If a baseline data element is not known, you assume the SOFA score for that individual parameter started at 0. The SOFA score's importance is that it predicts hospital mortality in patients presenting to an ICU. The higher the total SOFA score on presentation to the ICU the worse the hospital mortality **(Figure 4-3)**.

The qSOFA is a simpler marker of disease mortality to consider. You can probably remember the HAT variables even if you are sleep-deprived. The qSOFA will need to be further validated to confirm its clinical value – but qSOFA represents a good reminder of variables to assess in your infected patient to decide if the patient just might be sicker than you thought.

Early recognition and treatment in patients with sepsis saves lives. SIRS criteria, SOFA criteria, and qSOFA help the clinician to recognize that patients with an infection are at increased risk and warrant an early, aggressive intervention.

4.2 Sepsis and Shock

Shock is a life-threatening condition in which a generalized maldistribution of blood flow fails to deliver or utilize oxygen at the tissue level, leading to tissue dysoxia.[5] *Tissue dysoxia* is a state of abnormal tissue oxygen metabolism resulting from either a change in oxygen supply or oxygen utilization.[6] Shock produces an initial reversible injury, which, if not resolved, can lead to irreversible cellular damage. Logically, shock manifests clinically with signs of organ dysfunction. The clinical features of shock manifest in three "windows" to the body.[5] The exam features of shock are shown in:

1. The *Peripheral Window* – cold, clammy, pale or discolored skin and decreased peripheral pulses
2. The *Renal Window* – decreased urine output to < 0.5 ml/kg/hr
3. The *Neurologic Window* – altered mental status

The definition of shock does not mention a specific blood pressure. Hypotension occurs frequently in shock, but low blood pressure is not required for shock to be present.

Hypotension, in contrast to shock, is defined by blood pressure parameters including

- Systolic blood pressure (SBP) < 90 mm Hg
- Mean arterial blood pressure (MAP) < 60 mm Hg
- Decline in systolic blood pressure > 40 mm Hg from the patient's baseline

You can have shock without hypotension, and you can have hypotension without shock.

A key variable in shock resuscitation is restoring organ perfusion. So the theme for this section will be, *It's the flow stupid!!* Your assessment of the patient with shock involves two interacting components: a metabolic component (tissue oxygen delivery and oxygen consumption) and a hemodynamic or flow component (mean arterial blood pressure and cardiac output). To resuscitate a patient effectively, we need to assess parameters from both components. Let's introduce a few terms and the parameters that influence those terms in **Figure 4-4**.

Hemodynamic Parameters	
Mean Arterial Pressure (MAP) =	Cardiac Output (CO) x Systemic Vascular Resistance (SVR)
Cardiac Output (CO) =	Heart Rate (HR) x Stroke Volume (SV)
Metabolic Parameters	
Oxygen Delivery (DO_2) =	Cardiac Output (CO) $\times$ Arterial Oxygen Content (CaO_2)
Oxygen Consumption (VO_2) =	Cardiac Output (CO) $\times$ [Arterial Oxygen Content (CaO_2)-Venous Oxygen Content (CvO_2)]

Figure 4-4 Summary of hemodynamic and metabolic parameters that are components of shock assessment.

Let's get started with assessing hemodynamics using a septic ICU patient.

42 yo WM with progressive SOB, fevers, and chills presents to the emergency department. On initial presentation, he is noted to have tachypnea (respiratory rate 32 breaths per minute), tachycardia (heart rate 120 beats per minute) and mild hypotension (BP 100/60). He is febrile at 38.5. He is speaking in short sentences. His initial assessment reveals a pulse oximetry saturation of 85% (normal > 92%). His lungs have rales in the right lung base. He has tachycardia, but no gallop or murmur is appreciated. His abdomen is soft and non-tender. Bowel sounds are absent. His extremities are very cool, with a delayed capillary refill, and peripheral pulses are hard to palpate. His WBC is suppressed at 3.4 cells/mm³ with a shift to immature forms.

4.3 Initial Sepsis Management

Sepsis is a medical emergency, and three things must be achieved before you even consider going to the bathroom! To make this fun, you will need to try and do all three at the same time!! Be aggressive because early resuscitation improves patient outcomes!

1. Reverse hypoxemia and limited ventilation
2. Reverse hypotension and support organ perfusion
3. Provide immediate antibiotic administration and search for a source of infection

4.3.1 Reverse Hypoxemia and Limited Ventilation

Patients with sepsis and shock may simply require supplemental oxygen or in more severe cases intubation with mechanical ventilation. The need for mechanical ventilation may be due to an altered mental status (septic encephalopathy), marked hemodynamic instability (shock with borderline oxygenation and metabolic acidosis), or a more advanced mechanical workload due to pulmonary parenchyma disease (e.g., Adult Respiratory Distress Syndrome). The decision to immediately intubate these patients has risks and benefits. Intubation is often the best way to secure the airway and assure oxygenation. Yet, these patients often have a reduction in left ventricular preload (i.e., preload responsive) on presentation, so intubation and the shift to positive pressure ventilation could compromise venous return, lower cardiac output, lower blood pressure, and reduce tissue perfusion. Further, sedative medications required for intubation can also jeopardize cardiovascular status. Adequate vascular access to support the circulation with intravenous fluids and vasoactive medications is an immediate priority for any septic patient that might require intubation and mechanical ventilation. Caution must be employed not to compromise ventilation during the intubation process as these patients may suffer from a metabolic acidosis, and respiratory compensation for this acidosis may be lifesaving.

If intubation is not needed, supplemental oxygen should be provided to correct peripheral oxygen saturation to a target of 92-94%. The patient should receive continuous monitoring with pulse oximetry. Note that poor peripheral perfusion characterizes patients with shock, and this clinical finding can compromise the accuracy of pulse oximetry. An initial arterial blood gas is beneficial to confirm the blood partial pressure of oxygen (PaO_2), saturation of oxygen (SaO_2), and the blood pH. A chest radiograph is indicated to assess for pulmonary infiltrates that might suggest acute lung injury and the adult respiratory distress syndrome. Patients may have improvement of their oxygenation with supplemental oxygen yet demonstrate a high ventilatory workload. In this case, intubation and mechanical ventilation may be essential to stabilize the patient.

The sequence of these interventions can be challenging and requires expert judgment, as fixing one problem (respiratory system) can destabilize another (hemodynamics). In the ICU you will be working with a team and often provide these interventions in parallel. Move along quickly as the time to first dosing of the right antibiotic and completion of a sepsis bundle has been associated with an improved patient survival[7]

The clinical history suggests our patient may have pneumonia. He is not an immunocompromised host. Broad spectrum antibiotic coverage addressed at pathogens known to be associated with severe community-acquired pneumonia are administered immediately following cultures of his blood and sputum.

4.3.2 Reverse Hypotension and Support Organ Perfusion

You have ordered your initial antibiotic coverage for your patient's suspected infection. Make sure those get administered! You have stabilized the respiratory system. You must also focus your attention on the adequacy of organ perfusion. The most obvious sign of inadequate tissue perfusion will be hypotension. But even the normotensive patient can have evidence for organ hypoperfusion manifested by low urine output, abnormal mentation, or a metabolic acidosis (remember those windows!)

A major initial focus in sepsis management is to correct hypotension if present. This is achieved through either fluid administration, vasopressor support, or some combination of both interventions. A personalized approach to the mean arterial pressure (MAP) would adjust the MAP target based upon the

Parameter	Target
Hemodynamic	
Mean Arterial Pressure	$\geq$ 65 mm Hg
Capillary Refill	< 2 seconds
Oxygen Delivery	
Hemoglobin	> 7.0 gms / dL
Arterial Oxygen Saturation	= 92 – 94 %
Organ Dysfunction	
Lactate	< 2.2 mM/L
*ScvO$_2$	$\geq$ 70%
Urine Output	> 0.5 ml/kg/hour
Encephalopathy	Reversed
Renal and Hepatic Function	Normalized

*ScvO$_2$ is the central venous oxygen saturation (Keep reading!!)

Figure 4-5 *A checklist of goals to accomplish during resuscitation to reflect adequate organ perfusion.*

Two quick parameters to assess organ perfusion require no fancy equipment.

- Check for dorsalis pedis and posterior tibial pulses. If present and strong, – you generally have adequate global tissue perfusion.
- Check for capillary refill. Manually compress the nailbed or distal skin of an extremity to the point of blanching. Release and note the time to return to normal. A delayed return (> 3 sec) suggests abnormal regional or systemic circulation. Easy–no special training required!

patient's chronic blood pressure history and underlying pathophysiology.

Organ perfusion is regulated by the gradient between the organ inflow pressure (MAP) and the organ outflow pressure. Personalized blood pressure management recognizes that different pathophysiologic conditions can alter the perfusion pressure gradient by changing organ outflow pressure. Increased intracranial or intra-abdominal pressure would increase the organ outflow pressure, supporting the need for a higher MAP to maintain organ perfusion under these conditions. In addition, patients with chronic hypertension may need a higher minimal organ inflow perfusion pressure to maintain a constant organ blood flow.

Despite the logic of these physiologic principles, practical guidelines do not provide a personalized MAP target in the septic patient. A mean arterial pressure (MAP) $\geq$ 65 mm Hg is chosen as the most appropriate

initial target for patients with septic shock. Some evidence exists to suggest a higher target for patients with chronic hypertension may reduce the risk of acute renal injury, but this comes at the expense of greater arrhythmias associated with augmented vasopressor support.[8]

An arterial catheter may be inserted to allow continuous monitoring of blood pressure. A central venous catheter can also be employed to provide access for rapid fluid administration and vasoactive medications that cannot be safely infused into a peripheral vein. Recognize, however, that the time needed to place these catheters cannot delay the initial therapy for hypotension and hypoxemia. Most importantly, we now have evidence from three randomized clinical trials in the sepsis population that specialized catheters for hemodynamic management do not improve patient outcome.[9–11] So you can use your best judgment whether these catheters will help your patient assessment and management.

Figure 4-5 provides a set of goals or maybe a "checklist" for you to monitor as markers of adequate organ perfusion during your initial resuscitation.

While assessing our patient, we have ordered the empiric broad-spectrum antibiotics to cover possible community-acquired bacteria. Although our patient's blood pressure is only borderline reduced, he has markers of compromised systemic perfusion. He will need resuscitation and reversal of hypoperfusion within the first few hours of care to minimize his risk of organ failure. We will use his blood pressure as one marker of success but will need repeated assessment of his peripheral pulses, capillary refill, and urine output to reverse his hypoperfusion.

4.4 Fluid Administration in Sepsis

For the majority of patients, the initial step in hemodynamic management is fluid resuscitation. Fluid resuscitation is necessary to increase ventricular preload, compensate for any loss of plasma volume into the interstitial space, and overcome the myocardial depression of sepsis which requires a greater filling pressure to maintain cardiac function (i.e., a rightward shift in the Starling curve). Successful correction of fluid deficits will restore cardiac function, enhance tissue oxygenation, and may resolve metabolic acidosis.

The critical initial decision in treating the patient with sepsis and shock is to identify those patients who will respond favorably to fluid resuscitation. This category of patients is often termed *preload responsive*. Fluid resuscitation in *preload responsive patients* restores stroke volume, improves cardiac output, lowers HR, raises mean arterial pressure, and improves tissue oxygen delivery (DO_2). *Preload responsive* patients are functioning on the ascending limb of their Starling curve (**Figure 4-6**, blue triangle). If the patient is not preload responsive (**Figure 4-6**, red triangle), then aggressive fluid administration can only cause harm (*Think lung water!*).

House officers across the world, after an overnight call, have reported to their attendings they "tanked up" their hypotensive patient. Two problems here. First, patients do not come with a fluid gauge which tells you when the tank is appropriately filled but not

overflowing. Wouldn't that be nice! Second, increasing evidence from many clinical trials now suggests we can do as much harm with excess fluid as we can with under resuscitation.[12–14] So like Goldilocks… not too little… not too much… but just the right amount of fluid is your target. Remember, our best estimate suggests 50-60% of septic patients are fluid responsive at the time of clinical presentation. Time might be a very important variable, with early resuscitation more commonly associated with the patient being *preload responsive!* A significant fraction of septic patients are not fluid responsive. "Tanking up" these patients may actually be harmful.

How do we tell if fluid is beneficial to our patient? Fluid administration in sepsis is best provided in bolus form, meaning a volume of fluid over a short time interval. Bolus fluid administration provides an immediate effect on cardiac preload that allows your clinical reassessment of perfusion parameters to occur. Ongoing evaluation of organ perfusion parameters will guide the need for subsequent fluid boluses. The benefits of fluid resuscitation on hemodynamics are offset by potential adverse effects of fluid loading on the lung. Any co-existing capillary leak in the pulmonary vascular bed can worsen in severity during fluid resuscitation in direct proportion to the success of that resuscitation in raising left ventricular filling pressures.

Figure 4-7 outlines a simple clinical decision algorithm for interpretation of the response to a fluid bolus in septic shock.

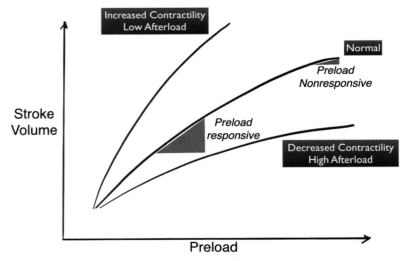

Figure 4-6 The Starling curve illustrates the relationship between cardiac preload and stroke volume for different degrees of contractility and afterload. A patient on the ascending portion of the curve will increase their stroke volume with an increase in preload (blue triangle). In contrast, a patient on the flatter portion of the curve will not increase their stroke volume with an equal increase in preload (red triangle).

Δ Mean Arterial Pressure (MAP)	Δ Urine Output/ Tissue Perfusion	Δ Oxygenation i.e., PaO₂ or SaO₂	Plan
increase	increase	No Δ	Effective fluid bolus. *Consider additional* fluid bolus resuscitation.
No Δ	No Δ	No Δ	Ineffective fluid bolus. Support circulation with a vasopressor as needed.
No Δ	No Δ	decrease	Ineffective fluid bolus and capillary leak in lung. Limit additional fluid bolus and support circulation with a vasopressor.
partial increase	partial increase	decrease	Effective fluid bolus with capillary leak in lung. Very cautious fluid administration and circulatory support with a vasopressor.

Figure 4-7 Clinical decision algorithm to interpret the response of your patient to a fluid bolus based upon three assessment variables.

Continue fluid boluses as long as the patient continues to improve hemodynamically (in blood pressure, pulse pressure, capillary refill, urine output or hopefully all parameters) and gas exchange is not adversely impacted.

A traditional fluid bolus is provided in the range of 250-500 ml of a crystalloid solution. If a clear hemodynamic benefit is not evident after ~30 ml/kg over the initial 6 hours of resuscitation, the patient is likely not preload responsive, and vasopressors are indicated to maintain MAP. But don't target a specific number (i.e., 30 ml/kg); target a measurable hemodynamic response. A patient with sepsis in the setting of significantly impaired left ventricular function will not tolerate the same level of fluid resuscitation as a healthy individual with community-acquired pneumonia. Know your patient!

Fluid management in sepsis is often supported by specific hemodynamic measurements including central venous pressure (CVP), bedside echocardiography, radial artery pulse pressure analysis, and aortic blood flow velocity. We will discuss these tools more extensively in *Chapter 7, Hemodynamic Monitoring*. Use your knowledge of the patient's history and your exam findings in making decisions about fluid administration. The ICU has all sorts of toys for estimating whether your patient will respond appropriately to a fluid bolus. But these toys all have limitations and should only serve to augment your clinical assessment – NOT replace it.

A commonly used adjunct to your clinical assessment of preload responsiveness is point of care ultrasound (POCUS) (See *Chapter 3, Point of Care Ultrasound*). Don't say POTUS—that is the President, and you will not sound cool—we are talking about ultrasound magic or Hocus-POCUS! POCUS uses imaging ·markers to try to estimate the potential benefits and risk of fluid administration. For example, POCUS looks for pulmonary edema in the lungs, represented as *B lines in* the lung window. POCUS also uses a wide range of parameters to predict the hemodynamic response

to a fluid bolus. One of the more common advocated parameters is the collapsibility (spontaneous breathing) or expandability (mechanical ventilation) of the inferior vena cava (IVC) seen just inferior to the liver in response to the different phases of the respiratory cycle. If the IVC shows significant variability between the inspiratory and expiratory phase, this "suggests" the patient will improve his or her cardiac output with a fluid bolus. In **Figure 4-7**, we could substitute the *Presence of B lines on POCUS for Δ Oxygenation and IVC volume variability for Δ Mean Arterial Pressure (MAP) and have a POCUS-based fluid challenge.*

We will talk more about POCUS and the range of tools to support your assessment of preload responsiveness in our *Chapter 7 Hemodynamic Monitoring*. But all the tools have *significant* limitations and need to be additive to a careful history and exam at the patient's bedside. Despite their sophistication, no patient outcome data exists to favor the use of these specific tools in your decision making over careful clinical assessment.[15] Most of these techniques also require specialized training.

Learning to assess a complex patient's response to a fluid challenge will be a valuable tool to be used throughout your career. Bolus your resuscitation fluid so you can observe the reaction of the patient. An order for "125cc NSS per hour and I will see you in the morning" is not going to tell you if your patient is preload responsive or non-responsive.

4.4.1 Crystalloids vs. Colloids

So what type of fluid should you choose for your initial resuscitation?

Crystalloids are a group of sodium-based electrolyte solutions. Crystalloid resuscitation uses saline, or more balanced electrolyte solutions including lactated ringers (sometimes abbreviated LR) and Plasma-Lyte. **Figure 4-8** outlines an electrolyte comparison of these solutions.

Electrolyte	Plasma	0.9% NaCl	Lactated Ringer's (Hartmann's Solution)	Plasma-Lyte
Sodium	140	154	130	140
Potassium	4	0	4	5
Chloride	103	154	109	98
Bicarbonate	24	0	0	0
Lactate	1	0	28	0
Acetate	0	0	0	27
Calcium	5	0	3.0	0
Magnesium	2	0	1	3.0

Figure 4-8 *Comparison of electrolyte composition in common resuscitation fluids.*

In comparison to plasma, normal saline (NS) has a higher sodium and chloride concentration. Infusion of large volumes of NS can produce a *hypochloremic metabolic acidosis*. The clinical significance of this metabolic acidosis relates to two outcomes. First, the metabolic acidosis from excessive saline administration is a non-anion gap metabolic acidosis and must be distinguished from an anion gap acidosis, such as lactic acidosis. Secondly, recent clinical trials suggest resuscitation with large volumes of hyperchloremic saline may have adverse effects on renal function.[16–19]

Lactated Ringer's (LR) solution, also called Hartmann's solution, contains potassium and calcium in amounts that approximate plasma (free or ionized) concentrations. Sodium lactate is added to provide a buffer for metabolic acidosis. This combination results in a lower sodium and chloride concentration in LR in comparison to NS. The calcium in LR could theoretically bind to certain drugs and the citrated anticoagulant in blood products so, to be safe, infuse LR without medications or blood products. Plasma-Lyte, like LR, is a buffered solution that contains acetate, as well as potassium and magnesium. Plasma-Lyte provides a second type of chloride-restricted crystalloid for fluid resuscitation. In contrast to LR, Plasma-Lyte is a calcium-free solution.

The appropriate crystalloid solution for resuscitation may depend on the expected volume needed and clinical condition. Larger volume resuscitation (> 1-2L) in septic patients is accomplished with chloride-restricted solutions to avoid a non-anion gap metabolic acidosis and possibly renal dysfunction.[16] However, if resuscitation involves smaller volumes (i.e., < 2L), we have less evidence to favor chloride-restricted solutions over normal saline.

The most common colloid solution currently in use for resuscitation is albumin. Albumin is responsible for the most significant component of colloid osmotic pressure in the blood (~80%) and plays a major role as an antioxidant, and as a transport protein for both drugs and hormones. Albumin for administration is a heat-treated preparation of human serum albumin. In the U.S., albumin is administered as either a 5% solution (50 g/L, oncotic pressure 20 mm Hg) or a 25% solution (250 g/L, oncotic pressure 70 mm Hg). The 5% albumin (often termed salt-poor albumin) is *iso-oncotic* to human plasma and will expand the plasma volume equal to the volume infused in healthy individuals. The 25% albumin product (sometimes called concentrated albumin) is *hyper-oncotic* and will expand the plasma volume by a greater fraction than the volume infused. The expansion of plasma volume with the 25% solution occurs due to shifts of fluid from the interstitial space. Standard teaching holds that three times the volume of crystalloid is required to achieve the same hemodynamic effect as the administration of the hyper-oncotic albumin. The volume ratio in clinical practice in the SAFE trial (4% albumin) suggested the ratio was closer to 1.4:1.[20]

Albumin may be added to the initial fluid resuscitation in severe sepsis or septic shock if a large fluid volume is required, but this is not advantageous over crystalloid solutions in randomized trials.[20,21] Albumin is not indicated for the resuscitation of traumatic head injury.[20] Hetastarches/Hydroxyethyl starches, which also have higher oncotic pressures, are not currently recommended for resuscitation due to a reported risk of renal dysfunction.[22]

At the current time, no specific fluid resuscitation has been defined to provide a clear survival benefit in patients with septic shock. Based on many large randomized trials and meta-analysis, crystalloid solutions (normal saline or lactated ringers) appear to be as effective as colloid solutions (albumin) in the initial treatment of the patient with sepsis. The only argument for colloid resuscitation over crystalloid is that 25% albumin will increase the plasma volume with 1/3 or less of the volume with crystalloid solutions. However, colloid solutions are significantly more expensive than crystalloid solutions.

Total fluid resuscitation in sepsis is based upon the patient's response to a given fluid load – and that requires monitoring at the bedside as you resuscitate your patient.

Once preload and cardiac performance are maximized from fluid resuscitation, patients with persistent hypotension may have residual systemic vasodilation from reduced vascular tone. These patients, no longer responsive to fluid administration or with complications from that fluid administration (i.e., non-cardiogenic edema), need to be supported with vasoactive medications to increase vascular resistance. Note the sequence is to restore preload first to maximize cardiac output for systemic perfusion before the use of vasopressors (Remember, it's the flow, stupid!).

Our patient has received four 500 ml fluid boluses of plasmalyte. His blood pressure transiently improved but has remained low with MAP ~ 55 mm Hg, and he is no longer responding clinically to the fluid boluses. His skin is still cool, pulses are stronger, and capillary refill is < 3 sec. His urine output is < 0.5 ml/kg/hr. His oxygen saturation is currently 92%, but we have increased his high-flow oxygen from 6 to 8L over the past hour. He has improved his perfusion by pulse indices, but his MAP is still below the therapeutic target, and urine output remains poor. Fluid administration has produced a slight decline in his oxygenation. We will stop our bolus fluid administration and use vasopressor support for his blood pressure. We will also attempt to get an additional assessment of his cardiac function to guide our resuscitation.

4.5 Vasopressors and Inotropes

You have a patient who has hit your unit with a low MAP, and you have run through your ABCs, stabilized gas exchange and assessed perfusion, made a diagnosis of septic shock, provided initial empiric antibiotic coverage, and have fluid resuscitated the patient to resolve preload dependence. But your patient has failed to achieve your target MAP of 65 mm Hg. Now what? You need to keep the MAP up (ideally ≥ 65 mm Hg) and maintain perfusion (cardiac output, the flow!). You will need drugs at this point.

Let's review basic physiology. Sympathomimetic agents (also called adrenergic drugs) stimulate receptors that mimic the effects of endogenous agonists on the sympathetic nervous system. The adrenergic receptors and their physiologic impact include:

- Alpha 1 = cause vasoconstriction
- Alpha 2 = cause vasoconstriction and feedback inhibition of norepinephrine release
- Beta 1 = cause an increase in HR, increase in cardiac contractility, peripheral vasodilation
- Beta 2 = cause vasodilation, bronchodilation

- Dopamine = causes a dose-dependent effect of vasodilation in the renal and mesenteric circulation, with vasoconstriction at higher dosing

Non-adrenergic agents mediate their hemodynamic effects through unique mechanisms from the sympathetic nervous system.

Figure 4-9 summarizes the agents used for hemodynamic support, the pharmacology of the receptors they activate, and the potency of the activation. Let's clarify a few terms:

- *Vasopressor* – an agent that causes blood vessel constriction (vasoconstriction) with an associated increase in blood pressure (sometimes called a "pressor" for short)
- *Inotrope* – an agent that affects the contraction of a muscle, most commonly referring to cardiac muscle
- *Chronotrope* – an agent that alters the rate of the heart

Dopamine is the most complex drug regarding the dose-effect relationship. At low doses, of 1-5 mcg/kg/min, dopamine activates the splanchnic dopaminergic receptors, vasodilates this bed, and causes the excretion of sodium in the urine (natriuresis). This level of dopamine administration was called "renal dose dopamine" for this reason. Low dose dopamine has diuretic effects, but despite long-standing lore has NOT been proven to protect the kidneys from injury. At intermediate doses of 5 -15 mcg/kg/min the drug has mostly beta-1 receptor effects, which increase cardiac inotropy and chronotropy. At higher doses, > than 15 mcg/kg/min dopamine has more α-receptor effects, but modest compared with norepinephrine.

A comparison of dopamine and norepinephrine as a treatment for septic shock demonstrated similar effects on survival with an increased risk of cardiac arrhythmias for dopamine.[23]

Phenylephrine is a synthetic catecholamine and is unique in that it has a pure α-receptor, modest 2+ vasoconstrictive effect. This is an ideal drug for a

> You are called to the bedside to address a patient who has a new PSVT running at 180 beats per minute and a MAP of 55 mm Hg on a dopamine drip. The nurse asks if you want to give adenosine or shock the patient. You calmly say no and ask the nurse to hang neosynephrine, rapidly increase the dose, and stop the dopamine. The nurse gives you a suspect look but changes the drips and in 30 minutes the patient is in a normal sinus rhythm! Keep in mind this pure alpha trick!

Drug	Receptor			Comments	Starting Dose
	Dopa	Beta 1/2	Alpha		
Adrenergic Agents					
Dopamine (≤ 3 mcg/kg/min)	1+	0	0	Diuretic at low dose	
Dopamine (5-10 mcg/kg/min)	1+	2+	1+	Inotrope at moderate dose	
Dopamine (>10 mcg/kg/min)	0	2-3+	2-3+	Inotrope/vasopressor at higher dose	
Phenylephrine	0	0	2+	Pure vasopressor; most common use in patients with tachyarrhythmias	0.5-2 mcg/kg/min
Norepinephrine	0	3-4+	3-4+	First-line drug for septic shock	0.01-3 mcg/kg/min
Epinephrine	0	5+	5+	Big gun, rocket fuel, not for the timid	0.05-2 mcg/kg/min
Dobutamine	0	2+/2+	0	First-line drug for pure cardiogenic shock with preserved blood pressure	2-20 mcg/kg/min
Non – Adrenergic Agents	**Mechanism**			**Comments**	**Starting Dose**
Vasopressin (0.03 units/ minute)	Increases intravascular cAMP levels			Vasopressor to be used in refractory septic shock	0.04 units/minute
Angiotensin II	Stimulates AT1 and AT2 receptors			Alternative vasopressor for treatment of septic shock	
Milrinone	Inhibits adenylate cyclase			Alternative agent for cardiogenic shock	0.375-0.75 mcg/kg/min

Figure 4-9 *Summary of adrenergic and non-adrenergic vasoactive medications.*

vasodilatory state with a low systemic vascular resistance (SVR) and high cardiac output (CO), such as neurogenic or anaphylactic shock. However, it is not a very potent drug, so often one needs to bring in some real muscle (God's own catecholamine: norepinephrine). It is also an ideal drug for a patient with hypotension and sepsis who also has a tachyarrhythmia such as atrial fibrillation/flutter or a paroxysmal supraventricular tachycardia (PSVT). This pure alpha agonist will increase systemic vascular resistance without the beta stimulation that is maintaining the PSVT.

Norepinephrine is an endogenous molecule, not a cheap synthetic imitation. And as you can see in **Figure 4-9**, it has 3-4 + alpha and 3-4+ beta effect. This drug typically will get the job done and increase blood pressure and cardiac output. In the last 20 years, with appropriate fluid resuscitation (remember that preload!), this drug has emerged as the first-line choice for shock resuscitation.

Epinephrine use is a move to ROCKET FUEL. This stuff is 5+ alpha and 5+ beta. We typically use this drug for "vasopressor refractory" septic shock and at this time would have already treated the patient with preload resuscitation and norepinephrine.

Vasopressin is a second-line agent again for patients with vasopressor refractory septic shock. It acts on

vascular cells at high concentrations to increase intracellular cAMP levels and calcium.

Angiotensin II has been reported to have a vasopressor effect in patients with primarily vasodilatory shock (i.e., sepsis). Additional clinical trials are needed to determine whether Angiotensin II offers any significant treatment advantage over available agents. Because of the limited studies to date, the risk profile for Angiotensin II is not well defined.

Dobutamine is an inotrope and should NOT be considered as a first-line drug for shock because it has no alpha activity. It is a pure beta agonist, and by acting on the cardiac beta-1 receptor increases cardiac inotropy and chronotropy. Dobutamine also works on beta-2 vascular receptors, which cause vasodilation. This drug can drop blood pressure! Dobutamine is an ideal drug for pure cardiogenic shock, with low cardiac output and high systemic vascular resistance. By increasing inotropy, chronotropy, and by lowering afterload it increases cardiac output and forward flow. Dobutamine is also used for right heart failure in patients with pulmonary hypertension. Dobutamine effectively treats patients with cardiac dysfunction suggested by high filling pressures and low cardiac output. Dobutamine is used when the patient has evidence for poor tissue perfusion despite restoration of blood pressure and adequate volume resuscitation.

Milrinone stimulates adenylate cyclase in the myocardium to also increase inotropy and chronotropy. It is also vasodilatory and is used in similar clinical situations to dobutamine. Again, it is not a first-line agent for your hypotensive patient with sepsis.

Most clinicians consider norepinephrine to be the first-line agent for sepsis resuscitation as the drug is found to be less arrhythmogenic than dopamine. Dopamine is a first-line agent for select patients where the risk of arrhythmia is very low, or the patient has bradycardia with or without a low cardiac output. For the patient with significant arrhythmias, phenylephrine, which features only α-adrenergic stimulation, may be preferred.

Norepinephrine should be started early during the resuscitation of patients with septic shock when depressed vascular tone (as opposed to volume contraction) is assumed to be the primary cause of hypotension. Both epinephrine and vasopressin are additional agents to be considered for the treatment of sepsis with shock, primarily for patients with an incomplete response to norepinephrine. Vasopressin provides an alternative mechanism of action to adrenergic stimulation and is useful, but not superior to adrenergic agents in patients with vasodilatory shock.[24]

Currently, we are limited by the lack of randomized trials to favor one vasopressor agent over the other, or to define a specific sequence of use. The dose of vasopressor is titrated to produce an appropriate blood pressure response or improved markers of organ perfusion. Add a second agent, if the maximal dose of an initial agent does not achieve the therapeutic target.

Logically we might select a vasopressor based upon the desired pharmacology. In a patient with tachycardia and high cardiac output, you might favor vasopressin or phenylephrine. In contrast, a patient with bradycardia and decreased cardiac function might benefit more from dopamine or epinephrine. Because the majority of patients will fit into a middle group, norepinephrine is a logical initial choice for most patients. A vasopressor titration may be used to best guide how your patient will respond to a drug. This approach may help you select agents that are most effective and avoid agents that do not appear to be working.

A few additional important key points to remember:

- Vasopressors will be ineffective or minimally effective in the setting of intravascular volume contraction.
- Hypoxemia and acidosis decrease adrenergic receptor affinity, so your vasopressor agents may be less active under these conditions.
- The response to vasopressors can decrease with time due to tachyphylaxis, requiring an increase in the administered dose or a different agent (i.e., non-adrenergic) to be considered.

4.6 Assessment of Tissue Oxygenation

In addition to the hemodynamic targets of blood pressure and flow (cardiac output), additional blood markers of tissue oxygenation are helpful to measure in your shock patient. These parameters include the blood lactate and the mixed venous oxygen saturation.

Global tissue oxygenation represents a balance between oxygen delivery (DO_2) to the capillaries and the oxygen uptake or requirement (VO_2) of the tissues. The DO_2 is the amount of oxygen delivered to the capillaries measured in mL/minute and is the product of cardiac output (CO) and arterial oxygen content (CaO_2). Arterial blood oxygen content (CaO_2) is determined by the level of hemoglobin (gms/dL) and the saturation of that hemoglobin by oxygen (SaO_2). The normal DO_2 in adults at rest is ~ 1000 mL/min or 500 mL/min/M^2.

The rate at which oxygen dissociates from hemoglobin and moves into the tissues is the tissue oxygen uptake (VO_2). The oxygen uptake into the tissues is also called the *oxygen consumption* of the tissues as oxygen is not stored in the tissues. The VO_2 is calculated as the product of the cardiac output and the difference between arterial and venous oxygen content (CaO_2-CvO_2). The normal VO_2 is ~ 250mL/min or 150 mL/min/M^2. **Figure 4-10** illustrates a summary of the normal global parameters of oxygenation.

The relationship between oxygen delivery (DO_2) and oxygen uptake by the tissues (VO_2), expressed as a ratio of VO_2 / DO_2, is termed the *oxygen extraction ratio* (O_2ER). The VO_2, sometimes referred to as the metabolic rate, in most ICU patients remains relatively constant and is mainly determined by lean tissue mass. Fever and activity will increase the VO_2.

Oxygen delivery (DO_2) must be adequate to meet the peripheral tissue oxygen uptake (VO_2). If DO_2 is 1000 ml/min and tissue VO_2 is 250 ml/min, then oxygen extraction at 25% (VO_2/DO_2) will be adequate. Venous blood, in this condition, will have an oxygen content of 15 mL/dL, which corresponds to a venous blood oxygen saturation (SvO_2) of 75%. The relationship between VO_2 and DO_2 is defined by:

$$VO_2 = DO_2 \times O_2ER$$

For the VO_2 to remain constant, O_2ER must adjust appropriately to changes in DO_2.

Figure 4-11 illustrates the impact of changing variables associated with DO_2 (PaO_2, hemoglobin, cardiac output, SaO_2) on tissue oxygenation indicators (extraction ratio and SvO_2). The figure assumes a constant VO_2 of 250ml/min and changes only one variable in each row. The adjusted variable is shaded in gray. The dependent variables are shaded in white. As oxygen delivery (DO_2)

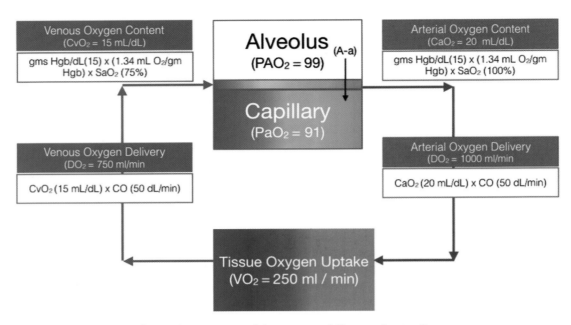

Figure 4-10 *A summary of systemic parameters of tissue oxygen delivery and extraction.*

PaO$_2$ (mm Hg)	SaO$_2$ (%)	Hgb (gms/dl)	CO (dl/min)	DO$_2$ (ml/min)	O$_2$ER	SvO$_2$
100	100	15	50	1020	0.24	74
50	87	15	50	882	0.28	62
100	100	7.5	50	518	0.48	27
100	100	15	25	510	0.49	26

Figure 4-11 *A comparison of oxygenation parameters. The initial line represents normal variables. In each subsequent line one variable (grey box) has been reduced by 50% and the impact on the other oxygenation parameters is demonstrated.*

decreases, the extraction ratio must increase to maintain a constant VO$_2$. Note the inverse relationship between the extraction ratio (ER) and SvO$_2$.

The ability to adjust O$_2$ER is a significant regulator of tissue oxygenation. However, the ability of the peripheral tissues to adjust the O$_2$ER is not limitless. Local factors, such as capillary density, peripheral oxygen affinity, and substrate utilization combine to influence tissue oxygen extraction.

A critical reduction in DO$_2$, which exceeds the ability of the tissues to counterbalance by maximizing the O$_2$ER, will produce a fall in VO$_2$. At this point, the rate of aerobic tissue metabolism is restricted by the DO$_2$, and cellular oxidative phosphorylation, generation of ATP, and cell function are altered, leading to tissue *dysoxia*.[6]

A decline in DO$_2$ from a reduced cardiac output will reduce SvO$_2$ and also produce an elevation in venous pCO$_2$. This leads to a widening of the arterial-venous CO$_2$ gradient (usually < 6 mm Hg).

Note that the O$_2$ER can be therapeutically modulated to help you manage a patient. Controlling fever and the use of paralytic drugs will reduce VO$_2$ and therefore reduce the demand on the O$_2$ER. You will learn later that this can help in a patient with severe Adult Respiratory Distress Syndrome and limited oxygen delivery to tissues.

4.6.1 Mixed Venous Oxygen Saturation

Assuming a constant VO$_2$ and a variable extraction ratio, the SvO$_2$ is inversely related to DO$_2$ and becomes a global indicator of the VO$_2$/DO$_2$ balance. To measure an accurate *mixed venous oxygen saturation (SvO$_2$)* requires a pulmonary artery catheter with the sample obtained from mixed venous blood in the pulmonary artery. However, an alternative measurement is the *central venous oxygen saturation (ScvO$_2$)*, which is obtained from a central venous catheter located within the superior vena cava. Since pulmonary artery catheters are much less commonly used to guide resuscitation currently, we will use the ScvO$_2$ as our index of venous blood oxygen saturation in our discussion. In general, the SvO$_2$ and ScvO$_2$ values agree within +/- 5%.

The $ScvO_2$ is a surrogate marker of the VO_2/DO_2 relationship, and a value $< 70\%$ can suggest an impairment of DO_2. The reduction in DO_2 can be caused by a reduction in cardiac output, hemoglobin, or blood hemoglobin saturation.

Thus, the $ScvO_2$ is considered a "poor man's" cardiac output as long as VO_2, blood hemoglobin levels, and saturation are within normal limits.

Should you monitor $ScvO_2$ in all your septic patients? Certainly not, especially if you must expose your patient to the risk of central venous access for the sole purpose of obtaining this value. *Consider $ScvO_2$ one additional tool in your resuscitation toolbox.* You don't use a screwdriver to fix every problem in your house. Use the tool when it can add information to your overall bedside assessment. A low $ScvO_2$ in your septic patient can suggest inadequate oxygen delivery, especially in the presence of an elevated lactate level (*see below*). A normal or high $ScvO_2$ in your septic patient is of limited value. A significant limitation of $ScvO_2$ is that normal or high values cannot discriminate between adequate oxygen delivery and limitations in local tissue extraction. The veno-arterial carbon dioxide partial pressure (pCO_2) difference is another marker of impaired tissue perfusion. A value > 6 mm Hg suggests inadequate tissue perfusion if the $ScvO_2$ is normal.[25]

Our patient has responded to volume resuscitation and low dose norepinephrine. He remains febrile at 38.8°C. He can maintain his mean arterial blood pressure > 65 mm Hg with the vasopressor support. His oxygen saturation is currently 92%. His $ScvO_2$ is 50%, and his lactate is 3.5. His hemoglobin is 7 gms/dL. He has evidence of residual hypoperfusion as manifested by low urine output and mildly elevated lactate. His low $ScvO_2$ can be a good sign in sepsis, confirming the peripheral tissues continue to utilize oxygen. However, a mismatch between supply (DO_2) and demand (VO_2) exists. We will decrease his oxygen demand by suppression of his fever with acetaminophen and consider transfusion of one unit packed red blood cells to improve his tissue oxygen delivery. We will also check a point of care ultrasound to assess his preload and ventricular performance.

4.6.2 Blood Lactate

The blood lactate level is considered a crude measure of tissue dysoxia, although in reality, this is a very simplified view of elevated lactate in the blood (hyperlactatemia). Multiple metabolic factors contribute to the measured blood lactate level, some of which are beneficial to the host. *Elevated blood lactate levels represent one of the best biomarkers to predict survival in patients with septic shock regardless of the cause.* Arterial and venous blood lactate levels are well correlated, so either can be measured.

Lactate arises from the metabolism of glucose. Glycolysis in the cytoplasm leads to the formation of the intermediate metabolite pyruvate. Under aerobic conditions, pyruvate is converted to acetyl CoA to enter the Krebs cycle. Alternatively, pyruvate is converted by lactate dehydrogenase (LDH) to (or from) lactic acid in the cytoplasm. In aqueous solutions, lactic acid dissociates almost entirely to lactate and H^+. Consequently, the terms *lactic acid* and *lactate* are used interchangeably.

An elevated blood lactate level (hyperlactatemia) results from an imbalance of lactate production and lactate clearance. Lactate production occurs primarily from glucose metabolism via the glycolytic pathway in skeletal muscle, skin, brain, bowel, and erythrocytes. Lactate clearance occurs in the liver (60%) via mitochondrial oxidation to carbon dioxide and water (70 to 80%), or through hepatic gluconeogenesis (15 to 20%). The kidney plays a lesser role in lactate clearance (30%) via similar metabolic pathways. The net result of the balance between lactate production and clearance is a normal plasma lactate level of < 2.2 mmol/L.

Hyperlactatemia is a persistent increase in blood lactate concentration (> 2.2 mmol/L) without metabolic acidosis. Lactic acidosis is a persistently increased blood lactate level associated with an anion gap metabolic acidosis.

The relationship between lactate production and acidosis is complicated. The hydrolysis of adenosine triphosphate (ATP) provides the energy source for protein synthesis at the cellular level as defined by:

$$ATP = ADP + Pi + H^+ + energy$$

where ADP is adenosine diphosphate and Pi is inorganic phosphate. When oxygen supply is adequate, the cells use ADP, Pi, and H^+ in the mitochondria to reconstitute ATP. In the setting of cellular hypoxia, the hydrolysis of ATP leads to the accumulation of H^+ and Pi in the cytosol. This ATP hydrolysis is the source of cellular acidosis during hypoxia and not the formation of lactate from glucose. The formation of lactate from glucose is defined by:

$$glucose + 2\,ADP + 2\,Pi = 2\,lactate + 2\,ATP$$

Note the formation of lactate from glucose neither consumes nor produces H^+. The hydrolysis of the 2 ATP molecules for energy leads to the generation of ADP, Pi, and H^+. If oxygen supply is adequate, the mitochondria recycle the ATP metabolites, and the lactate level will increase without an associated acidosis. In contrast, if cellular hypoxia exists, the ATP hydrolysis associated with lactate production leads to H^+ and the associated acidosis.

In any given patient, an acidemia may occur with an elevated blood lactate. The development of lactic acidosis depends on the magnitude of hyperlactatemia, the body's buffering capacity, and the co-existence of tissue hypoxia. Also, blood pH is influenced by co-existing conditions such as hyperventilation. Therefore, hyperlactatemia may be associated with acidemia, a normal pH, or alkalemia.

Hypoxia blocks the oxidative phosphorylation of pyruvate within the mitochondria, leading to accumulation of pyruvate. Pyruvate metabolism is then shifted to lactate formation. Intracellular lactate concentrations rise rapidly in the setting of tissue hypoxia, and lactate is excreted into the bloodstream, leading to elevated blood lactate levels. Lactate generation secondary to oxygen deficiency and the associated cessation of oxidative phosphorylation is often called *Type A lactate elevation*.

In conditions of accelerated glycolysis, lactate levels can also rise as the rate of pyruvate generation exceeds the capacity of the Krebs cycle to proceed with oxidative phosphorylation. In this state, lactate generation occurs in the setting of a fully functional mitochondrial electron transplant chain with no oxygen deficiency! Lactate production in the absence of tissue hypoxia is classified as *Type B lactate elevation*.

A transient increase in lactate production occurs following the tonic-clonic contractions of epilepsy or the vigorous muscle contractions of exercise. Both these conditions cause a profound transient elevation in serum lactate and reductions in blood pH. However, these values rapidly return to normal after the event has terminated, due to an accelerated lactate clearance.

In sepsis, the source of elevated lactate is multi-factorial. Lactate production is increased due to accelerated aerobic glycolysis, resulting from adrenergic-dependent stimulation of the B_2 adrenoreceptor. The administration of exogenous B_2-agonists (either intravenous or inhaled) can also further stimulate lactate production via accelerated glycolysis.

Sepsis impairs hepatic clearance of lactate due to poor hepatic or renal perfusion or intracellular acidosis. If tissue hypoxia also exists, impaired mitochondrial oxidation further impairs lactate clearance.

A current debate exists regarding the relative contribution of these individual mechanisms to the elevated lactate level seen in patients with septic shock. Does it reflect primarily tissue dysoxia, or is it a "stress" biomarker related to the high glucose oxidation rate associated with high-level adrenergic stimulation[26]? In the "stress" biomarker model, volume resuscitation serves to lower adrenergic tone, which reduces lactate generation. In this model, lactate generation would be a clinical marker similar to tachycardia or an elevated white blood cell count in the patient with sepsis and shock.

In most critically ill patients, lactate production is a combination of factors, including increased production and a decreased rate of clearance. In population studies, elevated blood lactate levels have provided an important biomarker of a shock state with a poor prognostic outcome. Less clear is whether a reduction in the lactate level (lactate clearance) is a useful marker of a successful resuscitation. Some investigators have demonstrated correlations between lactate clearance and patient mortality in sepsis.[27,28] Other investigators have challenged this hypothesis.[26]

An elevated lactate level is best considered a marker of disease severity, rather than a specific target to resolve.[27] There are many reasons a lactate level can be elevated, so each patient has to be carefully assessed. Look for other parameters of organ hypoperfusion, if your patient has an elevated lactate level on presentation. If poor perfusion is suspected, focus on those aspects of the resuscitation you can control including restoration of preload, maintenance of the mean arterial pressure, and correction of hypoxemia and deficits in tissue oxygen delivery. Shoot for those target values outlined in **Figure 4-5.** Currently, we have no evidence to suggest that targeting supernormal parameters to achieve very high levels of DO_2 during resuscitation are any more effective at reversing the mortality effect than standard resuscitation.

If your lactate levels fail to decrease or increases in the septic patient during resuscitation, reconsider impaired organ perfusion (e.g., gut or limb ischemia) and global tissue dysoxia as underlying etiologies. Avoid excessive beta-agonist stimulation and address hepatic insults such as medications or venous congestion to augment lactate clearance.

The combination of $ScvO_2$ and blood lactate provide crude measures of tissue metabolism to help guide resuscitation. All critically ill patients with elevated lactate do not suffer from a limited DO_2, and all patients with a limited DO_2 do not have an elevated lactate level. Consider each of these parameters and their limitations in your assessment of tissue oxygenation. The clinical interpretation of these indicators and possible interventions are outlined in **Figure 4-12.**

Our patient has stabilized in his resuscitation with IVF administration, and his MAP is now acceptable. We have provided acetaminophen, his fever is reduced, and his $ScvO_2$ is now 70%. We elected to transfuse one unit of packed red blood cells, and his urine output is now improving. A point of care ultrasound examination shows normal left ventricular function and no dynamic collapse of his inferior vena cava with respiration. Broad spectrum antibiotic coverage addressed at pathogens known to be associated with severe community-acquired pneumonia have been infused.

Lactate	ScvO$_2$	Assessment	Intervention
Normal	Normal	Normal O$_2$ER without tissue dysoxia	No specific intervention if other clinical markers of tissue perfusion are normal
Normal	↓	Increased O$_2$ER without tissue dysoxia	Control fever Consider transfusion of Hgb to ≥ 7.5 gms/dL Obtain an echocardiogram to assess cardiac function Consider an inotrope trial if evidence for reduced cardiac function
↑	↓	Increased O$_2$ER with tissue dysoxia	Control fever Consider transfusion of Hgb to ≥ 7.5 gms/dl Obtain an echocardiogram to assess cardiac function Consider an inotrope trial if evidence for reduced cardiac function
↑	Normal or high	Normal to low O$_2$ER with hyperglycolysis or tissue dysoxia	Treat underlying condition (i.e., sepsis) and consider additional causes for mitochondrial oxidative inhibition

Figure 4-12 Results of the tissue oxygenation parameters, lacate and mixed venous oxygen saturation (ScvO$_2$), and their assessment and possible interventions.

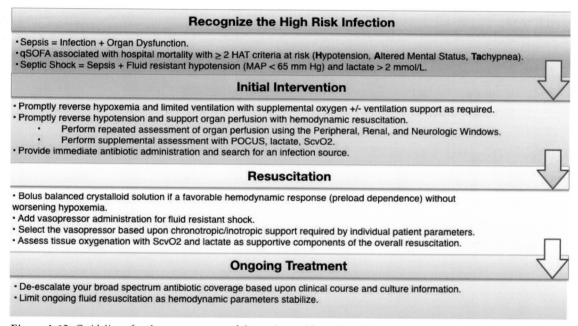

Figure 4-13 Guidelines for the management of the patient with sepsis and septic shock.

How do these parameters of hemodynamics and tissue oxygenation interact in your shock assessment? Consider the hypovolemic ICU patient. This patient suffers from a reduced end-diastolic volume of the left ventricle (reduced preload) leading to a reduction in stroke volume. The decrease in stroke volume can be partially compensated for by an increase in HR to maintain CO, explaining the frequent presence of tachycardia in the setting of volume contraction. However, a progressive fall in CO will eventually lead to a reduction in mean arterial pressure (MAP) and oxygen delivery (DO$_2$). The body will attempt to maintain MAP through systemic vasoconstriction (increased SVR) to compensate for the reduction in CO. In addition, the O$_2$ER will rise, and the ScvO$_2$ will fall. The patient may show evidence of a lactic acidosis.

While an appropriate response to the reduction in MAP, systemic vasoconstriction will compromise tissue oxygen delivery, potentially leading to systemic organ failure. Early application of vasopressors could also worsen DO$_2$. The correct initial therapeutic maneuver is volume resuscitation to restore preload, improve cardiac output, reduce the O$_2$ER, and increase the ScvO$_2$. This intervention will lead to optimal organ perfusion and hopefully is timely to limit the progression to sustained organ dysfunction.

A summary of the approach to the septic patient is shown in **Figure 4-13**.

4.7 Hydrocortisone and Septic Shock

In addition to volume resuscitation and vasopressor support, the administration of corticosteroids to patients with septic shock has been investigated in multiple clinical trials. The two largest trials have confirmed a beneficial effect of hydrocortisone (equivalent dose to hydrocortisone 200 mg IV q24 hours) treatment in septic shock on secondary outcome parameters of shock reversal and the duration of mechanical ventilation.[29,30] However, these trials differed in the primary outcome parameter of 90-day survival, leaving clinicians inconsistent data to support a survival advantage for adrenal axis treatment strategies in patients presenting with septic shock. This therapy might be considered for patients with vasopressor-resistant shock to improve hemodynamics when vasopressor titration is not effective. However, based on the inconsistent mortality effect, hydrocortisone administration should be discontinued when the patient is weaned off the vasopressors consistent with resolution of the shock state. Treatment with adrenal replacement therapy does not prevent the progression to shock.[31]

4.8 Antibiotics and Source Control

A critical aspect of sepsis intervention is source identification and prompt antibiotic administration. Carefully consider signs and symptoms that might suggest a respiratory, renal, or intra-abdominal source. Sample all available body fluids for gram stain and culture. All existing intravenous catheters in the unstable patient should be removed and replaced if still needed. Blood should be cultured from two independent collections.

Time is everything: Antibiotic administration should be prompt, and the timeliness may be the most critical intervention (< 1 hour of assessment).[7,32] Antibiotic selection should be based on the source assessment, Gram stain data, local resistance patterns, and knowledge of the patient's previous resistance patterns and specific immune defects. A review of past culture data and a history of prior hospitalization is critically important for patients with frequent hospitalizations that are at risk for methicillin resistant staph (MRSA) infection and multiple drug resistant (MDR) gram-negative infections.

Given the range of variables that influence antibiotic selection in the septic patient, a recommendation for a specific regimen is not possible. Antibiotic coverage initially should cover a broad range of Gram-positive and Gram-negative organisms. An extended-range penicillen/beta-lactamase inhibitor (e.g. piperacillen/tazobactam), a broad-spectrum carbapenem (e.g. meropenem), or third generation cephalosporin are often chosen. Your patient is at risk from any delay in antibiotic administration or the selection of antibiotics that are later proven to be ineffective for the patient's organism. The clinician should never limit the use of broad-spectrum antibiotic coverage in the initial management of sepsis, and especially septic shock. The antibiotic therapy can be tailored to cover the identified organism and susceptibility once cultures are reported. Antibiotics are selected from different classes to avoid overlapping mechanisms of action.

Know your own hospital's antibiogram data. Attention to your local antibiogram pattern can potentially inform decisions regarding the need for dual Gram-negative treatment and potentially reduce the need for empiric methicillin-resistant Staphylococcus aureus (MRSA) treatment for hospital-acquired and ventilator-associated pneumonia.[33] If your local antibiogram suggests < 10% exposure risk

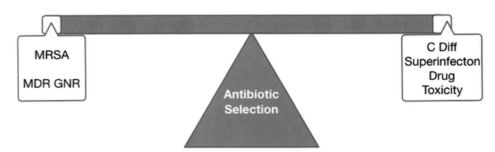

Figure 4-14 *Illustrates the balance clinicians must consider in their hospital based antibiotic selection. Hospitalized patients are at risk for complex hospital organisms such as methicillin resistant staphylococcus aureus (MRSA) and multi-drug resistant gram negative organisms (MDR GNR) favoring antibiotics with a broad spectrum of coverage. This need is offset by the risk of superinfection, Clostridium difficile infection (C Diff) and associated drug toxicities.*

to methicillin-resistant Staphylococcus aureus (MRSA) then vancomycin can be excluded from initial HAP coverage. Likewise, if your local antibiogram suggests < 10% risk of multi-drug resistant Gram-negative infection, then single coverage for these pathogens may be appropriate.

The initial use of combination antibiotic therapy for Gram-negative infections is logically justified based upon potential synergy between two classes of antimicrobial drugs and the prevention of resistance emergence during treatment. Although logical, the clinical evidence to support these hypotheses remains limited.[34] This potential benefit is offset by the incremental risk of drug toxicities including Clostridium difficile colitis, renal insufficiency (aminoglycosides), and superinfection with resistant organisms **Figure 4-14.** Currently, we have no clinical data that suggest combination therapy of a β-lactam plus a fluoroquinolone or aminoglycoside results in improved patient outcomes compared with a β-lactam antibiotic alone.[35] The initial empiric antibiotic coverage remains typically broad in scope (escalated) but should be narrowed in spectrum (deescalated) based upon the individual patient culture data available to the clinician.

OK. That should be a good start on key information for the initial management of a patient with sepsis. We will expand your knowledge base on all these topics as we move along in our other chapters.

Suggested Reading

- Rhodes A, Evans LE, Alhazzani W, et al. Surviving sepsis campaign: international guidelines for management of sepsis and septic shock. Crit Care Med. 2017;45(3):486–552.
- Semler MW, Kellum JA. Balanced crystalloid solutions. American Journal of Respiratory and Critical Care Medicine. 2018.
- Fang F, Zhang Y, Tang J, et al. Association of Corticosteroid Treatment With Outcomes in Adult Patients With Sepsis. JAMA Intern Med [Internet] 2019;179(2):213–23.

5

Management of Tachyarrythmias

In this chapter, we will review the approach to the diagnosis and management of the more common tachyarrhythmias you will encounter on the wards and ICUs, including atrial fibrillation/flutter and stable/unstable paroxysmal supraventricular tachycardia. Let's start with the general approach and then talk about the specific etiology, diagnosis, and management of each. Each time you encounter a tachyarrythmia you need to ask five questions.

1. Do I have time to think?
2. What is the diagnosis?
3. How do I stop the tachyarrythmia and prevent it from coming back?
4. What is the rhythm trying to tell me?
5. Do I need to consider anticoagulation?

5.1 Do I Have Time to Think?

The patient's hemodynamic stability is the first question to consider when you walk into the room. If the patient has significant hypotension or has no pulse, you *DO NOT HAVE TIME TO THINK, SO CHARGE, SYNCHRONIZE, AND SHOCK.* Note that for a narrow complex tachycardia you can deliver a low-energy synchronized cardioversion (50 – 100 J). The synchronization will prevent providing a cardioversion during ventricular repolarization, which can cause ventricular fibrillation.

If you have time to think, meaning the blood pressure is relatively stable, you can work on a diagnosis and treatment plan more carefully.

5.2 What is the Diagnosis?

A patient history, particularly concerning baseline rhythm and cardiac history, is very beneficial to characterize the type of rhythm abnormality in a given patient. Does the patient have a history of arrhythmia, and what type? This background information can be as valuable as the current 12 lead ECG in helping to characterize a specific rhythm abnormality. Pacemakers and implantable cardiac defibrillators can provide a "memory" of stored information from the patient to characterize past or current rhythm abnormalities.

*You are working on the rapid response team, and you are called to see a 76 yo female post-op day #2 from a right total hip replacement. The patient had noted a fluttering sensation in her chest and the nurse recorded vital signs with a HR of ~150, a blood pressure of 110/80, a RR 18, with an SaO2 on room air of 90%. The patient's lungs are clear to auscultation, and the cardiac exam reveals a regular tachycardia. The rate is rapid, but you do not appreciate a murmur. The patient is placed on the monitor, and the nurse hands you the rhythm strip in **Figure 5-1**.*

5.2.1 Narrow Complex Tachycardia

The narrow complex (QRS < 120 ms) suggests a rhythm originating from the atrium or AV bundle. The regular R-R interval narrows your differential to three principal causes for a rate of 150-180 with a regular rhythm **(Figure 5-2)**:

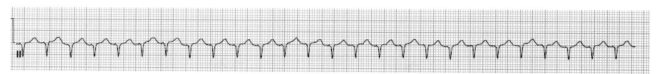

Figure 5-1 *Narrow complex tachycardia rhythm strip.*

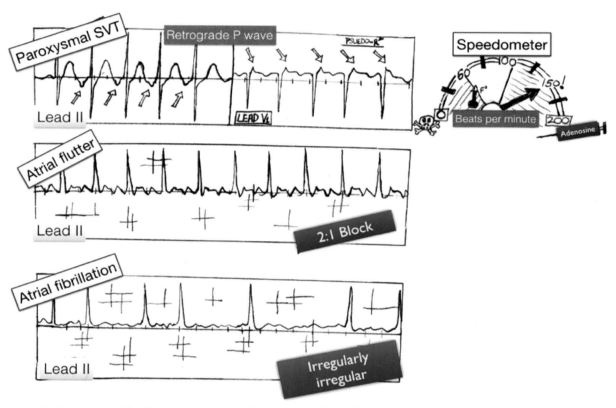

Figure 5-2 *Comparison of the three common causes of narrow complex tachycardia.*

1. Sinus tachycardia
2. Atrial flutter with a fixed 2:1 block
3. Paroxysmal supraventricular tachycardia (PSVT), meaning an arrhythmia with an origin above the bundle of His (this includes AV nodal and atrioventricular nodal reentry tachycardia)

Note that neither atrial fibrillation nor multifocal atrial tachycardia is on the list. Both these arrhythmias would typically have an irregularly irregular rhythm. So, you can ask two easy questions with any rhythm strip to get started

1. Narrow complex vs. wide complex?
2. Regular vs. irregular?

The first step is to get a full 12-lead ECG and a longer-running rhythm strip. The strip that is best to examine for P waves is lead II or V₁ to help distinguish

the three most common narrow complex arrhythmias. Uniform P waves with a fixed R-R interval suggest sinus tachycardia; absent P waves suggest PSVT; and sawtooth waves suggest atrial flutter. How else can you sort through the differential diagnosis of a narrow complex, regular tachycardia?

Pressing broadly on the carotid artery (if there is no bruit or history of stroke) at the same time the ECG strip is running performs a vagal maneuver. If you are in the ICU working with a ventilator patient, you might try suctioning, which can have the same effect. A vagal maneuver will slow down the A-V node and allow you to see more clearly if there are P waves and their relationship to the QRS complex. A vagal maneuver can help you see if the diagnosis looks like a sinus tachycardia, with one P wave preceding every QRS, or if there are atrial flutter waves, typically running at 300 beats per minute. Atrial fibrillation will not have a regular QRS rate, but the rate will be irregularly irregular, and with a vagal maneuver you may see the fibrillation background. For an AV nodal or atrioventricular reentrant tachycardia, the vagal maneuver may break the cycle and convert the rhythm, but this tends to be temporary. The vagal maneuver is most effective when there is no significant sympathetic tone present. Unfortunately, this is often *NOT* the case in the typical ICU patient with a rapid, narrow complex tachycardia.

Adenosine is an endogenous purine nucleoside that signals through four adenosine receptor subtypes (A1, A2A, A2B, and A3). When administered intravenously, adenosine activates the A1 receptor, as well as other receptors, to block the AV node. The different adenosine receptor subtypes can either stimulate or inhibit adenylate cyclase activity.

You will experience the power of adenosine signaling first-hand. Do a quick check to see if your patient has a history of asthma or obstructive lung disease, in which case you avoid adenosine due to the risk of aggravating bronchoconstriction. Also, adenosine is less useful in the presence of theophylline, as theophylline blocks the adenosine receptors.

If no asthma or theophylline, proceed. As a patient's heart races at a rate of 150 beats per minute in a paroxysmal supraventricular tachyarrhythmia, you will prepare 6-12 mg of adenosine while running a continuous electrocardiogram. You then push the drug as a bolus into an intravenous line to deliver the medicine to the heart. Since the half-life of the drug is so short, it is key to push the adenosine and flush behind it. There are few experiences as dramatic in medicine as watching the monitor expectantly until the racing QRS complexes suddenly stutter, slow, and then stop. Flat-line… **Figure 5-3**.

Time will seem to slow down as the 15-30 second heart block drags on, seemingly forever, while you move closer to the patient, contemplating chest compressions. Wait… And then the adenosine is degraded by the red cell and vascular adenosine deaminase, the A1 receptors clear, and the electrical activity recovers, often with conversion to normal sinus rhythm or back into the AV nodal re-entry tachycardia.

From a diagnostic standpoint, if you run a rhythm strip during the infusion of adenosine, you will have an opportunity to see the underlying problem, based upon the response of the rhythm to adenosine as outlined in **Figure 5-4**.[36] If the adenosine causes no change, then you did not give enough, or the arrhythmia is below the AV node that you attempted to block. Adenosine will be ineffective if the arryhthmia source is high in the ventricular conduction system, so it maintains a narrow complex. If it suddenly stops and then you see sinus P waves, this suggests that you had an AV nodal re-entry or atrio-ventricular nodal re-entry tachycardia (described below) that you blocked by inhibiting the circuit running through the A-V node. Finally, if the QRS complexes stop or gradually slow and reveal fast regular or irregular P waves, this suggests an atrial tachycardia, either sinus or ectopic (going at around 150) or atrial flutter (going at close to 300).

> If the patient has a history of structural heart disease, this greatly increases the probability that a wide complex tachyarrhythmia originates from the ventricle (V tach)! In the setting of significant heart disease, best to treat a wide complex tachycardia as VT until proven otherwise.

An alternative therapeutic option to adenosine for the control of supraventricular narrow complex rhythms would include the AV nodal blocking agents verapamil (2.5-5 mg IV over 2 minutes) or diltiazem (10-15 mg IV). In general, adenosine is used initially as a diagnostic agent due to its short half-life.

Or maybe the nurse handed you the rhythm in **Figure 5-5**:

This rhythm has a narrow complex (QRS < 120 msec) but is irregular without a pattern (i.e., irregularly irregular). A narrow complex rhythm with an irregular R-R interval would most likely be

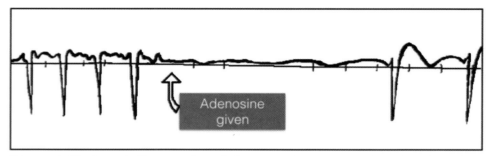

Figure 5-3 Rhythm strip illustrates the typical response of a suprventricular tachycardia to the administration of adenosine.

1. Atrial fibrillation (or atrial flutter with a variable block)
2. Multifocal atrial tachycardia

Multifocal atrial tachycardia will demonstrate multiple P waves morphologies with a variable P-R interval. Atrial fibrillation has no identifiable P waves.

5.2.2 Wide Complex Tachycardia

Alternatively, you might have been handed the rhythm in **Figure 5-6** by the nurse. (Hopefully, the nurse does not hand you all three rhythm strips!)

This rhythm is a little harder to sort out as the wide complex can be due to either ventricular tachycardia or aberrant conduction of a supraventricular rhythm. The most common arrhythmias associated with this ECG would include

1. Sinus tachycardia with aberrant ventricular conduction
2. Atrial flutter with a 2:1 block with aberrant ventricular conduction
3. Paroxysmal supraventricular tachycardia with aberrant ventricular conduction
4. Ventricular tachycardia

In this case, you still ask the same question, "Do I have time to think?" *No time to think – synchronize and shock!* Time to think – well, it gets a little tricky at this point.

Ventricular tachycardia can occur with uniform-appearing QRS complexes (monomorphic VT) and variable QRS morphology (polymorphic VT). The

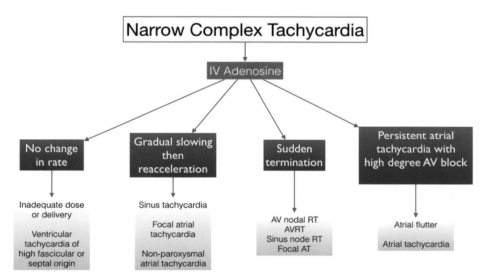

Figure 5-4 *Differential diagnosis of narrow complex tachycardia based upon the response to the administration of IV adenosine.*

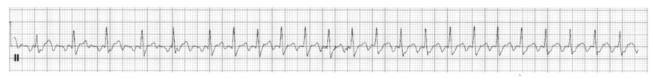

Figure 5-5 *Irregular narrow complex tachycardia rhythm strip.*

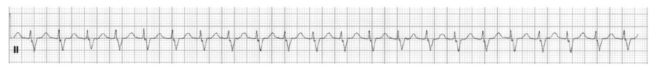

Figure 5-6 *Wide complex tachycardia rhythm strip.*

monomorphic VT can be very tough to distinguish from aberrantly conducted supraventricular arrhythmia. Aberrant conduction is conduction of a supraventricular impulse to the ventricles in a pattern different than the usual conduction pattern. The supraventricular impulse reaches the ventricle during the refractory period of the conduction system, leading to a prolonged QRS pattern seen as a bundle branch block pattern. Since the right bundle branch refractory period is longer than the left, the majority of aberrant conduction occurs with a right bundle branch pattern. Any supraventricular rhythm, including sinus tachycardia, can be conducted with an aberrant pattern.

The most important clues to favor ventricular tachycardia over an aberrant SVT are the presence of *fusion beats* and *AV dissociation*. In *AV dissociation*, there is no consistent relationship between the P waves and QRS complexes. *Fusion beats* is a "hybrid" QRS complex produced by a ventricular impulse that merges with a normal QRS complex (**Figure 5-7).** If either of these two features is present, this argues strongly that the wide complex tachycardia is ventricular in origin.

How should you approach a wide complex tachycardia? If the blood pressure is stable, you can consider the possibility the rhythm is SVT with aberrancy, using the vagal maneuver and adenosine to diagnosis and possibly treat the problem. If an aberrant SVT, the maneuvers may help you confirm AV association (atrial flutter/fib with aberrancy), or the rhythm may immediately terminate (AVNRT with aberrancy). Commonly in patients with cardiac disease, ventricular tachycardia will not respond to adenosine or vagal maneuvers. If the rhythm does not respond to these maneuvers, you can treat with amiodarone. Less commonly, an adenosine sensitive form of ventricular tachycardia does occur in patients with normal hearts.

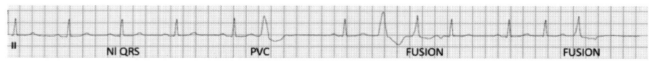

Figure 5-7 *ECG rhythm strip illustrates fusion beats.*

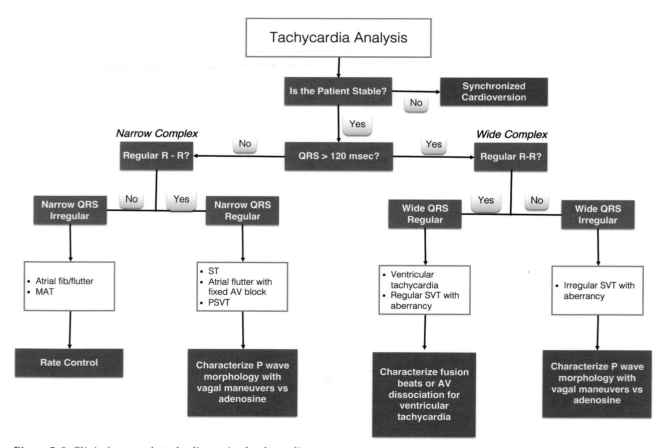

Figure 5-8 *Clinical approach to the diagnosis of tachycardia.*

If you suspect ventricular tachycardia from the beginning or the patient is older (age > 35) with a history of significant structural cardiac disease, then administer amiodarone.

The diagnostic approach to tachycardia is summarized in **Figure 5-8**.

5.3 How Do I Stop the Arrhythmia?

Now that you have a diagnosis or think you have a diagnosis, you can focus on a specific therapy. The big picture is: *Slow down the bad boy and then convert!* We will review for each specific disorder.

5.3.1 Sinus Tachycardia

Uniform P wave morphology and a constant P-R interval characterize sinus tachycardia. The key here is to identify and treat the underlying cause of the sinus tachycardia. The etiology can be hypotension, pain, or a cardiorespiratory problem. You need to assess fluid status, vital signs, and laboratory tests for evidence of sepsis, and evaluate the chest radiograph and ECG for congestive heart failure, pneumonia, or myocardial infarction. Rare etiologies for tachycardia include hyperthyroidism and pulmonary embolism. Therapy should address the primary cause, and the tachycardia will recover. The primary indication for pharmacologic treatment is evidence for myocardial ischemia in the setting of the tachycardia. A carefully titrated dosing of beta-receptor antagonists may be helpful for this condition.

5.3.2 Atrial Fibrillation and Flutter

Atrial fibrillation (AF) is the most common cardiac arrhythmia you will see in clinical practice. Atrial flutter is considered just another flavor of this same rhythm abnormality and treated in an identical manner. AF is a very common post-operative arrhythmia. The post-operative AF is typically self-limited with the clear majority of patients converting to NSR within 6-8 weeks post op.

How to approach AF/flutter in the acute hospital setting?

No time to think – go right to electrical cardioversion. Time to think—OK, you have a few choices to make. Does your patient have any evidence for pre-excitation (see below)? Important to know, because this requires special precautions. We will assume no evidence for pre-excitation and move forward.

The initial therapy is the intravenous administration of either a beta blocker or a non-dihydropyridine calcium channel blocker. You can treat with an IV bolus of diltiazem (0.25 mg/kg) or verapamil (0.075 to 0.15 mg/kg) administered as a bolus over 2 minutes. Currently, diltiazem is favored over verapamil as the first-line agent because it produces less myocardial depression. A second intravenous bolus dose of diltiazem may be administered after 15 minutes at a dose of 0.35 mg/kg over 2 minutes. The bolus dose administration will have a typical onset within 5 minutes and last a few hours. The bolus dose of diltiazem can be followed by a diltiazem infusion at 5-15 mg per hour targeting a heart rate of < 110 bpm if the arrhythmia persists or is recurrent. For patients with persistent symptoms, you may set a more aggressive target of < 85 bpm.

Alternatively, a beta-1 selective IV Beta-blocker such as metoprolol or esmolol may be administered. The initial dose for metoprolol is 2.5-5.0 mg every 2 to 5 minutes (maximum 15 mg in 15 min). An even shorter-acting, titratable Beta-blocker is esmolol. Esmolol is given as a 500 mcg/kg IV bolus over 1 minute, then 50-300 mcg/kg/min as a continuous infusion.

The decision to use a beta blocker vs. a calcium channel blocker in atrial fibrillation is guided by medical variables, physician preference, and patient response. For patients with reactive airways disease, a calcium channel blocker is preferred. For patients with an acute MI, post cardiac surgery or with hyperthyroidism (all hyperadrenergic states), a beta blocker may be more useful for rate control.

What should you do if your patient has borderline hypotension or heart failure? You have enough time to think – but you are a little nervous about the drug effects (impaired LV contractility) used for control of the rate. Remember, the rapid heart rate may be compromising ventricular filling, leading to your symptoms. The potential adverse drug effect on blood pressure can be offset by improved heart rate control and cardiac output. So, rate control solves the problem!! Just gradually titrate your medication up and observe both your HR and blood pressure response. If unstable – shock!

The third choice for rate control in critically ill patients is amiodarone. Remember, amiodarone is not only an anti-arrhythmic, it also has negative chronotropic activity and will slow down that bad boy. Amiodarone may offer similar rate control to diltiazem but avoids the risk of negative myocardial contractility associated with diltiazem. Amiodarone can be dosed as 150 mg IV over 10 minutes, followed by 1mg/min for 6 hours, then 0.5 mg/min over 18 hours. The potential adverse side effects include hypotension (15%), infusion phlebitis (15%), and bradycardia (5%).

Finally, digoxin can be administered for rate control at 0.25 mg IV, repeated every 2-4 hours over 24 hours to maximum dosing of 1.5 mg over 24 hours. Long the standard medication used for atrial fibrillation, digoxin is generally considered less effective than beta blockers and calcium channel blockers. The drug may have a more favorable role in the setting of atrial fibrillation and heart failure. The effect of digoxin can be additive to other medications, leading to its frequent combination with other rate control agents.

In patients with evidence for pre-excitation conditions, like WPW (read on below), adenosine, digoxin, the non-dihydropyridine calcium channel antagonists (i.e., diltiazem and verapamil) and amiodarone should not be administered. These agents may promote conduction down an accessory pathway and increase the ventricular response rate.

After controlling rate, or if the blood pressure starts to drop with rate control interventions, one can consider conversion of the atrial fibrillation or flutter. Elective cardioversion, either chemical or electrical, can be attempted if the rhythm is new (i.e., < 48 hours) and there is no risk of atrial clot formation (see below).

5.3.2.1 Chemical Cardioversion

Medications including flecainide, dofetilide, propafenone, and IV ibutilide can be used for chemical cardioversion of atrial fibrillation and to maintain sinus rhythm. The medications have individual contraindications and are usually selected by the cardiologist to help guide your decision making. However, only ibutilide has a recognized success rate. Infuse Ibutilide as 1 mg (weight > 60 kg) given slowly over ten minutes. If there is no conversion, this can be repeated as 1 mg over 10 minutes dosed again. Since this drug can prolong the QT interval and lead to torsade depointes, it is prudent to correct hypokalemia and hypomagnesemia before infusion of ibutilide. Pretreatment with IV magnesium sulfate may prevent increases in QT and QTc interval, 30 minutes after the last dose of ibutilide. Administer the drug in a highly monitored environment with personnel trained to address ventricular arrhythmias. Ibutilide appears to be most effective for cardioversion of atrial fibrillation in patients with coronary artery disease and in patients without mitral valve disease and a markedly enlarged left atrium.

Amiodarone can be given before electrical cardioversion in an attempt at chemical cardioversion, or to increase the probability of electrical conversion, as well as to maintain conversion if atrial fibrillation relapses after chemical or synchronized cardioversion. It is typically given as a 150 mg load over 10 minutes, and then at 1 mg per minute for 6 hours, and then 0.5 mg per minute for 18 hours. Amiodarone can then be given orally 600 to 800 mg per day in divided doses until a total of 10 g has been given; then 200 mg per day.

5.3.2.2 Electrical Cardioversion

Cardiac defibrillators provide two types of "shocking" experiences. In a monophasic shock, the shock is delivered in only one direction, passing from one electrode to the second. In a biphasic shock, the energy moves in two directions. Most newer model defibrillators provide a biphasic waveform. Biphasic cardioversion requires less energy (~ ½) and is considered more effective. Theoretically, the use of less energy for cardioversion can reduce damage to the heart muscle.

Atrial flutter will respond to a low-energy synchronized cardioversion (50-100 J), while atrial fibrillation may take more energy. The patient should undergo carefully monitored conscious sedation, after placing chest electrodes anteriorly and posteriorly. Conscious sedation can be accomplished using fentanyl for pain and versed or propofol for sedation while carefully monitoring oxygenation and ventilation by a physician trained in conscious sedation.

For atrial fibrillation, start with 200 joules (J) monophasic or 100 J biphasic. For atrial flutter, begin with 50 J monophasic or 25 J biphasic. Wait at least one minute between shocks and repeat if necessary. Increase the energy level with subsequent shocks to a maximum shock strength of 400 J monophasic or 200 J biphasic. If three efforts to cardiovert fail, you will need to load amiodarone, recheck electrolytes, and reconsider your diagnosis.

Everyone deserves a chance to be in sinus rhythm! A question arises in the case of a patient with chronic atrial fibrillation. Should one merely control the rate, anti-coagulate, and leave alone, or should one try to convert the patient to sinus rhythm? The consensus now is to attempt conversion because this will improve cardiac function and reduce the risk of stroke. However, a very high fraction of ICU patients have recurrent atrial fibrillation following initial successful cardioversion. For the ICU patient, initial rate control and stabilization of the underlying medical condition is favored, with delayed consideration for electrical cardioversion. In many cases, simple rate control and treatment of the underlying disease will result in spontaneous conversion to NSR. Patients who do not convert should be considered for electrical cardioversion prior to being discharged from the hospital.

5.3.3 Multi-focal Atrial Tachycardia

Three different P wave morphologies with variable P-R intervals suggest that ectopic atrial electrical foci are driving the rhythm **(Figure 5-9)**. The ventricular rhythm is irregular. MAT can be confused with AF if the P waves are not recognized. MAT is a problem in elderly patients

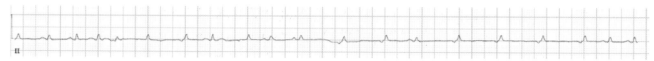

Figure 5-9 Multi-focal atrial tachycardia rhythm strip.

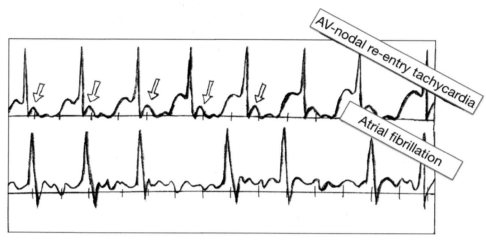

Figure 5-10 Comparison of AV-nodal re-entrant tachycardia and atrial fibrillation.

and frequently associated with chronic lung disease, such as a COPD exacerbation. The best approach to this problem is to treat the underlying cause of lung disease, and the problem corrects. Giving magnesium or potassium and stopping theophylline medications if present can sometimes resolve the abnormal rhythm. Alternatively, rate control with a Beta-blocker (if not contraindicated by lung disease) or a calcium channel blocker can sometimes help.

5.3.4 *Paroxysmal Supraventricular Tachycardia (PSVT)*

PSVTs are a narrow QRS complex tachycardia that results from an accessory pathway in the conduction system, such that a faster and slower conduction pathway "team up" to create a recurrent loop (called re-entrant) in the conduction system. The electrical impulse travels down one pathway, only to travel back up the second pathway. There are five different types of PSVT, characterized by the location of the accessory pathway. The re-entry pathways may be at the level of the low atrium, AV node or AV valve rings; and the P and QRS can be on top of each other; or more often the P wave follows the QRS buried in the ST segment (See **Figure 5-10**). These are fast rhythms running at 150-240 bpm, typically around 180.

Knowledge of the location and activity of the pathways is necessary for electrophysiologists to target

and radiofrequency ablate. You might need help from the electrophysiologist here, but we will review two common PSVT's.

5.3.4.1 AV Nodal Re-entry Tachycardia (AVNRT)

AVNRT is defined by a reentrant circuit (fast and slow pathways) that is in or next to the AV node in the right atrium. AVNRT is the most common regular supraventricular tachycardia and is more common in women than men (approximately 75% of cases occurring in females). Initial treatment is the same as above for SVT with specific vagal maneuvers, adenosine, or calcium channel blockers used to slow the rate or interrupt AV nodal pathways. Rarely, synchronized cardioversion is required. Frequent attacks may require radiofrequency ablation, to destroy the abnormally conducting tissue in the heart. There are two types of AVNRT:

1. The *common form AVNRT* has the slow pathway as the anterograde limb and the fast pathway as the retrograde limb of the reentry circuit (so-called slow-fast common AVNRT). Because the fast pathway is retrograde, the upside-down P wave is often buried in the QRS.
2. The *uncommon form AVNRT* is the opposite; fast is forward and slow is retrograde. This form of AVNRT usually gives an upside-down P wave after the QRS.

5.3.4.2 Atrioventricular Re-entry Tachycardia (AVRT)

AVRT also results from a re-entry circuit. One portion of the circuit is usually the AV node, and the other is an abnormal accessory pathway from the atria to the ventricle (**Figure 5-11** and **Figure 5-12**). The accessory pathways or bypass tracts are abnormal conduction pathways formed during cardiac development. An accessory pathway can conduct impulses either anterograde (toward the ventricle), retrograde (away from the ventricle), or in both directions.

The conduction through the AV node is slower than conduction through the accessory pathway. In sinus rhythm, any conduction over the accessory pathway leads to activation of the ventricles faster than if the impulse had traveled the AV node, leading to the condition of *pre-excitation*. The conduction pattern of pre-excitation leads to the classic ECG findings in sinus rhythm of a shortened PR interval (< 120 ms) and a delta wave (slow rise of the initial portion of the QRS **(Figure 5-13)**. Additional discordant ST segment and T wave changes are often present.

The features of pre-excitation may be present only intermittently and are more pronounced with increased vagal tone or pharmacologic therapy that promotes AV blockade. In patients with a retrograde-only accessory conduction pathway, antegrade conduction only occurs via the AV node, and no findings of pre-excitation are seen. These patients have a "concealed" bypass tract.

During tachyarrythmias, the features of pre-excitation no longer appear on the rhythm strip. An ECG taken after termination of the tachycardia will show evidence for pre-excitation, so always obtain an ECG after termination of an SVT.

Wolff-Parkinson-White syndrome (WPW) refers to an accessory pathway with associated tachyarrhythmia. Some patients may not manifest the tachyarrhythmia but only the characteristic ECG findings of a short PR interval and delta wave **(Figure 5-13).** These patients are diagnosed to have a "WPW pattern" or "WPW ECG" but no diagnosis or symptoms of a fast heart rhythm characteristic of WPW syndrome.

There are two types of AVRT seen in patients with WPW, which can influence the treatment approach:

1. *Orthodromic AVRT* has the supraventricular impulses conducted to the ventricle by the AV node / His-Purkinje system. The accessory pathway provides retrograde conduction. A characteristic of orthodromic AVRT is a P-wave that follows the QRS, caused by this retrograde conduction. The QRS will be a narrow complex in the absence of underlying conduction disease or aberrancy with a ventricular rate between 150-300 bpm. In sinus rhythm, wide QRS complexes may be seen caused by conduction over both the normal and accessory pathways, resulting in a fusion beat. Orthodromic AVRT is the most common variety of WPW syndrome, accounting for 90% of AVRT. Orthodromic AVRT can be initiated by atrial or ventricular premature beats.

2. *Antidromic AVRT* has the supraventricular impulses conducted *down through the accessory pathway* and re-enters the atrium retrogradely via the AV node. Because the accessory pathway initiates conduction in the ventricles outside of

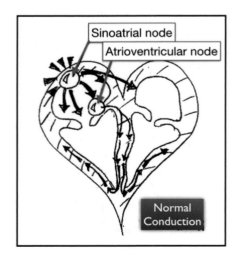

Figure 5-11 *Normal conduction through the AV node.*

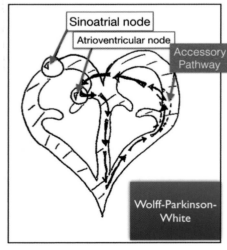

Figure 5-12 *Abnormal conduction through the AV node due to an accessory pathway.*

the bundle of His, the QRS complex in antidromic AVRT is wide. This arrhythmia can easily be confused with ventricular tachycardia. Again, antidromic AVRT can be initiated by atrial or ventricular premature beats.

If WPW is suspected, the traditional therapeutic approaches to rate control can be problematic. Patients with hemodynamic instability are the easiest – no time to think – shock!

For hemodynamically stable patients with orthodromic AVRT, antegrade conduction down the AV node is the component of the re-entrant circuit for therapeutic targeting. Pharmacologic interventions that lengthen AV nodal refractoriness and depress its conduction can block the impulse within the AV node and terminate the tachycardia. Vagal maneuver and agents that block AV nodal conduction, such as adenosine or calcium channel blockers, can be considered. Use DC cardioversion for patients not responsive to medical therapy.

For hemodynamically stable patients with antidromic AVRT, procainamide is considered the medication of choice. In patients with atrial fibrillation and pre-excitation, AV nodal-specific antiarrhythmic drugs used to control the ventricular rate in atrial fibrillation (adenosine, verapamil, amiodarone, digoxin) are contraindicated, as they may accelerate conduction via the bypass tract. Use DC cardioversion for hemodynamically unstable patients or those not responsive to medical therapy.

5.3.5 Ventricular Tachycardia

Ventricular tachycardia is caused by an electrical circuit within the ventricle with depolarization not following the His-Purkinje high-speed electrical highway. Slow depolarization of the ventricle results in a wide QRS not preceded by a P wave. When the ventricular rate is slow, the cardiac output and blood pressure may be stable, but when fast you get into trouble and do not have time to think (shocking events!). Ventricular tachycardia is usually caused by structural cardiac problems, most typically new or old myocardial infarction. *The management of this ventricular tachycardia is easy: amiodarone or electricity!*

5.4 What is the Rhythm Trying to Tell Me?

Remember that dysrhythmias happen for a reason. It is essential, after the dust settles, to think about the why's. For example, sinus tachycardia, atrial fibrillation, and atrial flutter can be caused by hypotension, pulmonary embolism, pulmonary hypertension and right heart failure, hyperthyroidism, and myocardial infarction. An AV-nodal re-entry tachycardia can suggest a chronic problem with the AV node that may need electrophysiological ablation. Ventricular tachycardia can arise from structural heart disease and myocardial infarction. Remember, the causes of SVTs can sometimes work together to cause more hypotension. For example,

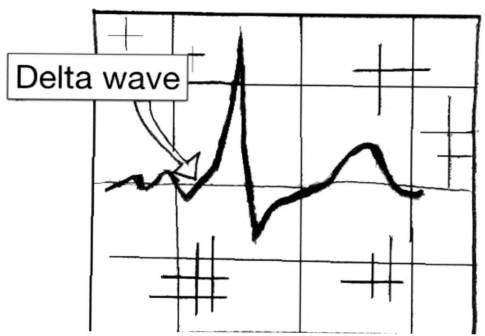

Figure 5-13 *Illustration of the short PR interval and delta wave which characterize Wolff-Parkinson White syndrome.*

if you are treating new atrial fibrillation that is producing hypotension at a relatively low heart rate (100-120), you should consider why the blood pressure is so low at a heart rate that would not be expected to drop cardiac output. Does this patient have an acute pulmonary embolism? Valvular or ischemic heart failure?

Don't forget the humility feedback loop; if your treatment is not working go back and re-evaluate the diagnosis! I (M.G.) will always remember a patient in the emergency room with a tachyarrhythmia of 180 bpm. After doing a vagal maneuver, then 3 doses of adenosine, and one synchronized cardioversion, we realized that we were actually treating a sinus tachycardia and sepsis! Only after one liter of fluid had run in did the hypotensive state correct and the heart rate slowed down enough to see the P waves!

Because atrial fibrillation is one of the most common rhythms you will see in the ICU, remember the mnemonic *PIRATES,* which summarizes the things that can precipitate atrial fibrillation. **Figure 5-14** shows the *PIRATE Blackbeard,* who has a swollen right leg with a DVT and a pulmonary embolism. He is smoking and has emphysema, he clutches his chest with his myocardial infarction, his valves are not normal from mitral regurgitation and endocarditis, his hand shakes, and he has goiter from his hyperthyroidism. Luckily, he has some amiodarone hanging!

Pulmonary: PE, COPD
Iatrogenic
Rheumatic heart: mitral regurgitation
Atherosclerotic: MI, CAD
Thyroid: hyperthyroid
Endocarditis
Sick sinus syndrome

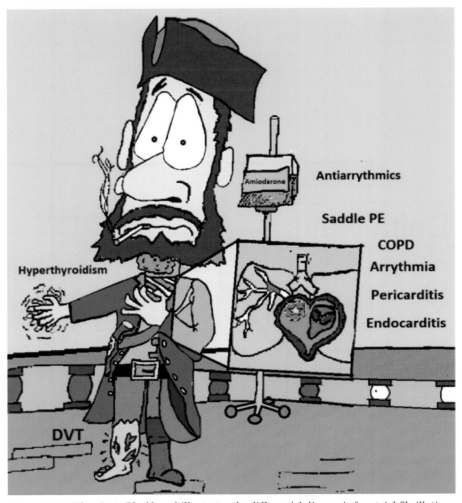

Figure 5-14 The pirate Blackbeard illustrates the differential diagnosis for atrial fibrillation.

5.5 Do I Need to Anticoagulate?

Atrial fibrillation (AF) of > 48 hours in duration carries an increased risk of an associated embolic event. The difficulty in most patients is that the duration of AF is not defined, so most AF is treated with anticoagulation. The decision to anticoagulate a patient with atrial fibrillation must consider the risk-benefit profile associated with anticoagulation, but a few general concepts apply.

For acute episodes of atrial fibrillation > 48 hours in duration with a plan for cardioversion, the patient should receive three weeks of anticoagulation before and four weeks after cardioversion. The need for anticoagulation applies to both chemical and electrical cardioversion. If patients begin immediate anticoagulation, a negative transesophageal echocardiogram (TEE) for atrial clot can avoid the three-week pre-anticoagulation requirement.

For patients with atrial fibrillation and a mechanical heart valve with no plan for cardioversion, warfarin is recommended, with a target international normalized ratio (INR) of 2.0 – 3.5, depending on the type and location of the prosthesis. In patients with non-valvular atrial fibrillation and no plan for cardioversion, the current suggestion is to assess stroke risk with the CHA_2DS_2-VASc score **(Figure 5-15)**.[37] Patients with a CHA_2DS_2-VASc score ≥ 2 should receive anticoagulant. Patients with a CHA_2DS_2-VASc score of 0 are very low risk, and anticoagulation may be omitted. Patients with a CHA_2DS_2-VASc score of 1 are an intermediate risk, warranting consideration of the risk-to-benefit ratio. Patients with atrial flutter are considered to have the same risk profile as patients with atrial fibrillation. For patients with advanced chronic kidney disease (CKD), warfarin remains the agent of choice. In patients without CKD, a direct thrombin or factor Xa inhibitor,

Variable	Points
Female Gender	1
Age 65 to 74 years	1
Age $\geq$ 75 years	2
Diabetes mellitus	1
Prior stroke, TIA, or thromboembolism	2
Vascular Disease (prior MI, PAD, or aortic plaque)	1
Hypertension	1
Congestive Heart Failure	1

Figure 5-15 *Scoring summary for the CHA_2DS_2-VASc score.*

CHA_2DS_2 – VASc Score	Unadjusted Ischemic Stroke Rate (% per year)
0	0.2 %
1	0.6%
2	2.2%
3	3.2%
4	4.8%
5	7.2%
6	9.7%
7	11.2%
8	10.8%
9	12.2%

Figure 5-16 *Ischemic stroke risk per year (%) based upon the CHA_2DS_2-VASc score.*

such as dabigatran, rivaroxaban, or apixaban may be considered.

The associated stroke risk increases progressively, based upon the total score as outlined in **Figure 5-16.**

If the score is > 1, you should receive anticoagulation if specific contraindications do not exist. The stroke risk rises each point value to 9.7% with a score of 6. The stroke risk above a CHA_2DS_2-VASc score of 1 exceeds the reported risk of bleeding associated with anticoagulation, which is typically in the range of 1-2%.

Suggested Reading

- Lip, GYH, Lane, DA. Stroke prevention in atrial fibrillation: a systematic review. JAMA: 2018;313(19), 1950–1962.
- Kusumoto FM, Schoenfeld MH, Barrett C, et al. 2018 ACC/AHA/HRS Guideline on the evaluation and management of patients with bradycardia and cardiac conduction delay. A report of the American College of Cardiology/American Heart Association Task Force on Clinical Practice Guidelines and the Heart Rhythm. JACC. 2018

6

Running a Code

In this chapter, we will not provide a detailed review of cardiac arrest management. We will focus on the basic tricks and approaches that you should learn to run the code right and save a life. Advanced Cardiac Life Support (ACLS) guidelines, developed in five-year intervals by the American Heart Association, provide a more comprehensive review.[38]

The moment the code is called, start analyzing. As you are running to the scene, consider the type of patient located on the floor. If this is a neurology floor, you might be ready for a seizure; if this is a cardiac floor, you want to be prepared for a conduction block or an arrhythmia.

If you are leading the code, *do not touch the patient!* As soon as you start to put in a line, do CPR, intubate the patient, etc., you will become distracted and forget how much time has elapsed, if you have made the right diagnosis, and if you have given the right drugs at the right interval. If you run the code and do not touch the patient but stand next to the bedside, you will find that you have a lot of time to think, are very clear-headed, and will not miss a beat.

Always be thinking: pulse – rhythm – blood pressure. We classify cardiac arrest into shockable and non-shockable rhythms. The shockable rhythms are ventricular fibrillation and ventricular tachycardia. The non-shockable rhythms are pulseless electrical activity and asystole.

If you have a pulse, you can relax, and you will have some time to think. Next, analyze your rhythm and measure the patient's blood pressure. If you do not have a pulse, then figure out if you have a shockable rhythm. Mainly, you need to decide if you have ventricular fibrillation/ventricular tachycardia (VF/VT) or asystole/pulseless electrical activity (PEA). Pulseless electrical activity is also called *electromechanical dissociation.* PEA is a non-shockable rhythm (i.e., sinus rhythm) that should produce a pulse, but does not. If you have VF/VT – *Shock!*

6.1 Chest Compressions

Your initial goals in the cardiac arrest patient should focus on excellent cardiopulmonary resuscitation (CPR) in the absence of a definitive pulse, and early defibrillation for shockable rhythms. ACLS guidelines have summarized the initial cardiac arrest management cycle as illustrated in **Figure 6-1**.

The quality of CPR is assessed based on the following targets:

- Chest compressions to a depth of 5-6 cm allowing for approximately equal compression and recoil times
- Chest compression rate at 100 - 120 /min
- Minimize interruptions in chest compressions. Rotate the person doing compressions every 2 minutes (~ 5 cycles at 30:2 compression: ventilation ratio)
- If no advanced airway, 30:2 compressions to ventilation ratio
- Achieve an end-tidal CO_2 ($P_{ET}CO_2 \geq 10$ mm Hg).
- Achieve diastolic blood pressure ≥ 20 mm Hg if invasive monitoring is present.

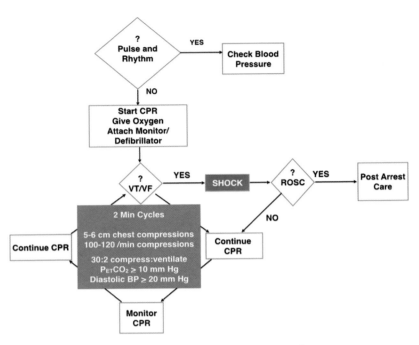

Figure 6-1* *Summary of the cardiac arrest management cycle.*

*Modified from Adult Advanced Cardiovascular Life Support: 2010.
American Heart Association Guidelines for Cardiopulmonary Resuscitation
and Emergency Cardiovascular Care. © 2010 American Heart Association, Inc.

End-tidal CO_2 is the partial pressure of CO_2 measured at the end of the endotracheal tube or artificial airway at the end of a breath. The value is expressed as a partial pressure or % of CO_2. The partial pressure of $ETCO_2$ is usually in the range of 35-45 mm Hg. The excretion of CO_2 at the airway during CPR helps affirm the airway is correctly placed in the trachea but also confirms that pulmonary blood flow is adequate to deliver CO_2 to the lungs.

CPR should be continued until the return of spontaneous circulation (ROSC), as evidenced by return of pulse and blood pressure, an arterial pressure waveform if invasive monitoring is present, and a sustained increase in $P_{ET}CO_2$.

6.2 Circulation: Take Charge and Shock

You will often hear colleagues talk about the *A, B, C* in resuscitation meaning *Airway, Breathing, Circulation*. But current thinking focuses on immediate cardioversion for patients with ventricular fibrillation. So, let's start with C!

Pulse-rhythm-pressure. You should be thinking about this sequence over and over. If there is any doubt about the presence of a pulse, initiate or continue chest compressions. You then need to get an immediate look at the rhythm. Your monitoring equipment will come in two flavors – pads or paddles.

6.2.1 Defibrillators

Paddles are the better-known interface electrode between the patient and the defibrillator, and are the usual method shown on every doctor TV show! They consist of a metal paddle with an insulated plastic handle. A gel pad is often used to reduce thoracic impedance when paddles are applied directly to the chest wall to deliver a shock. The gel pads come in a packet that must be newly opened to assure the pads have not dried out. The pads also serve to protect the skin. Placement of the two paddles in the correct position allows a "quick look" at the cardiac rhythm on the monitor. They are then held in place with approximately 25 lbs of pressure while a shock or series of shocks is delivered. The paddles are usually placed on the chest using an anterior-apex scheme as illustrated in **Figure 6-2,** top panel.

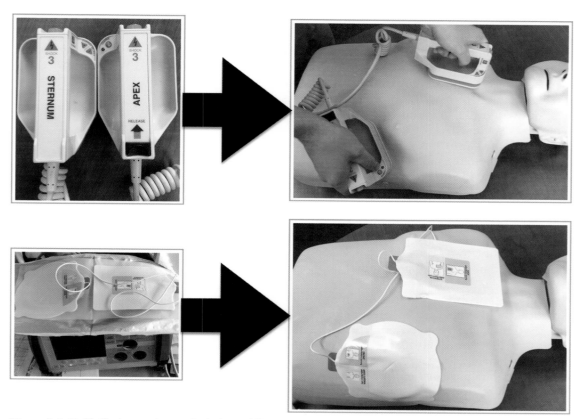

Figure 6-2 *Defibrillation equipment includes paddles with correct placement illustrated (top images). Alternatively, electrode adhesive pads can be used (bottom images).*

Alternatively, newer monitor-defibrillators use self-adhesive monitor-defibrillator electrode pads **(Figure 6-2,** bottom panel). The self-adhesive pads allow cardioversion and defibrillation – similar to paddles – but they also allow continuous ECG monitoring and external pacing. These adhesive pads include either a solid or wet gel. Remove the adhesive backing and place the pad on the patient like any other large sticker. No specific pressure requirement exists to accomplish defibrillation. These pads are single use, which may involve multiple shocks for one patient, but are replaced for each patient or each subsequent cardiac arrest event.

There are two commonly accepted positions for pad placement. The anteroapical position has one pad placed to the right of the sternum below the clavicle, and the second pad placed lateral to the cardiac apex in the anterior or midaxillary line. This apical pad position is adjusted to avoid direct placement on breast tissue **(Figure 6-2).**

The anteroposterior position places one pad over the precordium or apex and the second pad on the back in the left or right infrascapular region.

Place the pad/paddles in proper position; look at the rhythm. If the rhythm you recognize is ventricular

fibrillation or ventricular tachycardia—charge and shock!

So how much juice should you use? Defibrillation is classified as monophasic or biphasic. For many years, defibrillators used *monophasic waveforms*, meaning the current flow is unidirectional from one electrode to the other. Newer defibrillators are *biphasic*, where current flows are bidirectional. Monophasic defibrillators are typically charged to a maximum voltage of 360J, while biphasic defibrillators require less energy for equal efficacy and are charged to a maximum of 200J; however, maximum values may vary slightly based on the manufacturer. The lower energy biphasic shocks are felt to cause less myocardial injury and post-resuscitation myocardial dysfunction.

6.2.2 Pulseless and a Shockable Rhythm

Your first question in a pulseless situation is pretty simple. Is this rhythm shockable? If you are in doubt, shock. This is the most effective way to save a life. In the case of hospital-based cardiac arrest with ventricular fibrillation or pulseless ventricular tachycardia, this approach has the absolute best outcome. Note that pulseless ventricular tachycardia in cardiac arrest is four times more common than PSVT with aberrant conduction, and PSVT will also respond to a shock!

The successful termination of ventricular fibrillation/ventricular tachycardia with the initial shock approaches 90% in most series. Upon defibrillation, VF is often followed by a period of asystole or PEA, so CPR is continued for two additional minutes post defibrillation prior to the first rhythm check.

For patients with recurrent Vtach/Vfib following the initial defibrillation, the mnemonic *Shock, EVerybody Shock And Shock,* provides a sequence to consider in refractory cases. A second defibrillation follows 2 min of CPR (*Shock* - 360J monophasic or 200J biphasic), then 2 min of CPR to support the circulation, then *E*pinephrine (1 mg every 3-5 minutes), followed by 2 min of CPR, then *Shock.* For persistent Vtach/Vfib, consider *V*asopressin (40 units) or *A*miodarone (300 mg IV initial dose, then 150mg IV subsequent doses), then *Shock.*

The timing of epinephrine administration in cardiac arrest is critical. In-hospital cardiac arrest patients with shockable rhythms, who received epinephrine within two minutes of the first defibrillation, demonstrated a decreased survival and return of spontaneous circulation.[39] Use epinephrine after the second shock for a shockable rhythm. In contrast, early administration of epinephrine may be favored for patients presenting with non-shockable rhythms.

Half of patients with a persistent shockable rhythm received epinephrine within two minutes after the first defibrillation, contrary to current American Heart Association guidelines. The receipt of epinephrine within two minutes of after the first defibrillation was associated with decreased odds of survival to hospital discharge, as well as decreased odds of return of spontaneous circulation and survival to hospital discharge with a good functional outcome.

Note, however, that no specific drug therapy (vasopressor or antiarrhythmic) is associated with long-term survival or survival with favorable neurologic outcome. Further, the existing evidence suggests vasopressin alone or in combination with epinephrine offers no advantage as a substitute for epinephrine alone in the management of cardiac arrest. No interventions including vascular access, advanced airway management, or drug administration should interfere with effective CPR and timely defibrillation, which is associated with improved patient outcome in shockable rhythms.

There was a time when we used lidocaine or bretylium, but amiodarone is currently favored, making the CODE sequence easier to remember. If you are still not succeeding after many doses of amiodarone, you can try lidocaine 100 mg (1-1.5 mg/kg), magnesium (1-2 grams) and bicarbonate (1-2 amps), but things are not looking good at this point.

6.2.3 Pulseless Electrical Activity (PEA)

Pulseless electrical activity (PEA) represents a heterogeneous group of organized electrical rhythms with the absence of a palpable pulse. This is an ominous cause of cardiac arrest. In this case, the electricity is running but the pump is not responding.

PEA is usually caused by primary heart failure (as bad as asystole) or something reversible that is preventing blood from filling the left side of the heart. Clinical examples include hypovolemia (severe sepsis, dehydration, hemorrhage, etc.), tension pneumothorax, cardiac tamponade, severe dynamic hyperinflation in COPD or an asthmatic patient (auto-PEEP), or massive pulmonary embolism.

The approach to PEA is

- Establish excellent CPR
- Fluid resuscitation (hypovolemia so common)
- Give epinephrine (1 mg IV/IO every 3-5 minutes) with continuous CPR
- Look for reversible causes, often referred to as the 5 H's and 5 T's (**Figure 6-3 and Figure 6-4**)

The problem for you is whether you can remember the 5 *H*'s and 5 *T*'s in the middle of a cardiac arrest. Your memory seems (and is) unlikely to be this efficient under stress, so clinicians have been searching for a structured approach to PEA.

The availability of bedside Doppler-echocardiography (POCUS—Point of Care Ultrasound) has the potential to transform the therapy of PEA arrests *(see Chapter 3, Point of Care Ultrasound).*

Pulse checks by palpation of the carotid artery are potentially inaccurate during a code event.[40] The use of bedside ultrasound (POCUS) or central aortic pressure monitoring to define the presence or absence of cardiac contractility allows PEA to be divided into two categories:

- *True PEA – P*ulseless with a *R*hythm, but no cardiac contractility by echo motion = *e*cho *s*tandstill. This has been called *PRES* in the arrest literature.
- *Pseudo PEA – P*ulseless with a *R*hythm, with *e*cho *m*otion. This has been called *PREM* in the cardiac arrest literature.

H's	*T*'s
Hypoxia	Toxins
Hypovolemia	Tension pneumothorax
Hydrogen ion acidosis	Tamponade, cardiac
Hyperkalemia	Thrombosis, coronary
Hypothermia	Thrombosis, pulmonary embolism

Figure 6-3 Reversible causes of pulseless electrical activity.

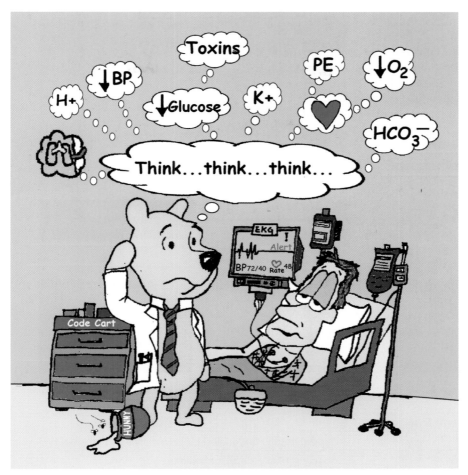

Figure 6-4 Attempting to remember the reversible causes of pulseless electrical activity.

Pseudo PEA (or PREM) is often associated with narrow QRS complex rhythms in the setting of hypovolemia or obstruction to the circulation (cardiac tamponade, dynamic hyperinflation, or tension pneumothorax).

True PEA (or PRES) is often associated with a wide QRS complex in the setting of factors that inhibit myocardial shortening, including hypoxemia, acidosis, or electrolyte abnormalities (potassium or calcium).

A modified PEA algorithm has been proposed based upon the ECG appearance alone to simplify the approach to PEA – because you probably will not remember all those *H*'s and *T*'s.[41] This modified algorithm is illustrated in Figure 6-5.

POCUS can directly recognize cardiac activity adequate to provide perfusion in association with an underlying rhythm. However, the incorporation of POCUS into cardiac life support cannot interfere with the provision of high-quality chest compressions. An apical four-chamber or subcostal view is preferred during CPR with the probe positioned without disturbing the CPR provider. This view, initially obtained during pulse checks, can remain available during chest compressions. In contrast, a parasternal view cannot be achieved without interfering with chest compressions. If this represents the only adequate window, preload the probe with gel and then place the probe during the pulse check. Count during the pulse checks to limit the duration to 10 seconds and record the images for review during the intervals of chest compression.

POCUS can also support your assessment for reversible causes of PEA. *MANY* ultrasound protocols with catchy names now exist in the literature for assessing the unstable patient. However, these protocols really focus on very similar basic components.

A focused echocardiographic evaluation in life support (FEEL) can be incorporated into the CPR algorithm with appropriate training.[42] A summary of the etiologies to address and the associated POCUS findings with this exam are outlined in **Figure 6-6.**

A few of the diagnoses for PEA deserve special consideration:

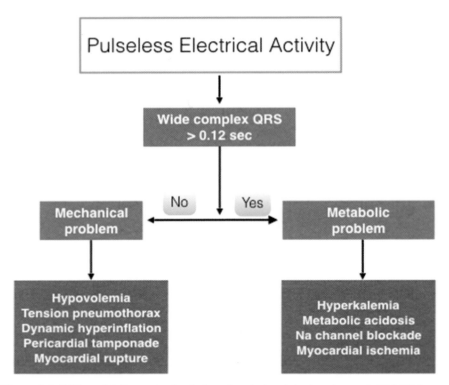

Figure 6-5 *Differential diagnosis of pulseless electrical activity based upon initial QRS complex.*

Etiology	POCUS Findings
Hypovolemia	Hyperdynamic underfilled LV with a small collapsible IVC
Tension pneumothorax	Absence of unilateral lung sliding
Tamponade	Pericardial effusion with a distended non-collapsible IVC
Thrombosis, pulmonary	Dilated RV with a RV/LV ratio > 1
Thrombosis, cardiac	Decreased ejection fraction with wall motion abnormalities

Figure 6-6 *Etiologies for pulseless electrical activity based on appearance of POCUS.*

6.2.3.1 Hyperkalemia and Acidosis

This prevalent problem in hospitalized patients occurs most frequently in patients with renal failure. After you have stabilized the C-A-B's and have given fluids and epinephrine, you want to ask about a brief history and send STAT labs. At this point during asystole or a PEA code, you might empirically give sodium bicarbonate and calcium chloride or gluconate. Severe hyperkalemia can progress from peaked T waves to a widened QRS to asystole or a wide complex PEA. Bicarbonate and calcium can remedy this quickly, allowing you to take more aggressive long-term measures (kayexalate and hemodialysis). Calcium stabilizes the cardiac membrane potential through a mechanism that is still unclear, thus restoring the abnormal gradient between threshold potential and resting membrane potential, which characterizes hyperkalemia. One ampule of calcium chloride has approximately 3 times more calcium than

calcium gluconate. Bicarbonate stimulates an exchange of cellular H^+ for Na^+, thus leading to stimulation of the sodium-potassium ATPase pump.

6.2.3.2 Hypothermia

A hypothermic patient will only recover when warmed up. A variety of warming maneuvers is available, from warming blankets to invasive warming catheters. NG lavages with warmed fluids or blood, and more aggressive pleural or peritoneal warming can be used.

Don't forget the golden rule with hypothermic arrests: The patient is not dead until warm and dead!

6.2.3.3 Dynamic Hyperinflation

With dynamic hyperinflation, a new breath begins before the lung has reached its static (or resting) equilibrium volume. Most commonly seen in patients

> The Lazarus effect! Case reports exist of patients with COPD who developed pulseless electrical activity (PEA) cardiac arrests not responsive to aggressive resuscitation, only to suddenly have the arterial line pick up a pulse after resuscitation efforts are halted. The code is started again, and PEA then recurs! The discontinuation of mechanical ventilation allows for full exhalation (long expiratory time) and intrathoracic pressures decrease, resulting in enhanced venous return and restoration of cardiac output. This may be a much more common event than we would expect. This potential etiology for PEA should be considered in any patient with obstructive lung disease.

with severe airflow obstruction, the incomplete expiratory phase leads to increased lung volume and intrathoracic pressure, venous return is impaired, and the right ventricle and pulmonary veins are mechanically compressed. The intrathoracic pressure changes act to reduce left ventricular preload and cardiac output. Continued severe dynamic hyperinflation may result in pulseless electrical activity (PEA) and cardiac arrest. The patient with COPD or severe asthma is at greatest risk for this complication immediately following intubation. The urgency of the arrest situation often leads to overzealous manual bag-mask ventilation prior to connection to the ventilator, and the resultant large tidal volumes and rapid respiratory rates increase lung volume and shorten expiratory time, preventing adequate exhalation and potentiating dynamic hyperinflation. In the setting of non-elective emergency intubation, the reduction in cardiac output associated with dynamic hyperinflation is often compounded by volume depletion and sedation.

So clearly, dynamic hyperinflation must be considered as a potential cause of hypotension in the mechanically ventilated patients with COPD, as well as in the setting of cardiac arrest with PEA. A 30-second interruption of positive-pressure ventilation can be diagnostic, as prolonged expiration and reduction in intrathoracic pressure relieve hemodynamic embarrassment.

6.2.3.4 The T's

If your efforts to correct PEA are not working, you will consider tension pneumothorax, cardiac tamponade, or massive pulmonary thromboembolism. If you hear decreased breath sounds on one side or see a shift of the trachea, you should place an angiocatheter in the chest to treat a possible tension pneumothorax. The catheter will convert the pneumothorax from a tension pneumothorax to an open pneumothorax. This will relieve the pressure on the heart and improve venous return. If the patient has a history that suggests tamponade or massive PE (such as metastatic cancer), you can consider placing a needle in the pericardium or giving tissue plasminogen activator empirically, but these are heroic measures that rarely are effective in the setting of PEA.

6.2.4 Pulseless and Asystole (Flat Line)

Asystole is the absence of any ventricular electrical activity. Asystole is a bad one to treat and a bad one to have. While accounting for about a third of in-hospital arrests, less than 10% of patients who present with asystole make it out of the hospital alive.

A few tricks to remember:

- Establish excellent CPR.
- Check more than one lead. A disconnected lead and fine V-fib can look like asystole.
- Consider a shock if in doubt about the diagnosis.
- Stabilize C, B, A's fast. Oxygenate and ventilate. Give epinephrine (1mg IV/IO every 3-5 minutes) and continue good CPR.
- Place a transcutaneous pacer, turn it up, and pace. Make sure you see the chest wall muscles tense up with every pace before you give up. Unfortunately, no good data exists to show that transcutaneous pacing improves survival.

Consider the 5 H's and 5 T's discussed under PEA (**Figure 6-3**), as many of these disorders can also cause asystole.

6.3 Breathing and Airway

Make sure you have an airway. Although ultimately this may be a supraglottic airway or endotracheal tube (advanced airway), this will take time. Advanced airway placement in cardiac arrest should not delay the initial CPR or defibrillation for a shockable rhythm. Overattention to endotracheal intubation early in the resuscitation can adversely impact patient outcome. *If you see a shockable rhythm – do it!*

A patent airway can be established with correct attention to patient positioning, use of appropriate airway adjuncts, and effective bag-mask ventilation (*see Chapter 12 Basic Airway Management*). Two trained providers best perform bag-mask ventilation. One provider seals the mask and opens the airway, and the second provider squeezes the bag. The target tidal volume is ~600 ml. During CPR, two breaths are provided during a brief pause to allow chest expansion after every 30 chest compressions.

Establish an airway and make sure you assure the following without interrupting chest compressions:

1. Good breath sounds exist on both sides of the chest.
2. The airway is showing a positive partial pressure of end-tidal CO_2 ($P_{ET}CO_2$).
3. The patient has no gas sounds in the stomach.

These three steps are essential to confirm the correct position of the endotracheal tube, and you need all three for confirmation. You will order a portable chest radiograph, but you will not see this until the game is decided. Remember, in an arrest situation a $P_{ET}CO_2 < 10$ mm Hg could mean the endotracheal tube is incorrectly placed *OR* the overall perfusion is poor. If the position of the ETT is confirmed by direct visualization and auscultation, improve the quality of the CPR provided. You can even use this idea in reverse!! In some patients such as those with peripheral vascular disease or morbid obesity, it becomes challenging to palpate a pulse. A sustained, strong $P_{ET}CO_2$ signal at the airway is pretty good evidence that you have sufficient circulation.

Current data in out-of-hospital arrests suggests bag-mask ventilation is not inferior to endotracheal intubation for survival or 28-day neurologic function.[43] The provider is encouraged to weigh the risk of interrupted chest compressions against the need for insertion of an advanced airway (endotracheal intubation or supraglottic airway). If placement of the advanced airway will lead to prolonged interruption of chest compressions, the airway insertion should be delayed until you provide initial resuscitation efforts including defibrillation.

6.4 Post-Arrest Care

Once the patient has return of spontaneous circulation (ROSC), the management shifts to a focus on achieving normal cardiovascular physiology, limiting organ injury from the arrest including brain injury, attempting to determine the cause of the arrest, and managing complications from post-arrest ischemia and reperfusion injury.

Fix the numbers. Oxygenation and ventilation are normalized, and electrolyte abnormalities are corrected. The patient's inspired oxygen concentration is titrated to maintain arterial oxygen saturation > 92-94% with the lowest possible inspired oxygen concentration (F_iO_2) to avoid hyperoxia ($PaO_2 > 300$). *Ventilate the patient just right.* The level of ventilation is targeted to avoid both marked hypercapnia and hypocapnia. $P_{ET}CO_2$ monitoring can be used to guide ventilation management. A target blood $PaCO_2$ of 40-45 mm Hg or a

$P_{ET}CO_2$ of 35-40 mm Hg is "just right" and an appropriate target range for adjusting ventilator support. Target glucose control to the more moderate range of 150-200 as the risk of hypoglycemia post-arrest is recognized.

From a hemodynamic perspective, the goal is to return the patient to a level of function equivalent to their pre-arrest condition. Volume and vasopressor support are titrated to achieve a target mean arterial blood pressure (MAP) of ≥ 65 mm Hg. Coronary reperfusion should be addressed promptly for the appropriate patient and having immediate access to coronary interventional therapy is a critical component of post-arrest management. Antiarrhythmic medications are reserved for patients with recurrent or ongoing unstable arrhythmias. At the current time, we have no data to support a protective role for antiarrhythmic medications after ROSC.

Immediate assessment to determine the arrest etiology is indicated as soon as cardiopulmonary physiology is stabilized. This comprehensive assessment will include an electrocardiogram (ECG), laboratory, and imaging studies. Review the 12 lead ECG for evidence to suggest the need for urgent coronary intervention (ST elevation or new onset left bundle branch block). Correct positioning of the endotracheal tube should be assured.

In patients with out-of-hospital cardiac arrest, a neurologic injury is the most common cause of death. The initial assessment post-arrest attempts to determine if the patient is responsive to verbal commands. If yes, the patient is merely monitored for neurologic recovery. If no, then temperature control is indicated to minimize neurologic injury.

Therapeutic or resuscitative hypothermia is employed in patients with ROSC who remain unresponsive post-cardiac arrest. Therapeutic hypothermia initially targeted active cooling of patients to 33 °C for several hours. In comparison to standard post-arrest care, clinical trials of therapeutic hypothermia, conducted primarily in patients following a ventricular tachycardia/ventricular fibrillation arrest, have shown that the neurologic injury from cardiac arrest may be attenuated.[44] A large randomized trial has shown equivalent outcomes with targeted temperature control following out-of-hospital cardiac arrest from a non-shockable rhythm using a target of 33°C or 36°C for a duration of 28 hours.[45] Since these two interventions are considered equivalent, many investigators are advocating 36°C for routine care post ROSC, and possibly reserving the more aggressive active temperature management (33°C) for patients with a defined poor neurologic prognosis for recovery. Hopefully, further clinical trials will better clarify this issue.

The findings that guide the clinician's assessment of the patient for neurologic recovery remain a dynamic area of active investigation, as post-arrest care is refined at experienced post-arrest centers. Neurologic prognostication for the patient is confounded by the influence of medications, metabolic abnormalities, or induced hypothermia.

As a general rule, delay neuro prognostication until after the window of therapeutic hypothermia has passed. Early findings associated with a poor prognosis include myoclonic electrical status in the initial 24 hours post-arrest, and evidence for brain death due to cerebral herniation at any time. The neurologic assessment post-therapeutic cooling typically incorporates a clinical neurological examination (including Glasgow Coma Scale [GCS], pupillary and corneal reflexes), somatosensory evoked potentials (SSEP), and the electroencephalogram (EEG).[46]

The neurologic exam focuses on five key areas:

1. Presence of spontaneous movement
2. Response to external stimulation
3. Pupillary size and reaction to light
4. Cranial nerve assessment, including corneal, gag, cough, and oculovestibular reflexes
5. Respiratory pattern

The Glasgow Coma Scale (GCS) is a neurological scale between 3 (unconscious) and 15. It was developed originally to assess the level of consciousness after head injury and is now used for acute medical and trauma patients for monitoring in the ICU (**Figure 6-7**). The score can be considered by the individual components or as the sum of all three portions.

Somatosensory evoked potentials (SEPs) are electrical signals that are generated by the nervous system in response to sensory stimuli. SEPs use electrical stimulation of peripheral nerves (most commonly the median nerve, common peroneal nerve, and the posterior tibial nerve) with the response measured by surface EEG electrodes. The evoked potentials are a series of waves that reflect sequential activation of the neural structures along the somatosensory pathways. The primary cortical SEP to a median nerve stimulation is recorded over the parietal area on the contralateral side and is called *N20*. N20 refers to a negative stimulus that occurs at 20 milliseconds after the stimulus.

From the comprehensive neurologic assessment, specific variables that predict a poor prognosis for neurologic recovery include

- Absent or extensor motor response on day #3
- Absent pupillary or corneal reflexes on day #3
- Persistent coma with a Glasgow Motor Score of 1-2 and bilateral absence of N20-peak on median nerve SSEP
- Persistent coma with a Glasgow Motor Score 1-2 and a treatment refractory status epilepticus
- Generalized myoclonic convulsions in face and extremities and continuous for a minimum of 30 min.
- Treatment refractory status epilepticus

The Pittsburgh group has defined a Post-Cardiac Arrest Category (PCAC) score which is predictive of survival to hospital discharge.[46] The PCAC combines two components (**Figure 6-8**):

- **F**ull **O**utline of **U**n**R**esponsiveness (FOUR) brainstem and motor sub-scores
- **S**erial **O**rgan **F**ailure **A**ssessment (SOFA) cardiac and respiratory subscales

The four PCAC levels that result from the score and their associated prognosis include

1. Awake (FOUR motor + brainstem = 8); 80% survival, 60% good outcome
2. Coma (not following commands but intact brainstem responses; FOUR motor + brainstem of 4–7) and mild cardiopulmonary dysfunction (SOFA cardiac + respiratory score < 4); 60% survival, 40% good outcome
3. Coma (as defined above) with moderate to severe cardiopulmonary dysfunction (SOFA cardiac + respiratory score ≥ 4); 40% survival, 20% good outcome
4. Coma with at least one absent brainstem reflex (FOUR motor + brainstem < 4); 10% survival, 5% good outcome

The FOUR score is obtained from the best neurological examination within 6 h after ROSC. Patients are

	Score 1	Score 2	Score 3	Score 4	Score 5	Score 6
Eye	Does not open eyes	Opens eyes in response to painful stimuli	Opens eyes in response to voice command	Spontaneous		
Verbal	Makes no sounds	Incomprehensible sounds	Utters inappropriate words	Confused	Oriented	
Motor	Makes no movements	Extension to painful stimuli (decerebrate response)	Abnormal flexion to painful stimuli (decorticate response)	Withdrawal response to pain	Localizing response to pain	Obeys commands

Figure 6-7 Glasgow Coma Scale by category and point value.

examined free of sedation and neurological blockade before consideration of hypothermia. Drugs should not cloud the exam. The worst SOFA score in the first 6 h after ROSC is used to derive the PCAC scores.

Suggested Reading

- Jentzer JC, Clements CM, Wright RS, White RD, Jaffe AS. Improving survival from cardiac arrest: A review of contemporary practice and challenges. Ann Emerg Med 2016;68(6):678–89.
- Nassar BS, Kerber R. Improving CPR performance. Chest 2017;152:1061–69.
- Newell C, Grier S, Soar J. Airway and ventilation management during cardiopulmonary resuscitation and after successful resuscitation. Crit Care [Internet] 2018;22(1):190.

SOFA Score	0	1	2	3	4
Cardiovascular	No hypotension	MAP <70	Dopamine <5	Dopamine >5 or Epi/Norepi <0.1	Dopamine >15 or Epi/Norepi >0.1
Respiratory (Pa02/Fi02)	>400	<400	<300	<200	<100
FOUR Score	**4**	**3**	**2**	**1**	**0**
Motor	Follow commands	Localizing Pain	Flexion to Pain	Extension to Pain	No Response
Brainstem	+ Pupil and Corneal reflex	One Pupil Fixed	Either Pupil or Corneal Reflexes Absent	Absent Pupil and Corneal Reflexed	Absent Pupil, Corneal, and Gag Reflexes

Figure 6-8 Post Cardiac-Arrest Category Score by category and point value.

7

Hemodynamic Monitoring

In this chapter, we focus on hemodynamic monitoring, how to estimate and measure cardiac output, vascular resistance, and oxygen delivery, and how to use all the tools in the toolbox to figure out if your patient needs fluid resuscitation.

You will learn why they teach the cardiac cycle in med school and why this is needed to save lives. You will learn the diagnosis and management of common problems using invasive monitoring: heart failure, septic shock, and ARDS; as well as unique problems like cardiac tamponade, pericardial constriction, right heart myocardial infarction, and pulmonary hypertension.

7.1 Arterial Blood Pressure

In a critically ill patient, as soon as you have established your *A*'s and *B*'s you must get to work on the circulation (*C*). There are only a few essential things to remember:

Check your pulse. Stay cool and think things out. Organize your steps so you can pull out your resuscitation algorithms during a hot firefight.

Check your patient's pulse. Start low tech. Does the patient have a palpable carotid and femoral pulse? Always make sure and don't trust the numbers on the wall, because your blood pressure cuff can be cycling every 5 to 30 minutes, and you might be looking at yesterday's stock prices. If you can feel a pulse, things are not all that bad, and you have some time to think. If there is no pulse, skip the next three sections and call a code. You might want to shift your reading to *Chapter 6, Running a Code.*

Measure a blood pressure non-invasively. Place a cuff on the arm or leg. Measure the blood pressure, at least systolic. Use a manual cuff if the automated cuff is not working. If the room is too loud, you can inflate the cuff until the radial pulse disappears, and that will be your systolic blood pressure. If over 100 mm Hg, you have a little more time to think. If using an automated cuff, make sure it is cycling every 3 minutes. Don't forget that when the automated cuff inflates the IVs, arterial lines, and pulse oximeters may be inaccurate as the device may shut off the blood flow to the patient's arm.

Measure cardiac output (It's the flow, stupid!) at the bedside using the Poor Man's method, the capillary refill and Foley catheter! After you have measured blood pressure, you want to know if the patient is well-perfused. Looking at capillary refill in the fingers can test this. Pinch the nail bed or skin and watch for how fast the capillaries flush red again. You can feel for warmth and color of extremities. Cold, cyanotic extremities with livedo reticularis suggest low flow. Finally, the best poor man's evaluation of flow is the Foley catheter. A urine flow of more than 60 mL (1 ml/kg/min) per hour suggests adequate flow to the kidneys. If the urine output is low, you don't know if the kidneys are failing or the cardiac output is low, so this is a sensitive test for adequate perfusion, but not specific for cardiac output.

The detailed physical exam may be all you need in a significant fraction of patients. If your rhythm is sinus with an appropriate rate, blood pressure is adequate for perfusion (traditionally a MAP > 60 mm Hg), and urine output is sufficient, then continue to treat the underlying condition. So, normal HR, normal BP, good urine output, and adequate capillary refill, you can probably rest easy. But sometimes you need more information and tools to assess organ perfusion.

7.1.1 The Arterial Catheter

Placement of an arterial catheter is one of the harder procedures in the ICU. If you have time, set up carefully, sit down and get comfortable, and use lots of lidocaine. If in a code and the radial artery is too hard to cannulate, move quickly to the femoral artery with ultrasound guidance. The arterial pressure wave will have an expected systolic and diastolic pressure, and sometimes the abscissa or dicrotic notch is visible. The dicrotic notch represents closure of the aortic valve and elastic recoil of the aorta to generate a dip-peak-and-drop in pressure. There are only a few things to know about arterial line hemodynamics.

- *Note any respiratory variation.* If you note variability in the blood pressure with the respiratory cycle, try to time whether the drop occurs in inspiration or expiration. This variation applies only to a patient in a regular sinus rhythm.
  - If the blood pressure drops during inspiration this suggests that the patient might have *pulsus paradoxus*, caused by a drop in cardiac output during inspiration. This change occurs with cardiac tamponade, constrictive pericarditis, and severe asthma. In these cases, the pressure around the heart is high so that increased venous return during inspiration increases right ventricular volume, which applies more pressure on the left ventricle and limits its filling (preload), dropping cardiac output and pressure.
  - If the blood pressure drops during expiration, especially in association with mechanical ventilation and the respiratory cycle, this suggests intravascular volume contraction. Reduced arterial pressures on expiration may be a sign of preload dependence and will be discussed later.
- *Note the pulse pressure.* High systolic pressure and low diastolic pressure occur with aortic insufficiency, anemia, distributive shock, and arteriosclerosis. We see this in our patients with aortic valve endocarditis and aortic regurgitation.

7.2 Pressure Transducers

We should probably have an introduction to pressure transducer systems and how we measure intravascular pressures. Then we will walk through the measurement of vascular system pressures using the pulmonary artery (PA) catheter.

Intravascular pressure measuring systems use a column of fluid to connect the vascular pressure waveform to a pressure transducer. These systems are used to measure all vascular pressures (arterial and venous). The transducer converts the pressure signal to an electrical signal. The electrical signal is converted into a visual display signal by a microprocessor (**Figure 7-1**).

The key components of the pressure monitoring system include

- Flush Bag

A bag of 0.9% saline or heparinized saline is connected to the monitoring system under pressure (typically ~ 300 mm Hg). This flush system provides a slow infusion of fluid (2-4 ml/hr) to maintain the patency of the cannula and prevent thrombosis. The slow infusion rate does not affect the pressure readings. The flush system also allows an intermittent high-pressure flush of the system.

- Transducer

The pressure transducer converts the pressure waveform to an electrical signal that can be measured, processed, and sent to the monitoring system for display. To function properly, a pressure transducer must be calibrated for two parameters:

  - *Zeroing* – Pressure measurements must be related to a reference value. The measuring device is adjusted so the baseline force or neutral value is equivalent to atmospheric pressure. The process of zeroing discounts atmospheric pressure from the pressure measurement. The transducer is exposed to atmospheric pressure by opening the stopcock on the transducer. The atmospheric pressure is calibrated to 0 by selecting the zero-pressure button on the monitoring system.
  - *Leveling* – Because the height of the fluid column adds to the pressure measurement, the measuring device must be set at a level which is considered the physiologic reference value in the body. A standard reference position is required so the pressures can be compared between two patients. In physiologic studies, the height of the transducer is positioned at the same level as the patient's heart (4th intercostal space, mid-axillary line), which approximates the mid-point of the right atrium. A transducer below the heart level will measure additional hydrostatic pressure from the fluid column and overestimate the vascular pressure. A transducer above the heart level will measure a reduced hydrostatic pressure from the measured vascular pressure and underestimate

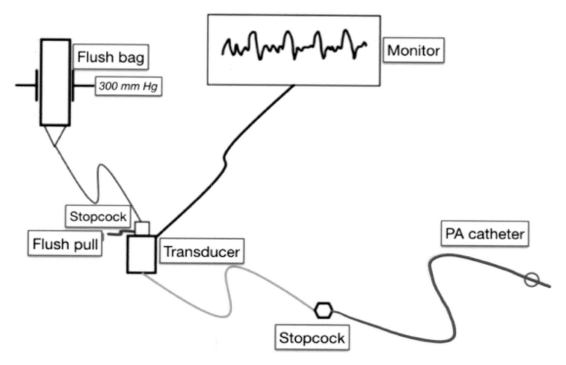

Figure 7-1 Hemodynamic monitoring components for a pulmonary artery catheter.

the vascular pressure. The conversion between height (cm) and pressure (mm Hg) establishes that a transducer 10 cm above or below the R heart position will change the vascular pressure by ± 7.4 mm Hg.

- *Catheter and tubing* – The catheter and tubing must be made of stiffer materials, so they do not absorb the pressure waves from the catheter tip to the pressure transducer.

Two variables that influence the performance of the pressure monitoring system are the resonant frequency and damping factor. The resonant frequency refers to the inherent frequency of oscillations in the system. When the oscillations of the signal (vascular pressures) approach the oscillations of the system, the signal can be amplified. The issue is called *underdamping*.

Underdamped systems are characterized by a brisk upstroke in the arterial pulse pressure waveform and may overestimate systolic arterial pressure as much as 25 mm Hg, leading to an overly wide pulse pressure. The mean arterial pressures are most often accurately represented, however.

If the monitoring system reduces the amplitude of oscillations in the system, this tends to attenuate the signal, leading to *overdamping*. Overdamping in a pressure monitoring system can be produced by multiple variables including

- Air bubbles or clots in the system
- Kinks in the vascular cannula or monitoring tubing
- Multiple partially closed stopcocks or long compliant tubing

Overdamped systems will demonstrate a gradual upslope and downslope of the waveform with a narrow pulse pressure. However, the mean arterial blood pressure will be relatively accurate.

The system performance can be assessed using a simple bedside maneuver called a fast Flush Test **(Figure 7-2)**. The Flush Test involves opening the one-way valve (flush pull), exposing the transducer to the pressurized fluid source in the flush bag. The pressure will rise immediately upon exposure to the pressure in the flush bag and exceed the normal upper limit of the scale, forming a square wave. When the flush valve is closed, the pressure falls, but the waveform initially is characterized by a few oscillations before returning to the baseline. After you flush you should see a perfect square wave, followed by a few brief oscillations (3-5 like **Figure 7-2**). If you see <3 oscillations, or the wave is not square, the system is overdamped, and you can begin working with your nursing staff to find the problem (bubbles, kinks, partially closed stopcocks, etc.). Think of the fast Flush Test as a quick check on your external system. You do not want to misinterpret your hemodynamic measurements because the external monitoring system is not working correctly.

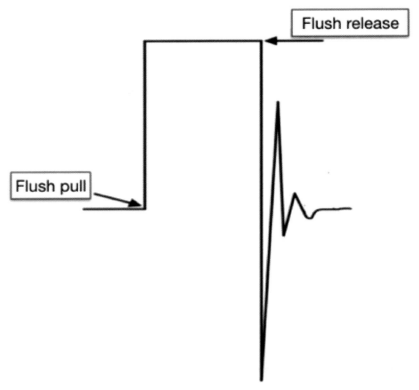

Flush release

Flush pull

Figure 7-2 *The monitoring waveform produced by a fast flush test.*

7.3 Vascular Pressures and the Pulmonary Artery Catheter

The gold standard for the measurement of intravascular pressures is the pulmonary artery catheter, also called the right heart catheter. Designed by Swan and Ganz, we still call this yellow balloon tip wonder the *Swan-Ganz catheter*. Typical situations where this catheter can help in diagnosis and management are pulmonary edema with renal failure (Is this ARDS with acute tubular necrosis or heart failure and cardiogenic pulmonary edema with pre-renal kidney failure?), pulmonary hypertension with cor pulmonale, left heart failure from acute myocardial infarction, valvular heart disease, and cardiac tamponade.

The PA catheter has 3-4 ports leading to separate lumens within the catheter **(Figure 7-3)**. The longest lumen runs to the tip (balloon tip) of the pulmonary artery catheter and is called the *distal port*. The pressure at the end of the distal port communicates via a sterile saline-filled channel to the pressure transducer. As you advance the catheter, you monitor the pressure at the end of the distal port. You can "see" where you are by the pressure waves the tip of the catheter is monitoring. A more *proximal port* is located within the central venous circulation when the pulmonary artery catheter is fully

inserted. This port is used to inject saline solution to measure cardiac output. An inflatable balloon is located at the tip, and a syringe can be used to inflate the balloon via the *balloon inflation port*. A thermistor, or temperature-sensing device, is located at the tip of the catheter but is connected to a measurement device at the proximal thermistor probe.

The PA catheter is introduced via a central vein in the right-sided circulation and then gradually passed with the balloon inflated (also called "floated") from the right atrium, to the right ventricle, to the pulmonary artery. In **Figure 7-4,** note the insertion point in the right internal jugular catheter for all images (green arrow). Alternatively, you could introduce the catheter via the subclavian or femoral vein. Once in the central venous circulation, the balloon is inflated. Inflating the balloon is like unfurling the sails on a sailboat, and the balloon is caught by flowing blood and is carried, while you push the catheter in, into the right atrium, through the tricuspid valve (where it takes a sharp turn and crosses the pulmonary valve), into the main pulmonary artery. The balloon-tipped catheter is then carried deeper into one of the main pulmonary arteries, usually the right, until it lodges or wedges into a distal pulmonary artery about 1/3 of the way out in the lung. Note the different positions of the pulmonary

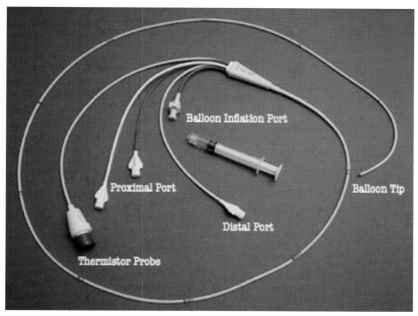

Figure 7-3 Components of the pulmonary artery (Swan-Ganz) catheter.

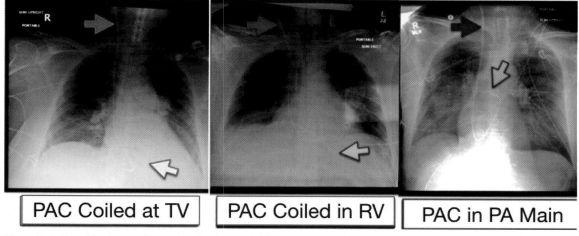

Figure 7-4 Portable chest radiographs showing variable position of pulmonary artery catheter inserted from the right internal jugular vein. Left and middle image are incorrect catheter placements. Right image is the catheter in the correct position.

artery catheter (PAC), coiled in the right atrium at the tricuspid valve (wrong!), coiled in the right ventricle (wrong!), positioned in the main pulmonary artery (right!) **(Figure 7-4)**.

Once located within the pulmonary artery, the balloon is inflated and the catheter "wedges" into a subsegment of the pulmonary artery, occluding flow. The "wedge" position, blocks forward flow from the right ventricle and the catheter provides a static measure of left atrial pressure, often called the wedge pressure or pulmonary artery occlusion pressure (PAOP).

Figure 7-5 illustrates the chambers of the heart and their associated pressure waveforms during the placement of a pulmonary artery catheter. Note the right atrium and pulmonary artery wedge or occlusion pressures are venous pressures in appearance. The pulmonary artery pressure is an arterial pressure. Note the transition you will see as the catheter

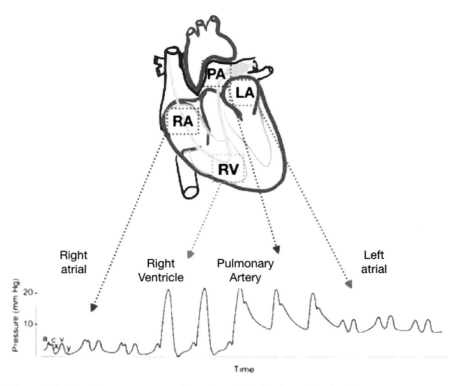

Figure 7-5 Vascular pressure waveforms from individual cardiac chambers.

floats from the right atrium, to the right ventricle, to the pulmonary artery, to the wedge or occlusion position.

So, let's take a closer look at all the information we can get from this advanced form of hemodynamic monitoring using the pulmonary artery catheter.

The waveforms obtained from a centrally placed pulmonary artery catheter have three basic shapes: 1) atrial, 2) ventricular, and 3) arterial. We will review each as a group.

7.3.1 Atrial Pressures and Waveforms

Pressures rise inside a heart chamber for two reasons: contraction of the chamber (squeeze-systole) or filling of the chamber with blood (diastole). We can measure the pressure in the right atrium by transducing the distal port of a venous catheter placed in one of the central veins (internal jugular, subclavian, or femoral vein) or in the left atrium by transducing the distal port of the pulmonary artery catheter **(Figure 7-3)**. The right atrial pressure is normally 0-6 mm Hg and with each breath often drops below zero. In an ICU patient who is fluid loaded on a ventilator with positive end-expiratory pressure, the normal value is more typically

5-10 mm Hg. The CVP waveform starts with an A wave, which is named for atrial contraction and occurs when the patient is in sinus rhythm **(Figure 7-6)**. The A wave will be the first pressure wave observed after the P wave of the ECG tracing. The atrial contraction pushes approximately 1/3 of the atrial blood into the ventricle at the end of ventricular diastole (squeeze that last drop of blood in before the ventricle lets go!). After the peak of the A wave, the ventricle contracts (ventricular systole), and the tricuspid valve closes and slams the tricuspid valve backward into the atrium, creating a second pressure peak in the atrial waveform, called the C wave. The C wave is like the dicrotic notch or abscissa in the pulmonary artery or systemic arterial waveform. After the A and C waves comes the X descent as the atrium relaxes (atrial diastole). The X descent is followed by the V wave caused by atrial filling during atrial diastole (note the ventricle is at the end of systole now). The ventricle relaxes and drops pressure, and at the point the ventricular pressure drop matches the atrial V wave peak, the tricuspid valve opens, and the atrium rapidly empties into the ventricle, creating the Y descent **(Figure 7-6)**. During this passive phase of atrial emptying (Y descent), about 2/3 of the atrial blood fills the ventricle. The fact that

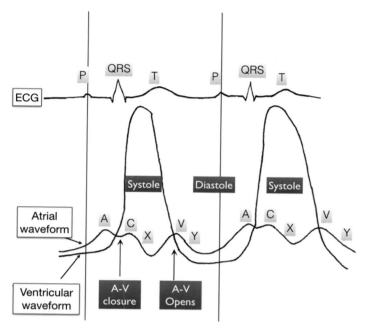

Figure 7-6 *Waveforms associated with vascular pressure measurements.*

most of the ventricle fills from passive atrial emptying explains why cardiac output can remain normal in a patient with atrial fibrillation. The magnitude of the V wave is determined by the amount of volume returning to the heart per beat and the compliance of the right ventricle and upstream venous vessels. The height of the A wave is determined by the force of contraction of the atrium and the compliance of the atrium, right ventricle, and upstream veins.

Note that the pulmonary artery occlusion pressure (PAOP) provides a measure of reflected pressures from the left atrium and will have the same A, C, V waves and X and Y descents. The cardiac cycle is the same except you are looking at the left atrium, mitral valve closing and opening, and left ventricular systole and diastole. The normal PAOP is higher than the CVP at about 8-12 mm Hg.

Key components of atrial pressure measurements include:

- A right atrial (RA) waveform is obtained from any catheter in the right atrium or great veins. No valves exist between the IVC and SVC, which provides an open pathway to the RA. The pressure obtained from a catheter in the great veins is termed a central venous pressure (CVP).
- A left atrial (LA) waveform is rarely obtained from a catheter placed directly into the LA. Rather, an LA waveform is usually obtained

from placing a pulmonary artery catheter in the pulmonary artery in a wedge position to reflect the LA pressure or pulmonary artery occlusion pressure (PAOP).

- To accurately interpret a CVP or PAOP waveform, a simultaneous waveform tracing and electrocardiogram (ECG) is beneficial. The V wave follows the peak of the T wave on the ECG. The A wave should be located within the PR interval of the ECG.
- The end-diastole pressure occurs just before the C wave. This would be the measurement point for the end-diastolic pressure. As this point is often difficult to identify, end-diastolic pressure is alternatively taken as the mean of the highest and lowest A wave pressure.
- CVP and PAOP represent filling pressures and not volume. A low filling pressure reflects a low volume, but a high pressure may also reflect normal to low filling volume with poor ventricular compliance. The trend in waveform pressure measurements may provide the most valuable information.

7.3.1.1 Cannon A Waves

A CVP tracing with *cannon A waves* refers to giant and tall A waves **(Figure 7-7)**. Cannon A waves are caused by the atrium contacting against a narrow

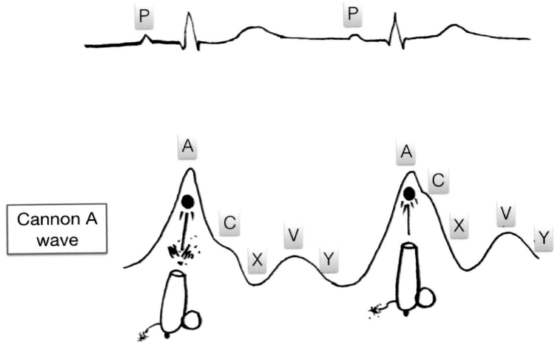

Figure 7-7 *Cannon A waves suggest stenotic or closed A-V valves.*

(stenotic) atrial-ventricular valve or a closed valve if there there is heart block and the atrium and ventricle are contracting out of synchrony. Stenosis of the tricuspid or mitral valve can occur with old rheumatic heart disease.

7.3.1.2 Giant V Waves

A *giant V wave* occurs when the A-V valve is leaky so that as the ventricle contracts, blood blasts backward into the atrium, augmenting the atrial filling pressure curves from all sides **(Figure 7-8).** Giant V waves are caused by tricuspid or mitral valve regurgitation (rheumatic heart disease, dilated heart, endocarditis, ruptured cordae tendinae). Typically, a Giant V wave is associated with an elevation in mean pressures, so the CVP or the PAOP will be increased. This is because the ventricular pressure is much higher, and if it chronically regurgitates, it will raise the right atrial or left atrial pressure.

7.3.1.3 Deep Y or X Descent

Sometimes the central venous pressure or pulmonary artery occlusion (left atrial) pressures are increased, but the pressure drops significantly during the Y descent or the X descent. This finding happens in cases of cardiac tamponade *(Why? Y? We will tell you later)* and during constrictive pericarditis *(X-plain? We will explain later).*

7.3.1.4 Increase in CVP or PAOP Pressures

The central venous pressure or pulmonary artery occlusion pressure is determined from the atrial waveform using one of two methods:

- Read the value at the Z point, which is the pressure just prior to the tricuspid or mitral valve closing (C wave). This tends to occur towards the middle or end of the QRS. The Z point is especially valuable when A waves are not apparent (i.e., atrial fibrillation).
- Read the high and low point of the A wave and sum the values – then divide by 2 **(Figure 7-9)**. The atrial contraction occurs during the opening of the valve, and the pressure should reflect the average equilibration of pressures during this time interval.

Another very important factor in measuring intrathoracic pressures relates to the time in the respiratory cycle the pressure is measured. The CVP value will appear to change with the respiratory cycle. Your goal of measuring the vascular pressure is to provide an estimate of ventricle preload. The transmural pressure or the gradient between the intravascular pressure and the extravascular pressure best estimates the volume of the chamber or preload. Transmural pressure is the actual distending pressure for the cardiac chambers. The extravascular pressure in the case of the heart is the pleural pressure, and this varies across the respiratory

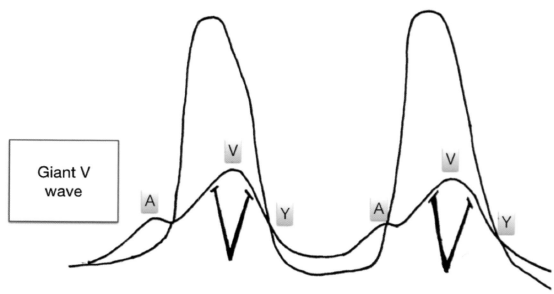

Figure 7-8 *Giant V wave suggesting "leaky" A-V valves.*

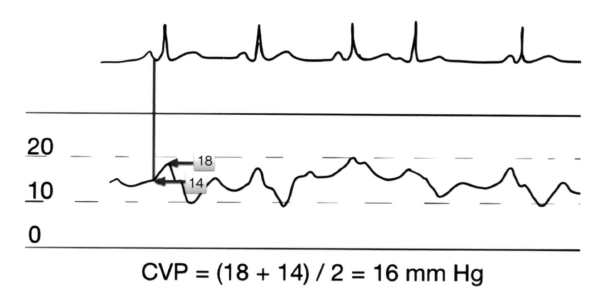

$$CVP = (18 + 14) / 2 = 16 \text{ mm Hg}$$

Figure 7-9 *Calculation of central venous pressure (CVP) from analysis of the pressure waveform.*

cycle. You could measure the pleural pressure with a catheter in the chest cavity, but this is not practical in the care of your ICU patient. So, to minimize the variability in vascular pressure measurements, all vascular pressures are measured at end-expiration. At end-expiration, the pleural pressure will be closest to the atmospheric pressure. During spontaneous ventilation, pleural pressure is slightly negative at end-expiration, and transmural pressure is slightly underestimated by the central venous pressure. In contrast, during positive pressure ventilation, pleural pressure usually is positive, in which case transmural cardiac pressure is overestimated by central venous pressure. In a patient on positive end-expiratory pressure (PEEP), the pleural pressure is even more positive and therefore the transmural pressure is again overestimated.

Patients who incorporate forced expiratory efforts into the respiratory cycle can raise the end-expiratory pleural pressure and produce a further artifact in the assessment of transmural pressure.

The variability produced from different CVP measurements in relation to the respiratory cycle is illustrated in **Figure 7-10**. Note: the CVP measurement baseline varies with the respiratory cycle (RESP). The blue and green arrows illustrate two different locations for measurement of the CVP, based upon the ECG tracing. Note, these measurements would provide two very different values! However, the respiratory trace (RESP) defines the end-expiratory position (red arrow) and the correct measurement (green arrow) for the CVP. To provide careful CVP measurements, either a respiratory trace on the monitor or simultaneous exam of your patient is required to define the exact point of end-expiration.

Ideally, the measurement of CVP would provide an indicator for the clinician of which patients may respond to an intravenous fluid bolus with an improvement in cardiac output. These patients are termed *preload responsive*. However, many studies have confirmed that a specific CVP threshold does not predict which patient will respond to a fluid bolus.[47]

The lack of a strong correlation between CVP (and PAOP) and a cardiac response to fluid administration should not be surprising. CVP is determined by the interaction of cardiac function and return volume.

The actual return volume can be influenced by several variables independent of fluid administration, including venous tone. CVP might not even increase with the administration of a fluid bolus. Cardiac function can also vary due to factors independent of venous return and preload, such as cardiac contractility and cardiac afterload. We can only reasonably expect that CVP might provide one indicator of the cardiac preload rather than one absolute value to define a patient who will be fluid responsive.

Right heart failure from right heart myocardial infarction, pulmonary embolism, or pulmonary hypertension would all be expected to increase the CVP. If the measured CVP is low, it would be unlikely any of these conditions would be the cause of hypotension and low cardiac output. Left heart failure, tamponade, or fluid overload can all increase the PAOP. An elevated PAOP tells you that the left atrial pressure is up but does not distinguish between left heart failure, left-sided valvular disease, cardiac tamponade, fluid overload, etc. You need the full hemodynamic profile to sort this out, so keep reading. If the CVP is very high, hypovolemia is unlikely to be the sole cause of shock, unless the pleural pressure is very elevated, leading to a reduced transmural pressure.

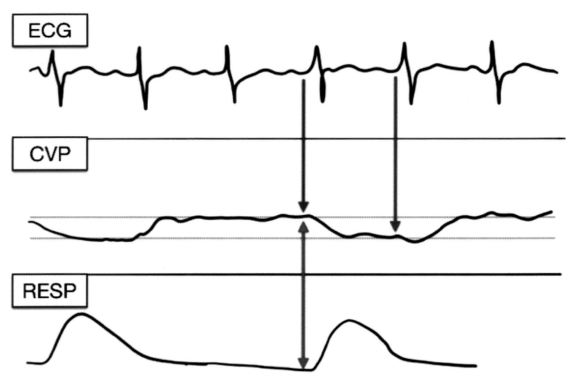

Figure 7-10 *The measurement of central venous pressure (CVP) requires the clinician to find the right waveform (follows P wave on ECG – blue and green arrows) and is measured at end inspiration (red arrow).*

7.3.2 Ventricular Pressures and Waveforms

Pressures rise inside the ventricle for two reasons: ventricular contraction (squeeze-systole) or filling (diastole). We can measure the pressures in the right ventricle by transducing the distal port of the pulmonary artery catheter as you are moving in from the atrium to the pulmonary artery. You have to pay close attention when you are inserting a PA catheter; you only have one quick opportunity to see the right ventricular pressure tracing, because you usually trigger ventricular ectopy or tachycardia as you pass the catheter inside the ventricle. You will need to move quickly from the right atrium to the pulmonary artery. The right ventricle waveform has a systolic and diastolic pressure. The diastolic pressure is the same as the central venous pressure when the A-V valve is open and usually is low at 0-4 mm H_2O. As mentioned earlier, for an ICU patient who is fluid loaded, on a ventilator with positive end-expiratory pressure, the normal value is typically 5-10 cm H_2O. During right ventricular systole, the pressure rises to 25-35 cm H_2O. Unlike the complicated CVP curve, the right ventricular pressure curve is simple; it just goes up and comes down. *Systole, diastole, systole, diastole, yawn....* Note that systole rises between the A and C wave and the diastole falls at the peak of the V wave. When the ventricular pressures rise above the atrial pressure (A wave), the A-V valve closes (and pushes in backwards with C wave); and when the ventricular pressure drops below the atrial pressure (V wave), the A-V valve opens.

With heart failure, whether right heart failure from pulmonary hypertension, or left heart failure from any cause, the RV pressures rise. Typically, both the systolic pressure and the diastolic pressure rise. Rarely a high RV pressure can occur from pulmonary artery stenosis.

Key components of ventricular pressure measurements include:

- A right ventricle (RV) waveform is obtained from any catheter passed through the right ventricle. The RV waveform is usually obtained from a PA catheter, either during the period of floating the catheter or from a port that remains in the RV after placement.
- A left ventricle (LV) waveform is similar in characteristics to the RV waveform but with higher pressures. An LV waveform is only obtained during left heart catheterization and not routinely in ICU care.
- When measured via the PA catheter, the rise in the right ventricular pressure is slightly delayed from the QRS onset of the ECG.

7.3.3 Pulmonary Artery Pressure and Waveforms

As soon as the PA catheter crosses the pulmonary artery valve, something new happens: you have a diastolic pressure (**Figure 7-11**)! As you pass the valve, the systolic pressure from the right ventricle to the pulmonary artery stays the same, but suddenly the closure of the pulmonic valve traps the pressure in the pulmonary artery, and we have a jump up in diastolic pressure. This sudden jump in diastolic pressure and the appearance of a dicrotic notch similar to the one seen in a systemic arterial pressure tracing tells you that you have successfully made it into the pulmonary artery. If you are advancing the PA catheter through the ventricle you can now relax; you got the catheter in, avoided ventricular arrhythmias, and can now slowly advance the catheter to the wedge position. The pulmonary artery waveform mirrors the top of the ventricular waveform but has a dicrotic notch and maintains a diastolic pressure. The PA waveform

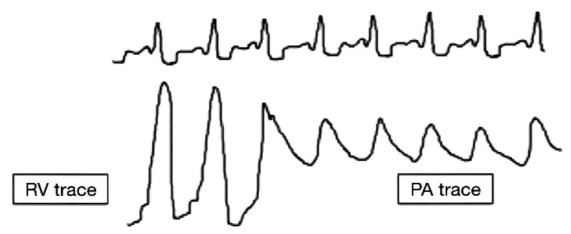

Figure 7-11 *Transition from right ventricular (RV) hemodynamic tracing to a pulmonary artery (PA) tracing.*

looks exactly like your arterial line tracing except that the pressures are lower. Instead of 120/80 in the systemic arterial circulation, the pressures in the pulmonary artery are approximately 25-35/10-15 mm Hg

The PA pressures rise because of pulmonary hypertension. This can occur because of resistance within the pulmonary vascular bed (called *pulmonary arterial hypertension)* or from increases in pressure from the left heart (called pulmonary venous hypertension).

The mean arterial pressure (MAP) is the pressure averaged over one cardiac cycle. Because systole is shorter than diastole, the MAP is less than the average of systolic and diastolic pressures. The mean pulmonary artery pressure is calculated as:

Mean arterial pressure (MAP) = [(2 x diastolic) + systolic]/3

You might also see the following equation, which uses the pulse pressure to calculate the mean arterial pressure. The pulse pressure is the difference between the systolic and diastolic pressure and is typically ~ 40 mm Hg. This alternative equation for calculating the mean arterial pressure is:

Mean arterial pressure (MAP) = [(diastolic) + (systolic-diastolic)/3]

The mean pulmonary artery pressures will rise behind any anatomical place where the pressure builds up. Pulmonary hypertension is like the water level building up behind a dam. Find the dam, and you know where the pressures will be elevated.

Key components of pulmonary arterial pressure measurements include:

- The pulmonary artery has a similar waveform morphology to arterial pressure waveforms.
- The upslope occurs as blood is ejected from the ventricle into the pulmonary artery or aorta.
- As the ventricles relax, the pressure in the great vessels will exceed the ventricular pressure, and the aortic and pulmonic valves will close. This produces a small rise in arterial pressures, producing a bump in the waveform called the dicrotic notch.
- The RV systolic and PA systolic pressures may be relatively equal, but the RV diastolic pressure is lower than the PA diastolic pressure.

Let's review a few conditions leading to pulmonary hypertension.

7.3.3.1 Left Heart Failure from Systolic Dysfunction

Left heart failure is caused by diseases such as myocardial infarction, cardiomyopathy, and aortic

or mitral valvular disease. In conditions of left heart failure, the left atrial pressure is high, the pulmonary artery occlusion pressure (PAOP) is high, the mean pulmonary artery pressure may be high, the RV diastolic and systolic pressures are high, and the CVP is high. Typically, the pressures are highest at the PAOP and drop as we move backward away from the left atrium. Because the elevated pressures are produced by high pressures in the left ventricular end-diastolic filling pressures, the gradient between the mean pulmonary artery pressure (mPAP) and the pulmonary artery occlusion pressure (PAOP) is small – both are elevated. This gradient is called the *transpulmonary gradient* (TPG) and is defined by

TPG = mPAP- PAOP

Key: TPG < 12 cm H_2O and PAOP elevated in left heart failure

7.3.3.2 Pulmonary Arterial Hypertension (PAH)

PAH is caused by progressive vasoconstriction, smooth muscle hypertrophy, intimal hyperplasia, and the development of complex vascular lesions referred to as *plexogenic vasculopathy*. PAH can arise for unknown reasons (idiopathic), secondary to hereditable mutations in the BMPRII receptor, endoglin-1 or alk-1, or secondary to many systemic diseases such as emphysema, lung fibrosis, congenital heart disease, sickle cell anemia, HIV infection, scleroderma and other auto-immune diseases, and many other disorders. In pulmonary arterial hypertension, the dam occurs in the pulmonary arterioles (or rarely in the pulmonary veins, referred to as *pulmonary veno-occlusive disease*). The key to diagnosing pulmonary arterial hypertension is that the blockage is between the pulmonary artery and the left atrium, so the transpulmonary gradient is large and the PAOP is normal. Note that similar findings can occur with a massive pulmonary embolism blocking the pulmonary vessels.

Key: TPG >12 cm H_2O and PAOP normal in PAH

7.4 Cardiac Chamber Pressures and Pericardial Disease

In cardiac tamponade, fluid fills the pericardial sac around the heart, applying constant hydraulic pressure on the heart chambers. Because all four chambers are inside the pericardium, the external hydraulic force pressurizes them all equally. The critical feature of tamponade is the development of *equalization of pressures*.

Under pressure!!! In tamponade, the heart is under massive pressure or stress; it can never relax! The internal hydraulic pressure makes all the diastolic pressures rise.

Don't be fooled. A few diseases can mimic cardiac tamponade and cause equalization of pressures:

- *Left heart failure with a big fluid bolus.* The PAOP is high with left heart failure, and after a significant fluid bolus, the CVP can rise acutely, leading to equalization of pressures.
- *Right ventricular myocardial infarction (RV MI).* An RV MI occurs when the right coronary artery is occluded. In a right-dominant system, the inferior part of the heart is perfused by the right coronary artery, which can involve both the right ventricle and inferior wall of the left ventricle. The combination can drop both left and right chamber cardiac output.
- *Increased intrathoracic pressures.* With severe dynamic hyperinflation from COPD or asthma (auto-PEEP), the pressures rise in the lung and apply pressure to the thoracic space, squeezing the heart. Dynamic hyperinflation can produce both equalization of pressures and pulsus paradoxus. Very high applied PEEP can also do this.
- *Constrictive pericarditis.* Like tamponade, the scarred pericardium squeezes all the heart chambers. So how do we distinguish constrictive pericarditis from tamponade?

In both cardiac tamponade and constrictive pericarditis, you will have a reduced cardiac output and equalization of pressures. The trick to telling the two apart is to look at the right ventricle pressure tracings for a square root sign and to look at the X and Y descents of the CVP tracing.

In constrictive pericarditis we have a RV square root sign and a prominent Y descent (X<<Y) **(Figure 7-12)**.

In tamponade, there is NO square root sign and the X descent is greater than or equal to the Y descent **(Figure 7-13)**.

7.5 Cardiac Output

The PA catheter can provide blood from the distal pulmonary artery port to measure the SvO_2, and you can directly measure cardiac output with a technique called *thermodilution*.

The concept of thermodilution is simple and derives from an age-old physiological concept of chemodilution. Thermodilution utilizes a very sensitive temperature probe, called a *thermistor*, located at the tip of the PA catheter. An injection of cold or room temperature saline in the central venous port hits the right atrium and is carried by the blood to the right ventricle and into the pulmonary artery, where the thermistor measures the change in temperature over time (thermodilution curve) **(Figure 7-14)**. A small, fast peak with rapid decay means a high cardiac output; while a larger, longer peak with a slower decay means a low cardiac output. A continuous cardiac output PA catheter has metal heating coils around the proximal catheter at about the level of the right atrium. These

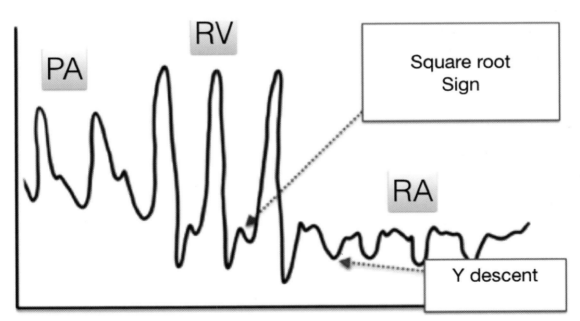

Figure 7-12 Hemodynamic waveform shows characteristic square root sign and prominent Y descent (> x descent) of constrictive pericarditis.

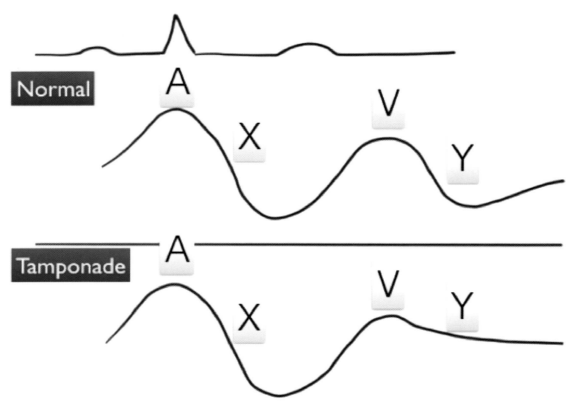

Figure 7-13 Hemodynamic waveform shows characteristic X descent > Y descent and no square root sign in cardiac tamponade.

coils heat in little bursts, and the thermistor detects the change in temperature in blood over time to calculate cardiac output continuously.

The limitation of using the PA catheter thermodilution method is that pulmonary artery flow can vary widely over the respiratory cycle. Variation over the respiratory cycle can produce non-artifact fluctuations in the thermodilution CO measurement with repeated measures. To compensate for this variability, multiple measurements (i.e., 3-5) are made with each assessment, and their values averaged to provide a reliable estimate of cardiac output.

The ability to measure cardiac output and stroke volume (cardiac output/heart rate) with the pulmonary artery catheter allows direct assessment of the patient's cardiac response to a fluid bolus, vasopressor support, or inotrope administration. In the case of fluid loading, measurement of cardiac output before and after a fluid bolus allows direct assessment of a patient's *preload responsiveness*. Although the definition is variable across the medical literature, generally a change in cardiac output of 12-15% between measurements pre- and post-fluid loading is required for the patient to be considered preload responsive.

When we measure cardiac output or flow, what we want to know is the delivery of oxygen to the body. Arterial blood oxygen content is calculated from hemoglobin levels from standard laboratory values and oxygen saturation from blood gas analysis. The oxygen content in arterial blood (CaO_2) is determined by:

$$CaO_2 = [Hgb\ (gms/dL) \times SaO_2\ (as\ fraction) \times 1.39\ ml\ O_2/gm\ Hgb \times 10] + (PaO_2 \times 0.0031\ ml/mmHg)$$

The equation illustrates the two most important variables in blood oxygen content: 1) the grams of hemoglobin (Hgb) and 2) the saturation of that hemoglobin (SaO_2). The constant of 1.39 converts grams of hemoglobin to mL of oxygen, and the value of 10 converts dL to liters of blood. Dissolved oxygen, primarily influenced by the partial pressure of oxygen (PaO_2), only accounts for a very minimal component of total blood oxygen content. For example, total arterial oxygen content for 15 g/dL hemoglobin and a PaO_2 of 100 mm Hg (SaO2 98%) is about 200 mL per liter of blood, yet only 0.3 ml of oxygen is dissolved in blood.

Arterial oxygen delivery (DO_2) is the product of cardiac output and arterial blood oxygen content. If

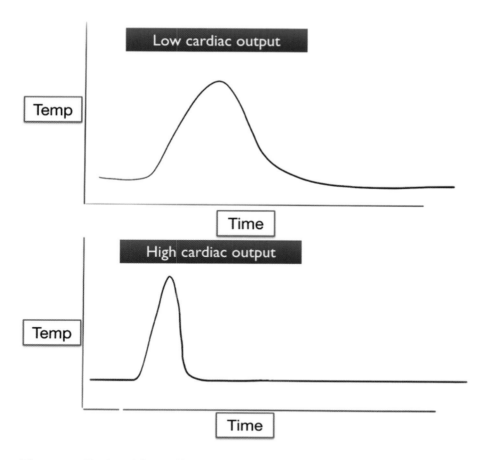

Figure 7-14 *Tracing of thermodilution cardiac output measurement.*

we took a sample of blood from the tip of a central venous catheter or a pulmonary artery catheter (see below), we could measure the venous hemoglobin oxygen saturation. A true mixed venous sample (SvO_2) is obtained from the pulmonary artery and includes all the blood returning from the head and arms (via superior vena cava), the gut and lower extremities (via the inferior vena cava), and the coronary veins (via the coronary sinus). Alternatively, venous blood is obtained from a central venous catheter in the internal jugular or subclavian veins providing a central venous oxygen saturation ($ScvO_2$). The $ScvO_2$ will reflect the average saturation of blood returning from the head and arms. In most clinical situations, the $ScvO_2$ will approximate the SvO_2, and the two values are considered interchangeable.

7.6 Vascular Resistance

Oxygen delivery to the vital organs, especially the brain and heart, is what you want to know about and maintain *(It's the flow, stupid!)*. The blood pressure is only one indicator suggesting that the flow is adequate. However, blood pressure alone is not enough, as a patient can often keep the systemic circulation clamped down to maintain blood pressure even in the setting of low cardiac output with little flow to vital organs. To understand this, we must understand the relationship between blood pressure, vascular resistance, and cardiac output.

For electrical currents, think

$V = IR$: Voltage (V) = Current (I) $\times$ Resistance (R)

For human physiology, think

$$P_1 - P_2 = Q \times VR$$

The pressure change across a vascular bed ($P_1 - P_2$) = Flow (Q) $\times$ Vascular Resistance (VR). When working with the *systemic circulation*, P_1 is mean blood arterial pressure (MAP), and P_2 is the central venous pressure; Q is the measured cardiac output (CO), and VR is systemic vascular resistance (SVR). We define the relationships for the systemic circulation as

$$MAP - CVP = CO \times SVR$$

For the *pulmonary circulation*, P_1 is the mean pulmonary artery pressure (mPAP) and P_2 is the left atrial pressure. The left atrial pressure is estimated by the pulmonary artery occlusion pressure (PAOP), also called the pulmonary capillary wedge pressure (PCWP). The VR is the pulmonary vascular resistance (PVR). We define the relationship for the pulmonary circulation as

$$mPAP - PAOP = CO \times PVR$$

These relationships tell us that we can have a severe drop in cardiac output during heart failure, myocardial infarction, cardiac tamponade, etc., and if we can clamp down our resistance vessels by producing epinephrine and norepinephrine, we can maintain blood pressure. Just looking at the blood pressure, without measuring the cardiac output, one would not know this was the case.

7.7 Shock and Hemodynamic Assessment

Now that we have the basics of vascular pressures, flow (cardiac output), and vascular resistance, let's look at how these pieces fit together in the management of the patient with shock. There are three major types of shock or hypoperfusion states that you need to figure out, as the treatment for each one is different:

1. Hypovolemic shock
2. Cardiogenic shock
3. Distributive shock

While all these disorders can present with low blood pressure (MAP), they will have different measures of CO and calculated SVR, which will help you diagnose them and apply the right treatments. For the majority of your ICU cases, you will not need the PA catheter, but understanding the measurements we have just discussed will help you understand the physiology of different types of shock.

7.7.1 Hypovolemic Shock

Severe bleeding or dehydration can lead to hypovolemic shock. The tank is empty, so there is no preload to fill the heart and the stroke volume drops. These patients have a low CO, or flow, due to the reduction in preload and are clamped down (high SVR) in an attempt to maintain MAP and perfusion to the vital organs, brain, and heart. Unlike cardiogenic shock, in these patients the filling pressures are low, with a low

PAOP, PA pressure, RV pressure, and CVP.

7.7.2 Cardiogenic Shock

Primary pump failure of either the left or right ventricle leads to cardiogenic shock. For all types of cardiogenic failure, the cardiac output drops, the MAP is sustained by systemic vasoconstriction with an SVR that is very high. These patients have low CO and flow and are clamped down (high SVR) to maintain MAP and perfusion to the vital organs, brain, and heart. In this case the filling pressures are high, with a high PAOP, PA pressure, RV pressure, and CVP. If the cause is right heart failure from pulmonary hypertension, the PAOP is normal, the TPG is >12, and the PA pressure, RV pressure and CVP will be high.

7.7.3 Distributive Shock

Severe infection, neurological injury, or severe anaphylaxis are clinical conditions that cause distributive shock. In this condition, there is a severe peripheral vasodilation that moves blood through arterial-venous anastomoses and away from organ tissues (maldistribution of flow). Distributive shock is different from the other types of shock, in that these patients classically have a high CO and flow and very low SVR, with a low MAP at time of diagnosis. In these patients, the filling pressures can be low or high depending on how much fluid resuscitation they have received.

In patients with sepsis, the hemodynamic manifestations are further complicated as the systemic inflammatory response syndrome can contribute a decline in cardiac contractility. In sepsis, multiple components can interact to produce a reduction in MAP and shock.

Figure 7-15 and **Figure 7-16** summarize the hemodynamic patterns associated with these three forms of shock.

Notice that in all of these forms of shock, the MAP can be variable. This is the last physiological variable to go as the body increases cardiac output, increases heart rate and stroke volume, and increases SVR in an effort to sustain the MAP.

7.8 Limitations of the Pulmonary Artery (PA) Catheter

Now that we have told you all the cool information the PA catheter can provide, we have to say why not to use it! Before 1983, almost all patients with shock in ICUs had PA catheters in place to measure hemodynamics, monitor cardiac output, and monitor oxygen delivery and consumption. These catheters

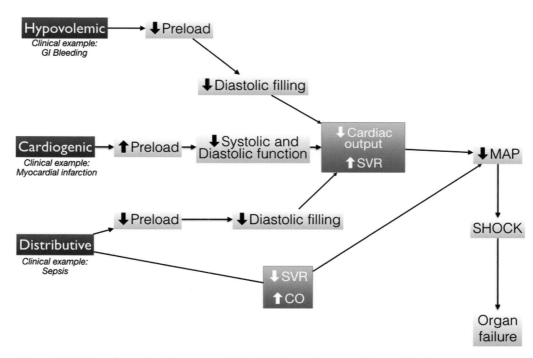

Figure 7-15 Hemodynamic patterns associated with the most common forms of shock.

Type	CO	SVR	MAP	Comments
Hypovolemic	↓↓↓	↑↑↑	↓	low PAOP, PA, RV, and CVP
Cardiogenic	↓↓↓	↑↑↑	↓	high PA, RV, and CVP RV failure: normal PAOP LV failure: high PAOP
Distributive	↑↑↑	↓↓↓	↓	low PAOP, PA, RV, and CVP, but may be variable based upon volume resuscitation and condition

Figure 7-16 Hemodynamic changes associated with different types of shock. CO = cardiac output. SVR = systemic vascular resistance. MAP = mean arterial presssure.

were believed necessary to establish correct diagnoses and manage interventions. A landmark study using retrospective data with careful patient matching to suggest an equal need for a pulmonary artery catheter, reported that patients managed with a PA catheter had an increased mortality rate, even after adjusting for severity of illness and the propensity for physicians to use a catheter in sicker patients.[48] Randomized trials followed in patients with cardiogenic shock, septic shock, and ARDS, all of which confirmed no mortality benefit to the use of a PA catheter in the study groups.[49] The result of these trials led to a dramatic reduction in the use of PA catheters.[50] A PA catheter remains a great tool to learn cardiac physiology, but now is reserved for the more complicated patient who requires an assessment of cardiac output when standard diagnostic and therapeutic interventions are not clear. The PA catheter can also be used for patients with known right or left ventricular failure not responding to initial inotropic and diuretic strategies.

7.9 Hemodynamic Assessment without the PA Catheter

As the PA catheter became less prominent in monitoring resuscitation, investigators turned to other less-invasive strategies to assess cardiac output or flow in critically ill patients. Let's remind you of some terminology from our Chapter 4 on *Sepsis and Resuscitation*. A critical decision in the patient with shock is to identify those patients who will respond favorably to fluid resuscitation. This category of patients is termed *preload responsive*. Fluid resuscitation in preload responsive patients restores stroke volume, improves cardiac output, lowers HR, raises mean arterial pressure, and improves tissue oxygen delivery (DO_2). Preload responsive patients are functioning on the ascending limb of their Starling curve (**Figure 4-6**, blue triangle). If the patient is not preload responsive (**Figure 4-6,** red triangle), then aggressive fluid administration can only cause harm (*Think lung water!*).

The tools used to define preload responsiveness can be grouped into static and dynamic measurements. Static measurements have been discussed above, including central venous pressure, pulmonary artery occlusion pressure, and LV and RV end diastolic dimensions. The most common static variable used to guide fluid resuscitation has been the central venous pressure (CVP). In theory, CVP should provide a reliable indicator of right ventricular preload. Unfortunately, the relationship between measured CVP and preload is complex, and no specific cutoff value has been shown to discriminate preload responders from non-responders.[51] We would expect complex ICU patients to follow their *individual* Frank-Starling curves, making a single CVP value for all patients illogical. We have some evidence to suggest the extremes of CVP (i.e., CVP < 6 or CVP > 15) might be more predictive. CVP is a "tool" to incorporate into your overall patient assessment but is most valuable when you recognize the limitations in the measured value.

Dynamic measurements attempt to create a change in cardiac preload and then assess the response to that change through some comparative assessment of cardiac output or stroke volume. A dynamic measurement consists of two variables: 1) an intervention to change preload, and 2) a measurement of how that preload change impacts cardiac output or flow.

7.9.1 Techniques to Change Preload

7.9.1.1 Fluid Challenge

The most common dynamic measurement used in clinical practice is a fluid challenge. Clinicians use a fluid challenge recurrently in resuscitation and continuously assess heart rate, blood pressure, urine output, and oxygenation. This technique works for the majority of patients.

A very simple clinical decision algorithm for interpretation of the response to a fluid bolus in your hemodynamically unstable patient is repeated from Chapter 4 in **Figure 7-17**.

Incremental fluid boluses could be continued as long as the patient continues to improve hemodynamically in blood pressure, pulse pressure, capillary refill, and urine output. Be cautious that pulmonary gas exchange is not adversely impacted during your fluid bolus resuscitation.

The major limitation of a fluid bolus is that it is not reversible. A fluid bolus does not "predict" fluid responsiveness; rather it "assesses" fluid responsiveness. Do we have any tools that could "predict" fluid responsiveness, so we could avoid administering fluid to ~ 40% of sepsis patients who do not need it?

7.9.1.2 Passive Leg Raising

A dynamic test to create a preload variation is the *passive leg raising (PLR) test*. The PLR test offers the advantage of being a reversible preload challenge to cardiac function. Lifting the legs above the horizontal position creates a gravitational transfer of blood from the lower limbs to the thorax, raising ventricular preload. Of note, the effects of PLR reach a maximum within 30-90 sec, are not prolonged, and are reversed by returning the patient to the supine position. PLR may be a more effective marker of preload dependence if the patient begins in the 45° thorax-elevated position and converts to the 45° leg-elevated position (**Figure 7-18**).[52]

PLR-induced changes in blood pressure alone are not as predictive of preload responsiveness compared to PLR-induced changes in measured cardiac output or stroke volume. Aortic blood flow velocity, pulse pressure variation, echocardiography indices, or end-tidal CO_2 measurements are required to accurately recognize the change in cardiac function associated with the PLR maneuver.[53,54]

7.9.1.3 Heart-Lung Interactions

A second alternative approach for manipulating preload is to use heart-lung interactions. Positive

Δ Mean Arterial Pressure (MAP)	Δ Urine Output/ Tissue Perfusion	Δ Oxygenation i.e., SaO₂	Plan
increase	increase	No Δ	Preload responsive. Continue fluid bolus resuscitation.
No Δ	No Δ	No Δ	Preload unresponsive. Support circulation with a vasopressor as needed.
No Δ	No Δ	decrease	Preload unresponsive and capillary leak in lung. Limit additional fluid bolus and support circulation with a vasopressor.
partial increase	partial increase	decrease	Preload responsive with capillary leak in lung. Very cautious fluid administration and circulatory support with a vasopressor

Figure 7-17 *Interpretation of the hemodynamic response to a fluid challenge.*

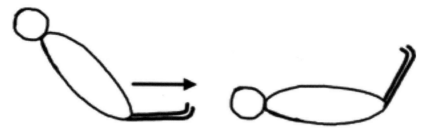

Figure 7-18 *Patient positioning for passive leg raising.*

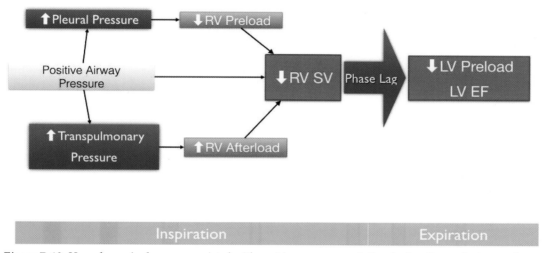

Figure 7-19 *Hemodynamic changes associated with positive pressure variation during the respiratory cycle. See text.*

airway pressure ventilation introduces a variable change in cardiac preload that can be used to change preload and then assess the hemodynamic response (**Figure 7-19**).

Venous return to the right ventricle (RV) varies with the ventilatory cycle. Mechanical lung insufflation decreases preload (reduced venous return) and increases afterload of the RV (increased transpulmonary pressure). These changes combine to reduce RV output, which will be at the minimum value at end inspiration. The reduction in RV stroke volume leads to a reduction in left ventricular (LV) filling after a few cardiac cycles determined by the pulmonary blood transit time. The reduction in LV filling lowers LV stroke volume, which tends to be at the maximum reduction during the exhalation phase. These changes in RV and LV stroke volume are best appreciated when the ventricle is underfilled or operating on the steep portion of the Starling curve. The magnitude of the respiratory cycle changes in left ventricular stroke volume is an indicator of biventricular preload dependence.

Despite the appealing physiology of using heart-lung interactions to manipulate preload, some very key limitations exist, including

- The patient must be in sinus rhythm to assess beat-to-beat changes in cardiac stroke volume.
- The patient cannot be spontaneously breathing, with or without the ventilator. Spontaneous respiratory effort introduces variable changes in intrathoracic pressure that can independently change preload and the associated stroke volume.
- A higher tidal volume is needed to cause intrathoracic pressure changes of significant magnitude to manipulate preload. Studies in the ARDS patient population suggest this tidal volume needs to be ≥ 8 ml/kg IBW (Ideal Body Weight) in patients with lung compliance < 30 ml/cm H_2O

The outlined limitations significantly restrict the utility of heart-lung interactions as a preload assessment tool to a small volume of ICU patients.

7.9.2 Techniques to Assess Stroke Volume

7.9.2.1 Pulse Pressure Variability (PPV)

Arterial pressure waveform analysis estimates stroke volume on a beat-to-beat basis using an indwelling arterial catheter and analysis of the arterial pressure pulse wave (**Figure 7-20**). Arterial pulse pressure is the difference between the peak systole pressure and the nadir diastole pressure.

Arterial pulse pressure is proportional to left ventricular (LV) stroke volume and inversely related to arterial compliance. If we assume the arterial compliance remains constant, cyclic changes in pulse pressure (termed *pulse pressure variation, PPV*), could provide a dynamic indicator of the change in stroke volume during a maneuver that changes preload.[55] PPV is calculated as the ratio of the difference in maximal and minimal values of pulse pressure averaged over two cardiac cycles and can be directly measured from an arterial pressure tracing (**Figure 7-21**).

In published trials using heart-lung interactions to vary preload and pulse pressure variation to assess stroke volume, the mean threshold to detect *preload dependence* for pulse pressure variation was 8% (range, 5%-12%) in low tidal volumes studies (< 7 ml/kg) and 11% (range, 4%-15%) in high tidal volumes ($\geq$ 7 ml/kg) studies.[47] A PPV higher than the specific threshold for each tidal volume was 5x times more likely to predict fluid responsiveness in the high tidal volume population and approximately 8x more likely in the low tidal volume population. Remember, patients must be in sinus rhythm and have no spontaneous respiratory efforts. These specific requirements limit the use of pulse pressure variation to a narrow spectrum of ICU patients.

Studies using change in pulse pressure following passive leg raising to predict fluid responsiveness found a mean threshold of 10% (range, 9%-12%). Patients with an increase in pulse pressure of 10% or greater had a 3.6x higher likelihood of being fluid responsive (summary specificity, 83%).[47] In general, PLR combined with an appropriate CO assessment tool can be predictive of preload responsiveness in both spontaneously breathing patients and patients on mechanical ventilation.

An alternative to pulse pressure variation is called *stroke volume variation (SVV)*. Several commercial monitors use analysis of the pulse contour to derive stroke volume. These devices employ proprietary calibration schemes to convert the arterial pulse pressure waveform to stroke volume, a technique called *pulse contour analysis*. Pulse contour devices come in two basic types: calibrated and uncalibrated. Calibrated devices use a transpulmonary dilution technique to calibrate their prediction models to the individual patient,

including transpulmonary thermodilution (PiCCO™ [Pulsion Ltd, Munich, Germany]) or transpulmonary lithium dilution (LiDCO™ LiDCO Ltd, London UK). Non-calibrated versions use patient-specific data for calibration (FlowTrac™ [Edwards Life Sciences, Irvine CA]). These devices show modest accuracy in the measurement of stroke volume, and they appear to trend the effect of medical interventions differently.[56] Do not use pulse contour analysis in the setting of aortic insufficiency, which alters the pulse wave contour and may decrease the accuracy of the assessment. Several non-invasive monitors have also been marketed that use analysis of the plethysmograph waveform or finger pulse pressure monitoring. Studies investigating the accuracy of stroke volume variation during positive pressure ventilation had a mean cutoff of 13% to predict preload responsiveness (range, 10%-20%). Stroke volume variation above the individual study cutoff predicted a ~ 5x greater likelihood of being fluid responsive.[47]

A meta-analysis has suggested the AOC curves are most favorable for pulse pressure variation as an indicator of preload responsiveness in comparison to systolic pressure variation and stroke volume variation. This analysis used a threshold value of 12.5 $\pm$ 1.6%.[57] Consistently, in mechanically ventilated patients, dynamic indices of arterial waveform-derived variables have been more accurate than static indicators, such as central venous pressure, in predicting a preload response to a volume challenge.

7.9.2.2 Esophageal Doppler

An alternative technique to measure stroke volume is the use of esophageal Doppler. Esophageal Doppler monitoring uses a small Doppler probe placed through the nose or mouth to measure the blood flow velocity in the descending thoracic aorta. The operator can position the probe blindly with some training to focus on the posterior thoracic descending aorta. The velocity time interval of moving blood through the aortic cross-sectional area provides an estimate of stroke volume. The descending aortic blood flow is converted to cardiac output by assuming that 70% of circulation goes to the caudal regions with 30% of blood flow to the cephalic and coronary artery regions. The esophageal Doppler can provide evidence for stroke volume variation as an indicator of volume responsiveness when preload is manipulated. Although results have been variable, in general, esophageal Doppler monitoring has shown correlations to CO measured by FICK or PA thermodilution with a small systematic underestimation.

7.9.2.3 Doppler Echocardiography

Cardiac output can be calculated using Doppler Echocardiography at any of the heart value orifices.

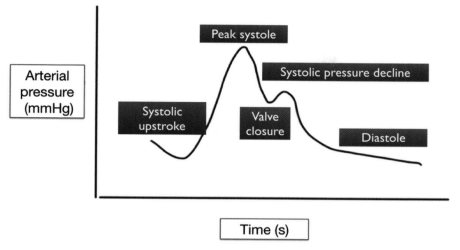

Figure 7-20 *Components of the arterial pulse pressure.*

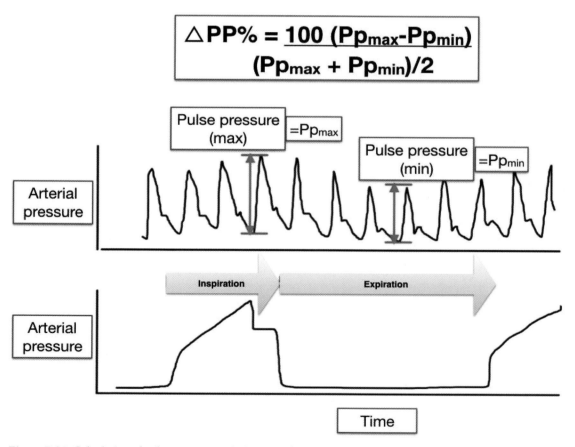

$$\triangle PP\% = \frac{100\ (Pp_{max} - Pp_{min})}{(Pp_{max} + Pp_{min})/2}$$

Figure 7-21 *Calculation of pulse pressure variation over the respiratory cycle.*

However, the most common technique is done at the left ventricular outflow tract (LVOT). Stroke volume is estimated based on the principle that flow through a vessel represents the average velocity x the cross-sectional area. The cross-sectional area (CSA) of the LVOT is calculated from a parasternal long axis view with the aortic valve leaflets wide open. A second five-chamber apical image is used to obtain a Doppler image of the LVOT and provides a calculation of a velocity time integral (VTI). Stroke volume is the product of LVOT CSA x LVOT VTI. Heart rate x the calculated stroke volume provides the measure of cardiac output. Modern POCUS machines automate these calculations. Although the technique correlates well with thermodilution cardiac output measurements, it remains very operator dependent.

An alternative Doppler technique to estimate stroke volume is the use of carotid Doppler imaging. A variety of carotid flow indices have been investigated as indicators of preload dependence during resuscitation.[58] While promising measurements due to their non-invasive nature and independence of mechanical ventilation, these carotid flow measurements are again operator dependent and need continued validation.

7.9.3 Inferior Vena Cava Diameter

A variation in vena cava diameter has also been used to predict preload responsiveness. The superior vena cava (SVC) is an intrathoracic vessel, while the inferior vena cava (IVC) is predominantly an intra-abdominal vessel. Ultrasound examination of the SVC requires transesophageal echocardiography, but a transthoracic subcostal approach can perform ultrasound examination of the IVC (*See Chapter 3 Point of Care Ultrasound [POCUS]*). Here again, we most commonly use heart-lung interactions to create a variation in preload.

The diameter of the IVC will normally show an inspiratory increase and an expiratory decrease in diameter during positive pressure ventilation. The theory behind the ultrasound assessment of IVC holds that in the setting of a high-volume status, the IVC is dilated and no respiratory variation is recognized. The *inferior vena cava distensibility index (dIVC)* is calculated according to the following equation:

dIVC = (maximum diameter on inspiration - minimum diameter on expiration)
([maximum diameter on inspiration + minimum diameter on expiration]/2)

In patients not on mechanical ventilation, the distensibility of the IVC across the respiratory cycle is reversed (smaller on inspiration). In a recent meta-analysis in ventilated patients without spontaneous respiratory efforts, the mean inferior vena cava distensibility index threshold was 15%. A high caval distensibility index predicted a 5x greater likelihood of the patient being fluid responsive. But the requirements of sinus rhythm, tidal volume $\geq$ 8ml/kg IBW, and no spontaneous respiratory activity significantly limit the accuracy of this tool in the broad range of ICU patients. The accuracy in patients receiving lung protective ventilation appears limited.

The IVC diameter should reflect the pressure gradient between intravascular (central venous) pressure and extravascular (intra-abdominal pressure). When the intra-abdominal pressure is negligible, the IVC diameter should reflect changes in the central venous pressure. Conditions which increase intra-abdominal pressure may also limit the interpretation of IVC diameter measurements.

7.9.4 Miscellaneous Methods for Preload Assessment

An ever-emerging list of techniques to assess preload responsiveness is being investigated. These techniques focus on the mechanically ventilated patient, but some apply to patients breathing spontaneously.[59] Clinical research into fluid resuscitation has focused on preload response as the key outcome parameter, measured as an increase in cardiac output ~ 15%. However, clinicians are focused on more direct outcome parameters in their patients, including heart rate, blood pressure, vasopressor requirement, urine output, or capillary refill. More clinical trials that focus on the incorporation of these measurement tools into relevant clinical outcome parameters are needed to advance the field. All these tools can be helpful. Incorporate them as your skill sets allow into your decision making, but don't mistrust your clinical judgment based on a single measurement device.

7.10 Hemodynamic Approach to Your ICU Patient

Whew! That was a lot of information. Need some rules of operation.

- Your resuscitations will be guided most frequently by a careful history and physical examination with attention to readily available parameters, including heart rate, blood pressure, capillary refill, urine output, gas exchange, and mentation.
- Bedside echocardiography provides a valuable, low-risk tool for assessment of left and right ventricular function to help guide resuscitation. For most patients, a bedside Doppler-echocardiogram is sufficient to suggest normal cardiac function.

- More complex patients, often with multisystem disorders, may require advanced diagnostic tools to guide resuscitation decisions. The pulmonary artery catheter can provide a detailed assessment of atrial, ventricular, and pulmonary artery pressures. Also, the thermodilution technique can be used to determine cardiac output. In very complex patients, integration of this information can help classify the type of shock and guide therapeutic decisions. However, no current data suggests this more comprehensive patient assessment will improve your patient outcome. Single or "static" measurements of central venous pressures from the PA catheter are less valuable than trending information over time.
- A more recent focus has emerged on the use of non-invasive dynamic indicators to guide resuscitation. Dynamic indicator assessments require two components:
  - An *intervention* is used to create a variable preload in the cardiovascular system. Both heart-lung interactions during positive pressure mechanical ventilation and straight leg raising have been used to manipulate preload.
  - An *assessment tool* is paired with the intervention to measure the hemodynamic or flow response (estimate of the change in biventricular stroke volume). Pulse pressure variation (arterial waveform analysis), aortic blood flow velocity (esophageal Doppler), vascular (IVC) dimensions by POCUS, have all been tested in critically ill patients. A decision about which tool to employ will often depend on local practice or your training skills.

Despite their appeal, all of the assessment tools have limitations. The tools require equipment and specialized skill training not uniformly available to all clinicians. Arrhythmias will cause beat-to-beat variability in stroke volume independent of heart lung interactions or leg raising maneuvers. This factor often restricts these interventions to patients in sinus rhythm. Small tidal volumes, frequently used in mechanical ventilation, minimize pleural pressure swings and the associated hemodynamic response.

No single measurement will provide the "answer." No formula works in all complex patients. The wise ICU physician incorporates all of these skills into his or her resuscitation practice to make smart treatment decisions.

Suggested Reading

- Atkinson PR, Milne J, Diegelmann L, et al. Does point-of-care ultrasonography improve clinical outcomes in emergency department patients with undifferentiated hypotension? An International Randomized Controlled Trial From the SHoC-ED Investigators. Ann Emerg Med 2018;72:478–489.

8

Acute Coronary Syndromes

Patients with acute coronary syndromes (ACS) most frequently present to the emergency department complaining of chest pain. ACS represents a spectrum of conditions in the coronary circulation that contribute to myocardial ischemia. The ACS syndromes include three clinical manifestations:

1. Unstable angina (UA)
2. Non-ST-segment elevation myocardial infarction (NSTEMI)
3. ST-segment elevation myocardial infarction (STEMI)

From a management standpoint, NSTEMI and UA are grouped together, as the management principles are similar. A *very large* number of clinical trials with a variety of entertaining abbreviations such as ISIS-3, TACTICS-TIMI-18, OASIS-6, NORDISTEMI, PRAMI, PROVE-IT have established the management principles of ACS. Whew!! Fortunately, those crazy cardiologists get together every few years and try to put it all together for you. Guidelines for the management of ACS are regularly updated by the American College of Cardiology and the American Heart Association. The most recent guidelines and a comprehensive set of references can be found at www.acc.org. We will try to summarize this information, so you have time to take care of the patient.

You will regularly be challenged to distinguish an acute coronary syndrome (myocardial infarction or unstable angina) from non-ischemic causes of acute chest pain, such as pulmonary embolism, aortic dissection, or esophageal rupture. The immediate (< 10 min) management is focused on an assessment of *ABC's (Airway, Breathing, Circulation)*, continuous monitoring of cardiac rhythm, and interpretation of the complete 12 lead ECG. If ACS is suspected based upon this initial prompt assessment, aspirin (325 mg) is administered to all patients unless there is a strong history of anaphylaxis. Discontinue non-steroidal medications other than aspirin if an agent was previously part of the patient's medication regimen.

Base your initial diagnosis on a combination of presenting symptoms, electrocardiographic (ECG) findings, and measurement of serum biomarkers. Because the efficacy of many interventions for acute coronary syndromes is time-dependent, patient evaluations must occur efficiently and mandate the availability of expertise to guide rapid decisions about appropriate interventions.

You will be challenged when ACS presents with atypical symptoms including dyspnea alone, weakness, nausea and vomiting, palpitations, or syncope. The absence of classic chest pain symptoms (which occur more often in women, diabetics, and the elderly) can delay prompt evaluation and intervention for ACS in these patients. In addition to atypical symptoms, the initial ECG may be unrevealing and should be repeated if a high clinical suspicion remains (q 20-30 min).

The diagnosis of chest pain etiology is approached using the OPQRST mnemonic. Although no chest pain characteristics are considered specific for ACS, some knowledge of the more common features in ACS can aid the clinician.

- **O**nset - gradual in onset which may include variable intensity
- **P**rovocation - classically related to exertion
- **Q**uality - discomfort rather than pain
- **R**adiation – typically to arms and rarely above the chin or below the abdomen
- **S**ite – diffuse
- **T**ime course – usually lasts > 30 min for ACS

We condense the approach to ACS into five big easy treatment steps **(Figure 8-1).**

1. Medical therapy to **cool down** the heart.
2. **Classify** the ACS syndrome (STEMI, unstable angina, NSTEMI)
3. **Crush** the platelets with dual antiplatelet therapy (DAPT)
4. **Bash** the coagulation system for unstable angina, NSTEMI, and STEMI

5. **Blast** open the obstruction for STEMI and high-risk NSTEMI

Acute myocardial infarction is classified into six subtypes:

1. Type 1—infarction due to coronary atherothrombosis
2. Type 2—infarction due to supply-demand imbalance without coronary athero-thrombosis
3. Type 3—infarction causing sudden death without ECG or biomarker confirmation
4. Type 4—infarction post-acute coronary intervention
5. Type 5—infarction post coronary artery bypass graft

In the ICU, you will most commonly need to distinguish between Type 1 and Type 2 myocardial

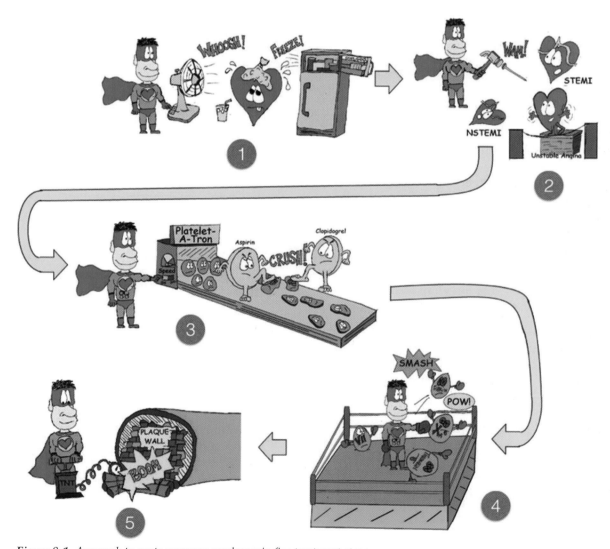

Figure 8-1 *Approach to acute coronary syndrome in five treatment steps.*

infarction in the management of your patients. Obviously, the treatment for these two conditions will be approached differently. For this chapter, we will focus on the intervention for Type 1 myocardial infarction.

8.1 Step 1: Cool Down the Heart

Initial cool-down management of ACS is standard for all the coronary syndromes:

- *Supplemental oxygen therapy if the measured peripheral oxygen saturation is < 90%.* Supplemental oxygen is not beneficial to patients with normal oxygen saturation.[60]
- *Control of chest pain with sublinqual or intravenous nitroglycerin* based upon the clinical response to therapy. If pain persists after three consecutive sublingual nitroglycerin doses (0.4 mg q 5 minutes), the patient is a candidate for intravenous nitroglycerin. Intravenous nitroglycerin is also favored in the absence of pain but in an ACS patient with uncontrolled hypertension or pulmonary edema. Nitrates are not administered (or used cautiously) in patients with
  - Systolic pressure < 90 mm Hg or > 30 mm Hg below baseline, due to the risk of worsening hypotension
  - Severe bradycardia (< 50 bpm)
  - Tachycardia (> 100 bpm) due to a risk of additional reflex tachycardia
  - Suspected right ventricular infarction due to preload dependence of the right ventricular for sustained cardiac output
  - Recent use of phosphodiesterase inhibitors (past 24 hours for sildenafil or vardenafil, or 48 hours for tadalafil). These medications prevent the breakdown of cGMP, and a drug interaction can lead to vasodilation with a risk of profound hypotension and or cardiogenic shock.
- Intravenous morphine sulfate (2-4 mg IV, repeated at 5-15-minute intervals) can also be administered to relieve chest pain and reduce catecholamine-induced stimulation from pain and anxiety. However, a potential inhibitory effect of morphine sulfate on $P2Y_{12}$ receptor blockers (platelet inhibitors like clopidogrel, prasugrel, and ticagrelor) has raised concern about its indiscriminate use.
- Administer a Beta-blocker within 24 hours in the absence of hemodynamic instability or a risk for hemodynamic instability. The early administration of Beta-blockers is associated with a reduction in infarct size and both short- and long-term mortality. Beta-blockers are contraindicated if ACS has been precipitated by cocaine use because

this would allow unopposed α stimulation from the cocaine effect. Early use of Beta-blockers, often via the intravenous route, is appropriate for patients with hypertension or tachycardia without evidence of CHF. Discharge patients on oral, Beta-blocker cardioselective agents, including metoprolol succinate, carvedilol, or bisoprolol. The following are clinical exceptions to the immediate administration of Beta-blockers:
  - Signs of heart failure, low perfusion, or risk factors for cardiogenic shock due to the negative inotropic effect of Beta-blockers
  - PR > 0.24, second- or third-degree heart block due to the risk of worsening the conduction delay
  - Asthma or reactive airways disease due to the risk of worsening bronchospasm

NOTE: As the clinical condition stabilizes, you should re-evaluate, as necessary, to determine subsequent eligibility for Beta-blocker therapy in patients with initial contraindications to their use.

As your patient stabilizes over the first few hours of admission, additional interventions may be added to cool down that heart.

- In patients with recurrent ischemia and a contraindication to Beta-blocker therapy, but normal left ventricular function and conduction, a non-dihydropyridine calcium antagonist (diltiazem or verapamil) may be considered as an alternative or adjunctive therapy to a Beta-blocker. Calcium channel blockers have not been shown to reduce mortality and may be harmful in patients with reduced left ventricular function or atrioventricular heart block. These medications are indicated with nitrate therapy for the treatment of coronary vasospasm.
- Administration of an angiotensin-converting enzyme (ACE) inhibitor following an acute myocardial infarction improves left ventricular function at one-year post procedure. The data is strongest for patients with STEMI. An angiotensin receptor blocker (ARB) is indicated in patients with similar criteria who are intolerant of ACE inhibitors. ACE inhibitor administration guidelines include:
  - Specially indicated for anterior wall STEMI location
  - Specially indicated for post-MI systolic dysfunction with an EF ≤ 0.40
  - Indicated for patients with hypertension, diabetes mellitus, or stable chronic kidney disease (CKD) unless contraindicated.
  - Contraindicated in the setting of renal failure, hyperkalemia, or hypotension due to the risk of potentially worsening these findings

- Administration of high dose statin therapy (atorvastatin 80 mg daily or rosuvastatin 20 or 40mg daily) is recommended for all patients with ACS before hospital discharge regardless of the low-density lipoprotein-cholesterol level. Statin therapy has been associated with a lower risk of 30-day adverse cardiac events. Previous guidelines titrated statin therapy to an LDL < 100 mg/dL or < 70 mg/dL, but new guidelines favor administration of high dose statin therapy to all patients without a specific contraindication. Monitor patients for myopathy or hepatic toxicity.

- Administration of a mineralocorticoid receptor antagonist or aldosterone blocker, such as spironolactone, is also recommended in a post-MI patient with an LVEF < 0.40, CHF, or diabetes mellitus. This treatment produces a reduction in subsequent all-cause mortality. These patients should already be receiving therapeutic dosing of an ACE inhibitor and a Beta-blocker and have the absence of the following contraindications:
  - Significant renal dysfunction (creatinine >2.5 mg/dL in men or > 2.0 mg/dL in women)
  - Hyperkalemia (K+ >5.0 mEq/L)

8.2 Step 2: Classify the ACS Syndrome (STEMI, Unstable Angina, NSTEMI)

8.2.1 The ECG

The ECG is used to classify ACS patients into two categories of disease:

1. *ST elevation myocardial infarction (STEMI).* The criteria include new ST elevation at the J point in two contiguous leads: ≥ 0.1 mV (1 mm) in all leads other than V2-V3, where the following diagnostic thresholds apply: ≥ 0.2 mV (2 mm) in men ≥ 40 years; ≥ 0.25 mV (2.5 mm) in men <40 years; or ≥ 0.15 mV (1.5 mm) in women of all ages.

2. *Non-ST elevation myocardial infarction (NSTEMI) or unstable angina.* The criteria include new horizontal or down-sloping ST depression ≥ 0.05 mV (0.5 mm) in two anatomically contiguous leads, and/or T inversion ≥ 0.1 mV (1 mm) in two anatomically contiguous leads with prominent R wave or R/S ratio > 1.

A paced rhythm or left bundle branch block (LBBB) pattern complicates the interpretation of the acute ECG. A new LBBB pattern is considered suggestive of a possible STEMI but not diagnostic. The majority of LBBB patterns on presentation are "not known to be old," meaning a baseline ECG is not available. Transthoracic echocardiography can provide evidence for focal wall injury to support the diagnosis of STEMI in these special cases. Q waves may be present in the ECG but do not predict the success of reperfusion therapy.

Define the anatomic location of the ischemia by the location of the ST elevation and/or increased T wave positivity (**Figure 8-2**).

Note **Figure 8-3** with ST elevation in V$_{4-6}$ and leads I and aVL. The red arrows illustrate the anterior lateral ST elevation. Reciprocal depression in the ST segments in leads I and III are also noted (green arrows).

Add V$_7$, V$_8$, V$_9$ leads when the initial ECG is non-diagnostic and the clinical suspicion for ACS is high. Position these leads after the V$_6$ lead extending across the back.

Note **Figure 8-4** with ST elevation in leads II, III, and aVF consistent with an inferior ST elevation myocardial infarction (STEMI) (red arrows).

In patients with an inferior wall infarction, right-sided leads may also be added to assess for a right ventricular infarction. For a right-sided ECG, V1 and V2 remain in the same place. V3 to V6 are placed in the same general location but mirrored on the right side of the chest.

In addition to inferior wall myocardial infarctions, a right-sided ECG should be considered in patients with clinical evidence of clear lungs but elevated right-sided heart pressures or echocardiographic findings of depressed right ventricular function. The importance of

Location	Leads
Anterior wall	Leads V$_1$ to V$_6$
Anteroseptal	Leads V$_1$ to V$_3$
Apical or lateral	Lead aVL and I, Leads V$_4$ to V$_6$ (Figure 8-3)
Inferior wall	Leads II, III, aVF (Figure 8-4)
Right ventricular	Right-sided precordial leads (V$_{4R}$, V$_{5R}$, V$_{6R}$)
Posterior wall	Leads V$_1$ to V$_2$ and posterior precordial leads (V$_7$, V$_8$, V$_9$)

Figure 8-2 Location of myocardial injury based on ECG changes.

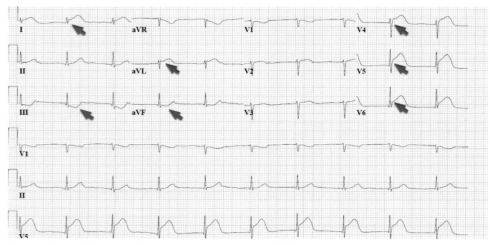

Figure 8-3 *ECG changes of anterior lateral myocardial infarction.*

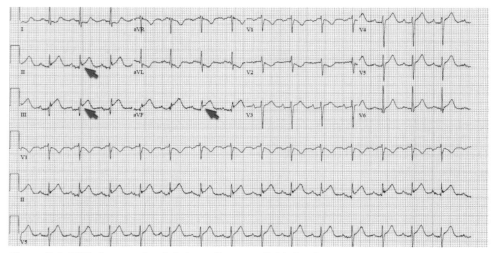

Figure 8-4 *ECG changes of an inferior wall myocardial infarction.*

recognizing right ventricular infarction is the need for preload (volume loading) to maintain cardiac output and to avoid nitroglycerin.

The clinician is expected to have the ECG completed and assessed within 10 minutes of the patient's arrival. Serial ECGs should be obtained at 15-30-minute intervals if the initial ECG is not diagnostic, but a clinical suspicion of ACS remains, or symptoms persist.

8.2.2 Cardiac Biomarkers

Cardiac troponin I (cTnI) and cardiac troponin T (cTnT) are cardiac regulatory proteins involved in actin-myosin contraction. cTnI has only been located in cardiac muscle, while cTnT has small components also located in skeletal muscle. A wide variety of assays exists in clinical practice with variable sensitivities. Higher sensitivity assays detect small amounts of circulating

cTn in "normal" patients. Each assay must provide a specific "cut-off" based upon the upper limit detection level in healthy individuals and the reported coefficient of variation for repeated samples. Patients with ACS suggested by biomarkers should have troponin levels that exceed the 99th percentile for normal individuals and also demonstrate a rise and fall on serial monitoring.

Cardiac troponin values begin to rise within 2-3 hours of acute MI and may persist for up to 10 days following the event. Elevations in cardiac troponin are not specific for ischemic heart disease, however. Troponin elevations are seen in moderate to severe pulmonary embolism with acute right heart overload, congestive heart failure, and acute myocarditis. Troponin elevations are also frequently seen in critically ill patients with sepsis.

Cardiac-specific troponin levels should be measured at presentation and repeated at 3 and 6 hours following symptom onset. Additional troponins are indicated beyond

6 hours if symptoms or ECG findings continue to suggest the diagnosis of ACS. If the actual symptom onset time is not known, then the presentation time is considered the time of onset. Creatine kinase (CPK) and myoglobin levels are no longer considered useful for the diagnosis of ACS.

8.2.3 ST Elevation Myocardial Infarction (STEMI)

Early identification of patients with STEMI is critical, as these patients benefit from prompt reperfusion therapy including both percutaneous coronary interventions (PCI) or systemic fibrinolytic treatment. This intervention benefit reflects the pathophysiologic mechanism of STEMI, which is the formation of *fibrin-rich clots* at the site of a ruptured atherosclerotic plaque. In contrast, NSTEMI is more characterized by *platelet-rich lesions*, with the primary therapy focused on platelet inhibitors. Successful intervention for patients with STEMI begins prior to the hospital.[61] EMS personnel should perform a 12-Lead ECG in patients with symptoms suggestive of STEMI at first contact. Reperfusion therapy is indicated within 12 hours of symptoms onset.

8.2.4 Non-ST Elevation Myocardial Infarction (NSTEMI) and Unstable Angina (UA)

Patients with an acute coronary syndrome, yet no findings to support an STEMI, are classified as unstable angina (UA) or non-ST elevation myocardial infarction (NSTEMI). UA and NSTEMI differ primarily in the duration of ischemia and whether actual myocardial injury has occurred, reflected in detectable levels of myocardial troponin. Because troponin may not be initially detectable, these two conditions often cannot be distinguished at presentation, and the initial treatment is identical.

Intravenous fibrinolytic therapy is not indicated for NSTEMI. Previous trials have suggested an adverse outcome for patients with NSTEMI who are provided fibrinolytic therapy. Immediate percutaneous intervention (PCI) is also not always indicated in the NSTEMI/UA patients.

8.3 Step 3: Crush the Platelets

For patients who meet the NSTEMI category, anti-platelet therapy remains the primary intervention. Divide your anti-platelet therapy into three components, and you will pick two for dual antiplatelet therapy (DAPT):

1. *Aspirin*, which blocks cyclooxygenase and inhibits the synthesis of prostaglandins and thromboxanes, including thromboxane A_2 from arachidonic acid.
2. *$P2Y_{12}$ receptor blockers or thienopyridines.* This category includes clopidogrel, prasugrel, and ticagrelor. These medications block the binding of ADP to the $P2Y_{12}$ platelet receptor and therefore inhibit the activation of the glycoprotein (GP) IIb/IIIa complex and platelet aggregation.
3. *Anti-glycoprotein (GP) IIb/IIIa antibodies and receptor antagonists.* This category includes abciximab, tirofiban, and eptifibatide. The platelet glycoprotein receptor plays an essential role in platelet adhesion and aggregation.

Aspirin should be administered as soon as feasible on initial presentation and continued indefinitely. An initial loading dose of 162 to 325 mg is favored, followed by a maintenance dose of 75 to 162 mg daily. Higher maintenance dosing (> 100 mg) is not associated with an incremental benefit but may be related to an increased rate of bleeding.

Patients with ACS are advised to receive one year of dual anti-platelet therapy (DAPT). In addition to aspirin, patients are prescribed an oral $P2Y_{12}$ inhibitor. The basis for DAPT comes from clinical trials finding better outcomes in ACS patients receiving clopidogrel and ASA in comparison to ASA alone. Daily maintenance of 75 mg clopidogrel follows a loading dose of 300 mg. Clopidogrel should also be administered in patients intolerant of aspirin. A 600 mg loading dose of clopidogrel is favored for patients who undergo PCI.

When aspirin or clopidogrel are administered to patients with a history of gastrointestinal bleeding, the use of medications to lower the risk of GI bleeding has been favored. However, proton pump inhibitors (PPI) alter the metabolism of clopidogrel to reduce formation of the active drug, leading to higher platelet reactivity in the setting of co-administration. The effectiveness of clopidogrel depends on its activation to an active metabolite by the cytochrome P450 (CYP-450) system, principally CYP2C19. About 25% of the population carries a CYP2C19*2 allele associated with lower levels of the metabolite at recommended doses, leading to a reduced effect on platelet function. A US Food and Drug Administration warning advises that poor metabolizers who received clopidogrel at standard dosing may exhibit higher cardiovascular event rates than patients with normal CYP2C19 function. Tests are available to identify a patient's CYP2C19 genotype and can be used as an aid in determining therapeutic strategy (called *pharmacogenomics testing*).

The significant individual variability in platelet response to clopidogrel has led to investigation of other agents. Prasugrel is a second $P2Y_{12}$ receptor blocker whose metabolism is not influenced by the presence of the allele. Prasugrel has a more rapid onset than clopidogrel, induces more intense platelet inhibition, and is associated with higher rates of bleeding. The use of prasugrel is contraindicated in patients with a history of stroke or TIA due to an increased bleeding risk. Patients older than 75 yo and weighing less than 65 kg may also show an increased rate of bleeding.[62]

Ticagrelor is an allosteric inhibitor of the $P2Y_{12}$ receptor, unlike the thienopyridines which act at the ADP binding site. Variations in the CYP450 allele do not alter the metabolism of ticagrelor. The drug has a rapid onset and induces more intense platelet inhibition than clopidogrel, but again is associated with higher rates of bleeding. Ticagrelor has a shorter duration of action that leads to a requirement for twice per day dosing but may offer an advantage to patients who need to undergo surgery. Ticagrelor is often favored over clopidogrel in patients with NSTEMI/UA who undergo an early intervention strategy. Unlike prasugrel, ticagrelor has not been linked with a higher bleeding rate in patients with a history of stroke or TIA, but this may reflect a smaller experience. Many clinicians also favor not using ticagrelor in these patients.

The primary concern for the use of $P2Y_{12}$ receptor blockers, in general, is the risk of bleeding. For patients at higher risk of bleeding, clopidogrel is favored as the agent of choice. The primary contraindication to the use of the thienopyridines is a short-term plan for cardiac surgery.

Potent inhibition of platelet function occurs with the administration of glycoprotein (GP) IIb/IIIa inhibitors, but these are currently reserved for very high-risk patients. These drugs target the final common pathway in platelet aggregation by blocking the binding of the GP IIb/IIIa integrin complex with fibrinogen and von Willebrand factor.

The glycoprotein (GP) IIb/IIIa inhibitors were initially studied before the routine use of DAPT. Their routine use in CAD syndromes has declined with the more routine use of DAPT therapy. Their current use is now restricted primarily to patients undergoing higher risk PCI, often with evidence for a high thrombotic burden or a low-flow condition.

In patients with NSTEMI/UA high-risk features (e.g., elevated troponin) and a low-risk bleeding profile who are not adequately pretreated with clopidogrel or ticagrelor, it may be useful to administer a GP llb/llla inhibitor at the time of percutaneous catheter-based intervention (PCI).

8.4 Step 4: Bash the Coagulation System for UA and NSTEMI

The hallmark of thrombosis is the conversion of soluble fibrinogen into insoluble strands of fibrin. This process is dependent on the activation of prothrombin to thrombin. So, in addition to anti-platelet therapy, the patient with Acute Coronary Syndrome is also treated with anticoagulation.

Anticoagulation therapy is administered as soon as feasible in patients with NSTEMI-ACS regardless of the management strategy selected. The selection of the actual agent is complicated by a diverse array of treatment options including

- *Unfractionated heparin*, a heterogeneous mixture of molecules that reversibly bind with antithrombin III, increasing antithrombin III's inhibition of factor Xa. Administer the drug with a 60-70 units / kg bolus followed by a 12 units/kg infusion, and then the continuous infusion is targeted to an aPTT 1.5-2.0 x control. The therapeutic effect of unfractionated heparin can be unpredictable and requires frequent monitoring of blood parameters.
- *Low molecular weight heparins (LMWH)* can provide a more predictable anticoagulation effect than unfractionated heparin but are more difficult to reverse and require adjustments for renal dysfunction. These drugs are absorbed when administered subcutaneously.
  - *Enoxaparin* – dosed at 1mg/kg subq q 12 hours. The dose is adjusted to 1 mg/kg q 24 hours for a creatinine clearance < 30 ml/min.
- *Factor Xa inhibitors* have a similar binding domain to heparin. The only available drug in this class is *fondaparinux*. Identical to the LMWH's, this medication is highly absorbed when given subcutaneously. The drug is cleared by the kidney and should be used with caution in patients with reduced creatinine clearance.
  - *Fondaparinux* – dosing is 2.5 mg subq once daily. If PCI is performed, the patient is converted to either unfractionated heparin (UFH) or bivalrudin.
- *Direct thrombin inhibitor* binds directly to thrombin, inhibiting conversion of fibrinogen to fibrin and thrombin-mediated platelet aggregation.
  - *Bivalirudin* – 0.1 mg/kg IV bolus followed by an infusion of 0.25 mg/kg per hour prior to angiography. Post angiography, an additional 0.5 mg/kg bolus, and the infusion rate is increased to 1.75 mg/kg per hour. In patients with NSTEMI/UA undergoing PCI who are at high risk of bleeding, it is reasonable to use bivalirudin monotherapy in preference to the combination of UFH and a GP IIb/IIIa receptor antagonist.

A considerable number of clinical trials have been conducted in the NSTEMI-ACS population to determine the optimal anticoagulation regimen. A few general principles are suggested by these trials:

- Anticoagulation of some form is recommended in all patients as soon as this can be accomplished.
- For patients where early PCI is expected, UFH or bivalrudin may be considered equivalent. Fondaparinux is not used to support PCI patients alone due to a risk of thrombosis but can be considered for patients at high bleeding risk on medical therapy.
- For patients where a conservative (non-PCI) strategy is planned, either enoxaparin or fondaparinux is favored over unfractionated heparin (UFH). Comparative trials have slightly favored enoxaparin (1mg/kg q12 hours) over UFH (aPTT 1.5-2.0 x normal) for patients who receive medical therapy only.

As a general rule, continue anticoagulation until a definitive coronary revascularization procedure occurs in the absence of contradictions or complications. For patients managed with a conservative medical strategy, continue anticoagulation for 2-5 days post presentation. Cautious attention to dosing adjustments is needed for elderly patients and patients with renal failure.

8.5 Step 5: Blast Open the Obstruction for STEMI and High-Risk NSTEMI

The timing of intervention in a patient with unstable angina or NSTEMI is complex. After initial stabilization, the decision focuses on an urgent/immediate invasive strategy vs. an ischemic guided strategy.

Immediate angiography with an attempt at revascularization is advised for very high risk NSTEMI populations based upon their recognized adverse outcomes. Clinical characteristics of this high-risk population include

- Hemodynamic instability +/- cardiogenic shock
- Severe left ventricular dysfunction or heart failure
- Recurrent or persistent rest angina despite medical therapy
- Mechanical complications (i.e., mitral regurgitation, ventricular septal defect)
- Sustained ventricular arrhythmias

An *invasive strategy* typically involves coronary angiography with intent for revascularization within the first 24 hours of presentation.[63] The early invasive strategy is not recommended for patients with extensive comorbidities where the risk of

revascularization exceeds the likely benefits. Risk stratification in NSTEMI seeks to identify patients at high risk for further cardiac events who would benefit from an early invasive strategy. Many risk models, including TIMI, GRACE, and PURSUIT, exist to guide the clinician. TIMI, as one example, consists of a seven-point scoring system assigning one point to each variable:[64]

1. Age $\geq$ 65 years
2. At least three risk factors for coronary heart disease (hypertension, diabetes, dyslipidemia, smoking, or positive family history of early MI)
3. Prior coronary stenosis of $\geq$ 50 percent
4. ST-segment deviation on admission electrocardiogram
5. At least two anginal episodes in prior 24 hours
6. Use of aspirin in previous seven days
7. Elevated serum cardiac biomarkers

Group patients into a risk level based upon their total score as follows:

- Low risk – score of 0-2
- Intermediate risk – score of 3-4
- High risk – score of 5-7

Patients with a high to intermediate risk TIMI score on presentation benefit from an earlier invasive strategy. For patients in the low-risk category, a *conservative approach* includes initial aggressive medical therapy. After a period of stabilization (chest pain free with low-level activity for 12-24 hours), the patient is further assessed using non-invasive stress and LV function assessment.

In contrast to the NSTEMI patient, an immediate invasive strategy is advised for all patients with STEMI, and time to intervention is an important outcome variable.

*68 yo with history of seizure disorder, anxiety, and obstructive sleep apnea developed chest pain and marked dyspnea at home over a 6-hour interval. He noted significant indigestion and "heartburn" overnight, which did not respond to antacid therapy. His wife called 911, and he became unresponsive during a period of aspirin administration. He was noted to be in ventricular fibrillation and was successfully cardioverted x 3 back to normal sinus rhythm. His pre-arrival ECG is shown in **Figure 8-5** (note acute findings illustrated by arrows). His presentation vital signs included a blood pressure of 154/115, HR 88 bpm and regular, RR 26 / min and shallow, oxygen saturation was 97% on room air. His lung exam showed bibasilar rales, and his cardiac exam revealed a normal sinus rhythm without a gallop or murmur. On arrival, the patient was immediately started on IV heparin and IV nitroglycerin.*

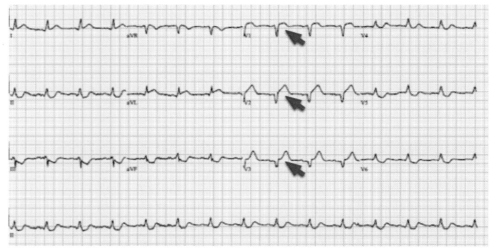

Figure 8-5 *Acute anterior wall STEMI (red arrows) noted in leads V_1, V_2, V_3.*

General principles for early intervention in STEMI include

- For patients initially evaluated at a non-PCI-capable hospital, immediate transfer to a PCI-capable hospital is preferred if a target first medical contact-to-device time of 120 minutes or less can be achieved. If the first medical contact-to-device time will exceed 120 min, then fibrinolytic therapy should be administered within 30 min of arrival in the absence of contraindications.
- All STEMI patients with cardiogenic shock or severe acute pulmonary edema, irrespective of the time delay from the first medical contact, should undergo PCI.
- PCI is advised for patients who have a contraindication to fibrinolytic therapy irrespective of the time delay from first medical contact.
- PCI is the recommended method of reperfusion in patients with STEMI and prolonged symptoms (> 12 hours).

A summary of the triage algorithm is outlined in **Figure 8-6**.

8.5.1 Treatment at a PCI-Capable Hospital

The interventional cardiologist will determine the type of intervention at the time of the PCI. Both bare metal stents (BMS) and drug-eluting stents (DES) are utilized. BMS are favored in patients who may be unable to tolerate 1 full year of DAPT due to a bleeding risk or need for an operative intervention.

PCI is supported with dual antiplatelet therapy (DAPT), as previously outlined, to minimize the risk

for thrombosis. Aspirin is administered as a 325 mg dose as early as possible before PCI. The patient is then maintained indefinitely on the 81 mg maintenance daily dose. The patient also receives a loading dose of a $P2Y_{12}$ inhibitor at the time of the PCI, and these medications are also continued for one year.

The patient was taken immediately to the cardiac catheterization laboratory on arrival. The left anterior descending artery had 100% occlusion with thrombus. Aspiration thrombectomy was performed to clear significant thrombus followed by successful PCI with placement of a drug-eluting stent. The patient was placed on daily ASA, received a loading dose of clopidogrel (300 mg) followed by daily maintenance therapy (75 mg per day), and was initiated on low dose metoprolol (25mg bid). He was also placed on atorvastatin (80 mg per day). His echo 24 hours after admission revealed apical akinesis and systolic dysfunction (EF ~35%). He was started on lisinopril prior to discharge. He demonstrated no evidence for volume overload.

Patients with STEMI undergoing PCI receive anticoagulation as previously outlined. Additional medical therapy recommended for treatment in STEMI was previously outlined for ACS in general and includes the big three in all patients without contraindications:

- Beta-blockers
- ACE Inhibitors
- High dose statin therapy

8.5.2 Pharmacologic Therapy for Non-PCI-Capable Hospital

In the absence of contraindications, fibrinolytic therapy should be given to patients with STEMI and

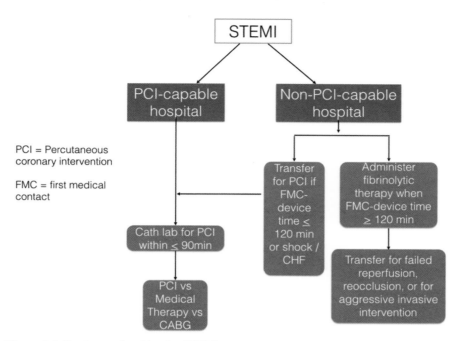

Figure 8-6 *Treatment algorithm for STEMI.*

Fibrinolytic Agent	Dose	Antigenic	Patency Rate
Tenecteplase	Single IV weight-based bolus not to exceed 50 mg < 60 kg: 30 mg 60 to < 70 kg: 35 mg 70 to < 80 kg: 40 mg 80 to < 90 kg: 45 mg ≥ 90 kg: 50 mg	No	85%
Reteplase	10U IV over 2 minutes followed by a second 10U IV bolus in 30 min if no significant bleeding or anaphylaxis	No	84%
Alteplase	90 min weight-based infusion If > 67kg: 100 mg over 1.5 hrs administered as a 15mg IV bolus over 1-2 min followed by 50mg over 30 min and then 35 mg over 1 hour If ≤ 67kg: administer a 15mg IV bolus over 1-2 min followed by 0.75 mg/kg (not to exceed 50 mg) over 30 min and then 0.5 mg/kg (not to exceed 35 mg) mg over 1 hour. Maximum total dose is < 100 mg		73-84%

Figure 8-7 *Fibrinolytic agents used for treatment of STEMI.*

onset of ischemic symptoms within the prior 12 hours when primary PCI cannot be accomplished within 120 minutes of first medical contact. The benefit of fibrinolytic therapy when symptom duration exceeds 12 hours is unproven but may be provided when a large area of myocardium is at risk or hemodynamic instability is present. Fibrin-specific agents are preferred and are summarized in **Figure 8-7**. Do not administer fibrinolytic therapy to patients with ST depression (NSTEMI) except when a true posterior MI is suspected. The absolute and relative contraindications to fibrinolytic therapy are outlined in **Figure 8-8**.

Hemorrhagic complications, particularly intracranial hemorrhage, are the most feared side effects of thrombolytic therapy and occur at a rate of approximately 0.5-1%. The decision to administer fibrinolytic therapy in STEMI must incorporate a careful risk-benefit analysis, considering time from symptom onset, hemodynamics at presentation, timely access to PCI, and risk of bleeding,

Absolute and Relative Contraindications to Thrombolytics for STEMI
Absolute Contraindications
• Active internal bleeding or bleeding diathesis (excluding menses)
• Recent spontaneous intracranial bleeding
• Recent intracranial or ocular surgery within 3 months
• Trauma or major surgery within 2 weeks
• Significant closed head or facial trauma within 3 months
• Any prior intracranial hemorrhage
• Known structural cerebral vascular lesion, or aortic dissection
• Known malignant intracranial neoplasm (primary or metastatic)
• Ischemic stroke within 3 mo
◦ EXCEPT acute ischemic stroke within 4.5 hours
• Suspected aortic dissection
• Intracranial or intraspinal surgery within 2 months
• Severe uncontrolled hypertension (unresponsive to emergency therapy)
• For streptokinase, prior treatment within the previous 6 months
Relative Contraindications
• Age > 75 years
• Chronic, severe, poorly controlled hypertension
• Significant hypertension on presentation with a SBP > 180 mm Hg or DBP > 110 mm Hg
• Non-compressive vascular puncture
• Recent traumatic or prolonged (> 10 min) chest compressions
• Major surgery, delivery of baby, organ biopsy, puncture of non-compressible vessel in last 10 days
• GI bleeding in last 10 days
• Ischemic stroke in last 3 months
• Serious trauma in last 15 days
• Platelet count <100,000
• Pregnancy
• Bacterial endocarditis
• Diabetic hemorrhagic retinopathy
• Active peptic ulcer
• Oral anticoagulant therapy

Figure 8-8 Contraindications to fibrinolytic therapy.

DAPT with aspirin and a PGY$_{12}$ inhibitor are indicated in patients who receive fibrinolytic therapy to limit the risk of rethrombosis. Patients should also receive anticoagulant therapy with unfractionated heparin (1.5-2.0 x control), enoxaparin, or fondaparinux for a minimum of 48 hours, and preferably for the duration of the index hospitalization up to a limit of 8 days or until revascularization is accomplished. Both enoxaparin and fondaparinux require adjustments for renal function and body weight. Bivalirudin may be substituted for UFH if HIT is a concern.

Following fibrinolytic therapy, transfer of a patient to a PCI-capable hospital for coronary angiography is reasonable for patients with STEMI who

- Demonstrate evidence of failed reperfusion or reocclusion after fibrinolytic therapy.
- Stabilize but warrant definitive angiography, based upon risk assessment, which can be performed > 2-3 hours following the administration of fibrinolytic therapy.

Chest pain resolution, resolution of ST elevations, or the presence of reperfusion arrhythmias suggests a successful post fibrinolytic therapy. The relatively sudden and complete relief of chest pain coupled with > 70% ST resolution (in the index lead showing the most significant elevation on presentation) is highly suggestive of restoration of normal myocardial blood flow.

8.5.3 Coronary Artery Bypass Grafting (CABG)

Urgent CABG is indicated for patients with STEMI and coronary anatomy not amenable to PCI in the setting of recurrent ischemia, cardiogenic shock, or severe HF. These patients often require bridging with mechanical assist devices in preparation for CABG. Ideally, the P2Y$_{12}$ inhibitors clopidogrel or ticagrelor are discontinued 24 hours prior to surgical intervention to reduce the risk of bleeding. In patients referred for elective CABG, clopidogrel and ticagrelor should be discontinued for at least 5 days prior to surgery (7 days for prasugrel). The short acting GP IIb/IIIa inhibitors (eptibatide or tiroban) should be discontinued for 2-4 hours before surgery. Abciximab is stopped for at least 12 hours prior to CABG to limit blood loss and transfusion.

8.6 Wrapping it up

Before discharge, several issues should be reviewed for consideration in the patient with STEMI:

- Reconsider Beta-blocker therapy in patients who demonstrated prior contraindications.
- Consider an implantable cardioverter-defibrillator in patients who develop sustained VT/VF more than 48 hours after STEMI, provided the arrhythmia is not due to transient or reversible ischemia, reinfarction, or metabolic abnormalities.
- Consider long-term anticoagulation with a vitamin K antagonist (*warfarin*) or novel oral anticoagulant (NOAC) for patients with atrial fibrillation with a CHADS2 score $\geq$ 2, mechanical heart valves, venous thromboembolism, or a hypercoagulable disorder. The duration of therapy with aspirin, P2Y$_{12}$ receptor inhibitor, and the oral anticoagulant should be minimized as soon as possible to limit the bleeding risk.

- Perform non-invasive testing for ischemia before discharge in patients without high-risk features who did not undergo coronary angiography.
- Refer patients to cardiac rehabilitation post-myocardial infarction.

To review the big-picture approach in five main steps:

1. **Cool down the heart** with medical therapy.
2. **Classify the ACS syndrome** (*STEMI*, unstable angina, NSTEMI).
3. **Crush the platelets** with dual antiplatelet therapy (DAPT).
4. **Bash the coagulation system** for unstable angina, NSTEMI, and STEMI.
5. **Blast open the coronary obstruction** if indicated for high-risk NSTEMI and all STEMI.

A summary approach to the patient with ACS is outlined in **Figure 8-9**. Key medication regimens are outlined in **Figure 8-10**.

Cool Down the Heart

- 12 Lead EKG within 10 minutes of arrival
- Use supplemental oxygen only to maintain oxygen SaO2 > 90%.
- Give 3 SL NTG (0.4mg) spaced 5 min apart until chest pain relieved, if no evidence for hemodynamic compromise and no recent use of phosphodiesterase inhibitors.
- Consider IV metoprolol for persistent tachycardia or hypertension with no evidence for heart failure, hemodynamic compromise, or severe reactive airways disease.
- Consider IV nitroglycerin for persistent chest pain, hypertension, or CHF if no evidence for RV infarction.
- Consider IV diuretics in addition to IV NTG for evidence of CHF. Consider additional use of non-invasive positive pressure ventilation in these patients to relieve dyspnea and reduce preload.
- Add atorvastatin (80mg) ASAP and administration of a B-blocker if no conduction block, CHF, or reactive airways disease

Classify the ACS

- Based upon ECG, troponin, +/- echocardiographic criteria classify syndrome as STEMI, non-STEMI, ACS.
- Associate STEMI with early acute intervention (lytic therapy vs PCI) to address coronary occlusion.
- Associate NTEMI with initial medical therapy to address platelet and coagulation systems.

Crush the Platelets

- Administer dual anti-platelet therapy with aspirin (325mg initial) (non enteric coated) ASAP if no allergy history.
- Give a P2Y$_{12}$ inhibitor or thienopyridine. Favor ticagrelor if no significant bleeding risk.
- For elderly patients (> 75yo), patients < 60 kg, or with hx of past stroke or TIA, favor clopidogrel.
- Consider a GP IIb/IIIa inhibitor (eptifibatide or tirofiban) in patients at very high risk (ie. recurrent ischemia or hemodynamic instability) with a low bleeding risk

Bash the Coagulation System

- Give **anticoagulation** to all patients. Favor unfractionated heparin or bivalrudin for patients that undergo an early invasive strategy. Favor enoxaparin for patients that undergo a conservative management strategy

Blast Open the Obstruction

- Target early reperfusion strategy with either PCI (preferred) within 120 minutes of first medical contact (FMC) or fibrinolysis if PCI target cannot be achieved with no CHF/shock and symptoms < 12 hours
- Target PCI for all patients with cardiogenic shock, CHF, or contraindication to fibrinolysis, regardless of time of presentation, or for patients with delayed presentation (> 120 minutes)

Figure 8-9 *Treatment algorithm for acute coronary syndrome.*

Medical Class	Medication	US Brand Name	Dosing
Anti-platelet Agents	Aspirin		Loading Dose 162-325mg Maintenance Dose 75-162 mg daily
	Clopidogrel	Plavix	300mg loading dose followed by 75 mg per day. Reduce loading dose to 75 mg if > 75 yo. For patients that undergo PCI, the loading dose may be increased to 600mg given as early as possible before or at the time of PCI.
	Ticagrelor	Brilinta	180mg loading dose followed by a maintenance dose of 90mg twice daily initiated 12 hours post loading dose
	Prasugrel	Effient	60mg loading dose administered after coronary anatomy is known, followed by a maintenance dose of 10mg once daily
Anticoagulation	Unfractionated Heparin (UFH)		60-70 unit/kg bolus (maximum 5000 units) followed by a 12 unit/kg infusion targeted to aPTT 1.5-2.0 x control
	Enoxaparin	Lovenox	1 mg/kg subq q 12 hours. Adjust dosing for renal impairment to 1mg/kg q24 hours (creatinine clearance < 30 ml/min)
	Fondaparinux	Arixtra	2.5 mg subq daily. Avoid medication in patients with reduced renal function (creatinine clearance < 30 ml/min)
	Bivalirudin	Angiomax	0.75 mg/kg IV bolus prior to procedure, followed by an infusion of 1.75 mg/kg per hour

Figure 8-10 Summary of drug interventions for acute coronary syndrome.

Suggested Reading

- Howard JP, Antoniou S, Jones DA, Wragg A. Recent advances in antithrombotic treatment for acute coronary syndromes. Expert Review of Clinical Pharmacology 2014;7(4):507–21.
- Anderson JL, Morrow DA. Acute myocardial infarction NEJM 2017;376(21):2053–64.

9

Acute Decompensated Heart Failure

Acute decompensated left heart failure refers to a condition characterized by an acutely elevated left ventricle filling pressure leading to respiratory distress. The respiratory distress can range from mild dyspnea to fulminant respiratory failure. The etiology of this condition is typically systolic or diastolic cardiac dysfunction in association with a cardiac illness (i.e., acute myocardial infarction or valvular heart disease). Alternatively, acute decompensated heart failure can be secondary to fluid overload in the setting of relatively normal left ventricular dysfunction due to renal failure, severe hypertension, or transfusion-associated circulatory overload (TACO).

45 yo with end-stage renal disease secondary to diabetes mellitus and hypertension was receiving hemodialysis scheduled on Monday-Wednesday-Friday. The patient missed her most recent dialysis treatment and presents to the emergency room with extreme dyspnea. Her presentation vital signs include a RR of 28, HR 120 in normal sinus rhythm, JVP ~ 12 cm H_2O, BP 215/110 mm Hg, and oxygen saturation on room air of 82%. Her exam reveals an S4 with no murmur, bibasilar rales, and 1-2+ peripheral edema. She is immediately placed on supplemental oxygen via a 100% non-rebreather mask, and her oxygen saturation improves to 95%.

"Flash" pulmonary edema refers to a condition in which elevated left ventricular diastolic pressure is associated with very rapid fluid accumulation in the lung, presenting as sudden "white-out" of the chest radiograph and acute hypoxemia. Flash pulmonary edema is often considered a subcategory of acute decompensated heart failure, because this more rapid deterioration has been associated with specific clinical conditions, including myocardial ischemia +/- infarction, hypertensive crisis, acute mitral regurgitation, and stress-induced (Takotsubo) cardiomyopathy. *Takotsubo cardiomyopathy*, or the *"broken heart syndrome,"* is an acute systolic heart failure thought to be caused by a surge in catecholamines released during emotional, neurological, or systemic stress (discussed more below).

Another popular term, primarily in the emergency medicine literature, is *SCAPE*. SCAPE stands for *Sympathetic Crashing Acute Pulmonary Edema*. SCAPE refers to a hyperacute condition with fulminant pulmonary edema in the setting of significant systemic hypertension (sympathetic overdrive). The primary pathophysiology in these patients is excessive left ventricular afterload rather than significant volume expansion. Your therapeutic attention will focus on vasodilator administration in SCAPE.

Most acute decompensated heart failure is secondary to a reduced cardiac ejection fraction, also called *systolic heart failure* or *heart failure with reduced ejection fraction* (HFrEF). Alternatively, acute decompensated heart failure can occur in the setting of a normal ejection fraction, often called *diastolic heart failure* or *heart failure with preserved ejection fraction* (HFpEF). Let's move forward with the term *acute decompensated heart failure* (ADHF) to group these various syndromes under a single heading.

9.1 Diagnosis of Decompensated Left Heart Failure

In patients with acute decompensated heart failure, exam findings might include elevated jugular venous pressure (JVP), bibasilar rales, and peripheral edema. Wheezing may occur in some patients (termed *cardiac asthma*) as part of their clinical presentation.

9.1.1 Imaging

Radiographic evidence for hydrostatic edema can support your clinical findings in acute decompensated heart failure. Chest radiographic findings that support your diagnosis might include cardiomegaly with vascular redistribution and bilateral perihilar edema in milder disease (**Figure 9-1**). More severe disease may present with extensive bilateral airspace infiltrates (**Figure 9-2**). Unilateral pulmonary edema is not typical in advanced decompensated heart failure in the absence of eccentric mitral regurgitation and should suggest another diagnosis. A common clinical challenge is to distinguish hydrostatic from pulmonary permeability edema or the adult respiratory syndrome (ARDS). Hydrostatic edema, which includes CHF and volume overload from other causes, more characteristically has vascular congestion with redistribution to the upper lung zones, peribronchial cuffing, thickening of the interlobular septa (Kerley B lines), and progression to "bat-wing" perihilar consolidation. A widened vascular pedicle is often reported as a sign of hydrostatic edema (**Figure 9-3**). The vascular pedicle extends from the right-sided superior vena cava to the left subclavian artery origin. A vascular pedicle width less than 60 mm on a PA chest radiograph is characteristic of a normal chest x-ray. As the vascular pedicle widens above 60 mm, this correlates with an expanding intravascular volume. A large azygous vein may be associated with the widened vascular pedicle. Cardiomegaly with a cardiothoracic ratio > 0.55 and bilateral pleural effusions are also more typical findings in hydrostatic pulmonary edema.

The primary limitation to the use of the vascular pedicle and cardiothoracic ratios in the ICU is the everyday use of portable film radiography. Patient position, inspiratory level, ventilator parameters, film distance, and patient size are all factors that influence

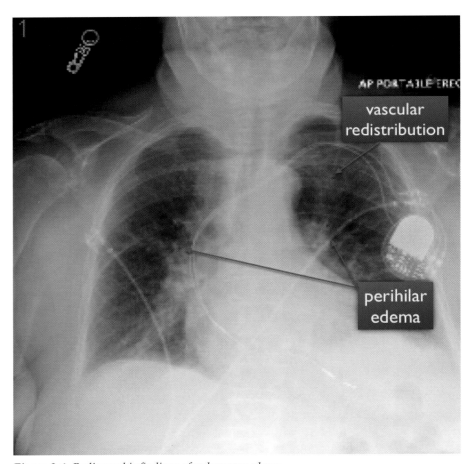

Figure 9-1 Radiographic findings of pulmonary edema.

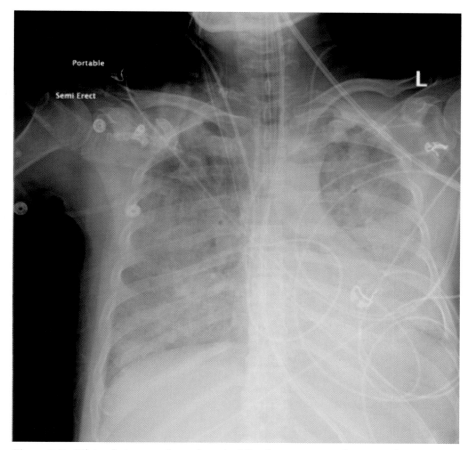

Figure 9-2. Bilateral airspace edema characteristic of more severe pulmonary edema.

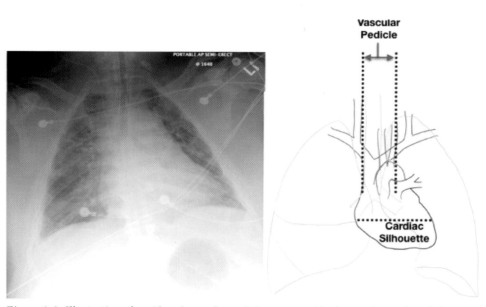

Figure 9-3 Illustration of a widened vascular pedicle on a portable chest radiograph and the associated vascular landmarks.

the width measurements. These variables must be considered when interpreting the portable images for these parameters.

An alternative to plain film radiography is a point of care ultrasound (POCUS). As a reminder from Chapter 3, the classic combination that suggests pulmonary edema would be lung sliding with B lines present **(Figure 9-4)**. B lines, also called *lung rockets* or *comet tails*, reflect thickening of the lung interstitium due to alveolar edema. More than three B lines per field are considered abnormal. Multiple anterior diffuse B lines with lung sliding indicated pulmonary edema (n= 64) with 97% sensitivity and 95% specificity in one series.[65]

Your bedside echo can also be used to assess cardiovascular function to help distinguish cardiogenic vs. non-cardiogenic pulmonary edema.

9.1.2 Brain Natriuretic Peptide

The measurement of natriuretic peptides may also support your diagnosis of ADHF. In humans, brain natriuretic peptide is produced in the heart cells (cardiomyocytes). When the heart undergoes pressure overload from heart failure or fluid overload, cardiomyocytes are stretched and release a pre-pro-hormone called pre-pro-brain natriuretic peptide.

Pre-pro-BNP is metabolized to pro-BNP and then cleaved to form the active 32 amino acid BNP hormone and a clipped N-terminal amino acid fragment, NT-proBNP (Figure 9-5). Commercial assays can measure both the NT-proBNP and the BNP, and their increase correlates with heart failure or fluid overload. Note, this process is compensatory since the BNP binds to atrial natriuretic peptide receptors and stimulates vasodilation (afterload reduction to help the heart) and acts on the kidney to cause diuresis (actually sodium excretion or natriuresis; thus the name). BNP also interacts with the renal-angiotensin-aldosterone system (RAAS). BNP reduces renin release and decreases circulating levels of angiotensin II and aldosterone. Decreased angiotensin II further contributes to systemic vasodilation and decreased systemic vascular resistance. These peptides counteract the tendency for salt retention and vasoconstriction that characterizes acute decompensated heart failure. Assays for NT-pro-BNP and BNP were developed as diagnostic tests for left heart failure, but also will increase in the case of right heart failure. BNP and NT-proBNP concentrations vary based upon the assay used, age, gender, and body mass index. BNP levels increase with renal failure, as they are cleared by the kidney, and they go up with anemia, two common ICU conditions. The normal values tend to increase in women and older patients but decrease in the setting of obesity. A high BNP level is, therefore, not specific for acute decompensated heart failure. A normal or low BNP does tell you that heart failure is likely not a problem for your patient (a sensitive test that can be used to rule *out* disease, but not specific so it cannot be used to rule *in* a disease).

Atrial natriuretic peptide (ANP) is another hormone released from the heart, primarily in the atria. The clinical experience is much greater with the use of BNP

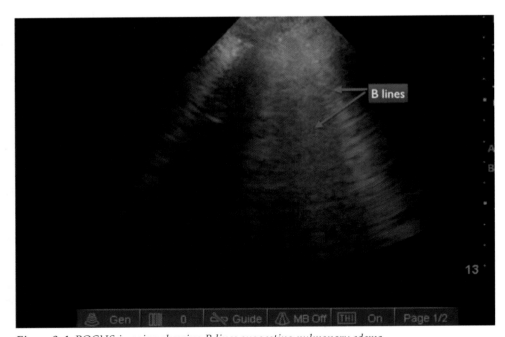

Figure 9-4 POCUS imaging showing B lines suggesting pulmonary edema.

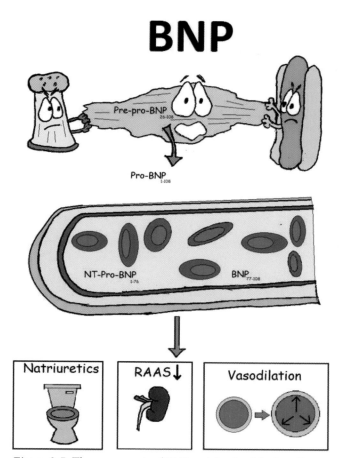

BNP

Pre-pro-BNP
Pro-BNP
NT-Pro-BNP
BNP

Natriuretics   RAAS↓   Vasodilation

Figure 9-5 *The components of BNP and its physiologic actions.*

and NT-proBNP as biomarkers compared to ANP in ADHF. In general, BNP and NT-proBNP values are reasonably correlated, and either can be used in clinical practice as long as their cutoff values are not used interchangeably. For this discussion, we will focus on the BNP measurement in ADHF.

In general, patients with decompensated heart failure from either the left or right ventricle, have an elevated BNP (> 400 pg/mL). Very low values (< 100 pg/mL) should raise concern that an alternative diagnosis may be the cause of the patient's respiratory distress. However, BNP levels are considered an adjunct to patient management, not a substitute for accurate clinical assessment. In some patients with acute decompensated HF, BNP levels may not be markedly elevated. In contrast, many pulmonary conditions, particularly those associated with right heart dysfunction, including pulmonary embolism and acute pneumonia, can be associated with elevated BNP with normal left ventricular function.

You will support your diagnostic and therapeutic efforts related to left heart failure with an assessment of myocardial ischemia with an ECG and serial troponin

assessment. However, troponin elevations are recognized in acute decompensated heart failure in the absence of significant epicardial coronary heart disease. This condition is often called *Type II* or *demand ischemia* and is attributed to an increased myocardial oxygen demand or decreased supply in the absence of an acute primary coronary occlusion. Many clinical conditions are associated with increased troponins in the absence of coronary artery thrombosis, including acute decompensated heart failure, as well as noncardiac conditions, including sepsis, atrial tachyarrhythmia, hypovolemia, and hypotension.

9.1.3 Echocardiography

Transthoracic echocardiography is a valuable tool to confirm the diagnosis of acute decompensated heart failure and to classify for etiology. Decompensated heart failure is classified as heart failure with reduced ejection fraction (HFrEF) when the ejection fraction is ≤ 40%, or heart failure with preserved ejection fraction (HFpEF) when the measured ejection fraction is greater than 40%.[66] This classification will be helpful in selecting intervention strategies. The syndrome of HF can also result from disorders of the heart valves, pericardium, or great vessels. The echocardiogram will also assist with the identification of these specific etiologies for HF.

Reserve advanced hemodynamic monitoring with a pulmonary artery catheter for patients with uncertain hemodynamics or those who fail to respond to initial therapy (*See Chapter 7, Hemodynamic Monitoring*). The PA catheter is not indicated routinely in patients with ADHF who are normotensive and respond to initial treatment with diuretics and vasodilators.

Identify the ADHF patient with an acute coronary syndrome through a combination of ECG, troponin, and echocardiographic parameters. Urgent coronary angiography is indicated when active ischemia is contributing to acute decompensated heart failure.

9.2 Treatment of Acute Decompensated Left Heart Failure

You have confirmed your diagnosis of left heart failure by using a combination of diagnostic tools. Now what to do? You have to get fluid out of the lungs and oxygenate the blood, and you have to reduce the work of the heart (increase cardiac oxygen delivery and reduce oxygen consumption) and improve cardiac performance (contractility, inotrope, etc.). Sounds like a lot to remember. But let's simplify this to four main assignments:

1. Reduce preload (left ventricular filling pressure).
2. Reduce afterload (systemic vascular resistance).

3. Increase cardiac function (minimize ischemia and improve contractility).
4. Find the cause.

Think of the broken heart as a dam **(Figure 9-6)**. Behind the dam the fluid is accumulating in the lungs. You have three primary interventions to fix this problem: fix preload, afterload, and cardiac inotropy (contractility). You can suck the fluid out from behind the dam using diuretics and venodilators, such as nitroglycerin. You can increase flow through the dam (putting pipes in the dam to increase passive flow), using afterload-reducing vasodilators such as nitroprusside, high dose nitroglycerin (NTG), and the peripheral β-2 vasodilating effects of dobutamine. You can improve the broken heart contractility (lower the height of the dam), using inotropic agents such as dobutamine and milrinone. Fixing the problem causing the broken heart in the case of ischemia is also vital. As described below, the use of continuous positive airway pressure (CPAP) will both decrease the preload and the afterload, and an intra-aortic balloon pump (IABP) can reduce afterload at the same time it increases blood flow (cardiac output) to the heart and body. Dobutamine also has dual effects of increasing inotropy and lowering afterload.

9.2.1 Reduce Left Ventricular Filling Pressure (Preload)

Patients with acute decompensated heart failure most typically have either systolic or diastolic heart dysfunction. Long-term treatment strategies for these conditions depend on the etiology, but the acute goals of treatment are relatively similar. Respiratory distress is immediately addressed with the administration of supplemental oxygen to maintain the oxygen saturation (SaO_2 > 90%). For patients with a normal oxygen saturation, supplemental oxygen is not required. For patients with significant respiratory distress, assisted ventilation may be needed.

A strategy to acutely lower left ventricular end diastolic pressure involves the application of positive airway pressure delivered via either invasive or non-invasive ventilation. Positive airway pressure accomplishes important hemodynamic changes through heart-lung interactions.[67] Positive airway pressure

1. *Reduces right ventricular preload* by increasing intrathoracic pressure and reducing venous blood flow to the right atrium.
2. *Increases right ventricular afterload* by potentially increasing lung volume, leading to compression of alveolar vasculature, and raising pulmonary vascular resistance.
3. *Decreases left ventricular preload* through reduced pulmonary venous return resulting from decreased RV preload and increased RV afterload with a possible additional contribution from a shift of the septum to compromise LV filling.
4. *Reduces left ventricular afterload* by creating a favorable gradient between increased intrathoracic pressure and lower atmospheric pressure in the

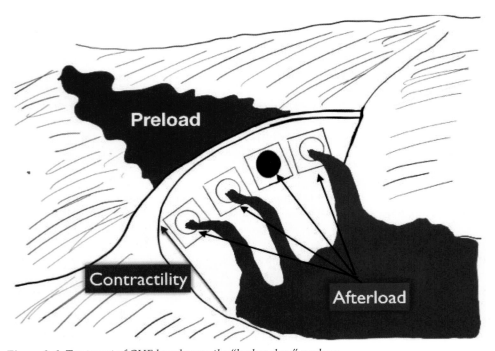

Figure 9-6 *Treatment of CHF based upon the "broken dam" analogy.*

extrathoracic cavities. This leaves most of the systemic vasculature at a lower pressure than the left ventricle and intrathoracic aorta.

The hemodynamic effect of positive airway pressure, therefore, becomes a summary of these multiple interacting variables and is not easy to predict. The effect can be very different in patients, based on their underlying cardiac condition. In patients with volume contraction or reduced preload, the application of positive airway pressure often leads to a reduction in cardiac output as the negative effect of positive airway pressure on preload dominates. In contrast, the use of positive airway pressure in the setting of elevated left ventricular filling pressures produces favorable hemodynamic effects, including a reduced venous return, reduced left ventricular preload, reduced left ventricular afterload, and sustained cardiac output.

Positive airway pressure can be provided in many forms, but continuous positive airway pressure (CPAP) has been most studied in the setting of acute congestive heart failure. CPAP is associated with relief of dyspnea in CHF patients and in some trials, but not all, a reduction in the need for mechanical ventilation, ICU days, and hospital days. CPAP is initiated via a non-invasive face mask in the range of 6-8 cm H_2O and is rapidly titrated to 10-12 cm H_2O in the acutely ill patient. This non-invasive ventilation allows an early, immediately effective treatment strategy during the period when additional therapeutic interventions are being implemented. Bilevel pressure (i.e., inspiratory pressure > expiratory pressure), sometimes called BIPAP, has been less effective than CPAP in comparative trials of ADHF. The specific reason for this variability between CPAP and Bilevel pressure has not been established and may merely represent variations in the machine settings and titration.

Our patient is placed on continuous positive airway pressure (CPAP) at 10 cm H_2O and supplemental oxygen at 40% FiO_2. The patient historically is anuric and therefore diuretics are not expected to be helpful. The patient is placed on intravenous nitroglycerin, starting at 50 mcs/min which is titrated to achieve a diastolic blood pressure ~ 90 mm Hg and can be easily titrated off as dialysis removes fluid. Beta-blockers are not administered despite the tachycardia and hypertension, due to the presence of ADHF. Arrangements are made for urgent dialysis.

We can also use venodilators to reduce left ventricular filling pressure. The most common agent is nitroglycerin (NTG). In the setting of ADHF, intravenous NTG, rather than oral or transdermal therapy, is used for the speed of onset and rapid titration. In the absence of hypotension, intravenous nitroglycerin can lead to early improvement in symptoms in combination with diuretics. The medication is often initiated at 5-10 mcg/min and titrated in 5 mcg/min increments based upon clinical response and repeated hemodynamic assessment (dose range of 5–400 mcg/min). In your acutely ill patient with pulmonary edema and hypertension, titration can be more rapid, often starting at an initial dose of ~ 100 mcg/min with rapid titration. Note that higher doses are used with aggressive upward titration to achieve both venodilation (preload) and arteriolar vasodilation in the patient presenting with systemic hypertension. Also, nitroglycerin can improve coronary blood flow, making it the ideal vasodilator medication for patients with acute coronary syndromes. The potential adverse effects of nitroglycerin include headache and hypotension. The drug is contraindicated in patients who have recently taken PDE-5 inhibitors.

A focus in both systolic and diastolic acute decompensated heart failure is to lower left ventricular filling pressure through the administration of loop diuretics. Withhold urgent diuretic administration only in the setting of significant hemodynamic instability and hypotension. In addition, patients with pulmonary edema in the setting of hypertensive emergency are not volume expanded, and the initial focus should be on afterload reduction. But for all other clinical conditions, the loop diuretics furosemide (Lasix), bumetanide (Bumex), or torsemide (Demadex) are the preferred agents to lower left ventricular preload due to their rapid onset. Administer these agents as an intravenous bolus (not oral) in the acute setting or as a continuous infusion in patients who are resistant to the initial therapy. The rate of diuretic filtration to the ascending loop of Henle determines the efficacy of loop diuretics. The natriuresis response is linear only after a rate of filtration threshold is achieved. The initial approach to therapy is to determine the effective diuretic IV bolus dose. Dosing begins at 20-40 mg of furosemide bid or the equivalent dose of bumetanide (1 mg), depending on the patient's history of prior diuretic exposure. A dosing table based on the patient's home diuretic dosing is outlined in **Figure 9-7.**

A dose of 40 mg of furosemide is considered equivalent to 1 mg of bumetanide or 20 mg of torsemide. A dose of 50 mg hydrochlorothiazide bid or chlorthalidone 50 mg po qday can be substituted for metolazone.

An alternative approach is to use 2.5 x the home dose of furosemide for selection of the urgent IV dose for administration in ADHF. Current evidence does not suggest greater efficacy from continuous infusion in comparison to intermittent dosing, but comparative studies are limited.[69]

A response to drug administration is expected within 30 minutes and a maximum effect within 1-2 hours. If a diuretic response is not evident, the dose is usually doubled to achieve the threshold excretion required, as reflected clinically by diuresis. The maximum single dose

Previous Oral Furosemide Dose	Suggested Furosemide IV Bolus in ADHF	Suggested Furosemide IV Infusion Rate	Adjunctive Metolazone Dose (Oral)
≤ 80 mg	40 mg	5 mg/hr	NA
81-160 mg	80 mg	10 mg/hr	5 mg
161-240 mg	80 mg	20 mg/hr	5 mg bid
≥ 240 mg	80 mg	30 mg/hr	5 mg bid

Figure 9-7* *Acute diuretic dosing based upon the patient's previous oral furosemide dose.*

*Adapted from Felker MG, Lee KL, Bull DA, et al. Diuretic strategies in patients with acute decompensated heart failure. NEJM 2018;364(9):797–805.

of furosemide is 40-80 mg for patients with normal renal function but may range up to 200 mg for patients with renal insufficiency. Patients in acute decompensated heart failure are recognized to have a higher threshold for diuretic response, due to decreased drug delivery to the tubule and compensatory mechanisms, which favor sodium reabsorption (called *cardio-renal syndrome*).

In addition to the effect on lowering intravascular filling pressures through natriuresis, the loop diuretics can also induce transient venodilation, which leads to a reduction in filling pressures prior to the onset of natriuresis.

Monitor your patient closely during a period of aggressive diuresis. Serum potassium and magnesium levels should be monitored at least daily and maintained in the normal range. Worsening renal function may complicate diuretic therapy. Hyponatremia may occur in response to natriuresis and require fluid restriction (≤ 2 liters/day). Excessive diuresis or too-rapid diuresis can also lower preload such that systemic blood pressure is compromised. This can occur more commonly in patients with diastolic heart failure or HFpEF in the setting of left ventricular hypertrophy or restrictive physiology. Unpredictably, in some patients with compromised renal function, continued diuresis may improve renal function despite reduced filling pressures.

Morphine sulfate administration has been used in the treatment of acute decompensated heart failure for many years. Morphine is believed to have a mild preload-reducing effect and relieves anxiety, possibly blunting catecholamine production. Very limited prospective data exist to support the use of morphine in acute decompensated heart failure, and recent retrospective reviews have suggested increased mortality in patients receiving this medication.

9.2.2 Reduce Systemic Vascular Resistance (Afterload)

In patients with decompensated CHF, afterload can be reduced using vasodilator therapy. Nitroglycerin, as discussed, at higher doses provides an effective arterial

vasodilator that also acts to reduce preload. In patients with significant hypertension, nicardipine or nitroprusside offers an alternative choice of vasodilator therapy. Clinical conditions where these medications are urgently indicated include hypertensive emergency, aortic dissection (in combination with a Beta-blocker), or acute valvular (mitral or aortic) regurgitation. The initial dose of nicardipine is 5 mg/hour and can be increased to a maximum dose of 15 mg/hour. Intravenous nicardipine has a more favorable safety profile than nitroprusside, but a longer onset of action and longer elimination half-life, meaning the drug effect on blood pressure is slightly less titratable.

Nitroprusside is initiated at a dose of 0.25 to 0.5 mcg/kg/min and titrated based upon the hemodynamic response to a maximum dose range of 8-10 mcg/kg/min. The main concern with the use of nitroprusside is toxicity from the metabolites, leading to cyanide or thiocyanate toxicity. This occurs primarily in patients on long-term dosing, at high doses, or in the setting of renal failure. Nitroprusside is avoided in patients with symptoms to suggest acute coronary insufficiency, as the arteriolar vasodilation can reduce coronary perfusion pressure.

In summary, we can accomplish our goals of reducing preload and afterload rapidly via one (or a combination) of three mechanisms:

1. *Mechanical* – continuous positive airway pressure
2. *Diuresis* – intravenous loop diuretics
3. *Vasodilator* – intravenous nitroglycerin, nicardipine, and nitroprusside

Rapid application of non-invasive ventilation and intravenous nitroglycerin therapy can often avoid imminent intubation in the patient presenting with acute pulmonary edema, particularly in the setting of hypertension.

9.2.3 Fix the Broken Heart (Dam)— Increase Cardiac Output

You are working in the hospital and your patient is admitted from the ER with severe shortness of breath, blood pressure of 100/79, heart rate of 130 bpm, oxygen saturation of 92% on face mask, with lower extremity edema, elevated neck veins, hepatojugular reflux and bibasilar rales on examination. The chest X-ray suggests early pulmonary edema. Your echo shows a severely dilated and hypokinetic left ventricle. You increase the inspired oxygen to a 100% non-rebreather mask, but the patient remains markedly tachypneic. You give the patient an initial dose of furosemide, but the blood pressure falls slightly to 85/60.

So what now? You try to oxygenate the patient with 100% CPAP and rapid delivery of diuretics. But the low blood pressure on presentation makes you appropriately concerned about the use of vasodilators. Because of the respiratory distress, you may have to intubate the patient. You need to be careful with your anesthesia for intubation to avoid deleterious hemodynamics during intubation. All induction agents may be associated with a blood pressure decline in the setting of hypotension. You might choose etomidate for sedation during the intubation process, as it has limited cardiodepressive effects and a short half-life of 3-5 minutes. Alternatively, ketamine causes sympathetic stimulation and is the most hemodynamically stable of all the available sedative-induction agents. Some concern has been raised about using ketamine in the setting of coronary disease, but hypotension may be the more significant risk compared to a theoretical risk of coronary vasoconstriction. *(See Chapter 12 Basic Airway Management).* The dissociative dose of ketamine used for intubation is 1-2 mg/kg.

Despite your best intentions, the hypotensive patient will often deteriorate during intubation. You should attempt to support the blood pressure before intubation to improve cardiac function. However, in this hypotensive patient, inotropes can be a challenge to use because they increase cardiac contractility but also act as peripheral vasodilators. Blood pressure remains preserved if the increase in cardiac output offsets the reduction in systemic vascular resistance. However, if the blood pressure starts low, you might be appropriately nervous about starting a medication (i.e., inotrope) that could lower the blood pressure. In these situations, a mixed alpha/Beta-1 active medication is chosen, and norepinephrine is a favored agent. In all cases, you must carefully monitor for the induction of arrhythmias or cardiac ischemia. As your blood pressure improves, you

can convert to the purer inotrope medications. **Figure 9-8** lists the intravenous medications commonly used in the management of acute decompensated heart failure.

Intravenous inotropes (milrinone or dobutamine) are appropriate for patients with advanced decompensated heart failure characterized by decreased ejection fraction, left ventricular dilation, and evidence for end-organ dysfunction (low output syndrome). Inotropes are acceptable for patients with marginal systolic blood pressure and adequate filling pressure, or those patients unresponsive to intravenous vasodilators. There is little evidence to support the use of inotropic agents in patients with acute decompensated heart failure not in a low output condition. Inotropes may be contraindicated in the setting of heart failure due to ischemic conditions.[70]

Inotropic agents to increase cardiac output include intravenous dobutamine at 3 mcs/kg/min, increasing to 5-7 mcs/kg/min if no dysrthythmias develop. The inotropic response to dobutamine is highly variable and requires careful drug titration. Alternatively, you can use milrinone as an inotrope. Milrinone generally has a lesser effect on heart rate than dobutamine and induces significant pulmonary arterial vasodilation. The effects of milrinone are not mediated by stimulation of Beta-receptors, which may offer a pharmacologic advantage in patients with advanced heart failure who have been receiving Beta-blocker therapy.

Inotropes must be used cautiously in the setting of myocardial ischemia as they can increase myocardial oxygen demand. If progressive hypotension and tachyarrythmias develop during the administration of inotropic agents, these medications should be discontinued.

You place the patient on CPAP, which appears to improve the respiratory distress, but the blood pressure remains tenuous. You start a low dose norepinephrine infusion, and the blood pressure improves. You call your CCU attending and together place a PA catheter. The mixed venous saturation is 40%, the cardiac output is 1.9 liters/minute, and mean pulmonary artery pressure is 50/30, while the central venous pressure is 25 cm H_2O. The pulmonary artery occlusion pressure is 29 cm H_2O, so you know this is left heart disease and not pulmonary arterial

Drug	Mechanism	Indication
Norepinephrine (0.01-3 mcg/kg/minute)	Mixed α/ Beta-1 stimulation	First-line drug for septic shock
Dobutamine (2-20 mcg/kg/minute)	Mixed α/ Beta stimulation	Inotrope for improved contractility and afterload reduction
Milrinone (0.375 to 0.75 mcg/kg/minute)	Inhibits adenylate cyclase	Inotrope for improved contractility and afterload reduction

Figure 9-8 Intravenous medications commonly used in the management of acute decompensated heart failure.

hypertension. The ECG shows no acute changes, and the troponin is minimally elevated. You place the patient on dobutamine and wean off the norepinephrine as the blood pressure improves.

What if the patient did not respond to your interventions or has increasing cardiac ischemia at the same time as cardiac failure? A significant challenge is the patient with cardiogenic shock and an acute coronary syndrome. This is the patient at highest risk of death. This patient should go immediately to the cardiac cath laboratory for a therapeutic intervention to try to restore blood flow to the heart if an acute coronary syndrome is suspected. Consideration can be given to the use of a mechanical device to assist cardiac function. An intra-aortic balloon pump can be inserted in the cardiac catheterization lab. This device is a particularly valuable tool in the patient with acute decompensated heart failure and ischemic heart disease.

The *intra-aortic balloon pump (IABP)* is a device that is placed via the femoral artery and positioned in the descending aorta **(Figure 9-9)**. It is a long tube (looks a lot like the kids' balloons that are used to twist and stretch into animal shapes at the zoo), and the tip of it should rest just below the aortic arch. If it goes into the arch, it could block the great arteries (carotid, subclavian, etc.) when it inflates. The balloon inflates at exactly the beginning of ventricular diastole at the time when the aortic valve closes (at the dicrotic notch or abscissa). The balloon

inflation is called *counter-pulsation* and *diastolic pressure augmentation*. The timing is automated by detection of either the ECG (starting at about the middle of the T wave and ending before the next QRS) or by detecting the aortic pressure drop. The balloon inflation is thus occurring after the aortic valve closes during ventricular diastole. The expanding balloon both pushes blood around it into the coronary arteries (which sit at the base of the aorta) to perfuse the heart, and to the systemic circulation (brain, kidneys, liver, etc.). When the balloon deflates, before ventricular systole, it leaves behind a relatively empty aorta so it dramatically reduces afterload as well. Intra-aortic balloon counterpulsation increases both coronary blood flow and cardiac output without dropping blood pressure. This is something our medical vasodilator drugs cannot do! **Figure 9-10** illustrates the correct radiographic position of the IABP.

IABP increases both oxygen supply (coronary flow) and decreases cardiac oxygen demand (reducing afterload).

This timing of balloon inflation is critical: If it inflates too early, it causes a high systolic afterload; and if it dilates too late, it has limited effects on augmenting diastolic perfusion. The timing for balloon inflation can be set to pump with every heart contraction or at lower ratios of 1:2 or 1:3. Changing the ratio can be used to wean the patient off the IABP pump or test for stability before turning it completely off. The proper diastolic

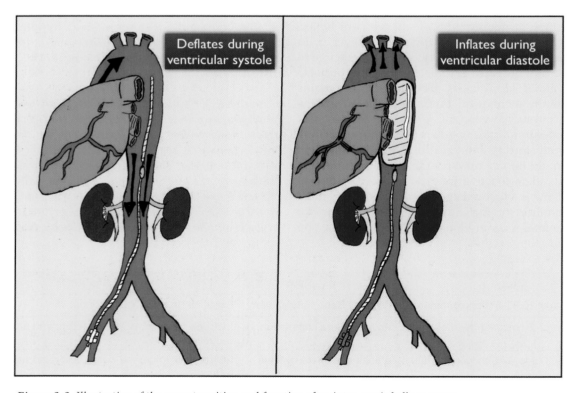

Figure 9-9 *Illustration of the correct position and function of an intra-aortic balloon pump.*

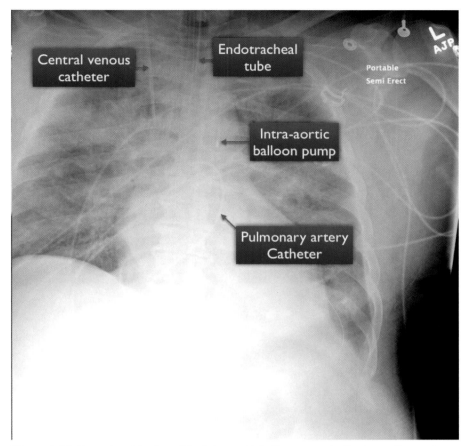

Figure 9-10 *Correct positioning of the intra-aortic balloon pump in the descending aorta just below the aortic arch confirmed by portable chest radiograph.*

augmentation of the IABP is evident on the arterial line tracing. **Figure 9-11** illustrates (A) The normal aortic pressure profile and (B) The correct timing of diastolic augmentation at the dicrotic notch, lasting through most of the ventricular diastole.

What if your hypotensive patient with cardiac disease has a normal ejection fraction? In these patients, the use of inotropes is contraindicated. These patients may require a vasopressor to support the blood pressure. Patients with left ventricular outflow obstruction may require the administration of a Beta-blocker to sustain left ventricular filling. Also, gentle fluid administration may be needed to optimize cardiac output.

A suggested algorithm for approaching the critically ill patient with left heart failure is shown in **Figure 9-12.**

9.2.4 Find the Cause

A key component in the treatment of ADHF is to identify the specific cardiac pathology, such as cardiac arrhythmias, coronary artery disease, or valvular dysfunction. Alternatively, factors exogenous to the heart such as hypertensive urgency, fluid overload in the setting of renal dysfunction, or acute pulmonary edema secondary to blood product administration (transfusion-associated circulatory overload = TACO) may precipitate ADHF. The introduction of new medications which act as negative inotropes including verapamil, Beta-blockers, or nonsteroidal anti-inflammatory agents must be recognized along with other cardiotoxic agents, including alcohol, cocaine, and some chemotherapeutic agents. Immediately after the initial steps to stabilize gas exchange and reduce left ventricular pressure, a thorough diagnostic evaluation should be undertaken to address reversible components of ADHF.

9.2.5 Arrythmia Management

Atrial fibrillation is one of the most common arrhythmias to occur in the setting of ADHF. Atrial fibrillation can both cause ADHF and be induced by ADHF. The sequence may not be clear, but the approach will be consistent as the focus will be on rate control. Attempts at cardioversion to normal sinus rhythm should be reserved for the hypotensive patient with

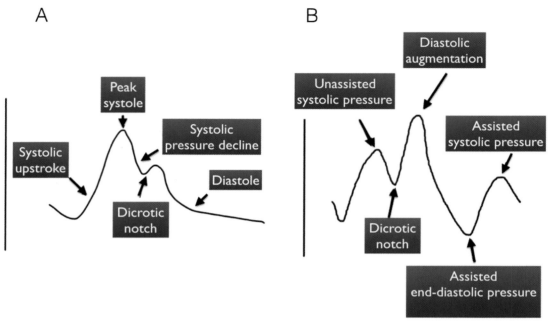

Figure 9-11 A. *Normal arterial pressure curve. B. Arterial pressure curve in the setting of an intra-aortic balloon pump with diastolic augmentation.*

PROVIDE SUPPORTIVE CARE

- Use supplemental oxygen only to maintain oxygen SaO2 > 90%.
- Initiate continuous EKG monitoring.
- Treat precipitating factors such as atrial arrhythmia, hypertension, ischemic heart disease, anemia, progressive renal disease.
- Bedside echo to assess for cardiac function and valvular dysfunction.

NORMOTENSIVE TO HYPERTENSIVE PATIENT

- Use non-invasive ventilation (CPAP) in patients with significant respiratory distress.
- Administer IV nitroglycerin for rapid relief in patients with pulmonary edema and severe hypertension.
- Administer IV loop diuretics including furosemide 20-40 mg IV or bumetanide 1mg IV.
- Monitor weight, fluid balance, electrolytes including magnesium, and renal function.
- Sodium restriction (< 2g/d) in all patients + fluid restriction (< 2L/day) if hyponatremia.

BORDERLINE TO LOW BLOOD PRESSURE PATIENT

- Consider intravenous inotropes with or without an IV vasopressor (norepinephrine) in patients with reduced ejection fraction (EF) and low output syndrome.
- Consider mechanical support (IABP, extracorporeal ventricular assist device) for patients with reduced EF unresponsive to inotropes especially in the setting of ischemic heart disease.
- Consider an IV vasopressor, +/- fluid administration, +/- B blocker treatment for low output syndrome with normal or preserved EF.

SPECIAL SITUATIONS

- Consider invasive hemodynamic monitoring in patients that fail initial therapy or when the volume status and cardiac filling pressures are unclear.
- Use early aggressive vasodilator therapy for patients with severe hypertension, and valvular regurgitation.

Figure 9-12 Clinical approach to the patient with advanced left heart failure.

cardiogenic shock, as the arrhythmia tends to recur until ADHF is resolved. Rate control for acute atrial fibrillation traditionally focuses on the use of Beta-blockers or non-dihydropyridine calcium channel blockers (*diltiazem*). These drugs can be problematic in ADHF patients due to their negative inotropic effect, unless the arrhythmia is clearly contributing to the decline in cardiac function. If the arrhythmia is adding to ADHF, then effective rate control may offset the negative inotropic effect of these medications. If the arrhythmia is secondary to ADHF, shorter-acting medications such as IV esmolol or medications without negative inotropic effects, such as digoxin or amiodarone, are preferred for effective rate control in the setting of ADHF.

In contrast, ventricular arrhythmias such as ventricular tachycardia in the setting of ADHF are usually life threatening and require prompt electrical cardioversion.

9.2.6 Hypertension Management

The majority of patients presenting with acute heart failure are hypertensive on initial assessment. Like atrial fibrillation, hypertension may be the inciting event with secondary myocardial dysfunction, or alternatively, hypertension in these patients may be a secondary component due to a sympathoadrenal response to hypoxemia, increased work of breathing, and anxiety. Regardless of the mechanism, efforts to control elevated systemic arterial pressure in this setting are essential, as high systemic arterial blood pressure in the patient with acute pulmonary edema contributes to an increased myocardial workload and diastolic dysfunction.

For the hypertensive patient with acute heart failure, *intravenous vasodilators* including nitroglycerin and nicardipine permit rapid titration of blood pressure and are preferred. Patients with acute pulmonary edema may be initially hypertensive secondary to high initial catecholamine levels. With effective treatment or control of hypoxemia and anxiety, blood pressure may fall rapidly, especially in the setting of concomitant diuresis. Avoid longer-acting medications such as ACE inhibitors or ARB therapy early in the treatment period. Patients with hypertensive emergencies may have suffered a natriuresis with elevated renin levels by the kidney and, hence, increased circulating levels of the potent endogenous vasoconstrictor, angiotensin II. Further reduction in intravascular volume and renal perfusion can lead to an increase in circulating angiotensin II levels. Therefore, aggressive diuresis before blood pressure control may not be advised for this population. Medications that increase cardiac work due to a reflex tachycardia (e.g., hydralazine) or impair cardiac contractility (e.g., labetalol) are contraindicated as

primary therapy for hypertension in the setting of ADHF.

In addition to the more traditional intravenous vasodilators, the intravenous calcium channel antagonists have demonstrated efficacy in the treatment of acute hypertension in the setting of left ventricular dysfunction. The dihydropyridine calcium antagonists nicardipine and clevidipine have been associated with reduced systemic arterial pressure with preservation of coronary blood flow.

You have a lot of tools in your toolbox to treat the patient with acute decompensated left heart failure **(Figure 9-13)**. Keep the four principles in your head to organize your treatment approach.

1. *Reduce preload* (left ventricular filling pressure).
2. *Reduce afterload* (systemic vascular resistance).
3. *Increase cardiac function* (minimize ischemia and improve contractility.
4. Find the cause.

9.3 Diagnosis of Pulmonary Hypertension and Right Heart Failure

Pulmonary hypertension (PH) is an elevation of vascular pressure in the pulmonary artery, rather than an elevation in the pressure in the aorta and systemic arteries. Pulmonary hypertension is classified as pulmonary arterial hypertension (PAH) or pulmonary venous hypertension (PVH). Direct occlusion of the pre-capillary arterioles results in a pressure elevation within the pulmonary arterial system causing PAH. In these patients, the blockage in flow through the pulmonary vasculature occurs in the small arteries and arterioles. Elevated pulmonary pressure results from a decrease in the arterial lumen through a combination of

- Endothelial dysfunction and increased contractility of small pulmonary arteries, termed *vaso-constriction*
- Proliferation and remodeling of endothelial and smooth muscle cells
- In situ thrombosis (secondary clotting in narrowed and blocked low-flow vessels). This increasing vascular resistance causes the mean pulmonary artery pressures to rise, but the left ventricular filling pressures are normal.

In patients with PVH, the problem arises in the left ventricle, caused by left heart failure. These patients have high mean pulmonary artery pressures but also a high left ventricular filling pressure. The diagnosis of PAH versus PVH often requires a right heart or pulmonary artery catheter to measure the individual vascular pressures.

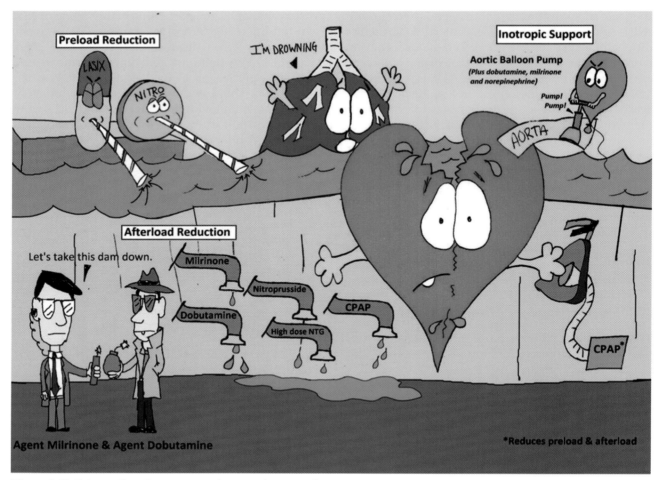

Figure 9-13 Interventions for treatment of acute pulmonary edema.

Figure 9-14 illustrates that the normal mean pulmonary pressure is less than 25 mm Hg, and the normal pulmonary artery occlusion (wedge) pressure is less than 15 mm Hg. In pulmonary arterial hypertension (PAH), the mean pulmonary artery pressure is greater than or equal to 25 mm Hg, and the wedge pressure is less than 15 mm Hg. In pulmonary venous hypertension (PVH) caused by left heart disease, the mean pulmonary artery pressure is greater than or equal to 25 mm Hg, and the wedge pressure is greater than 15 mm Hg.

In the ICU or in the hospital, you will often see patients with PAH and right heart failure that arise secondary to other common diseases. Clinical examples include pulmonary thromboembolism (see *Chapter 11 Pulmonary Thromboembolic Disease*), acute respiratory distress syndrome (ARDS), and severe chronic advanced lung diseases like COPD or interstitial lung disease (ILD, such as idiopathic pulmonary fibrosis). Patients who develop PAH and right heart failure are always at a significantly higher risk of death and are

more challenging to oxygenate and to wean from the ventilator.

Screening studies of Doppler-echocardiography have suggested that up to 29% of patients in the ICU have an elevated pulmonary pressure, estimated by echocardiography. Importantly, the presence of PAH represents an independent risk factor for death in ICU patients.[71] In a population of ARDS patients, the risk of death rose proportionally to the elevation in the transpulmonary pressure gradient (TPG = mean PAP − PAOP).[72]

The diagnosis of PH requires recognition and special diagnostic testing. Include PH and pulmonary embolism in your differential for the hypotensive, hypoperfused, or hypoxemic ICU patient. Let's run through the basics of diagnosis, pathogenesis, and treatment of both PAH, right ventricular failure, and acute thromboembolism in the ICU patient. Let's start with a blood test, move to Doppler-echocardiography, CT scanning, and then the invasive right heart catheterization.

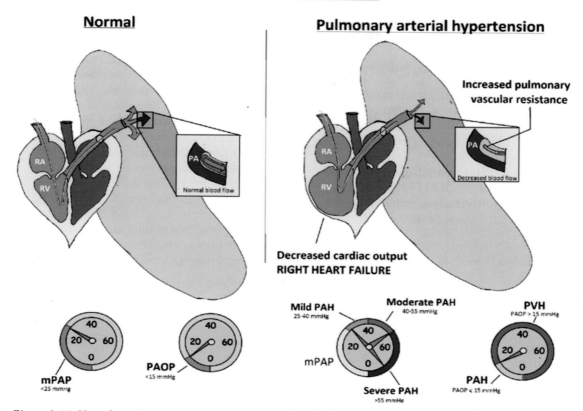

Figure 9-14 *Hemodynamic pressure measurements associated with normal and elevated pulmonary artery pressures of pulmonary hypertension.*

9.3.1 Pulmonary Hypertension Classification

Diseases that lead to pulmonary hypertension are shown in **Figure 9-15**. The Group I classification is important as these are the types of PAH for which available drugs have been approved. Group I includes 1) idiopathic disease where the cause is unknown; 2) familial disease related to hereditable germ-line mutations in the bone morphogenic receptor 2 (BMPR2), endoglin 1, and the activin-receptor-like kinase-1 (alk-1); 3) disease induced by drugs and toxins, especially the diet drugs; 4) PAH associated with connective tissue diseases, human immunodeficiency virus, portal hypertension, congenital heart diseases, schistosomiasis and chronic hemolytic anemia (sickle cell disease); 5) persistent pulmonary hypertension of the newborn; and 6) the very rare veno-occlusive disease.

There are other pathologies in which pulmonary hypertension presents as a secondary disease. Some examples include left heart disease, which is referred to as pulmonary venous hypertension (Group II);

chronic lung diseases and/or hypoxemia, which we see frequently in the ICU (Group III); chronic thromboembolic disease (Group IV); or pulmonary hypertension related to other miscellaneous diseases.

9.3.2 Pulmonary Hypertension Diagnosis

9.3.2.1 Brain Natriuretic Peptide

Similar to left heart failure, NT-proBNP and BNP are typically elevated in right heart failure. The levels can be falsely elevated in the setting of renal failure or anemia, and falsely low in the setting of obesity. A normal or low BNP suggests that hemodynamically significant PH and right heart failure are likely not a problem for your patient.

You have a 500 kg morbidly obese male with sleep apnea in the ICU. You are concerned about cor pulmonale (right heart failure from secondary PH) and order a screening NT-proBNP test. The result comes back at 99 pg/mL, with a

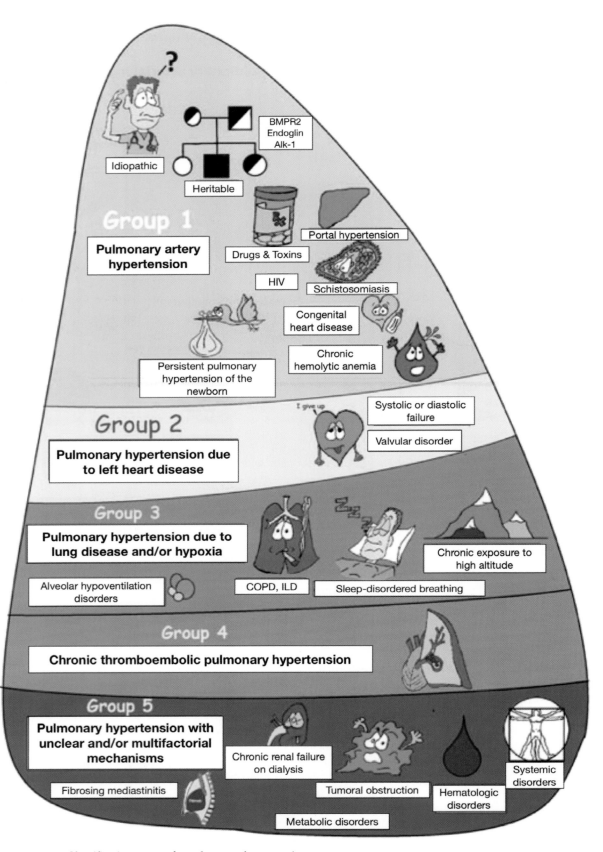

Figure 9-15 *Classification system for pulmonary hypertension.*

normal value of less than 100. You suggest to your attending that you don't need to work his heart failure up further since this test has more than a 90% sensitivity, so it is doubtful that he has PH and right heart failure. "NOT SO FAST!," says your brilliant ICU attending. "Haven't you read the study by Khan and colleagues in the Journal of Clinical Endocrinology and Metabolism, 2011?[73] Analysis of more than 7700 patients in the Framingham Heart Study and the Malmo Diet and Cancer study show that patients with either obesity or insulin resistance have 10-30% lower levels of BNP. So, we really cannot trust this borderline level. Let's check the echocardiogram!"

9.3.2.2 Doppler-Echocardiography

The most readily available test to detect PH is the echocardiogram. This test can be used to directly measure the size and function of the right atrium and right ventricle and can also be used to estimate the systolic pulmonary artery pressure. The finding of a large and dilated right atrium and ventricle, especially with evidence of bulging of the intraventricular septum into the left ventricle (so-called "D shaped left ventricle" or paradoxical septal motion), is relatively specific for PH and RV failure, but the measure of the pulmonary systolic pressure is an estimate that must be taken with a grain of salt (sensitivity and specificity of only approximately 70-80%).

The RV should typically be a half-moon shape, and mostly an empty ventricle stuck to the side of the large, thick, donut-shaped left ventricle. With severe PH, the RV dilates into a donut and pushes in the left ventricle. During diastole, when the left ventricular pressure drops, this is more apparent, resulting in a diastolic shift in the ventricular septum into the LV called *paradoxical septal motion*.

Figure 9-16 illustrates an echocardiogram of systole and diastole in a four-chamber view of a PH patient

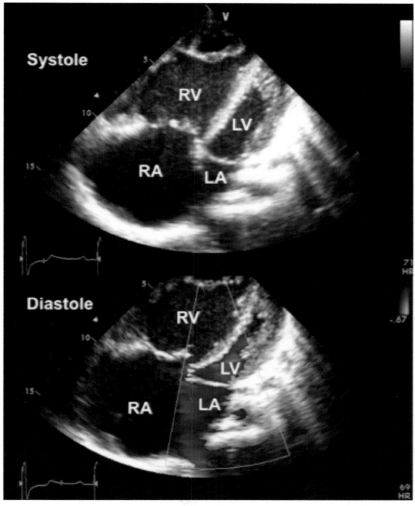

Figure 9-16 *Echocardiographic findings with right ventricle (RV) and right atrium (RA) enlargement consistent with pulmonary hypertension. LA= left atrium. LV = left ventricle.*

with very severe disease and severe right heart failure. This view of the heart in systole shows a massive right ventricle (RV) and massive right atrium (RA) that is actually bigger than the right ventricle as it balloons up. The RA almost obliterates the left atrium (LA) secondary to no blood filling it. During diastole the left ventricle has a D-shape to it. Note the septum is moving from the right side (large right ventricle) into the left ventricle) during diastole. This patient's Doppler-echo, right heart catheterization, and CT scan are all shown in subsequent figures to show the effects of severe PAH with all diagnostic modalities.

One can use Doppler-echocardiography at the bedside to estimate pulmonary artery pressures **(Figure 9-17)**. This technique uses Doppler-ultrasound to quantify the regurgitant flow velocity of blood across the closed tricuspid valve. The tricuspid is a floppy valve, and close to 90% of people have a leak that can be quantified. In patients with significant pulmonary hypertension, this leak will increase. The tricuspid regurgitant flow velocity (TRVmax) is proportional to the pressure gradient from ventricular systole (peak RV pressure) to right atrial pressure based on Bernoulli's principle. The right atrial pressure (RAP) can be estimated by the size and collapsibility of the inferior vena cava. The tricuspid regurgitant jet velocity (TRVmax) is used to estimate the right ventricle systolic pressure (RVSP), which is considered equal to the pulmonary artery systolic pressure, assuming there is no pulmonary artery stenosis. The pressure relationships are defined by the equation

$$RVSP = 4(TRVmax)^2 + RAP$$

A normal TRV is less than or equal to 2.5 m/sec (2 SD above the normal mean) and a level of $\geq$ 3.0 m/sec (3 - SD above the normal mean) is highly suspicious for pulmonary hypertension. If your TRV is $\geq$ 3.0 m/sec and you see RV dilation, then you need to consider PH as a diagnosis.

9.3.2.3 CT Angiogram

The thin-cut CT angiogram measures 0.5-5 mm cuts of the lung during contrast infusion, which can be timed so the image is taken when the contrast is in the arteries. Pulmonary hypertension can be diagnosed, or at least suggested, by findings on a regular CT scan, especially with IV contrast. The CT will show large pulmonary arteries. The normal pulmonary artery trunk is smaller than the aorta. In pulmonary hypertension, the right and left main pulmonary arteries are sometimes bigger than the aorta, and the right main pulmonary vessel can bulge out after it passes the aorta **(Figure 9-18)**. The contrast may show a big dilated inferior vena cava (IVC) meeting a huge dilated right atrium (RA) and big right ventricle.

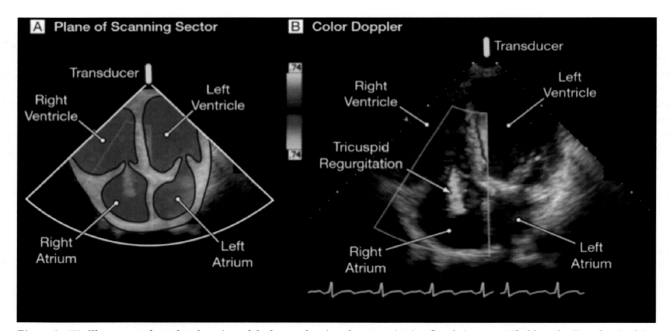

Figure 9-17 Illustrates a four-chamber view of the heart, showing the regurgitation flow being quantified by echo-Doppler. In this figure, the left panel A shows an illustration of the four chambers of the heart and the right panel B shows the tricuspid regurgitant jet across the tricuspid valve from right ventricle backwards to the right atrium. This patient had sickle cell disease and severe PAH.*

*Reproduced with permission from Barnett CF, Hsue PY, Machado RF. Pulmonary hypertension: an increasingly recognized complication of hereditary hemolytic anemias and HIV infection. JAMA 2008;299(3):324–31.

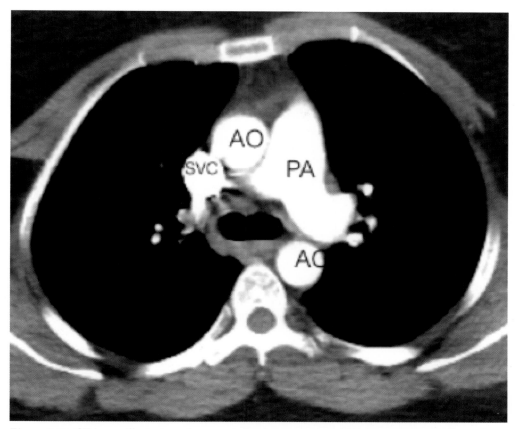

Figure 9-18 *CT image illustrates enlargement of pulmonary artery (PA) in comparison to the aorta (AO). SVC = superior vena cava.*

The lung parenchyma can be normal, or in severe cases (especially in cases of chronic thromboembolic pulmonary hypertension) can show a "mosaic" perfusion pattern (**Figure 9-19**). Areas of absent flow (from a clot or severe proliferative vascular disease) produce the mosaic pattern. The white areas are areas of normal or high flow, increasing blood volumes, and CT attenuation. The black areas are areas of low blood volume with only air (low attenuation).

9.3.2.4 Pulmonary Artery or Right Heart Catheter

Definitive diagnosis of PH requires direct measurement of the mean pulmonary artery pressure with a pulmonary artery catheter (Swan-Ganz catheter) (*See Chapter 7, Hemodynamic Monitoring*).

Pulmonary arterial hypertension (PAH), referred to as *pre-capillary pulmonary hypertension,* is a disease that predominantly affects the pulmonary capillaries or arterioles. The diagnosis of PAH requires right heart catheterization to establish a mean pulmonary artery pressure at rest greater than or equal to 25 mmHg, a left heart pressure (pulmonary artery occlusion pressure) that is normal at < 15 mmHg, and a high

pulmonary vascular resistance (typically greater than 3 Woods units). A *Woods unit* is a simplified system for measuring pulmonary vascular resistance that is made by subtracting pulmonary capillary wedge pressure from the mean pulmonary arterial pressure and dividing by cardiac output in liters per minute. *PAH is notable for the large pulmonary vascular resistance and large transpulmonary pressure gradient referred to as the TPG (Transpulmonary gradient).*

$$TPG = mPAP - PAOP \text{ (Pulmonary artery occlusion pressure)}$$

Pulmonary Arterial Hypertension = TPG > 12 mm Hg

In pulmonary venous hypertension (PVH), the pulmonary artery occlusion pressure is higher than 15 mmHg, suggesting that the high pressure originates from elevations in the left atrial pressure, not from a disease of the pulmonary arterioles.

Sometimes the pulmonary vascular resistance and the transpulmonary gradients are high, but the PAOP is also high. In fact, in patients with a chronically elevated PAOP from poorly controlled left ventricular heart failure (systolic or diastolic failure), the pulmonary vessels

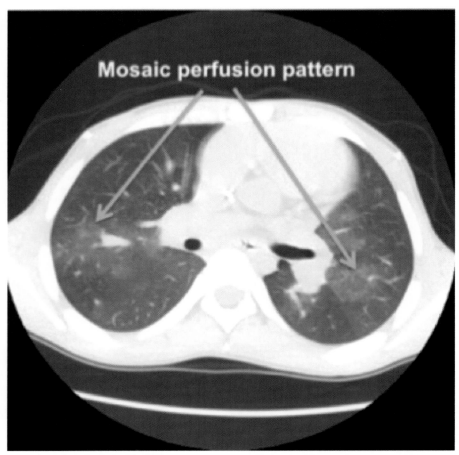

Figure 9-19 *CT image in patient with pulmonary hypertension showing a mosaic perfusion pattern.*

that are subjected to chronically elevated pressures can constrict and remodel. The remodeling process involves a smooth muscle and intimal proliferation that over time increases the pulmonary vascular resistance and transpulmonary gradient. So now the high mean PAP is determined by both a high PAOP (pulmonary venous hypertension) AND a high pulmonary vascular resistance (pulmonary arterial hypertension).

9.3.3 Why Pulmonary Hypertension Matters

The normal pulmonary vasculature is a low resistance, high-flow system. Progressive occlusion of the pulmonary arterioles in PAH increases pulmonary vascular resistance and pulmonary pressures, ultimately leading to a drop in cardiac output as the right heart fails. A progressive reduction in cardiac output results in exercise intolerance, shortness of breath, fluid retention, and likely death from right heart failure.

The relationship between vascular obliteration, vascular resistance, pulmonary pressures, and cardiac output (flow) are related to Ohm's law and reviewed in *Chapter 7 Hemodynamic Monitoring*. When working with the pulmonary circulation, the vascular pressure gradient is between the mean pulmonary artery pressure (mPAP) and the left atrial pressure, measured by the pulmonary artery occlusion pressure (PAOP), also called the *pulmonary capillary wedge pressure (PCWP)*. The vascular resistance is the pulmonary vascular resistance (PVR):

$$mPAP - PAOP = CO \times PVR$$

This relationship is particularly important in the patient with severe pulmonary hypertension and right heart failure, because as the right heart fails, it also fails to maintain a strong pressure. One can paradoxically see a lowering of pulmonary pressure in the setting of catastrophic right heart failure, and you might think the patient is getting better! This relationship is shown in **Figure 9-20**. As the figure illustrates, as PAH progresses, the vasculature of the pulmonary arterioles is progressively obliterated, and the pulmonary vascular resistance (PVR) rises over time. At first, the right

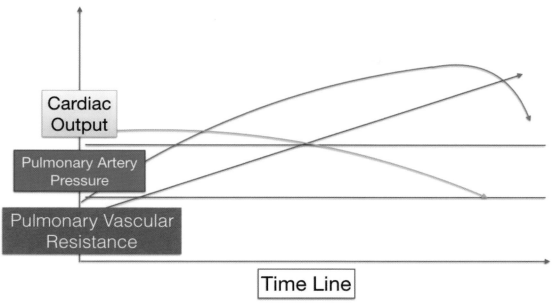

Figure 9-20 *Relationship between pulmonary artery pressure, pulmonary vascular resistance, and cardiac output. A progressive increase in pulmonary vascular resistance can lead to a reduction in pulmonary artery pressure and cardiac output.*

ventricular cardiac output is stable, and so the mean PAP rises proportionally to the rise in PVR (PAP = CO x PVR). However, as the right heart starts to fail and the CO drops, the PAP will drop. In this case, one needs to try to dilate the pulmonary arteries and decrease the PVR, but also improve cardiac output using an inotropic agent (dobutamine, milrinone) to save and stabilize the patient!

Patients at the highest risk of death are those with evidence of progressive right heart failure, elevated right atrial pressures, low cardiac outputs, and episodes of systemic hypoperfusion or syncope (sudden loss of consciousness). "Sudden death" can occur with a profound failure of the right ventricle, resulting in loss of blood flow to the brain followed by cardiac asystole.

9.4 Treatment of Pulmonary Hypertension in the Hospital

A central mechanism of pulmonary hypertension is a dysregulation of the balance of vasoconstrictors and vasodilators by the pulmonary blood vessels. This disequilibrium results not only in chronic vasoconstriction and impaired vasodilation but also down-stream "malignant" smooth muscle and intimal proliferation into the vascular lumen that blocks flow. The low flow through the pulmonary vessels is followed by in-situ thrombosis, further interrupting the flow. Based on the upstream failure

of the vasodilator/vasoconstrictor balance, all current FDA-approved medications for treatment of PH are based on stimulating the vasodilators or blocking the vasoconstrictors.

The three major pathways for the treatment of pulmonary hypertension are outlined in **Figure 9-21,** including targeting the nitric oxide pathway, prostacyclin pathway, and endothelin pathway. Nitric oxide (NO) activates vasodilation of smooth muscle cells via a cGMP-dependent mechanism. Examples of drugs targeting this pathway include inhaled NO, nitrite, nitrate, soluble guanylyl cyclase stimulator (riociguat), phosphor-diesterase 5 inhibitors (sildenafil and tadalafil), and tetrahydrobiopterin analogs (6R-BH4).

All currently available FDA-approved drugs for pulmonary hypertension are for PAH only. In fact, many of these drugs, such as the endothelin-1 receptor blockers and prostacyclin, were first developed for use in left ventricular heart failure with a high PAOP and actually worsened outcome in clinical trials. When used for PAH with a low PAOP, they improved survival and exercise tolerance. This actually makes sense as these drugs vasodilate the pulmonary arterioles, which should only help if the resistance problem is at the level of the pulmonary arterioles.

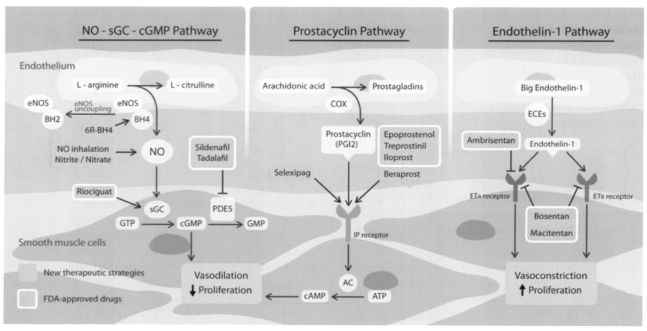

Figure 9-21*. *Therapeutic pathways for the treatment of pulmonary hypertension.*

*Reproduced with permission from Lai YC, Potoka KC, Champion HC, Mora AL, Gladwin MT. Pulmonary arterial hypertension: the clinical syndrome. Circ Res. 2014 Jun 20;115(1):115–30)

Prostacyclin activates vasodilation of smooth muscle cells via a cAMP-dependent mechanism. Prostacyclin and its derivatives (epoprostenol, treprostinil, iloprost, and beraprost) and I-prostanoid receptor agonist (selexipag) are approved or in development for PAH. Endothelin-1 stimulates vasoconstriction and proliferation via activation of receptors on smooth muscle cells. ETA blockers (ambrisentan, bosentan and macitentan) are approved for the treatment of PAH.

The drug categories and characteristics are further summarized in **Figure 9-22.**

9.4.1 Nitric Oxide

Nitric oxide (NO) is a diffusible free radical gas molecule that is produced by an enzyme in our endothelial cells called NO synthase. The NO then diffuses as a paracrine mediator from the endothelium

Drug	Characteristics
Prostacyclin and its derivatives	Effects on the pulmonary vasculature, including inhibition of smooth muscle cell constriction and proliferation, as well as platelet aggregation. Examples of this group are intravenous epoprostenol and treprostinil, and inhaled treprostinil and iloprost.
Phosphodiesterase 5 inhibitors	Sildenafil (trade name Viagra or Revatio): Recommended for patients with advanced PAH and dosed 3 times a day. Tadalafil (trade name Adcirca): The first once-daily phosphodiesterase type 5 inhibitor has shown favorable results.
Nitric oxide gas	NO gas can be given starting at 20-40 ppm in line with the ventilator. Monitor methemoglobin levels.
Endothelin receptor antagonists	Bosentan: ET-A and ET-B receptor blocker Ambrisentan: Selective ETA receptor blocker Sitaxentan: Selective ETA receptor
Inotropes	Dobutamine or milrinone for right ventricular failure
Surgical heroics	Atrial septostomy, extracorporeal membrane oxygenation (ECMO), lung transplantation

Figure 9-22 *Interventions to treat pulmonary hypertension with right ventricular failure.*

to the smooth muscle, where it binds to the heme-containing enzyme, soluble guanylate cyclase. This process in turn converts GTP to cGMP, which activates downstream kinases and relaxes smooth muscle. The cGMP is chewed up by an enzyme called *phosphodiesterase 5 (PDE5)* to turn off the vasodilation. A PDE5 inhibitor called *sildenafil* (Viagra or Revatio) was being developed as a blood pressure medication based on its ability to block PD5 and increase cGMP levels. During the early clinical trials of this drug, both patients and their doctors noticed a funny side effect, increased penile erections. This led to the discovery that PDE5 was highly expressed in the penile vasculature. Now many PDE5 inhibitors are FDA approved for erectile dysfunction. After sildenafil was clinically available, people began to try it for patients with PH, and it turns out that PDE5 is also highly expressed in pulmonary arterial circulation. Sildenefil therapy lowers pulmonary pressures and pulmonary vascular resistance while increasing cardiac output and exercise capacity in patients with PAH. Other PDE5 inhibitors are also now FDA approved for PAH therapy, including tadalafil, which can be dosed once a day. Side effects include color vision changes, myalgias, and headache.

A unique class of drug that is a small molecule that directly binds to and activates the soluble guanylate cyclase to make cGMP. This drug is called *riociguat* and has been approved for both PAH and chronic thromboembolic pulmonary hypertension.

Inhaled NO gas (or inhaled iloprost) is often used in patients with lung disease and severe PAH with right heart failure. These agents will maintain V/Q matching and prevent hypoxemia while vasodilating the pulmonary arteries and increasing right heart cardiac output. Inhaled NO will work for short periods of time (1-3 days) and often requires the addition of other drugs, such as sildenafil or prostanoids.

9.4.2 Endothelin A and B Receptor Blockers

Endothelin-1 is a small 21-amino acid peptide (protein) that is produced by endothelial cells and causes vasoconstriction. It is one of the more powerful vasoconstrictor molecules known. In fact, there are snakes (the burrowing asps or *Atractaspis*) that make a 21-amino acid peptide in their venom that mimics endothelin-1, called *sarafotoxin*. A bite of *Atractaspis* species causes coronary artery constriction and myocardial infarction. In humans, the endothelin-1 molecule binds to two classes of receptors, endothelin A and B receptors (ETA and ETB), to regulate vascular tone systemically and in the lung. Under normal physiological conditions, the ETB receptor

is expressed in the endothelium and promotes vasodilation, while the ETA receptor is expressed in the smooth muscle and promotes vasoconstriction. In PAH both receptors are expressed in the smooth muscle, and both promote vasoconstriction. For this reason, drugs that block both receptors (*bosentan*) and drugs that more selectively block the ETA receptor (*ambrisentan* and *sitaxsentan*) are efficacious. All three drugs reduce pulmonary pressures and pulmonary vascular resistance and increase cardiac output and exercise capacity in patients with PAH. Side effects include lower extremity edema, hepatitis, and anemia. Note that these drugs will increase left ventricular filling pressures (increase PAOP) so must only be used in PAH patients.

The PDE5 inhibitors are among the few systemic drugs that do NOT cause V/Q mismatch. In fact they tend to improve V/Q matching and oxygenation in patients with lung disease (COPD, IPF, ARDS) and PAH. This is because the NO synthase enzymes need oxygen to make NO (L-arginine + Oxygen + NOS makes NO + citrulline). So more NO is made in areas with good ventilation and good oxygen levels, so more cGMP.

9.4.3 Prostanoids

Prostacyclin (PGI2) binds to endothelial G-protein coupled prostacyclin receptors and activates adenylyl cyclase to produce cAMP levels in the cytosol. This cAMP then activates protein kinase A (PKA), which phosphorylates and inhibits myosin light-chain kinase, which leads to smooth muscle relaxation and vasodilation. The most potent and effective agent for the treatment of PAH is prostacyclin, called *epoprostenol (Flolan)*. Epoprostenol was the first FDA-approved therapy and the only drug shown to improve survival compared to a placebo-treated group. Prostacyclin derivatives such as treprostinil (IV and inhaled) and iloprost (inhaled) are also FDA-approved for the treatment of PAH. These drugs can cause facial flushing, jaw pain, body aches, abdominal pain and diarrhea, and hypotension as doses are increased. Both epoprostenol and treprostinil can be given intravenously to patients with severe PAH and right heart failure. A pulmonary artery catheter should be in place to monitor cardiac output and the dose started at 2 ng/kg/min, and every 15 minutes increased by 2 ng/kg/min. Dose-limiting side effects typically occur at 6-10 ng/kg/min in awake patients (abdominal pain, aches) and 15-20 in sedated patients (hypotension). As discussed below, this drug can cause diffuse pulmonary vasodilation, V/Q mismatch, and hypoxemia. Inhaled remodulin or iloprost can better match V/Q and can be used in these cases but is less potent than IV.

9.4.4 Inotropes

Remember *"It's the flow, stupid"*? The critically ill ICU patient with severe PAH and right heart failure will often require inotropic support to improve right ventricular function. Dobutamine is a perfect first-line drug as it has inotropic effects (beta 1) that increase RV contraction and also has pulmonary vasodilator effects (beta 2). Milrinone has similar ability to increase inotropy and vasodilate. Both drugs can increase V/Q mismatch and worsen oxygenation.

9.4.5 Heroics

When your PAH patient is failing despite inotropes and IV prostenoids and inhaled NO or iloprost, the only options are emergent extracorporal membrane oxygenation and cardiopulmonary bypass to maintain cardiac output. This should only be done in patients on the lung transplant waiting list in a high-volume center. Some centers can also place a right ventricular assist device to maintain cardiac output. Another bridge to lung transplant is an emergent atrial septostomy. This is a procedure where a catheter is placed into the right atrium and across the intra-atrial septum, and a balloon is inflated to create a large atrial septal defect. This allows blood from the failed right atrium/ventricle to go to the left atrium and pump to the body, since the left ventricle function is normal. While this creates an intracardiac shunt and hemoglobin oxygen saturation will drop, this is offset by the increase in cardiac output, which increases oxygen delivery.

9.5 Pulmonary Hypertension with Shock

You are working in the hospital, and the patient is admitted from the ER with severe shortness of breath, blood pressure of 100/79, heart rate of 130 bpm, oxygen saturation of 92% on face mask, with lower extremity edema, elevated neck veins, hepatojugular reflux, and clear lungs to examination and by chest radiograph. Your echo shows a severely dilated and hypokinetic right ventricle. You increase the oxygen to 100% non-rebreather mask, call your ICU attending, and together place a PA catheter. The patient's mixed venous saturation (SvO_2) is 40%, cardiac output 2.5 liters/minute, mean pulmonary pressures is 120/80, and central venous pressure 18 cm H_2O.

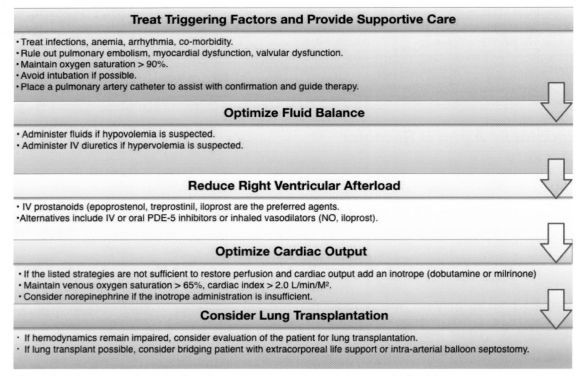

Treat Triggering Factors and Provide Supportive Care
- Treat infections, anemia, arrhythmia, co-morbidity.
- Rule out pulmonary embolism, myocardial dysfunction, valvular dysfunction.
- Maintain oxygen saturation > 90%.
- Avoid intubation if possible.
- Place a pulmonary artery catheter to assist with confirmation and guide therapy.

Optimize Fluid Balance
- Administer fluids if hypovolemia is suspected.
- Administer IV diuretics if hypervolemia is suspected.

Reduce Right Ventricular Afterload
- IV prostanoids (epoprostenol, treprostinil, iloprost are the preferred agents.
- Alternatives include IV or oral PDE-5 inhibitors or inhaled vasodilators (NO, iloprost).

Optimize Cardiac Output
- If the listed strategies are not sufficient to restore perfusion and cardiac output add an inotrope (dobutamine or milrinone)
- Maintain venous oxygen saturation > 65%, cardiac index > 2.0 L/min/M².
- Consider norepinephrine if the inotrope administration is insufficient.

Consider Lung Transplantation
- If hemodynamics remain impaired, consider evaluation of the patient for lung transplantation.
- If lung transplant possible, consider bridging patient with extracorporeal life support or intra-arterial balloon septostomy.

Figure 9-23 Treatment algorithm for pulmonary hypertension and right ventricular failure.

So what now? The critical first step is to avoid intubating her as the drugs and sedation will likely result in cardiac arrest. If you must intubate, select an agent with limited cardiodepressive effects and a short half-life. Fluids will not help as her filling pressures on the right side of the circulation are very high. The most important thing is to get her cardiac output up by increasing right ventricular inotropy and lowering afterload. Since her lung fields are clear, she is at a lower risk of shunting, so one might start with intravenous dobutamine at 3 mcs/kg/min, increasing to 5-7 mcgs/kg/min if no dysrhythmias develop. After this, the first-line agent to start is intravenous epoprostenol to attempt to vasodilate her pulmonary circulation. You can also consider either inhaled NO or inhaled iloprost if the patient develops worsening hypoxemia secondary to V/Q mismatch. If cardiac output begins to increase and you have a stable blood pressure, start therapy with furosemide to try to lower her right-sided central venous pressure.

Why is this happening? It is important to remember that acute right ventricular decompensation in a patient with baseline right heart failure may develop from conditions that lead to either an acute increase in cardiac demand, such as sepsis, or to an increase in ventricular afterload, including interruptions in medical therapy, arrhythmia, or pulmonary embolism.[74] At the same time you are stabilizing the patient, you should determine any history of drug interruptions or acute medical illness, check an ECG, send cultures, start empiric antibiotics (especially if the patient has a central line and is on chronic prostanoid infusion therapy), and assess anticoagulation and risk of PE or DVT.

It is key to consult cardiac surgery and cardiology early and determine the patient's lung transplant status. If the patient is a lung transplant candidate, you could offer more aggressive bridging strategies, like extracorporal membrane oxygenation (ECMO) and cardiopulmonary bypass. Atrial septostomy can be considered in experienced centers if central venous pressure is not too high (<20 cm H_2O) and oxygen saturations are greater than 80% on room air. *She will be the most dangerous patient you will treat, and she may not make it. Get help and be aggressive.*

A suggested algorithm for approaching the critically ill patient with right heart failure is shown in **Figure 9-23**, modified from an excellent review.[74]

Suggested Reading

- Kato T, Suda S, Kasai T. Positive airway pressure therapy for heart failure. World Journal of Cardiology 2014;6(11):1175–91.
- Humbert M, Sitbon O, Simonneau G. Treatment of pulmonary arterial hypertension. NEJM. 2004 Sep 30;351(14):1425–36.
- Barnett CF, Hsue PY, Machado RF. Pulmonary hypertension: an increasingly recognized complication of hereditary hemolytic anemias and HIV infection. JAMA. 2008 Jan 23;299(3):324–31. Review. PMID: 18212317
- Lai YC, Potoka KC, Champion HC, Mora AL, Gladwin MT. Pulmonary arterial hypertension: the clinical syndrome. Circ Res. 2014 Jun 20;115(1):115–30.
- Gelsomino S, Johnson DM, Lorusso R. Intra-aortic balloon pump: is the tide turning? Crit Care [Internet] (2018) 22(1):345.

10

High Systemic Arterial Blood Pressure

A hypertensive crisis is an acute elevation in systemic blood pressure. Hypertensive crisis is classically divided into two conditions:

- *Hypertensive urgency (HU)* is characterized by a severely elevated blood pressure (> 180/110 mm Hg) without evidence for acute and progressive dysfunction of target organs. The problem is urgent because this degree of blood pressure elevation has the *potential* to cause organ injury. Blood pressure should be reduced over 24-48 hours.
- *Hypertensive emergency (HE).* Now we have an emergency! Hypertensive emergency is characterized by a severe elevation in systemic blood pressure <u>and</u> new or progressive end-organ damage most frequently in the cardiac, renal, or central nervous systems.[75] Hypertensive emergency is the less common form of HC but requires immediate (within one hour!), titrated, blood pressure reduction. The patient's clinical signs and symptoms determine the diagnosis of HE, rather than a specific blood pressure elevation, although hypertensive emergency is typically associated with a blood pressure elevation > 180/110 mm Hg. Clinical conditions associated with HE might include hypertensive encephalopathy, intracranial hemorrhage, acute coronary syndrome, acute pulmonary edema, aortic dissection, acute renal failure, and eclampsia (**Figure 10-1**). HE is a *medical emergency* and requires reduction of MAP by 10-20% in one hour.

Some investigators have characterized a third category of hypertensive crisis as *hypertensive pseudocrisis.*[76] Hypertensive pseudocrisis describes transient elevations of blood pressure in the setting of any emotional, painful, or uncomfortable event. Clinical examples of hypertensive pseudocrisis might be seen in a patient with a migraine headache, acute urinary retention, or a panic disorder. Treatment for hypertensive pseudocrisis is directed to the primary disease process, as the hypertension is solely present due to the underlying disorder.

All forms of hypertensive crisis are typically associated with untreated hypertension, often with underlying noncompliance or poor management. The correct classification determines the type and urgency of treatment.

10.1 Pathophysiology of Hypertensive Urgency

Fundamentally, an acute elevation in systemic arterial BP involves an increase in systemic vascular resistance. A complex interplay of vasoconstrictor and vasodilator mediators determines vascular resistance. The release of proinflammatory cellular mediators promotes endothelial injury, leading to endothelial permeability and activation of the coagulation cascade. This combination of events leads to the pathologic changes of obliterative vascular lesions. A state of relative ischemia results in affected organs, leading

CATEGORY	CLINICAL CONDITIONS
Cardiovascular	• Acute coronary syndrome • Acute left ventricular dysfunction • Acute aortic dissection
Cerebrovascular	• Hypertensive encephalopathy • Acute ischemic stroke • Intracerebral hemorrhage • Subarachnoid hemorrhage
Renovascular disease	• Acute glomerulonephritis • Renovascular hypertension • Scleroderma renal crisis • Post kidney transplantation
Endocrine	• Pheochromocytoma • Cushing syndrome • Primary hyperaldosteronism
Drug Related	• Cocaine • Amphetamine • MAOI-tyramine interaction • Antihypertensive withdrawal • Alpha – stimulant intoxication
Miscellaneous Conditions	• Eclampsia/Preeclampsia • Post-operative hypertension • Systemic vasculitis • Autonomic hyperactivity (Guillain-Barre syndrome) • Burns

Figure 10-1 *Clinical conditions associated with hypertension emergency.*

to end-organ dysfunction. The advanced stages of hypertensive encephalopathy are characterized by a thrombotic microangiopathy with associated organ dysfunction.

The treatment involves effective blood pressure control, but this must proceed with some element of caution. A rapid decrease in blood pressure necessary to reduce brain edema and ischemia can drop brain blood flow and make the clinical features worse. For this reason, it is key to understand the relationship between blood pressure, blood flow, and the resistance settings of the pre-capillary arterioles

Remember our discussion of Ohm's law from *Chapter 7 Hemodynamic Monitoring*. Remember the equation that defines the relationships between mean arterial pressure (MAP), central venous pressure (CVP), flow (cardiac output [CO]), and resistance (systemic vascular resistance [SVR]) is

$$MAP - CVP = CO \times SVR$$

which can obviously be rewritten to

$$CO = (MAP - CVP) / SVR$$

Over a defined range of blood pressures, the precapillary arterial tone (SVR) is adjusted to maintain

a constant organ blood flow (CO) **(Figure 10-2)**. This is called *auto-regulation* and has been most extensively studied in relation to cerebral blood flow. An increase in arterial pressure is offset by an increase in vascular tone to maintain a constant blood flow. Alternatively, a reduction in arterial blood pressure is compensated by a decrease in vascular resistance to maintain the same flow. If the mean arterial pressure (MAP) falls below a critical minimum value, the vascular resistance cannot drop enough to sustain organ perfusion. Below this minimum MAP value, organ ischemia results from a reduction in blood flow. Alternatively, if the MAP rises above a certain upper inflection point, the resistance cannot rise enough to limit the increase in blood flow, and potential organ edema develops.

In patients with longstanding hypertension, a rightward shift of the MAP and cerebral blood flow relationship occurs, resulting in a higher transition point for the lower limit of autoregulation.[77] So, a chronically hypertensive patient is at risk for organ ischemia below a higher MAP value than a normotensive patient. The lower limit of autoregulation is about 20% below the resting MAP. These data form the standard recommendation that blood pressure reduction in hypertensive emergency be restricted to a 10-20% reduction of the MAP from the highest values on initial presentation.

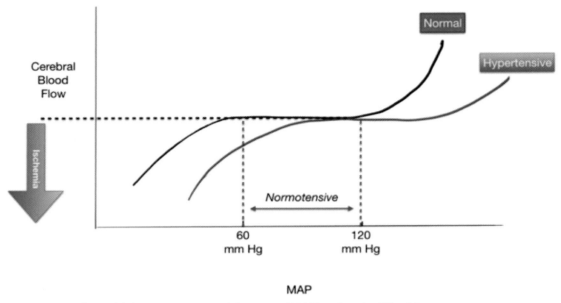

Figure 10-2 *Relationship between mean arterial pressure (MAP) and cerebral blood flow.*

In patients with CNS injury in addition to hypertension, the physiology is even more complex. Cerebral perfusion pressure (CPP) is the pressure gradient acting across the cerebrovascular bed. CPP can be defined as

$$CPP = \text{mean arterial pressure (MAP)} - \text{mean intracranial pressure (ICP)}$$

A sufficient CPP is required to maintain cerebral blood flow. Cerebral blood flow is maintained constant over a range of CPP's due to autoregulation as mentioned previously **(Figure 10-2)**. A very low CPP, below the autoregulatory reserve, would lead to a reduction in cerebral blood flow and the risk of brain ischemia. The lower limit of CPP is considered a threshold of 60-70 mm Hg in adults.

The skull provides a rigid case for its three main compartments, including the volume of the brain parenchyma (80%), the cerebral spinal fluid (10%), and the cerebral blood volume (10%). Any variable that increases the volume of one of the compartments requires the displacement of other structures, or an increase in the intracranial pressure. Anti-hypertensive medications that increase cerebral blood flow could increase cerebral edema and raise intracranial pressure. The combination of reducing MAP (blood pressure control) and increasing intracranial pressure (brain edema) would significantly lower CPP and could extend brain injury. These changes may not be apparent to the clinician without the advantage of invasive monitoring.

The "gold standard" for intracranial pressure monitoring is an intraventricular drain connected to an external pressure transducer. Intracranial pressure is usually ≤ 15 mmHg in adults, and pathologic intracranial hypertension is present at pressures ≥ 20 mmHg. Empiric treatment for presumed elevated ICP is less than optimal because CPP cannot be monitored reliably without measurement of ICP. The goal of ICP monitoring is to maintain the CPP at 60 mm Hg or higher. This can be accomplished by increasing (or maintaining) the MAP or decreasing the ICP.

For patients with hypertension in the setting of acute cerebrovascular disease, brain edema or hemorrhage can lead to an increase in ICP. Increased ICP narrows the gradient between MAP and ICP, leading to a progressive reduction in CPP for a given MAP. In addition to strategies directed at lowering ICP (i.e., osmotic diuretics), employ caution in the management of hypertension in the population. Aggressive blood pressure control to lower MAP can create a low CPP, which compromises CBF. Intracranial pressure monitoring is not required for the vast majority of patients presenting with acute cerebrovascular disease, but the physiologic principles are important to keep in mind as you make your treatment decisions. Invasive ICP monitoring is helpful for complex patients, especially those with closed head injury.

10.2 Patient Assessment

Patients with hypertensive emergency frequently have a history of chronic or current medication noncompliance. A detailed account of prescription drug use and recreational drug use is essential, as a substance abuse history is very common in these patients. No specific blood pressure level defines hypertensive emergency, but the median systolic blood pressure in a hypertensive registry was 200 mm Hg (interquartile range 186 – 220 and the median diastolic blood pressure was 110 mm Hg (interquartile range 93 - 123).[78]

The physical examination is focused on repetitive measurements of blood pressures since a patient frequently resolves hypertension quickly after presentation. Measure blood pressure in both arms with an appropriately sized cuff. Physical examination should focus on identification of signs suggesting end-organ dysfunction and include a funduscopic exam to identify papilledema.

10.3 Drug Therapy

Treat patients without hypertensive urgency using oral agents and allowing a gradual reduction in the blood pressure over 24-48 hours. Rapid declines in blood pressure may compromise organ blood flow. In contrast, a patient with hypertensive emergency requires a more immediate decrease in blood pressure but, again, hypotension and compromised organ perfusion should be avoided. Therefore, *short-acting titratable medications* provided in a highly monitored environment are preferred for the treatment of hypertensive emergency. Avoid the sublingual and intramuscular routes due to unpredictable pharmacokinetics. Maintain the patient on titratable medications until the blood pressure readings are stable and there is no further evidence of organ dysfunction.

A summary of the standard titratable medications for the treatment of hypertensive emergency is outlined in **Figure 10-3**. There is no single preferred medication for the treatment of all hypertensive emergencies. The patient's clinical condition determines the optimal prescription. We will start with a review of the medications by drug classification and then outline their specific use based upon the clinical syndrome of your patient.

10.3.1 Calcium Channel Blockers

The dihydropyridine calcium channel blockers (CCB) (e.g., nicardipine and clevidipine) are selective for vascular smooth muscle and have little activity in cardiac muscle or the sinoatrial node. These medications are considered the first line agent for treatment of most hypertensive emergencies with some exceptions.

Nicardipine hydrochloride acts primarily as a systemic, cerebral, and coronary artery vasodilator. The intravenous drug administration has a short onset (5-15min) and duration of action, and, therefore, easy titration to a therapeutic effect. Nicardipine readily crosses the blood-brain barrier and relaxes vascular smooth muscle, especially in regions of ischemic tissue. The medication acts as a vasodilator of small resistance cerebral arterioles but does not change intracranial volume or intracranial pressure, with preservation of cerebral oxygenation.

Nicardipine offers the advantage of avoiding the toxic metabolites of nitroprusside, requires less frequent dose adjustments, and has a decreased risk of increased intracranial pressure as reported with nitroprusside, with equal efficacy for blood pressure control. Nicardipine has been shown to increase coronary blood flow with a favorable effect on myocardial oxygen demand. For all these reasons, nicardipine has replaced nitroprusside as the titratable medication of choice for controlling hypertension.

Clevidipine, a second titratable calcium channel blocker administered by continuous infusion, also reduces afterload without adversely affecting cardiac-filling pressures or causing reflex tachycardia. Clevidipine has a rapid onset (~2–4 minutes) and offset of action (~5–15 minutes), making it even more titratable then nicardipine. The drug has poor water solubility, so the drug is administered by continuous IV infusion in a lipid emulsion. The drug has been most extensively investigated in patients with acute perioperative or postoperative hypertension in the setting of cardiac surgery, where the drug is effective for blood pressure control with limited toxicity.

Clevidipine is contraindicated in patients with allergies to soybeans, soy products, eggs, or egg products. Clevidipine is also contraindicated in patients with defective lipid metabolism. Due to lipid-load restrictions, no more than 1000 mL or an average of 21 mg/hr of clevidipine infusion is recommended per 24-hour period. Clinicians must account for the calories infused from the lipid emulsion and adjust the nutrition regimen as needed and monitor triglyceride levels during prolonged administration.

10.3.2 Nitric Oxide Vasodilators

Sodium nitroprusside (SNP) had previously been the gold standard for the treatment of hypertensive emergencies due to a short duration of action allowing careful titration. The blood pressure response to nitroprusside infusion is rapid and requires that this medication is administered in a monitored setting. SNP is a potent arterial and venous vasodilator that reduces preload and afterload. SNP has two recognized limitations:

1. The potent arterial vasodilation with SNP can redistribute oxygenated blood flow from nonresponsive ischemic regions to vasodilated nonischemic regions. In the coronary circulation, nitroprusside can reduce coronary perfusion

Medication (Route)	Pharmacology	Dosing	Indication	Contraindication
Nicardipine (IV infusion)	Onset: 5-15 min Duration: 4-6 hrs	Init: 5 mg/h Max: 30 mg/h	Most hypertensive emergencies	
Nitroglycerin (IV infusion)	Onset: 2-5 min Duration: 5-10 min	Init: 5 mcg/min Max: 200 mcg/min	Acute coronary syndromes	Contraindicated in pregnancy. Caution with use in a volume-contracted patient
Labetalol (intravenous, IV infusion, oral)	Onset: 2-5 min Duration: 2-4 hrs	Init: IV bolus 10-20mg Repeat bolus 20-80 mg q 10 mins Infusion: 1 to 2 mg/min	Pregnancy Neurologic injury Aortic dissection	Contraindicated in airflow obstruction, acute heart failure, or in patients non-tolerant of Beta-blockers.
Esmolol (IV infusion)	Onset: 2-10 min Duration: 10-30 min	Init: 0.5 mg/kg over 1 min Infusion: 50 mcg/kg/min titrated to 300 mg/kg/min May repeat bolus with each infusion increase	Aortic dissection	Cautious use in airflow obstruction, acute heart failure, or in patients non-tolerant of Beta-blockers.
Nitroprusside (IV infusion)	Onset: 2-3 min Duration: 1-10 min	Init: 0.25 to 0.5 mcg/kg/min Max: 2 mcg/kg/min	Select hypertensive emergencies with normal renal function	Contraindication in pregnancy. Caution with use in the settings of cerebral edema, acute coronary syndrome, or renal dysfunction
Clevidipine (IV infusion)	Onset: 2-4 min Duration: 5-15 min	Init: 1-2mg /hr Max: 32mg/hr	Most hypertensive emergencies	Contraindicated with allergy to soybean or egg products Contraindicated with defective lipid metabolism
Fenoldopam (IV infusion)	Onset: < 5 min Duration: 30 min	Init: 0.1 mcg/kg/min Max: 1.6 mcg/kg/min	Most hypertensive emergencies	Caution in patients with glaucoma and risk of increased cerebral blood flow
Phentolamine (intravenous, IV infusion)	Onset: 1-2 min Duration: 10-30min	1-5 mg bolus with a maximum dose 15 mg May start infusion at 1mg/hr	Pheochromo-cytoma. Catecholamine withdrawal or excess	

Figure 10-3 *Titratable medications for the treatment of hypertensive emergency.*

pressure, resulting in a "coronary steal" syndrome. A similar "cerebral steal" syndrome has been suggested with the use of SNP due to preferential vasodilation in systemic vascular beds vs. cerebral vessels. Through dilation of large capacitance vessels, SNP can also increase cerebral blood volume, leading to an increase in intracranial pressure. For these reasons, SNP is not favored for blood pressure control in patients with coronary or cerebrovascular disease.

2. SNP may also rarely be associated with the risk of cyanide, or thiocyanate toxicity. Cyanide toxicity from nitroprusside is uncommon and occurs primarily in patients receiving infusions for greater than 24 to 48 hours in the setting of underlying renal insufficiency. Another determinant is infusion doses that exceed the capacity of the body to detoxify cyanide (more than 2 µg/kg per min).

For this reason, SNP is not favored in patients with renal disease.

Nitroglycerin (NTG) is primarily a venodilator that promotes coronary vascular dilation. NTG influences arterial vascular effects only at higher dose infusions. The drug is contraindicated in patients with volume depletion, as venodilation in these patients will lower preload and cardiac output, compromising systemic perfusion. The drug has a short duration of action when administered by the intravenous route, so it is given as a constant infusion. The primary indication for the medication is hypertension in association with cardiac disease. The drug reduces myocardial oxygen demand by decreasing preload and afterload, and augments coronary artery oxygen delivery. Headache is the most common adverse effect of NTG, and methemoglobinemia is a rare complication of prolonged nitroglycerin therapy. Tolerance to the medication is recognized and may limit the overall effectiveness in longer-term infusions.

10.3.3 Beta-Blockers

Labetalol is an oral and parenteral agent that acts as an alpha- and nonselective beta-adrenergic blocker with an alpha-to-beta blocking ratio of 1:7. The blood pressure lowering effect is produced through a reduction in systemic vascular resistance without a compensatory increase in heart rate. In contrast to traditional Beta-blockers, labetalol is associated with preservation of cardiac output with minimal negative effects on heart rate. The hypotensive effect of labetalol has an onset of 2-5 min, peak effect at 5-15 min and duration of ~2-6 hours. Labetalol has minimal effect on the cerebral circulation and is thus not associated with an increase in intracranial pressure in the normal brain. The drug has minimal placental transfer and has been used effectively in pregnancy-associated hypertension. The primary contraindication to the use of the medication relates to its nonselective beta-blocking properties. The drug should be used cautiously in patients with reactive airways disease and heart block. Although appealing for its combined nonselective B-adrenergic blocker and α-blockade, labetalol is a less potent medication than comparable drugs for those specific indications.

Esmolol is a short-acting, cardioselective Beta-blocker with a rapid onset (< 1 min) and short duration of action of 10-20 min when administered by continuous infusion. Esmolol reduces blood pressure, heart rate, and cardiac output, and must be avoided in patients with bradycardia or impaired left ventricular function. Esmolol is optimally used in patients with tachycardia, hypertension, and normal to elevated cardiac output. Red blood cell esterases rapidly clear esmolol independent of renal or hepatic function. Esmolol offers a rapidly titratable medication for indications where negative intropy is indicated (i.e., aortic dissection).

10.3.4 Miscellaneous Medications

Intravenous *fenoldopam* is a postsynaptic dopamine-1 receptor antagonist with short-acting vasodilator properties. Fenoldopam lowers blood pressure by decreasing peripheral vascular resistance. The medication causes slight heart rate elevation with an increase in renal blood flow. The preservation of renal blood flow is attributed to the drug's mechanism as a dopamine-1 receptor agonist.

A dose-related tachycardia can occur with the administration of fenoldopam, especially at infusion rates > 0.1 mcg/kg/minute. The drug should be used with caution in patients with angina, since a reflux

tachycardia could increase myocardial oxygen demand. Fenoldopam should also be used with caution in patients with open-angle glaucoma or intraocular hypertension. The drug has not been investigated in the setting of increased intracranial pressure and should be used with caution in these patients.

Phentolamine is a rapid-acting, alpha-adrenergic blocker. Phentolamine is often considered the drug of choice for hypertensive emergencies secondary to pheochromocytoma, MAO-tyramine interactions, and clonidine rebound hypertension.

Many medications are used in the hospital setting to control blood pressure. However, these medications are *not favored* for a hypertensive emergency because they are not easily titratable. *Enalapril* is an intravenously administered angiotensin-converting enzyme (ACE) inhibitor. The medication reduces renin-dependent vasopressor activity, blocks the conversion of angiotensin I to angiotensin II (vasoconstrictor), and blocks the degradation of bradykinin (vasodilator). The drug is effective in patients with low to normal renin levels and hypertension. ACE inhibitor administration is associated with a decrease in systemic vascular resistance, with minimal change in heart rate, cardiac output, or left ventricular filling pressures. The peak effect of enalapril, however, may be delayed for up to 4 hours with a duration of 12-24 hours. These pharmacokinetic parameters limit the drug titration in the acute setting of hypertensive emergency. ACE inhibitors are contraindicated in the setting of renal artery stenosis and pregnancy.

Clonidine and *hydralazine* are long-acting medications with *limited titratability*. These medications are more appropriate for patients with hypertensive urgency than hypertensive emergency. Hydralazine is a direct-acting vasodilator with an onset (5-15 min) and prolonged effect (~12-hour ½ life), which can be highly variable. Because of hydralazine's prolonged and unpredictable antihypertensive effects, the medication is best avoided in the management of hypertensive emergency.

Diuretics should be avoided in the acute management of hypertensive emergency in the absence of pulmonary edema or renal parenchymal disease. Volume depletion is typical in HE patients, and these patients are susceptible to hypotension and compromised perfusion if vasodilators and diuretics are initiated together.

10.4 Hypertensive Emergency Clinical Syndromes

Patients with a hypertensive emergency present with a broad range of clinical signs and symptoms. But we will focus on the "big 3" clinical syndromes (**Figure 10-4**) and still discuss a few less common ones.

10.4.1 Cardiovascular Disease

10.4.1.1 Acute Coronary Syndrome

Patients presenting with acute coronary syndromes may suffer from elevated systemic arterial pressure. In many cases, hypertension may be a secondary event due to the crushing substernal chest pain. Pain control is an essential initial step in the management of the patient presenting with an acute coronary syndrome.

The increased afterload from hypertension in this setting raises myocardial oxygen demand as will tachycardia. A reduction of high systemic arterial pressure is needed in this setting, but proceed cautiously, as systemic arterial vasodilation without coronary vasodilation can lead to a reduced coronary artery perfusion pressure and infarct extension. For this reason, nitroglycerin (NTG), a potent coronary vasodilator, is the antihypertensive agent of choice in acute coronary syndromes. NTG infusion is rapidly titratable, and dosing can be adjusted as the patient responds to treatment. NTG can be administered in combination with beta-blocker therapy to reduce myocardial oxygen demand by controlling heart rate and reducing LV afterload if required. Careful monitoring of hemodynamic indices during the intervention is paramount.

10.4.1.2 Acute Left Ventricular Dysfunction

A significant fraction of patients presenting with acute heart failure and pulmonary edema are hypertensive on initial assessment. The clinical challenge is to determine if the hypertension is the inciting event with secondary myocardial dysfunction or if hypertension occurs secondary to the catecholamine surge associated with acute pulmonary edema. This syndrome has been called *SCAPE* for *Sympathetic Surge Crashing Acute Pulmonary Edema* in the ED literature.

Intravenous vasodilators, preferentially nitroglycerin and, to lesser degree, calcium channel antagonists, are the preferred agents for this condition as they permit rapid titration of blood pressure. NTG dosing is required in the higher dose range for this condition.

The dihydropyridine calcium antagonists nicardipine and clevidipine have been associated with reduced systemic arterial pressure while preserving coronary blood flow. Avoid longer-acting medications such as angiotensin-converting enzyme inhibitors or angiotensin II receptor blocker therapy early in the treatment period. *Use titratable medications!*

Patients with hypertensive emergencies may have experienced a natriuresis resulting in elevated levels of renin production by the kidney and, hence, increased circulating levels of the potent endogenous vasoconstrictor, angiotensin II. Therefore, aggressive diuresis prior to blood pressure control is not advised. Medications that increase cardiac work (e.g., hydralazine) or impair cardiac contractility (e.g., labetalol) are also contraindicated as primary therapy for hypertension in the setting of acute left ventricular dysfunction.

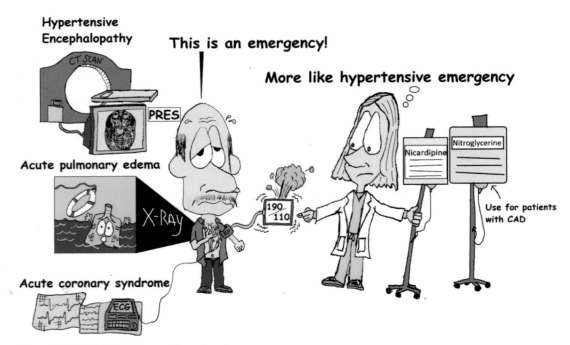

Figure 10-4 *Clinical features of hypertensive emergency.*

10.4.1.3 Acute Aortic Dissection

Aortic dissection results from an intimal tear in the aortic wall. Extension of that tear is promoted by factors that increase the rate of change of aortic pressure (dp/dt), including elevation in blood pressure, heart rate, and myocardial stroke volume. The classic triad of chest pain, BP differential between the right and left arm, and widened mediastinum is present in only ¼ of cases, so a high clinical suspicion is required. A new aortic regurgitation murmur can be another clinical clue to a proximal aortic dissection that extends to the aortic valve.

Unlike most cases of hypertensive emergency, promptly reduce blood pressure in aortic dissection to near normal levels. This requires initial control of the heart rate (~ 60 beats per min) followed by blood pressure control with a vasodilator. Isolated treatment with a vasodilator alone could precipitate a reflex tachycardia with an increase in the left ventricle ejection force. Combined modality therapy to promote vasodilation (nicardipine) and control cardiac contractility (Beta-blocker), is needed for this disorder. Labetalol can be given as a bolus (20 mg initially) or as an infusion (0.5 to 2 mg/minute). As an alternative, esmolol has a very short half-life and a favorable ability to titrate to effect. This might be a preferred medication for patients potentially intolerant of beta-blockers due to asthma or heart failure. If the blood pressure remains elevated after the administration of beta blockade and heart rate control, add nicardipine. The vasodilator medication should NOT be administered first, to avoid a reflex tachycardia and increase in wall stress.

10.4.2 Cerebrovascular Disease

10.4.2.1 Hypertensive Encephalopathy

Hypertensive encephalopathy presents with a headache, confusion or a depressed level of consciousness, nausea and vomiting, visual disturbances, or seizures (generalized or focal). Focal neurologic deficits are possible but much less frequent than in cerebrovascular accidents. Rarely, hypertensive encephalopathy can present with brainstem involvement manifesting as ataxia and diplopia. The MAP on presentation is significantly above the patient's baseline blood pressure. Retinal findings (including arteriolar spasm, exudates or hemorrhages, and papilledema) may be present but are not a requirement.

Magnetic resonance imaging studies classically show characteristic edema involving the subcortical white matter of the parieto-occipital regions (posterior brain regions) best seen on T2 and FLAIR imaging; a finding termed *Posterior Reversible leukoEncephalopathy Syndrome*

(*PRES*).[79] Approximately 2/3 of patients will also have hyperintense lesions on T2, and FLAIR imaging in the frontal and temporal lobes; and 1/3 will have brainstem, cerebellum, or basal ganglia involvement. The imaging findings are typically bilateral but can be asymmetric. Hypertensive encephalopathy is the most common cause of PRES, but it can also be caused by calcineurin inhibitors, like cyclosporine and tacrolimus, often associated with hypertension. Improvement or resolution of the radiographic findings often is delayed in comparison to the clinical improvement. Seizures can occur in patients with PRES and may include both focal and generalized features.

Hypertension as the etiology of the patient's clinical symptoms is confirmed by the absence of other conditions and the prompt resolution of symptoms and neuroimaging abnormalities with adequate blood pressure control. The failure of a patient to improve within 6 to 12 hours of blood pressure reduction should prompt an investigation for an alternative cause of the mental status changes. In the majority of cases, the condition is entirely reversible with no observable adverse outcomes.

The preferred agent for the treatment of hypertensive encephalopathy is *nicardipine*.

10.4.2.2 Acute Stroke

The majority of patients with acute stroke have elevated blood pressure on presentation, but this finding returns to normal within 48 hours of presentation. Several clinical features complicate the management of hypertension in acute stroke. First, during acute stroke, cerebral auto-regulation may be compromised in ischemic tissue and lowering of blood pressure may further compromise cerebral blood flow and extend ischemic injury. Second, medications used to treat hypertension may lead to cerebral vasodilation, augmenting cerebral blood flow and leading to progression in cerebral edema. Ideally, a "correct" level of mean arterial pressure should be targeted in each patient to maintain cerebral perfusion pressure without worsening cerebral edema or progression of the lesion, but the clinical determination of this "correct" value is often difficult.

Consensus guidelines recommend that blood pressure not be treated acutely in the patient with ischemic stroke unless the hypertension is extreme (systolic blood pressure >220 mmHg or diastolic blood pressure >120 mmHg) or the patient has active end-organ dysfunction in other organ systems.[80] Only cautious lowering of blood pressure by approximately 15% during the first 24 hours after stroke onset is suggested if absolutely needed. Antihypertensive medications can be restarted at about 24 hours after stroke onset in patients with preexisting hypertension who are neurologically stable, unless a specific contraindication to restarting treatment exists.

Special considerations apply to patients with extracranial or intracranial stenosis and candidates for thrombolytic therapy. The former group may be critically dependent on perfusion pressure, so blood pressure therapy may be further delayed. In contrast, before lytic therapy is started, treatment is recommended so that systolic blood pressure is ≤185 mmHg and diastolic blood pressure is ≤110 mmHg. The blood pressure should also be stabilized and maintained below 180/105 mmHg for at least 24 hours after intravenous lytic therapy.

The agent of choice for patients with these neurologic syndromes is nicardipine based upon titratability, safety, and favorable effects on cerebral blood flow.

Blood pressure is frequently elevated in patients with acute intracranial hemorrhage. Theoretically, hypertension worsens intracranial hemorrhage by creating a continued force for bleeding. *However, the increase in arterial pressure may also be necessary to maintain cerebral perfusion in this setting, and aggressive blood pressure management could lead to worsening cerebral ischemia.* For patients with suspected elevated intracranial pressure (ICP), ICP monitoring may be indicated to help maintain cerebral perfusion pressure during therapeutic interventions. However, based upon the INTensive Blood Pressure Reduction in Acute Cerebral Hemorrhage Trials (INTERACT 1 and 2), many investigators advocate acute blood pressure reduction to a target systolic blood pressure of 140 mm Hg as a reasonable option for patients with spontaneous intracerebral hemorrhage.[81]

10.4.3 Subarachnoid Hemorrhage (SAH)

Rupture of a saccular aneurysm most commonly causes SAH. The patient classically presents with the sudden, severe onset of headache. The diagnosis is based upon a non-contrast head CT +/- a spinal tap. The patient with SAH presents the challenge of both the initial bleed and the subsequent complications of hydrocephalus, rebleeding, and vasospasm. Blood pressure management has competing goals of lowering blood pressure to reduce the rebleeding risk, and elevating blood pressure to minimize the risk of cerebral vasospasm and infarction. In general, hypertension is not aggressively treated in this population for fear of precipitating cerebral ischemia. For the patient with a normal neurologic picture, small reductions in blood pressure can be accomplished to minimize the risk of rebleeding. For the neurologically impaired patient, aggressive control of blood pressure is avoided to maintain cerebral perfusion pressure.

To date, no well-controlled studies exist that answer whether blood pressure control in acute SAH influences outcome.

Patients with intracranial hemorrhage, especially with traumatic brain injury, may benefit from the monitoring of cerebral perfusion pressure. This allows direct monitoring and goal-directed titration of antihypertensive therapy in these high-risk conditions.

10.4.4 Renovascular Disease

Elevated systemic arterial pressure should be regulated in patients with underlying renal insufficiency and a comprehensive work-up initiated to determine the cause and effect relationship. Traditional vasodilator medications are preferred to ACE inhibitors in the acute setting because ACE inhibitors can compromise renal function. The risk of ACE inhibitor-induced renal dysfunction is particularly great in patients with hyperkalemia and acute uremia.

10.4.4.1 Scleroderma Renal Crisis

Scleroderma renal crisis is acute renal failure in the patient with scleroderma associated with moderate-to-severe hypertension and a normal to minimally abnormal urine sediment. The most significant risk factor for scleroderma renal crisis is the presence of diffuse skin involvement characteristic of the disease and recent treatment with high dose corticosteroids. The disorder results in marked activation of the renin-angiotensin system. Aggressive control of blood pressure using ACE inhibitors, particularly early in the disease process, can control blood pressure in up to 90% of patients and promote a greater rate of recovery in renal function.

10.4.4.2 Post-Kidney Transplantation

Hypertension following renal transplantation is prevalent. Hypertension in these patients is a manifestation of volume overload, graft rejection, ischemia, or drug effects (glucocorticoids and calcineurin inhibitors). Treatment is directed primarily at the underlying mechanism. Evaluate for renal artery stenosis in any patient post-renal transplant with resistant hypertension. This complication typically occurs from 2 months to 3 years post-transplantation. In the immediate post-transplant period, blood pressure should be regulated at the upper limits of normal to preserve graft function. In the later postoperative period, stricter control of blood pressure is favored. The goal blood pressure is typically 140/90 mmHg in patients without diabetes or proteinuria, and 130/80 mmHg in those with diabetes or proteinuria. Calcium channel blockers are frequently used to treat hypertension post-renal transplantation based upon their antagonism of cyclosporine-induced renal vasoconstriction. ACE inhibitors have the potential to exacerbate renal dysfunction and augment the hyperkalemia induced by calcineurin inhibitors. When a calcium channel blocker is used, a drug interaction with calcineurin inhibitors must be recognized with careful monitoring of drug levels.

10.4.5 Excess Catecholamine States

10.4.5.1 Pheochromocytoma

Pheochromocytoma leading to excess circulating catecholamines presents with hypertension, diaphoresis, tachycardia, and paresthesias of the hands and feet. These attacks can last from minutes to days and occur as frequently as several times a day or as infrequently as once per month. Operative manipulation of the tumor can result in perioperative hypertension. The treatment of hypertension in this disorder must avoid the use of isolated therapy with a beta-blocker, a strategy that can lead to unopposed alpha-adrenergic stimulation with the risk of further vasoconstriction and blood pressure elevation. The preferred agent for treatment of hypertension due to pheochromocytoma is *phentolamine*, a potent alpha-adrenergic antagonist. If necessary, combine this medication with a beta-blocker, or a combined alpha/beta-blocker, such as labetalol, can be used safely. Labetalol is not advised as first-line therapy in pheochromocytoma due to its differential blockade of the alpha and beta receptor.

10.4.5.2 Pharmacologically Mediated Hypertension

Clonidine withdrawal can mimic the crisis of pheochromocytoma. Clonidine is a centrally acting stimulant of α-adrenergic receptors, which reduces peripheral adrenergic system activation. Rapid withdrawal or tapering of therapy of this agent produces a hyperadrenergic state, characterized by hypertension, diaphoresis, headache, and anxiety. The syndrome can be best treated by restarting treatment with clonidine. If the symptoms are extreme, treatment can be initiated as outlined for the patient with pheochromocytoma. Hypertension can also occur during the withdrawal phase of alcohol abuse.

Monamine oxidase (MAO) inhibitors, like phenelzine and tranylcypromine, can be associated with a marked elevation in the systemic arterial blood pressure if the patient consumes foods or medications containing tyramine or other sympathomimetic amines. Tyramine-containing foods include champagne, avocados, smoked or aged meats, and fermented cheeses. The MAO inhibitor interferes with degradation of the tyramine in the intestine, leading to excess absorption and tyramine-induced catecholamine activity in the circulation.

Medications (including metoclopramide, a dopamine agonist; the calcineurin inhibitors cyclosporine and tacrolimus; and drugs of abuse, such as cocaine, phenylpropanolamine, phenylcyclidine, and methamphetamine) must all be considered as possible factors in the intensive care patient with elevated systemic arterial pressure.

Autonomic dysreflexia occurs in spinal cord injury and may manifest as a hypertensive state that follows stimulation of dermatomes and muscles below the level of the spinal cord injury. Patients with hypertension in this setting typically have lesions above the level of the thoracolumbar sympathetic neurons. The blood pressure elevation is believed to result from excess stimulation of sympathetic neurons. The hypertension is accompanied by bradycardia through stimulation of the baroreceptor reflex. Focus treatment on minimizing stimulation and providing medical therapy as necessary. Patients with Guillain-Barre can manifest a similar syndrome.

10.4.6 Miscellaneous Conditions

10.4.6.1 Preeclampsia / Eclampsia

Acute onset, severe systolic ($\geq$ 160 mm Hg) or diastolic ($>$ 110 mm Hg) hypertension can occur in pregnant women or women in the postpartum period. Acute severe hypertension in the second half of gestation may occur in preeclampsia, gestational hypertension, or HELLP (hemolysis, elevated liver enzymes, and low platelet count) syndrome. Preeclampsia/eclampsia remains the second most common cause of maternal death in the United States following thromboembolic disease. Hypertension occurs as one manifestation of preeclampsia in the pregnant patient; the other key features are proteinuria and edema. Severe hypertension, particularly systolic hypertension, in pregnancy can be associated with central nervous system injury, including cerebral infarction and hemorrhage.

When possible, the optimal treatment of preeclampsia is delivery of the fetus, an approach that prevents progression to eclampsia. However, blood pressure should be regulated in order to avoid end-organ damage. The treatment goal is to achieve a range of 140-50/90-100 mm Hg. Close maternal and fetal monitoring are required during the treatment of acute-onset, severe hypertension.[82] Intravenous (IV) labetalol and hydralazine had been considered the first-line medications for the management of severe hypertension in pregnant and postpartum women. More recent guidelines, however, have suggested nifedipine is a safe first-line therapy in pregnancy.[82]

Magnesium sulfate is not an anti-hypertensive agent, but rather is administered for seizure prophylaxis in severe preeclampsia and eclampsia. Avoid sodium nitroprusside (fetal defects), ACE inhibitors (renal dysfunction in fetus), and trimethaphan (meconium ileus) in pregnancy due to associated toxicities.

10.4.6.2 Postoperative Hypertension

Postoperative hypertension, commonly seen in the ICU, occurs most often following vascular surgery procedures in patients with a background history of hypertension. The duration of postoperative hypertensive crisis is often brief (2-6 hours), but untreated hypertension has been linked to postoperative cardiac and renal complications, including bleeding from suture lines, intracerebral hemorrhage, stroke, and left ventricular dysfunction. Hypertension in the postoperative period can be seen in up to 80% of patients post cardiac surgery, and 25% of patients undergoing major noncardiac surgery. Post hoc analysis of the ECLIPSE trials has demonstrated that perioperative systolic blood pressure variability is associated with an increased 30-day mortality and prolonged hospitalization.[83]

Patients with postoperative hypertension must be investigated thoroughly to rule out reversible causes prior to the institution of drug therapy. Factors such as pain, anxiety, hypervolemia, hypoxemia, hypercarbia, and nausea can contribute to postoperative hypertension. Postoperative hypertension is often limited in duration (i.e., 2 to 12 hours), and aggressive attempts to lower blood pressure acutely can lead to delayed hypotension.

A summary of medication use by disease type for patients with hypertensive emergency is outlined in **Figure 10-5**. The treatment algorithm for hypertensive emergency is summarized in **Figure 10-6**.

Organ System	Clinical Manifestation	Suggested Treatment
Cerebrovascular Disease		
	Acute Ischemic Stroke	nicardipine, labetalol
	Acute Intracerebral Hemorrhage	nicardipine, labetalol
Cardiovascular Disease		
	Acute Coronary Syndrome	nitroglycerin
	Acute LV Dysfunction	nitroglycerin, nicardipine
	Acute Aortic Dissection	Beta-blocker followed by nicardipine
	Acute Myocardial Infarction	clevidipine, nicardipine, nitroglycerin
Renovascular Disease		
	Acute Renal Failure	labetalol, nicardipine, nitroglycerin
	Scleroderma renal crisis	ACE inhibitor
Miscellaneous Disorders		
	Pheochromocytoma	phentolamine, labetalol
	Catecholamine toxicity	phentolamine
	Perioperative Hypertension	clevidipine, nicardipine, nitroglycerin
	Preeclampsia or Eclampsia	hydralazine, labetalol

Figure 10-5 *Suggested medications for hypertensive emergency by disease.*

Classify Hypertensive Crisis

• Hypertensive urgency = hypertension without evidence of acute and progressive target organ dysfunction.
• Hypertensive emergency = hypertension with new or progressive organ dysfunction.
• Hypertensive pseudocrisis = hypertension due to transient elevations of blood pressure due to pain or stress.

Initial Assessment

• Evaluate patient for end-organ damage primarily in the cardiac, renal, and CNS organ systems.
• Obtain a careful medication history including substance abuse disorders.
• Use titratable medications for emergent blood pressure reduction in hypertensive emergency conditions.
• Use oral medications for more gradual blood pressure reduction in hypertensive urgency conditions.
• Treat underlying disorder in hypertensive pseudocrisis.

Treatment of Hypertensive Emergency

• Target 10-20% reduction in mean arterial pressure in hypertensive emergency with the possible except of acute stroke.
• Delay treatment of hypertension in acute stroke unless extreme elevation (ie systolic blood pressure > 220 mm Hg or diastolic blood pressure > 120 mm Hg) or use of fibrinolytic medications planned.
• Favor titratable nitroglycerin for acute cardiac conditions including acute coronary syndrome, pulmonary edema, MI.
• Favor titratable nicardipine for acute neurologic conditions including acute stroke and intracerebral hemorrhage.

Figure 10-6 *Treatment algorithm for hypertensive emergency.*

11

Pulmonary Thromboembolic Disease

Massive pulmonary embolism (PE) is a thromboembolic event leading to right heart failure and a drop in cardiac output and blood pressure. Massive PE is defined by a pulmonary embolism producing a symptomatic systolic blood pressure of less than 90 mm Hg for at least 15 minutes or a sustained drop of blood pressure more than 40 mm Hg. Massive PE is a medical emergency with an associated mortality rate as high as 50% even with aggressive therapy. In the International Cooperative Pulmonary Embolism Registry (ICOPER), the 90-day mortality rate for patients with acute PE and systolic blood pressure < 90 mm Hg at presentation (108 patients) was 52.4% vs. 14.7% in the remainder of the cohort.[84] Similarly, in the Management Strategy and Prognosis of Pulmonary Embolism Registry (MAPPET) of 1001 patients with acute PE, in-hospital mortality was 8.1% for hemodynamically stable patients vs. 25% for those presenting with cardiogenic shock and 65% for those requiring cardiopulmonary resuscitation.[85]

To save your patient with massive PE, you must rapidly make the diagnosis, start a stiff dose of heparin, assess risks and benefits of thrombolytic therapy with tissue plasminogen activator (TPA), and consider other interventional or surgical approaches. The use of TPA requires careful consideration of ~ 3% risk of intracranial bleed with TPA, and an even higher risk of death.

11.1 Pathophysiology

Two significant problems will bring a massive PE patient to your intensive care unit:

1. Right heart failure
2. Marked gas exchange abnormality

11.1.1 Right Heart Failure in PE

Acute decompensation of pulmonary hypertension with right heart failure is the same whether caused by pulmonary arterial hypertension (PAH) or massive PE. In the case of PE, > 50% of the pulmonary vasculature must be occluded, or two large lobar pulmonary arteries, to increase the pulmonary artery pressure by the > 40 mm Hg necessary to cause the right ventricle to acutely fail in a previously healthy person.

50% clot occlusion → 40 mm Hg pressure rise → RV failure

As little as a 25% blockage can increase pulmonary artery pressures in a person with co-existing heart or lung disease who already has tenuous RV function, especially chronic lung diseases like COPD or idiopathic pulmonary fibrosis, who have baseline pulmonary hypertension.

The *right heart failure spiral of death is* a vicious cycle initiated by increased pulmonary vascular resistance leading to increased right ventricular afterload → right ventricular dilation and dysfunction with elevated intracardiac pressures → decreased right ventricular cardiac output, which reduces blood filling the left ventricle → enlargement of the right ventricle with septal shift that reduces left ventricular compliance and further prevents filling of the left ventricle → decreased left ventricular cardiac output → increased right

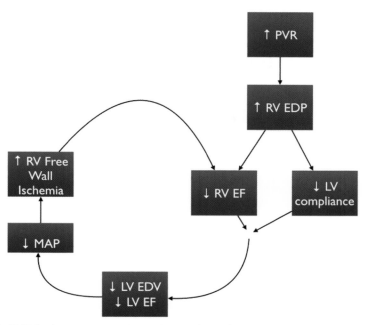

Legend: PVR (pulmonary vascular resistance), RV (right ventricular, LV (left ventricular), EDP (end-diastolic pressure), EDV (end diastolic volume), EF (ejection fraction)

Figure 11-1 *The hemodynamic changes associated with the right heart failure spiral of death. PVR=pulmonary vascular resistance. RV=right ventricle. LV=left ventricle. EDP=end-diastolic pressure. EDV=end-diastolic volume. EF=ejection fraction.*

ventricular wall tension and oxygen consumption (from afterload pressure) coupled with decreased blood flow (cardiac output) to the right ventricular coronary arteries producing ischemia → more right heart failure → all culminating in hypotension and death (**Figure 11-1**).

11.1.2 Gas Exchange in PE

If you think about the physiology, a large clot in a pulmonary artery should block blood flow to normal alveoli and should thus only cause a pure increase in physiologic dead space. This would cause the $PaCO_2$ levels to rise but maintain normal oxygen levels. However, this is not what we see clinically in patients with pulmonary thromboembolic disease. Instead, we most frequently see a low $PaCO_2$ and a low PaO_2. *Why???* The low $PaCO_2$ occurs in association with a characteristic increase in minute ventilation. Patients with pulmonary thromboembolic disease breathe fast to compensate for any dead space effect, and also in response to hypoxia, pain, and chemoreceptor activation. So, hyperventilation overcomes the dead space impact on $PaCO_2$ in pulmonary embolism.

Patients with pulmonary embolism patients frequently have hypoxemia. The drop in PaO_2 is caused by many mechanisms. The blockage of flow in one area results in a redistribution of flow to lower ventilation regions of the lung. Pulmonary hypertension and elevated right heart pressures can augment flow through a patent foramen ovale, creating a R to L shunt. PE may cause direct infarction of the lung, with lung tissue ischemia producing lung injury and edema, again dysregulating V/Q in the affected areas (**Figure 11-2**). Finally, the acute PE activates platelets and creates local red cell hemolysis, releasing platelet-derived vasoconstrictors (such as serotonin, thrombospondin, and thromboxane) and red cell vasoconstrictors (such as arginase 1 and cell-free hemoglobin). These vasoconstrictors further dysregulate V/Q relationship. Any time V and Q are not equal and balanced the oxygenation falls. Low cardiac output results in more peripheral oxygen extraction from hemoglobin and a lower mixed venous hemoglobin oxygen saturation, so now the effect of any V/Q imbalance or shunt will be worsened by a lower venous hemoglobin saturation.

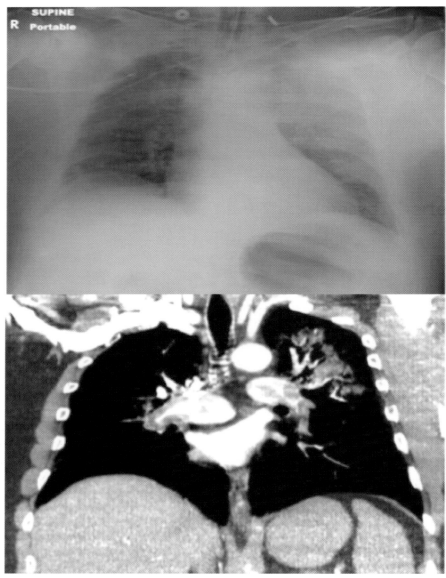

Figure 11-2 *A chest radiograph from a patient with a submassive pulmonary embolism (top image) and infarction of his left upper lobe. The bottom image shows the same patient's CT angiogram with multiple thromboemboli in the main pulmonary arteries and segmental pulmonary arteries that connect with infarcted lung tissue in the left upper lobe. This appearance is referred to as a wedge-shaped infiltrate caused by lung infarction.*

Hypoxia makes everything worse by causing more right ventricular ischemia and by causing hypoxic pulmonary vasoconstriction (back to that spiral – **Figure 11-1**).

11.2 Diagnosis and Risk Stratification

Because of the nonspecific nature of the clinical presentation and the variable therapeutic interventions for treatment, pulmonary thromboembolic disease has been extensively investigated with a broad range of risk stratification models. Risk stratification in pulmonary embolism comes in two flavors: 1) diagnostic risk (i.e., Does your patient have a pulmonary embolism?) and 2) mortality risk (i.e., Does your patient with a PE have a high risk of death?). Let's start with diagnostic risk.

25yo with history of polycystic ovarian syndrome presents to the emergency department complaining of progressive dyspnea on exertion for 6-8 weeks with intermittent *wheezing. She was assessed by her PCP as having asthma and was recently started on an inhaled bronchodilator. She denies any history of prolonged immobilization or lower extremity swelling. She is taking oral contraceptives. She has no family history of a clotting disorder. On presentation to the emergency room, her exam is notable for a HR 108 bpm, RR 32 per min. Her oxygen saturation was recorded at 88% and corrected to 96% with 3L supplemental oxygen. Her electrocardiogram showed sinus tachycardia with an $S_1T_3Q_3$ pattern.*

11.2.1 Diagnostic Risk – PE Clinical Decision Rules

The majority of patients with pulmonary embolism will present in a clinically stable condition, but nonspecific clinical symptoms often characterize the patient history. Therefore, several clinical decision rules (CDR) have been developed to predict the likelihood of pulmonary embolism based on the presenting clinical features. These CDRs can be helpful in stable patients to guide decisions regarding the need for diagnostic testing. Ideally, a CDR, if useful, either alone or in combination with other diagnostic criteria, eliminates the need for additional diagnostic testing in a significant fraction of patients. In the case of pulmonary embolism, CDRs are used to limit patient exposure to unnecessary radiation or contrast exposure.

The two most commonly applied clinical decision rules for patients with suspected pulmonary embolism are the *Wells and Geneva Criteria*. These rules were

developed primarily for outpatients (i.e., emergency room patients).

The Wells rule uses six objective and one subjective criterion, while the Geneva rule uses eight objective criteria (**Figure 11-3 and Figure 11-4**). The original rules have been modified in subsequent reports to minimize calculations for the user.

As an alternative to CDRs, physicians can use "gestalt" estimates, based on their clinical impressions, to identify low-risk patients. The gestalt estimate for the diagnosis of pulmonary thromboembolism has equal sensitivity with a lower specificity for the diagnosis of pulmonary embolism compared to the CDRs.[86]

Either gestalt or CDR-based *low risk* or *PE unlikely* patients can then be assessed with the *Pulmonary Embolism Rule out Criteria (PERC) rule* and a blood test called a *D-dimer*. The PERC criteria use an 8-factor decision rule which can be applied ONLY to *low risk patients* (**Figure 11-5**). If all requirements are met, the patient is considered PERC (-), and no additional diagnostic testing is needed.[87]

D-dimer is a fibrin degradation product, which can be measured in the blood after fibrinolysis degrades a clot. A positive test for D-dimer can have many explanations in addition to ongoing thrombus formation and is considered insufficient for the diagnosis of PE. However, a low D-dimer value (< 500 ng/L) in combination with a low clinical suspicion effectively excludes PE, and, therefore, no further testing is required. In patients with a high clinical suspicion, a negative D-dimer is not

Variables Included in Wells Criteria	
Previous PE or DVT	1.5
Heart rate > 100 beats/ min	1.5
Surgery or Immobilization ($\geq$ 3 days) within 4 weeks	1.5
Hemoptysis	1
Active cancer	1
Clinical symptoms of DVT (leg swelling, pain with palpation)	3
Alternative diagnosis less likely than PE	3
Wells Traditional Probability	
Wells Criteria Traditional Assessment	Wells Score
Low Probability	< 2.0
Moderate Probability	2.0 to 6.0
High Probability	> 6.0
Modified Wells Criteria Assessment	Modified Wells Score
PE Likely	> 4
PE Unlikely	$\leq$ 4

Figure 11-3 Wells criteria for clinical assessment of pulmonary embolism risk.

Variables Included in Modified Geneva Score	
Previous PE or DVT	3
Heart rate 75-94 beats/min	3
Heart rate ≥ 95 beats/min	5
Surgery or fracture within 1 month	2
Hemoptysis	2
Active cancer	2
Unilateral lower limb pain	3
Pain on lower limb deep venous palpation and unilateral edema	4
Age > 65 yo	1
Modified Geneva Score Probability	
Low Probability	0 to 3
Moderate Probability	4 to 10
High Probability	11 to 22

Figure 11-4 Modified Geneva criteria for clinical assessment of pulmonary embolism risk.

PERC Criteria
Age < 50 years
Pulse < 100 beats / min
SaO_2 ≥ 95%
No hemoptysis
No estrogen use
No surgery or trauma requiring hospitalization or intubation in past 4 weeks
No prior venous thromboembolism
No unilateral leg swelling

Figure 11-5 PERC criteria used to further assess patients with a suspected low risk for pulmonary embolism.

helpful, as significant positive diagnostic findings for PE are reported in these patients. Comparative analysis suggests the "PE unlikely patients" identified with any of the clinical decision rules can be combined with a negative D-dimer (< 500 ng/L) to determine a patient group that does not require additional diagnostic evaluation. The D-dimer thresholds for pregnancy are elevated and based upon the trimester.

The CDRs outlined provide a diagnostic approach for the patient when a pulmonary embolism is suspected:

- Use a CDR (Wells or Geneva) or gestalt impression to classify the patient as *PE unlikely* or *PE likely* for a PE diagnosis.
- For patients with a *PE unlikely* probability of PE, PERC criteria should be applied.

- ○ For PERC (-) patients, no further diagnostic testing is indicated.
- ○ Per PERC (+) patients, obtain a D-dimer.
- ○ If D-dimer is < 500 ng/mL, no additional diagnostic imaging is indicated.
- For *PE likely* patients, proceed directly to diagnostic imaging.

Using the CDRs as outlined above, diagnostic testing is reserved for two categories of patients:

1. All patients with clinical symptoms who have a *PE likely* probability
2. Patients with a *PE unlikely* probability of PE but are PERC (+) or with a D-dimer > 500 ng/dL

Our patient was assessed by Geneva and Wells CDRs to be low risk for PE. However, she failed PERC criteria due to her persistent tachycardia and 90% oxygen saturation. A D-dimer was recorded at 735 ng/mL, and she was sent for a CT angiogram to evaluate for possible pulmonary embolism.

For most patients, the computed tomographic pulmonary angiogram (CTPA) will be the procedure of choice, based upon favorable sensitivity and specificity for the diagnosis of pulmonary embolism. A ventilation/ perfusion (V/Q) nuclear imaging study is generally reserved for patients with contraindications to the CTPA (i.e., renal insufficiency or contrast allergy).

A smaller fraction of patients will present hemodynamically unstable. For patients who stabilize after initial resuscitation with a high suspected clinical probability, CTPA remains the diagnostic procedure of choice. *Do not delay treatment waiting for this procedure, however.*

For patients who remain unstable despite resuscitation, a bedside echocardiogram (transthoracic or transesophageal) can be used to confirm right heart dysfunction consistent with a hemodynamically significant PE. If established, severe right heart dysfunction in a shock setting may warrant empiric treatment for PE if the patient cannot be stabilized for a CT angiogram and no alternative diagnosis is likely.

11.2.2 Mortality Risk

In patients with acute pulmonary embolism, mortality risk stratification estimates patient mortality at the time of diagnosis to guide appropriate therapeutic interventions. Risk stratification can identify low-risk patients who might be appropriate for early hospital discharge or even home-based therapy. In contrast, risk

stratification can also help to identify higher-risk patients suitable for more aggressive therapeutic interventions, such as thrombolysis.

The *Pulmonary Embolism Severity Index Score (PESI)* uses clinical parameters to estimate 30-day mortality and has been extensively validated **(Figure 11-6)**.[88] The PESI consists of 11 parameters that are used to stratify patients into five categories of increasing short-term mortality risk. The original PESI score has been modified to a simplified version known as the *sPESI*, which has been equally validated.

The total PESI score is calculated as the patient's age + the points for each applicable predictor. Patients are then divided into specific classes:

- Class I   ≤ 65   Mortality risk 0-1.6 %
- Class II   66-85   Mortality risk 1.7-3.5%
- Class III   86-105   Mortality risk 3.2-7.1%
- Class IV   102-125   Mortality risk 4.0-11.4 %
- Class V   > 125   Mortality risk 10.0-24.5 %

For the sPESI score, patients are grouped into two categories:

- 0 points = 30-day mortality risk of 1.0% (95% CI 0.0%-2.1%)
- > 1 point = 10-day mortality risk of 10.9% (95% CI 8.5%-13.2%)

Patients in PESI Class I and II have a low mortality risk of ~ 2.0% and may be candidates for outpatient therapy or early hospital discharge.

As an alternative to the PESI score, the European Society of Cardiology (ESC) classifies patients with PE based upon the presence or absence of shock on presentation.[89] In this model, *HIGH- RISK PE* presents

Variables Included in PESI and Simplified PESI scores		
Predictors	PESI points	Simplified sPESI points
Age in years	Age in years	1 (if age > 80 years)
Male sex	10	-
History of cancer	10	1
History of heart failure	10	1
History of chronic lung disease	10	1
Pulse > 110 /min	20	1
Systolic blood pressure < 100 mm Hg	30	1
Respiratory rate ≥ 30 / min	20	-
Temperature < 36°C	20	-
Altered mental status	60	-
Arterial oxygen saturation < 90%	20	1

Figure 11-6 Pulmonary Embolism Severity Index Score (PESI) scoring parameters.

with shock, defined by a systolic blood pressure < 90 mm Hg or a drop of > 40 mm Hg for 15 minutes, if not caused by new-onset arrhythmia, hypovolemia, or sepsis. This patient group is at high risk for short-term mortality and frequently requires primary revascularization therapy.

Non-HIGH-RISK PE has a spectrum of severity ranging from patients who present with small asymptomatic PEs, to patients with borderline hypotension that may respond to an initial fluid resuscitation. Echocardiography and humoral biomarkers (troponin and BNP) are frequently utilized in this subgroup to identify an intermediate to higher-risk subgroup within the not-high-risk spectrum that presents with signs of right ventricular overload. The role of primary revascularization in this intermediate-risk group is currently controversial.

The American Heart Association uses a slightly modified version of the ESC criteria:[90]

- *Massive PE* is characterized as a PE associated with sustained hypotension (systolic blood pressure < 90 mm Hg for at least 15 minutes or requiring inotropic support). The hypotension is not due to a cause other than PE, such as arrhythmia, hypovolemia, sepsis, or left ventricular (LV) dysfunction, pulselessness, or persistent profound bradycardia (heart rate <40 bpm with signs or symptoms of shock).
- *Submassive PE* is without systemic hypotension (systolic blood pressure ≥ 90 mm Hg) but with either RV dysfunction or myocardial necrosis. RV dysfunction means the presence of at least one of the following:
  - RV dilation (apical 4-chamber RV diameter divided by LV diameter >0.9) or RV systolic dysfunction on echocardiography
  - RV dilation (4-chamber RV diameter divided by LV diameter >0.9) on CT
  - Elevation of BNP (>90 pg/mL)
  - Elevation of N-terminal pro-BNP (>500 pg/mL)
  - Electrocardiographic changes (new complete or incomplete right bundle branch block, anteroseptal ST elevation or depression, or anteroseptal T-wave inversion)

Myocardial necrosis is defined as either of the following:

  - Elevation of troponin I (>0.4 ng/mL) or
  - Elevation of troponin T (>0.1 ng/mL)
- *Low-Risk PE* is *without* systemic hypotension, normal RV dysfunction on imaging, and normal biomarkers. Short-term mortality rates in this population approach ~ 1%

A critical assessment of the patient with PE, both hemodynamically stable and unstable, is a measure of right ventricular failure or ischemia. *"It's the flow, stupid!"* means that any measure of right heart failure, low cardiac output (flow), and low blood pressure are *BAD* signs.

11.2.2.1 Brain Natriuretic Peptide (BNP) and Troponin Release

The failing right ventricle releases BNP, and elevated levels indicate a poor prognosis in patients with pulmonary thromboembolic disease. Similarly, elevations in troponin indicate right ventricular ischemia and a poor prognosis. High levels suggest that you are at high risk of right heart failure and should consider more aggressive therapy (more on this later).

11.2.2.2 Doppler-Echocardiography

Some patients with PE will show echocardiographic evidence for right ventricular dilation, dysfunction, paradoxical septal motion, high tricuspid regurgitant jet velocity, and sometimes even a clot extending backward into the right ventricle. RV dysfunction identified by echo is associated with an elevated short-term mortality risk in patients without hemodynamic instability. *McConnell's sign* is a finding more specific for right ventricular failure in the setting of massive PE. This is a pattern of right ventricular mid-wall hypokinesis but normal motion at the apex of the heart.

11.2.2.3 CT Pulmonary Angiogram

A CT scan with rapid image acquisition timed with intravenous contrast injection can give an excellent study of the pulmonary arteries and show clots and RV size. This study has good sensitivity and specificity compared to traditional pulmonary artery angiography, especially for segmental PEs. These studies will show the contrast in the pulmonary arteries and a black flow void within them. This suggests PE if the black flow void is seen in more than one cut following the internal course of a vessel with contrast-enhanced blood above and below the void. A meniscus of contrast-enhanced blood along the side of the flow void is particularly supportive of the PE diagnosis. A variety of terms are used to describe images from the CT angiogram. A *saddle embolus* refers to a large pulmonary embolism that straddles the bifurcation of the pulmonary arteries, extending into the left and right pulmonary arteries **(Figure 11-7)**.

Although dramatic in appearance, the designation as a "saddle" embolus has no specific prognostic value or therapeutic need for the patient's management independent of the effect of that embolus on right heart function.

Other common radiographic terms to describe pulmonary emboli are *segmental (SPE)* and *subsegmental*

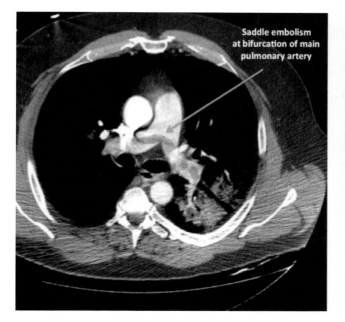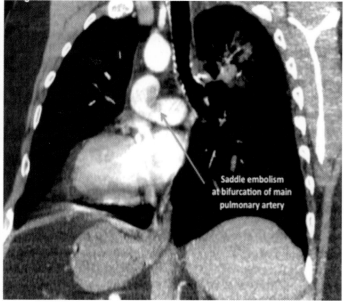

IMAGE A   IMAGE B

Figure 11-7 illustrates a "saddle" PE with a large thrombus extending across the bifurcation of the pulmonary artery in the cross-sectional (Image A) and sagittal projections (Image B).

pulmonary emboli (SSPE). The segmental and subsegmental pulmonary arteries parallel the segmental and subsegmental bronchi, running along their course. In contrast, the pulmonary veins course independent of the bronchi within the intralobular septa. There is a high concordance between radiologists in the identification of the more proximal SPE and a consensus for treatment **(Figure 11-8)**. In contrast, the more distal SSPE create a greater disagreement rate amongst radiologists with a concordance rate of ~ 70% **(Figure 11-9)**. The need for treatment of isolated subsegmental emboli in all cases remains controversial.[91]

In addition to the clot burden, examine your CT for evidence of right ventricular enlargement and vascular overload due to the clot obstruction. How do you know the right ventricle (RV) is big? Because the RV diameter is usually much less than the LV diameter. A ratio of the RV/LV of > 0.9 using a four-chamber view on echocardiography or CT imaging is an adverse prognostic sign **(Figure 11-10)**. Additional vascular enlargement of the RA, PA, SVC, and IVC are also confirmatory of acute right heart dysfunction **(Figure 11-11)**.

The patient's CT angiogram showed acute pulmonary thromboembolism extending from both main pulmonary arteries into the segmental and subsegmental arteries of all lobes. She demonstrated an RLL wedge-shaped pulmonary infiltrate consistent with a pulmonary infarction. She had evidence of right heart strain with RV5 LV dimensions.

Contrast reflux to the hepatic veins and inferior vena cava was noted. Her BNP was measured at 258 pg/mL, and her troponin was , 0.10 ng/dL . Let's move on to treatment.

11.3 Treatment of Massive PE

The treatment of massive PE is very similar to the suggested approach for the critically ill patient with pulmonary arterial hypertension and right heart failure, but in the case of PE we want to try and lyse the clot rather than give pulmonary vasodilator therapy. A treatment protocol for massive PE is shown in **Figure 11-12**. Note that many of these therapies and consultations are initiated at the same time to save lives.

While you are diagnosing and risk-stratifying your PE using BNP, troponins, Doppler-echocardiography and CT-angiogram, you will also be stabilizing the patient's hemodynamics (cardiac output and blood pressure) and gas exchange (oxygenation and ventilatory support if needed).

11.3.1 *Oxygenate and Ventilate*

Titrate face-mask oxygen or CPAP as needed to reduce work of breathing and increase oxygenation. Like severe PAH, intubation is very risky as the drugs will drop blood pressure and inhibit adrenaline surges that are maintaining blood pressure. If you have to intubate, use anesthesia with limited cardio-depressive effects and a short half-life (i.e., ketamine).

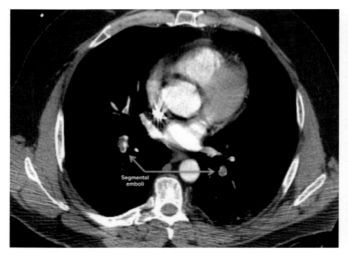

Figure 11-8 *Proximal segmental pulmonary emboli in right and left lower lobes (arrows)*

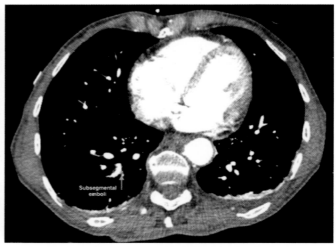

Figure 11-9 *Subsegmental pulmonary emboli in distal right lobe (arrow)*

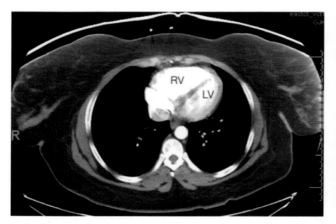

Figure 11-10 *CT imaging shows right ventricle (RV) to left ventricle (LV) ratio > 0.9.*

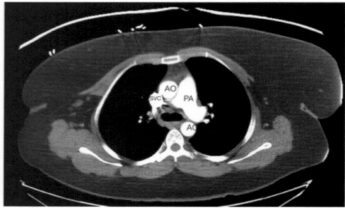

Figure 11-11 *CT imaged with enlarged pulmonary artery (PA) and superior vena cava (SVC) consistent with right heart dysfunction. AO= aorta.*

11.3.2 Optimize RV Cardiac Output

Patients with a massive PE may respond to a fluid bolus, especially if the central venous pressure is low (< 12 mm Hg). The fluid bolus should be limited in steps of 250-500 mL so as not to produce more right heart stress. If the patient is persistently hypotensive, norepinephrine is the favored vasopressor agent to provide both β1- and α1-receptor stimulation. An inotrope, such as dobutamine can be used for right ventricular inotropic support if the blood pressure is not too low. Inhaled vasodilator agents such as NO or prostacyclin therapy can be used but remain investigational.

11.3.3 Reduce RV Afterload with Anticoagulation

Start heparin fast and hard! If you even think of the PE diagnosis, start it, don't worry about complications (you

are going to do worse things soon), and give a stiff dose. Large volumes of the clot will suck up the heparin, so you need a reliable weight-based dose: Use real body weight and give 80U/kg bolus and 18 U/kg/hour, titrate to PTT> 80 seconds. Heparin works because it prevents new clots from forming while the body's natural fibrinolytic system (TPA) lyses the clot. For patients with heparin-induced thrombocytopenia (HIT), a non-heparin-based anticoagulant, such as lepirudin, argatroban, or bivalirudin, should be used.

11.3.4 To Lyse or Not to Lyse

To remember the steps to consider, think of the new *Hip-Hop Clot Rap: "Bust a move."* Imagine a team of doctors around a patient with a PE and blood pressure less than 90 mm Hg on the monitor. One doctor holds an IV bag with 100 mg TPA written on the side, another one has a suction catheter, behind him is the

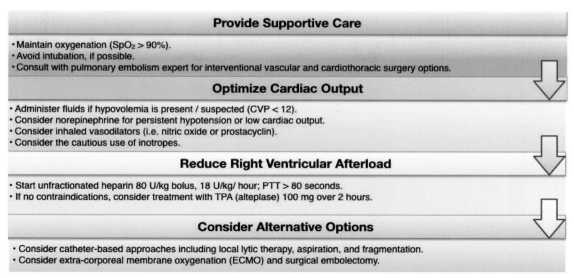

Provide Supportive Care

- Maintain oxygenation (SpO$_2$ > 90%).
- Avoid intubation, if possible.
- Consult with pulmonary embolism expert for interventional vascular and cardiothoracic surgery options.

Optimize Cardiac Output

- Administer fluids if hypovolemia is present / suspected (CVP < 12).
- Consider norepinephrine for persistent hypotension or low cardiac output.
- Consider inhaled vasodilators (i.e. nitric oxide or prostacyclin).
- Consider the cautious use of inotropes.

Reduce Right Ventricular Afterload

- Start unfractionated heparin 80 U/kg bolus, 18 U/kg/ hour; PTT > 80 seconds.
- If no contraindications, consider treatment with TPA (alteplase) 100 mg over 2 hours.

Consider Alternative Options

- Consider catheter-based approaches including local lytic therapy, aspiration, and fragmentation.
- Consider extra-corporeal membrane oxygenation (ECMO) and surgical embolectomy.

Figure 11-12 *Treatment algorithm for massive pulmonary embolism.*

cardiopulmonary bypass pump and a surgeon with a scalpel ready to crack the chest. They are all singing the *Hip-Hop Clot Rap: "Lyse it - suck it - pump it - crack it. Lyse it—suck it—pump it—crack it. Lyse it—suck it— pump it—crack it… Bust a move, bust a clot, bust a move, bust a clot…."*

11.3.4.1 Thrombolysis

The goal of this therapy is to rapidly reduce pulmonary vascular resistance, pressure, and RV strain; increase right ventricular cardiac output and systemic perfusion; and try to minimize clot burden that could lead to future chronic thromboembolic pulmonary hypertension. If you have a massive PE, defined by low or dropping systolic blood pressure (<90 mm Hg) with proven PE, all current guidelines recommend giving thrombolytic therapy if there are no absolute contraindications. On the other hand, the use of thrombolytics for all PEs (including non-massive) has NOT been shown to improve mortality in a meta-analysis and will lead to intracranial hemorrhage in up to 3% of patients.[92] A subgroup analysis of all trials restricted to only massive PE shows a significant reduction in recurrent PE or death from 19.0% with heparin alone to 9.4% with fibrinolysis. So, if you have a *massive PE*, you must first review the absolute and relative contraindications to giving thrombolytics, outlined in **Figure 11-13**. If there are no contraindications, you should talk to the patient and family about risks of intracranial hemorrhage, balanced by the risk of death, and then give the therapy.

Why take the risk? The reason to consider giving a clot buster is that patients treated with a fibrinolytic agent have faster restoration of lung perfusion. For example, by 24 hours patients treated with only heparin have no substantial improvement in pulmonary blood flow, whereas patients treated with a fibrinolytic drug have a 30% reduction in the perfusion defect. The more rapid clot lysis is probably why survival appears to improve in the subgroup of PE patients who have massive PE.

So why not give the drug to everyone? Well, by seven days, the blood flow improves similarly in all groups with an approximate 70% reduction in the total perfusion defect. Thrombolytics, therefore, do not improve survival for all patients with PE. We only give these drugs, which carry a high risk of serious complications, to patients who cannot afford to wait seven days for a therapeutic effect on heparin alone. These are the patients who have low blood pressure and right heart failure.

Once you decide to "pull the trigger" and administer thrombolytics the protocol is quite easy: A) Hold the heparin, B) give 100 mg of TPA (alteplase) as an infusion over 2 hours, C) check PTT every 4 hours and restart heparin when it drops below 60 seconds. Now you say your prayers. 8% of patients do not respond, up to 3% have an intracranial bleed, and 21% have a major bleed. Your hot potato can easily go out of the frying pan and into the fire!

Note that all fibrinolytic drugs approved by the US Food and Drug Administration (FDA) are enzymes that convert or activate the patient's native circulating plasminogen into plasmin (thus, *tissue plasminogen activator*). Plasmin is a serine protease that cleaves fibrin at several sites, liberating fibrin-split products, including the D-dimer fragment, thus dissolving the clot.

Absolute and Relative Contraindications to Thrombolytics for PE

Absolute Contraindications
   • Active internal bleeding
   • Recent spontaneous intracranial bleeding
   • Recent intracranial or ocular surgery
Relative Contraindications
   • Age > 75 years
   • Major surgery, delivery of baby, organ biopsy, puncture of non-compressible vessel in last 10 days
   • GI bleeding in last 10 days
   • Ischemic stroke in last 2 months
   • Serious trauma in last 15 days
   • Neurosurgery or eye surgery in last 1 month
   • Recent cardiopulmonary resuscitation with chest compressions
   • Platelet count <100,000
   • Pregnancy
   • Bacterial endocarditis
   • Diabetic hemorrhagic retinopathy

Figure 11-13 Contraindications to thrombolytic therapy in the treatment of pulmonary embolism.

11.3.4.2 Contraindication to Systemic Thrombolysis?

This will be your most challenging situation. You can assess your risk of death (based on blood pressure, measures of RV dysfunction, high BNP and troponin), and weigh these against your risk of major bleeding and stroke. Frank discussions with patient and family are critical. This group of patients may also benefit from alternative procedures with a lower risk of bleeding. The alternative procedures, such as catheter-based procedures, have limited outcome information from clinical trials about efficacy and safety,. Similar to thrombolytic therapy, the goals of these catheter-based therapies are to rapidly reduce pulmonary vascular resistance, pressure, and RV strain; increase right ventricular cardiac output and systemic perfusion; and try to minimize clot burden that could lead to future chronic thromboembolic pulmonary hypertension. Several procedures are available to consider.

11.3.4.3 Catheter-Directed Thrombolytics

Lyse it! A catheter is placed directly upstream or into the clot, and low dose TPA is infused at 0.5 - 1 mg per hour. Smaller randomized studies suggest that this works with a significantly lower risk of systemic thrombolysis and CNS bleeding rates of < 0.2%.

11.3.4.4 Catheter-Based Embolectomy

Suck it, roto-rooter it, blast it. New devices use aspiration via suction to pull out the clot, fragmentation via balloon angioplasty, pigtail rotational or impeller mechanical disruption (roto-rooters), or rheolytic fluid jet disruption of the clot. The rheolytic fluid method involves the introduction of a pressurized saline jet stream through the directed orifices in a catheter distal tip. This creates a mechanical effect to remove removing the clot debris into an evacuation lumen. In a systematic review of available cohort data comprising a total of 348 patients, clinical success with catheter-based therapy alone for patients with acute massive PE was 81% (aspiration thrombectomy 81%; fragmentation 82%; rheolytic thrombectomy 75%) and 95% when combined with local infusions of thrombolytic.[93] There are limited available randomized trials to compare these therapies to heparin alone or thrombolytics, so clinicians must use their best judgment.

11.3.4.5 ECMO and Direct Surgical Thromboembolectomy

The most aggressive step involves placing the patient on *extracorporal membrane oxygenation (ECMO)*, cracking the chest, and surgically extracting the clot in a procedure called *surgical thromboembolectomy*. It should be mentioned that anticoagulation with heparin is still required during this procedure. **Figure 11-14** reveals a case of sub-massive saddle pulmonary embolism diagnosed by CT pulmonary angiogram with a large saddle embolism, which looks like a horse saddle straddling the bifurcation of the main pulmonary artery and going down into the right and left main pulmonary arteries and segmental pulmonary arteries. This case destabilized despite thrombolytic therapy and required emergent extracorporeal membrane oxygenation and bypass surgery to remove the clots (**Figure 11-15**).

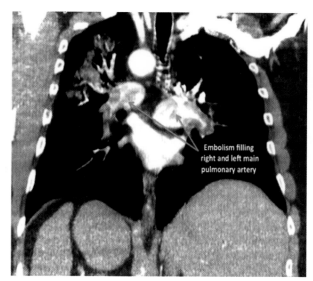

Figure 11-14 *Pulmonary embolism filling right and left main pulmonary arteries (arrows).*

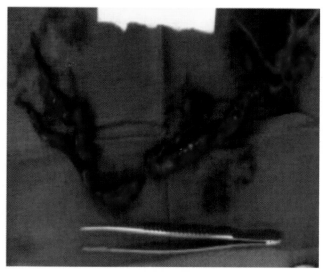

Figure 11-15. *Clot removed from patient in Figure 11-14 at surgical embolectomy.*

11.4 Treatment of Submassive PE

Data from PE registry studies indicate that the short-term mortality rate directly attributable to submassive PE treated with heparin anticoagulation is probably < 3.0%. Thus, even if adjunctive fibrinolytic therapy had extremely high efficacy, the effect size on mortality due to submassive PE would be minimal. For this reason, the main reason to consider lytic therapy for submassive PE is to reduce bad secondary outcomes, such as persistent right heart failure, chronic thromboembolic pulmonary hypertension (CTEPH), and shortness of breath. Studies vary in their reporting but estimate a significant fraction of patients with submassive PE demonstrate persistent RV dysfunction and exercise limitation post treatment with anticoagulation alone. Treatment of submassive PE with TPA (alteplase) reduced estimated pulmonary systolic pressures and improved 6-minute walk distance and dyspnea scores at 6-month follow-up.[94] Based on this limited data, the decision to use thrombolytics for patients with submassive PE requires clinicians to use their best clinical judgment. The risks of bleeding must be weighed against evidence of impending respiratory or circulatory collapse.[95]

A few tidbits of important clinical information can be pulled from the limited available clinical trials. Patients at highest risk of intracranial hemorrhage are frequently > 70 years of age, suggesting a much safer profile in younger patients. Secondly, patients more likely to decompensate have higher respiratory rates, suggesting that this could be used to stratify patients at higher risk. We currently reserve intravenous systemic thrombolysis for patients with hypotension (massive PE) or submassive PE with signs of right ventricular strain with positive biomarkers (troponin and BNP) and respiratory distress and age less than 70 years. We continue to be aggressive about using catheter-based lysis for other patients in this submassive category, since most studies indicate a low risk of hemorrhagic stroke (0.2%) and faster thrombolysis.

It will be critical to follow these patients up at two years to determine if early thrombolysis reduces the risk of late chronic thromboembolic pulmonary hypertension and respiratory decline.

Figure 11-16 outlines our current approach to PE therapy for low-risk PE, submassive PE with RV strain, and massive PE. Patients with low-risk PE (submassive without RV strain) are treated with heparin anticoagulation. Patients with massive PE are evaluated for fibrinolysis as primary therapy based upon assessment of the risk:benefit profile. Patients with submassive PE with RV strain are assessed for signs that suggest higher risk. Persistent respiratory distress, intermittent shock, younger age, or prolonged time to interventional radiology (IR) are all indications to proceed to systemic lytic therapy. The shock index (SI) refers to the heart rate in beats per minute divided by systolic blood pressure in millimeters of mercury (a value >1 is bad). Patients with these high-risk features are evaluated for systemic lysis. Alternatively, for all other submassive populations, we consider a role for catheter-based therapy.

Our patient did not manifest overt shock, but her exam was notable for persistent tachycardia without hypotension. Her PESI score was calculated at 85 points

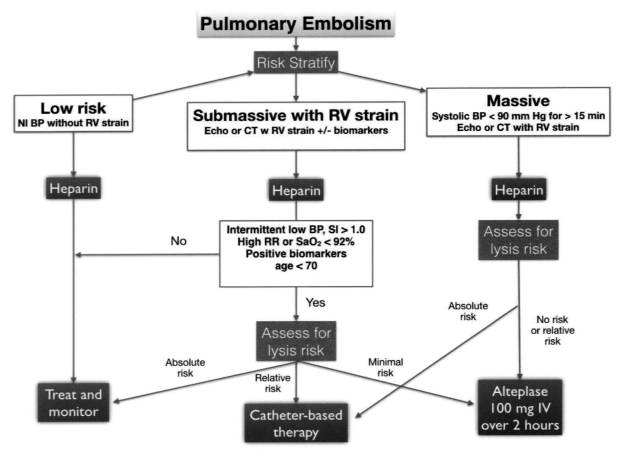

Figure 11-16 *Treatment algorithm for pulmonary embolism.*

or Class II (low risk 1.7-3.5% 30-day mortality). She received IV heparin bolus in the emergency room and was admitted for continued monitoring. She underwent a bedside echo with findings of right ventricular hypokinesis with preserved apical function (McConnell's sign). She remained hemodynamically stable after admission, and her tachycardia promptly resolved. The patient was assessed as a submassive PE by echocardiogram with 1 of 2 unfavorable biomarkers. After consideration of the risk:benefit variable for thrombolytic therapy, the patient and her physicians elected to treat with heparin. Four days following admission and therapy with heparin, her right ventricular dysfunction had resolved.

Suggested Reading

- Rali PM, Criner GJ. Submassive pulmonary embolism. Am J Respir Crit Care Med [Internet] 2018;198:588–598

12

Basic Airway Management

The management of the difficult airway is an advanced skill often left to anesthesiologists, intensivists, or otolaryngologists. But the basic skills are needed for all patients and should be a fundamental component in your toolbox. Your initial focus should be on stabilizing the airway and ventilation status with less focus on getting a "tube" in. If you do the steps right, the patient will remain stable and the "tube" will go in safely.

A ventilatory effort in the absence of airflow suggests airway obstruction. In the conscious patient, this frequently occurs from a foreign body in the airway, most often related to eating. Foreign body airway obstruction requires prompt resolution and relief. If mild obstruction is present, do not interfere with the patient's spontaneous coughing and breathing efforts. The rescuer should attempt to relieve the obstruction only if a severe obstruction is present, suggested by progression to a silent cough, respiratory difficulty with stridor, or the victim becomes unresponsive. For responsive adults and children >1 year of age, back blows or "slaps," abdominal thrusts, and chest thrusts are all effective. More than one technique may be needed. Abdominal thrusts should be applied first unless the patient is < 1 year of age, too obese to allow appropriate positioning, or pregnant. If not effective or possible, the rescuer should move from abdominal to chest thrusts to relieve the airflow obstruction.

In contrast, the complete absence of ventilatory effort is consistent with a respiratory system arrest in the unconscious patient. Immediate airway management will be needed to establish a patent airway with assisted bag-mask ventilation and progression to intubation.

12.1 Establish a Patent Airway with Ventilation

Is the patient a victim of trauma? Does the patient have a history of rheumatoid arthritis or ankylosing spondylitis? These questions are essential to consider in the setting of airway management to avoid aggravating an existing cervical spine injury with airway maneuvers.

Two maneuvers are used to provide a patent airway in the unconscious patient, and these maneuvers should be familiar to all health care personnel working in a hospital:

1. The *head tilt-chin lift (HT-CL) maneuver* is the primary maneuver used in any patient in whom cervical spine injury is NOT a concern (**Figure 12-1, left panel**). In this technique, the clinician uses two hands to extend the patient's neck and open the airway. While one hand applies downward pressure to the patient's forehead, the tips of the index and middle finger of the second hand lift the mandible at the mentum, which lifts the tongue from the posterior pharynx.

2. The *jaw thrust (JT) maneuver* has the clinician standing at the head of the bed. The technique is performed by placing the heels of both hands on the parieto-occipital areas on each side of the patient's head, then grasping the angles of the

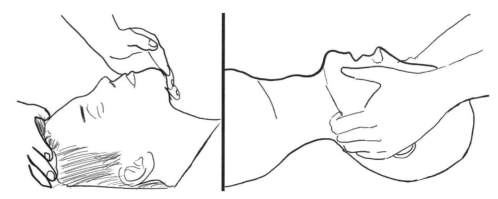

Figure 12-1 *Two maneuvers to achieve a patent airway in an unconscious patient. Left = head tilt-chin lift. Right = jaw thrust (JT) maneuver.*

mandible with the index and long fingers, and displacing the jaw anteriorly (**Figure 12-1,** right panel). The jaw thrust is considered the safer maneuver in the setting of a suspected neck injury because, when correctly performed, it can generally be accomplished without extending the neck. However, all maneuvers can provide a risk of cervical spine injury in the susceptible patient, so cervical spine immobilization is indicated for the jaw-thrust maneuver when cervical spine injury is suspected.

The HT-CL and JT maneuvers are supplemented by the use of artificial airways when necessary. Both oropharyngeal (OPA) and nasopharyngeal airways (NPA) can help maintain or accomplish a patent airway. For the semiconscious or arousable patient with intact protective reflexes, nasopharyngeal airways are preferred due to the risk of gagging or vomiting with OPAs (**Figure 12-2,** right panel). Also use NPAs when the patient has a limited airway opening or clenched jaw. Consider an OPA in any unconscious patient with absent protective reflexes (**Figure 12-2,** left panel). Both airways come in variable sizes. The appropriate airway size is determined by externally measuring the distance between the specific airway opening (nose or mouth) and mandible in the patient. Insert the OPA by starting with the curve of the OPA inverted (i.e., directed cephalad) or aimed laterally. The airway is rotated appropriately as its tip reaches the posterior pharynx. If there are problems ventilating the patient after insertion, the OPA should be removed and reinserted. If ventilation problems persist, the clinician should verify the size of the airway.

Coat the NPA with a water-soluble lubricant or anesthetic jelly prior to insertion. Insert the device along the floor of the naris into the posterior pharynx behind the tongue. The floor of the naris inclines in a caudad

orientation only approximately 15 degrees. The tube can be slightly rotated if resistance is encountered. The most common complications of NPA insertion include nasal mucosal bleeding (up to 30% of patients) and using an airway that is too long; this may cause the tip to enter the esophagus, increasing gastric distention and decreasing ventilation during rescue efforts.

Often the clinician with limited airway experience fails to implement the most critical phase of preintubation care, which is a patent airway and adequate bag-mask ventilation. *All care providers in a hospital should acquire this skill.* Effective bag-mask ventilation can be used to stabilize a patient for long intervals until more experienced personnel can get to the bedside.

Once an effective airway has been accomplished, the patient is assisted with bag-mask ventilation. The mask should be carefully positioned to cover the bridge of the nose but avoid allowing ventilation on the eyes. Establish a firm seal across the malar eminences and the mandibular alveolar ridge in addition to the nasal bridge. Accomplish bag-mask ventilation using a single-hand or two-hand technique.

The single-hand technique requires only one individual. Place one hand on the mask, with the web space between the thumb and index finger resting against the mask connector (**Figure 12-3, left panel**). The other three fingers (i.e., middle, ring, and little) are placed along the mandible and pull the mandible up into the mask in a chin-lift maneuver, allowing the airway to open further. Those with larger hands can put the little finger posterior to the angle of the mandible and perform a jaw-thrust, although this is tiring to the hand. Lift the mandible to the mask with the middle, ring, and little fingers, while holding the mask tightly against the patient's face with the thumb and index finger.

The two-hand technique requires two personnel to accomplish bag-mask ventilation but is considered the more effective technique. The two-hand technique

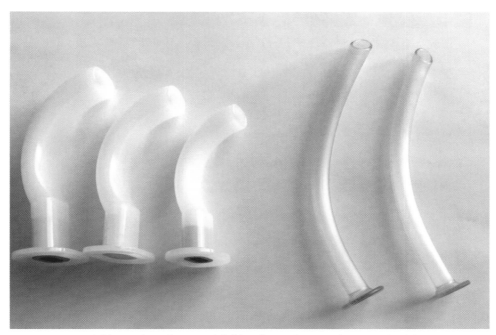

Figure 12-2 *Variably sized oropharyngeal (left) and nasopharyngeal airways (right).*

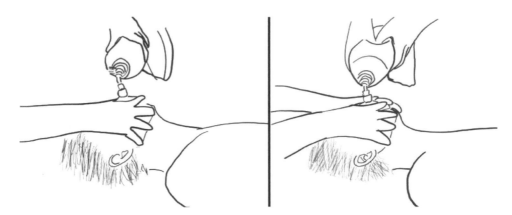

Figure 12-3 *Bag-mask assisted ventilation using a one hand (left panel) or two hand (right panel) technique.*

(**Figure 12-3,** right panel) is used when the single-hand technique is not effective. One provider uses both hands to create a good mask seal and to maintain an open airway. Another provider squeezes the bag to ventilate the patient. The thenar eminences are positioned parallel to each other along the long axis of each side of the mask, allowing the four remaining fingers to provide a chin-lift and jaw-thrust maneuver.

Failure to achieve sufficient ventilation with the two-hand technique, as reflected by a lack of chest rise or persistent airflow obstruction, should prompt the provider to:

- Reassess proper positioning and size of the nasal or oropharyngeal airway
- Reassess mask seal and consider KY jelly or water applied to improve the seal; edentulous patients should have their false teeth reinserted if necessary to accomplish a better seal
- Reassess airway maneuvers to achieve a patent airway

Provide bag-mask ventilation with a tidal volume just large enough to make the chest rise. Large tidal volumes should be avoided, and the bag should not be squeezed

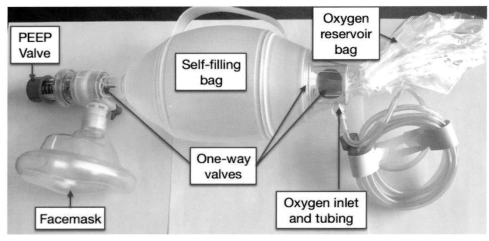

Figure 12-4 *Bag-mask components.*

explosively. Smaller tidal volumes and flow rates are favored to reduce the likelihood of creating sufficient pressure to open the gastroesophageal sphincter or to produce markedly increased intrathoracic pressures, which compromise both coronary and cerebral perfusion pressures. A standard bag-mask system is shown in **Figure 12.4.**

12.2 Clinical Clues for a Difficult Intubation

The management of the airway in the emergent ICU setting is very different than the more elective anesthesia setting. Complication rates are much higher, preoxygenation is less effective, and drug administration is associated with hypotension and arrhythmia in critically ill patients.

You must anticipate the physiologic changes that can occur with the transition from spontaneous ventilation to invasive mechanical ventilation. These changes occur in three major categories:

1. *Oxygenation issues.* Maintaining oxygenation with the transition to invasive mechanical ventilation will require both preoxygenation and maintaining saturation during the period of apnea.
2. *Ventilation issues.* Carefully consider ventilation for the patient with a metabolic acidosis that is being "compensated" with augmented ventilation. Your patient with Kussmaul respirations in the setting of DKA may be ventilating very well! Your transition to mechanical ventilation may decrease the patient's total effective alveolar ventilation and compromise his or her acid-base status.
3. *Hemodynamic issues.* Patients at high risk for post-intubation hypotension will often have underlying

conditions associated with volume depletion (collapsible IVC). Pre-intubation hypotension is a strong predictor of an adverse hemodynamic response to intubation.

ICU intubations are classified into three categories:

1. *Crash Intubation.* This includes the cardiorespiratory arrest patient or the patient with a rapid decline in cardiopulmonary status. The patient has limited cardiovascular or respiratory activity and is unlikely to respond to laryngeal stimulation. Airway management proceeds rapidly often without the need for induction medication. The time for careful assessment of risk is not available.
2. *Rapid Sequence Intubation (RSI).* This patient is adequately oxygenating with supplemental oxygen and is not judged to be a problematic bag-mask ventilation (BVM) or intubation. Endotracheal intubation proceeds after administration of induction and paralytic medications simultaneously. Preoxygenation may occur without bag-mask ventilation in a spontaneously breathing patient with high-flow oxygen administration or non-invasive mechanical ventilation.
3. *Difficult Intubation.* Several clinical clues suggest airway management will involve difficulties. Cautious use of induction and paralytic agents is employed to support spontaneous respirations until successful intubation is assured. These patients may be a candidate for an awake intubation.

The initial step in preparation for intubation, if time allows, is an airway history, physical exam, and review of available records whenever feasible. Conduct the airway exam even if only a quick and cursory examination is possible. This assessment attempts to predict difficulty with bag-mask ventilation, orotracheal intubation, and/or patient cooperation and consent. The examination may reveal anatomic variations of the face, the presence of a beard, significant obesity, or limited cervical spine mobility, all of which suggest the possibility of a difficult intubation.

Assess for potential difficulty with mask ventilation. Difficult mask ventilation is seen with Mallampati Class III or IV airways (see below); prior neck radiation; a history of obstructive sleep apnea; a short, thick neck; and the presence of a beard. Edentulous patients are also considered difficult to ventilate, and dentures can remain in during the period of bag-mask ventilation and then removed for intubation. Bag-mask ventilation often improves in edentulous patients if the mask is moved to the lower lip.

The Mallampati classification (**Figure 12-5**) is used to describe the oropharyngeal cavity size. This classification divides the airway into four categories based on the appearance of the posterior pharynx. Class I and II Mallampati classification is usually associated with an easier laryngoscopy.

The Mallampati classification is sensitive but not specific for airway complications. So the score should be considered with additional assessments of the airway.

- Size of the airway opening graded as good with > 3 cm fingerbreadths
- Thyromental distance graded favorably if three fingerbreadths **(Figure 12-6)**
- Hyoid to thyroid distance graded favorably as two fingerbreadths
- Assess mandibular protrusion
- Assess cervical mobility

During your anatomic assessment, identification and palpation of the cricothyroid membrane is advised in the event a subglottic airway management strategy becomes necessary.

The presence of severe cardiopulmonary disease will compromise tissue oxygen delivery during bag-valve mask ventilation. Hypoxemia occurs especially in patients with shunt physiology (borderline PaO_2 on FiO_2 = 1.0). Even with adequate preoxygenation, the time from apnea to oxygen desaturation (SpO_2 < 90%) can be short in these patients. Morbid obesity is also associated

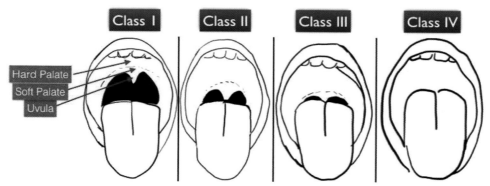

Figure 12-5 *The modified Mallampati score to predict the ease of endotracheal intubation.*

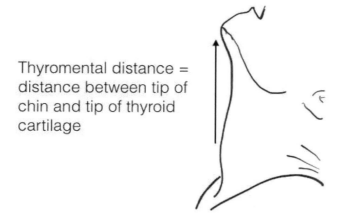

Thyromental distance = distance between tip of chin and tip of thyroid cartilage

Figure 12-6 *Illustration of the thyromental distance measurement.*

with decreased time from apnea to desaturation when the patient is placed in the supine position. Obesity creates a restricted residual capacity from compression on the lung volume by abdominal obesity. The time to desaturation is a critical component to consider in the analysis of the difficult airway.

Although many algorithms exist to predict a difficult airway, up to 90% of difficult airways are not anticipated. During your bedside assessment, you are asking three questions:

1. Will this patient be difficult to bag-mask ventilate?
2. Will this patient be difficult to intubate?
3. Will this patient be difficult to rescue if the initial intubation attempt fails?

Patients with multiple unsuccessful attempts at intubation (>3) have a significant incidence of cardiac arrest (2%) and a very high rate of desaturation, frequently require a surgical airway, and have a very high rate of gastric intubation. *Best to plan a maximum of 2 attempts at laryngoscopy, and if unsuccessful, move to Plan B or C or D!*

12.3 Key Steps to a Successful Airway

- Have two individuals present and preferably one with experience.
- Use induction medications judiciously in the setting of hypotension.
- Do not paralyze until you are sure you can mask-ventilate the patient.
- Have readily available instruments for advanced airway management.
- Use NIV and have nasal oxygen administration available for preoxygenation.
- In difficult airways, consider an awake intubation with topical anesthesia to avoid sedatives until the airway is secure.
- Have push dose vasopressors readily available to address post-intubation hypotension.
- Initiate positive pressure ventilation carefully to avoid hemodynamic compromise.

12.4 Endotracheal Intubation

Intubation in most patients is approached using a *Rapid Sequence Intubation (RSI)* to overcome the patient's gag reflex. The RSI technique involves the simultaneous administration of a rapidly acting sedative (induction) and neuromuscular blocking agent (paralytic). The primary goal is to minimize the risk of stomach content aspiration. Two significant contraindications to RSI include:

- *Crash (Arrest) Intubation.* Intubation in the unresponsive patient with absent or compromised cardiopulmonary function
- *Difficult Intubation.* Intubation in the patient with a high-risk airway when mask ventilation is expected to be difficult

In the Crash airway, the patient's gag reflex is absent, and the delay associated with medication administration is not likely to facilitate the procedure. On occasion, a high dose of neuromuscular blocking agent (i.e., 2mg/kg of succinylcholine) is administered to overcome muscle rigidity in this patient group. Patients with impaired mentation but intact cardiopulmonary function do not fit this category. These patients may suffer from an intracranial process. In these patients, RSI is still preferred to avoid adverse reflexes that might further increase intracranial pressure.

In the difficult airway patient, maintaining spontaneous ventilation by avoiding the use of a paralytic agent is preferred. If assessment suggests a problematic intubation or difficult bag-mask ventilation is expected, then alternatives to RSI (such as awake intubation with light or moderate sedation, or the use of topical anesthesia only) may be preferred.

Modifications to the RSI approach for intubation are discussed extensively in the emergency medicine and ICU literature.

Delayed Sequence Intubation refers to the use of induction agents with an attempt to preserve ventilation and airway reflexes.[96] This is followed by a brief period of preoxygenation before the administration of the paralytic agent. Consider this technique in the highly agitated patient with borderline oxygenation status. Uncoupling induction and paralysis allows preoxygenation and appropriate patient positioning and preparation. Favored sedative agents for this technique include ketamine (dissociative dose of ~ 1 mg/kg with repeat dosing of 0.5 mg/kg to goal) and dexmedetomidine (1 mcg/kg over 10 minutes).

Rapid Sequence Airway is similar to RSI but replaces the endotracheal tube with an extraglottic airway.[97] The patient receives an immediate induction and paralytic agent identical to RSI. The presumption is that the extraglottic airway will be easier and more efficient to place. This technique is described in EMS service delivery more frequently than ICU environments.

Awake Intubation avoids the induction and paralytic agent to maintain spontaneous ventilation.[98] This technique also allows the patient to be intubated in the upright position. Aggressive use of topical anesthesia is combined with the use of video laryngoscopy or fiberoptic bronchoscopy to allow an awake intubation. This technique is reserved for patients with very high-risk airways.

12.4.1 The Tools

Preparation for intubation requires equipment and supplies. *Anticipating* problems based on your assessment of patient risk helps you build your checklist. A checklist for intubation would include the items in **Figure 12-7**, grouped by timing for your organization. Get them all out and ready to go if your patient is stable.

Always prepare as if the intubation will be complicated and the patient will need some form of resuscitation. *Have a backup plan.* Have all of your equipment and drug needs readily available on an adjacent table **(Figure 12.8)**. A mnemonic often used for the intubation equipment is *SOAPME.*

S = Suction
O = Oxygen
A = Airway equipment
P = Pharmacology
ME = Monitoring equipment

12.4.2 Pre-oxygenation

Pre-oxygenation is a fundamental component of the pre-intubation airway management.[99] The patient is provided high-flow oxygen at the highest possible concentration. High-flow supplemental oxygen corrects any deficiencies in the patient's oxyhemoglobin saturation; displaces alveolar nitrogen in the lung's residual capacity, creating an oxygen reservoir in the lung (called *denitrogenation*); and increases the oxygen stores in the blood and tissues. The time to desaturation during the apnea period will vary with the clinical characteristics of the patient, but pre-oxygenation will extend this time regardless of the clinical circumstances. The patient is ideally provided a period of pre-oxygenation for a prolonged time interval (3-5 minutes) independent of the patient's pulse oximeter saturation. An alternative technique to support denitrogenation is to require a cooperative patient to take multiple vital capacity breaths.

Pre-oxygenation can be provided by

1. High-flow nasal cannula oxygen at 15 L/min
2. 1.0 FiO_2 non-rebreather face mask at 15 L/min
3. Bag-valve mask ventilation with or without the addition of a CPAP valve
4. Non-invasive ventilation

During the pre-oxygenation interval, the SaO_2 should be maintained $\geq$ 95%. The oxygen delivery system can be advanced from #1 to #4 to achieve the target saturation. Patients who are not responsive to high-flow oxygen ($FiO_2 = 1.0$) by definition have shunt physiology and will require positive pressure to support lung recruitment (option 3-4). A high-flow nasal cannula (#1) should be used in addition to methods #2-4 to support pre-oxygenation and then remain in place to maintain oxygenation during the period of apnea (termed *apneic oxygenation*).[99-100] A pulse oximeter with an appropriate waveform should be visible to the physician during the entire period of pre-oxygenation to post intubation.

Assessing the risk of aspiration is also a key component in planning your airway management. Mechanical drainage of gastric contents should be

Preparing for Intubation
Pre-intubation • Intravenous access • Supplemental oxygen devices including high-flow nasal cannula and high-flow oxygen • Suction • Bag valve mask with PEEP valve • End tidal CO_2 monitor • Oropharyngeal and nasopharyngeal airways
Intubation Equipment • Laryngoscopes – include a video laryngoscope as backup, if possible, to be available • Endotracheal tubes of various sizes • Stylet
The Backup Plan • Bougie • Supraglottic airway • A scalpel
Medications (all carefully labeled) • Induction and paralytic medications • Post-intubation analgesia/sedation • Push dose vasopressor (epinephrine or phenylephrine)

Figure 12-7 The steps to prepare your equipment for intubation.

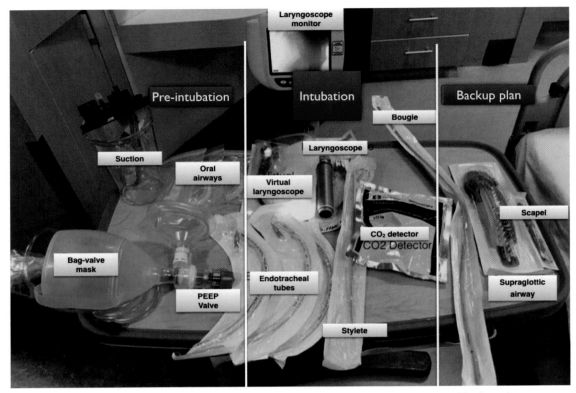

Figure 12-8 *Equipment for intubation procedure grouped by pre-intubation, intubation, and backup plan.*

considered in patients with residual gastric volume or delayed gastric emptying due to intestinal obstruction.

12.4.3 Intubation Pharmacology

Induction or sedative agents are essential for the RSI technique. Sedative use prevents the patient from being fully aware at the time the paralytic agent is administered. The commonly employed sedative agents for RSI are summarized in **Figure 12-9.**

Note that medication onset can be delayed in the setting of shock. The dosing of the sedative agent should be reduced a minimum of 50% in patients with compensated or non-compensated shock due to the risk of further hemodynamic compromise. A greater reduction for propofol in shock (10-20% of the dose) is indicated due to the risk of worsening hemodynamic compromise.

Select the most appropriate sedating agent for RSI based on the patient history. In patients with a risk for elevated intracranial pressure (ICP), adequate cerebral perfusion must be maintained. Agents are favored that do not further augment cerebral blood flow or cause hemodynamic instability. For these reasons, ketamine and etomidate are favored. Ketamine is favored for the hypotensive patient, while etomidate may be favored for the hypertensive patient. Pretreatment

with fentanyl can occur with etomidate to block any unfavorable effects from the lack of analgesic properties. The concern with the use of midazolam and propofol is the risk of hypotension.

For the patient with seizures, ketamine is avoided because of the stimulant properties of the medication although this remains controversial. Propofol and midazolam may be the favored agents as they also represent agents used in the treatment of status epilepticus.

For the patient with reactive airways disease, the bronchodilation properties of propofol or ketamine are favored. Thiopental is avoided due to the release of histamine. The selection of induction agents by clinical condition is summarized in **Figure 12-10**.

The neuromuscular blocking agent (NMBA) is administered immediately following the induction agent in RSI. Numerous clinical studies have confirmed that administration of NMBAs improves the success rate of endotracheal intubation. NMBAs do not have analgesic or sedating properties, and failure to provide adequate sedation can lead to adverse consequences, including tachycardia, hypertension, and increased intracranial pressure. The NMBAs are classified as depolarizing and non-depolarizing based upon their mechanism of action. A summary of the commonly used neuromuscular blocking agents for RSI is included in **Figure 12-11**.

Medication	Dose	Dose (70 kg)	Time to Effect	Comments
Etomidate	0.3 mg/kg	20 mg	15-45 seconds	• Minimal hemodynamic changes • No histamine release
Ketamine	dissociative dosing 1-2 mg/kg	70-140 mg	45-60 seconds	• Analgesic • Bronchodilator • Stimulates catecholamine release • Hypersecretion • Reemergence phenomena
Midazolam	0.2 mg/kg	14 mg	30-60 seconds	• Anticonvulsant • No analgesia
Propofol	1.5-3.0 mg/kg	150 mg	30-60 seconds	• Anticonvulsant • Neural suppressant • Hypotension

Figure 12-9 Commonly prescribed sedative agents during rapid sequence intubation.

Clinical Condition	Preferred Induction Agent (s)
Elevated intracranial pressure	Etomidate, ketamine Consider narcotic for analgesic effect
Hypotension	Ketamine
Seizures	Propofol, versed
Bronchospasm	Propofol, ketamine
Hypertension, tachycardia aortic dissection	Etomidate

Figure 12-10 Clinical conditions and the preferred intubation agent.

Agent	Dose	Onset	Comments
Succinylcholine	1.5 mg/kg	Rapid onset (45-60sec) Short duration (6-10 min)	• No histamine release • Contraindicated with a personal or family history of malignant hyperthermia • Hyperkalemia • Trismus, Fasciculations • Bradycardia
Rocuronium	1 mg/kg	Rapid onset (45-60sec) Moderate duration (45 min)	• Stimulates catecholamine receptors • Reemergence phenomena • Avoid with high ICP or hypertension
Vecuronium	0.01 mg/kg, then 0.15 mg/kg		• Amnestic • No analgesia properties • Hypotension (10-25%) • Anticonvulsantproperties

Figure 12-11 Commonly used neuromuscular blocking agents for rapid sequence intubation.

Succinylcholine (Sch) is considered the NMBA of choice in RSI due to rapid onset and short duration of action and predictable therapeutic success. However, Sch is contraindicated in several clinical conditions for which a non-depolarizing NMBA is preferred. Succinylcholine can cause malignant hyperthermia and is contraindicated in any patient with a personal or family history of this disorder. The second major contraindication to succinylcholine is any disorder with a risk of hyperkalemia. Patients with cell death (rhabdomyolysis) and conditions associated with upregulation of acetylcholine receptors are at risk of hyperkalemia. Upregulation of acetylcholine receptors occurs in chronic denervating diseases, such as multiple sclerosis, amyotrophic lateral sclerosis, inherited myopathies, or prolonged immobilization. Acute denervating injuries can also be associated with hyperkalemia following succinylcholine administration, including stroke, spinal cord injury, burns, crush injuries. The risk of hyperkalemia appears to begin approximately 72 hours after an acute injury. Succinylcholine is associated with nicotinic activation that can produce muscle fasciculation and bradycardia in selected patients, especially children.

Following appropriate administration of the induction and paralytic medication, RSI progresses with the actual intubation. If adequate preoxygenation has occurred with continued apneic oxygenation, bag-mask ventilation is not required if the oxygen saturation remains higher than 90%.

Following successful placement of the endotracheal tube, confirmation of correct placement is best confirmed using end-tidal CO_2 detection, either colorimetric or quantitative. CO_2 detection is considered the most definitive method in comparison to auscultation, endotracheal tube condensation, or direct visualization. The primary limitation to CO_2 detection is the cardiac arrest condition, where CO_2 detection may be absent due to the lack of circulation despite accurate endotracheal tube placement.

12.4.4 Post-intubation Hemodynamics

Post-intubation management must address several factors. The endotracheal tube must be appropriately secured either with tape or a tube holder. A post-procedure chest radiograph is obtained to confirm the depth of endotracheal tube placement. Hemodynamic assessment post-intubation frequently reveals hypotension. This hypotension may be due to a prolonged effect of the induction agents, or more commonly due to the hemodynamic effects of positive pressure ventilation. The need for additional long-acting sedative agents must also be appreciated. The agents used for RSI are short-acting and will wear off quickly.

Hopefully, you expected the possibility of post-intubation hypotension. You are ready to respond quickly with a plan.

- *Fluid resuscitation.* Remember your patient's preload was just shifted by the conversion from spontaneous to positive pressure ventilation.
- Push-dose vasopressor (PDP) support.
  - Use *diluted* epinephrine for patients without tachycardia to provide both alpha and beta (1/2) effects. Dilute 1ml of 1:10,000 epinephrine (cardiac arrest amp) with 9ml of normal saline to create a 1: 100,000 dilution. This mixture provides 10 mcg/mg of epinephrine to be

administered in 0.5-1cc dosing units. Onset should be within 1-2 minutes, so you can dose every 2-5 minutes.
  - Use *diluted* phenylephrine for patients with tachycardia to provide alpha-only effects. Use 1 ml from a 10mg/ml vial of phenylephrine diluted into 100 ml NSS to provide a 100 mcg/ml solution. Draw up 10cc of this solution. This provides 100 mcg/ml of phenylephrine to be administered in 0.5-1cc dosing units. Onset should be within 1-2 minutes, so you can dose every 2-5 minutes.
- *Watch your PEEP and tidal volume.* Remember, PEEP further impairs venous return, so go slowly—especially if oxygenation is satisfactory.

12.5 The Difficult Airway

For a young house officer with limited experience, *the most important goal is to recognize the difficult airway and call for the most experienced provider as a backup.* Starting your plan for a difficult airway after 2-3 failed intubation attempts is *TOO LATE!*

The clinician should consider a primary and alternative airway management strategy during the pre-intubation assessment period. Several simple questions can help outline the plan.

Is the patient best approached as a rapid sequence or awake intubation? Remember to ask these three questions:

1. Will this patient be difficult to bag-mask ventilate?
2. Will this patient be difficult to intubate?
3. Will this patient be difficult to rescue if the initial intubation attempt fails?

If the initial assessment suggests a potentially difficult airway and airway control is less urgent, consideration should be given to awake airway management using topical or local anesthesia. An awake, ventilating patient is often preferred in conditions that include

- *Oral route not possible* (i.e., wired jaw or angioedema)—nasal or surgical airway required
- *Laryngotracheal pathology,* such as an upper airway lesion
- *Difficult laryngoscopy or BVM anticipated* – morbid obesity or limited neck mobility

Recognize these conditions early and *GET HELP.*

If rapid sequence intubation (RSI) and direct laryngoscopy is chosen, outline your backup plan. The ability to achieve successful mask ventilation in the sedated and paralyzed patient will determine the next step in your algorithm if your initial attempt at intubation is not successful. Bag-valve-mask ventilation preferably involves two individuals with an optimal nasal pharyngeal (NPA) or oropharyngeal airway (OPA). The possibility of restoring spontaneous ventilation must also be considered if possible in a patient who fails the initial attempt at RSI.

What is your anticipated plan for *failure to intubate but able to ventilate?* If the initial airway attempt with RSI is unsuccessful, but you can successfully ventilate the patient with the BVM, then the subsequent steps might include changing patient position, changing modality (i.e., video laryngoscopy), or changing operator (experienced attending).

What is the anticipated plan for *failure to intubate and not able to ventilate?* If mask ventilation is not successful after the initial failed RSI attempt, emergent airway management with the use of rapidly performed alternative techniques must be considered. The approach may include a supraglottic airway, transtracheal ventilation, or cricothyrotomy and this should proceed directly.

Many treatment algorithms have been published for management of the difficult airway. Few randomized trials exist to confirm the benefit or limitations of these individual algorithms. Your local algorithm might be modified by your backup resources, available equipment, and skill set. But you should expect your environment to have the needed resources to advance through the clinical scenarios. A graphic summary of a common management algorithm is shown in **Figure 12-12.**

Time with simulation training and preferably a cadaver lab is helpful to gain skill with the variety of techniques. A variety of excellent online instructional videos are available to demonstrate basic techniques for airway management. A small sample of available videos is listed below. Explore widely to find your favorite instructional videos.

Basic airway management	https://www.youtube.com/watch?v=wZ2fbBOTvac
Face mask ventilation	https://vimeo.com/34883844
Laryngoscopy	https://player.vimeo.com/video/17542057
Supraglottic airway (iGel)	https://www.youtube.com/watch?v=ae1Yr0fbz98
Cricothyroidotomy	https://youtube/TveIsbjmakU

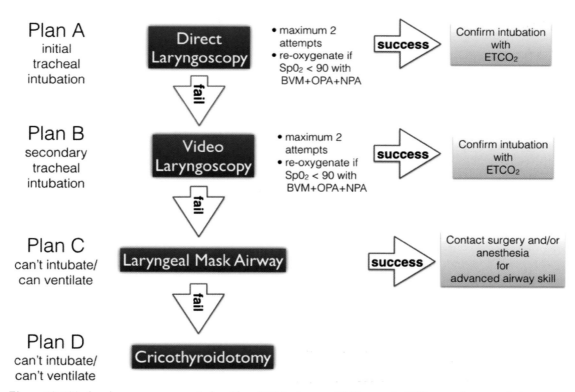

Figure 12-12* *An airway management algorithm. BVM= bag ventilation mask. OPA= oropharyngeal airway. NPA= nasopharyngeal airway.*

*modified from Douras et al. http://www.das.uk.com/files/simple-Jul04-A4.pdf

12.6 Changing the Endotracheal Tube

The nurse calls you to report a cuff leak in a patient with an endotracheal tube or tracheostomy tube. What steps should you take?

1. Check your end-tidal carbon dioxide with either recorded capnography or a capnometer. This will help you know if the tube is located within the patient's airway.
2. A video laryngoscope or bronchoscope can help you determine if the ETT is located appropriately below the glottic opening. An ETT may be high in the airway and continue to leak with a functional cuff despite overinflation. A tracheostomy tube may be too short to reach the trachea and be located barely within the trach lumen.
3. If the ETT is appropriately positioned in the airway, a persistent cuff leak requires a new ETT placement. A tube changer, which essentially changes the tube over a place-holding stylet device, can assist with changing a tube.
4. Prepare for a tube change like your preparation for a fresh endotracheal intubation. The procedure always incurs some risk of losing control of the original airway.

Be prepared!

Suggested Reading

- Sakles JC, Mosier JM, Patanwala AE, et al. First pass success without hypoxemia is increased with the use of apneic oxygenation during rapid sequence intubation in the emergency department. Academic Emergency Medicine 2016;23(6):703–10.
- Jabre P, Combes X, Lapostolle F, et al. Etomidate versus ketamine for rapid sequence intubation in acutely ill patients: a multicentre randomised controlled trial. The Lancet 2009;374(9686):293–300.
- Higgs A, McGrath BA, Goddard C, et al. Guidelines for the management of tracheal intubation in critically ill adults. British J Anesthesia 2018;120:323–352.
- Katz J, Greenberg S. Etomidate Is NOT a first-line induction agent in critically ill patients: primum non nocere—Above all, do no harm. Crit Care Med [Internet] 2018;46(9):1495. *Debate with* Lynde GC, Jabaley CS. Etomidate is a first-line induction agent in critically ill patients. Crit Care Med [Internet] 2018;46(9):1492.
- Driver BE, Prekker ME, Klein LR, et al. Effect of Use of a Bougie vs Endotracheal Tube and Stylet on First-Attempt Intubation Success Among Patients With Difficult Airways Undergoing Emergency Intubation: A Randomized Clinical Trial. JAMA [Internet] 2018;319(21):2179–89.

13

Acute Respiratory Failure

The principal function of the lung is to "pass gas" or, more properly stated, to facilitate the exchange of oxygen (O_2) and carbon dioxide (CO_2). When the lung fails to "pass gas" adequately, the patient has the clinical features of respiratory failure. Logically, two pathways lead to respiratory failure: 1) failure to oxygenate, and 2) failure to ventilate.

We define respiratory failure as the inability of the respiratory system to maintain the partial pressure of arterial oxygen (PaO_2) or carbon dioxide ($PaCO_2$) within their normal range. We further classify respiratory failure as acute, chronic, or acute on chronic based on the duration of the gas exchange defect. Acute respiratory failure (ARF), which implies a short-term change in gas exchange function, is one of the most common reasons for admission to an intensive care unit.

A reduction in the blood PaO_2 is termed *hypoxemia,* and an elevation in the blood $PaCO_2$ is termed *hypercapnia.* But deciding on the "normal" values for these parameters in a given patient can be a little tricky. A reasonable starting point is to consider an arterial oxygen tension (PaO_2) of less than 60 mm Hg, or a $PaCO_2$ of greater than 50 mm Hg, breathing room air, as values consistent with the concept of respiratory failure. But recognize that multiple factors, including age, environmental altitude, inspired oxygen concentration, as well as the presence or absence of underlying chronic lung disease influence the normal blood gas values for an individual. Therefore, always compare the measured PaO_2 and $PaCO_2$ in the blood to the patient's "normal" or expected state to identify an acute change in respiratory status.

Acute respiratory failure is typically characterized by marked derangements in arterial gas partial pressures and acid-base status. Acute hypercapnia is associated with a more dramatic pH change (i.e., < 7.3), while in chronic respiratory failure, the pH usually is only slightly decreased because the kidney has time to retain buffer to compensate for the hypercapnia. In addition to the pH marker, more chronic hypoxemia is suggested by the presence of polycythemia and cor pulmonale.

13.1 Assessment of Arterial Blood Oxygenation

Arterial blood oxygenation in the hospitalized patient refers to the measurement of blood oxygen levels either as the partial pressure of oxygen (PaO_2) or the saturation of hemoglobin by oxygen (SaO_2). These measurements can be obtained from an arterial blood gas (ABG) sample or non-invasively in the case of SaO_2 by the use of pulse oximetry (SpO_2).

Obtain your arterial blood gas from a small (1mL) sample of blood taken by puncture of the radial artery or from an indwelling arterial catheter. ABG analysis includes the direct measurement of PaO_2, $PaCO_2$, and pH in the sample. The SaO_2 can be estimated knowing the PaO_2, based upon the standard oxygen-hemoglobin dissociation curve, or measured if the blood gas analyzer includes a co-oximeter. Bicarbonate concentration is calculated using the Henderson-Hasselbalch equation. Base excess (BE), which is the amount of base necessary to return pH to 7.40, is also reported as a calculated value.

Hypoxemia is a decrease in the blood PaO_2 in comparison to expected values; whereas *hypoxia* is a decrease in the PO_2 in the tissues. *Hypoxemia* is defined as a PaO_2 low enough to reduce the hemoglobin oxygen saturation (SaO_2) below 90% (i.e., $PaO_2 < 60$ mm Hg).

Although the blood gas can report both the PaO_2 and SaO_2, these parameters are considered complementary and not equal in the assessment of oxygenation. With the widespread availability of pulse oximetry to assess oxygenation, the need for ABGs may be less frequent, but ABGs remain a critical tool for the assessment of gas exchange efficiency, ventilation, and metabolic disturbances.

13.1.1 Partial Pressure of Oxygen (PaO₂)

Oxygen and carbon dioxide move across the alveolar-capillary membrane due to the partial pressure gradient between the alveolus and capillary blood. So, the overall efficiency of oxygen transfer in the lung is determined by comparing the partial pressure of oxygen we expect to have in the alveolus (P_AO_2) and the measured partial pressure in arterial blood (PaO_2). This comparison of the Alveolar (Big A) to arterial (Little a) partial pressure difference is traditionally made using a calculation of the (A-a) gradient.

The (A-a) gradient allows you to interpret whether the measured PaO_2 is "normal" for your patient, based upon an understanding of the environmental oxygen and the patient's level of ventilation. Because it is not practical to take a sample of gas from the alveolus, Big A is calculated from measured variables using the Alveolar Gas Equation

$$P_AO_2 = FiO_2 (P_{ATM} - P_{H2O}) - P_aCO_2 / RQ$$

with the parameters for this equation defined in **Figure 13-1**.

An elevated (A-a) gradient only suggests parenchymal lung disease, without being specific for cause or mechanism. The recognized physiologic causes of an elevated A-a gradient with (clinical examples) include:

1. *V/Q mismatch* (pneumonia, CHF, COPD exacerbation) → elevated (A-a) gradient
2. *Shunt* (atrial septal defect, ARDS, atelectasis) → elevated (A-a) gradient
3. *Diffusion limitation* (interstitial lung disease) → elevated (A-a) gradient
4. *Hypoventilation* (CNS depressant, neuromuscular disease) → normal (A-a) gradient
5. *Low inspired oxygen concentration* (high altitude) → normal (A-a) gradient

A normal (A-a) gradient *breathing room air* is < 10 but can range from 5-20 mm Hg and varies with the age of the patient. The normal PaO_2 for a 20-year-old breathing room air with a normal level of ventilation is about 90 mm Hg. In contrast, the normal PaO_2 for an 80-year-old breathing room air with a normal level of ventilation is about 60 mm Hg. The normal PaO_2 for an 80-year-old is hypoxemia for the 20-year-old! To estimate the normal (A-a) gradient for a given age of a patient breathing room air you can use

$$\text{Age expected } (P_AO_2 - PaO_2) = (AGE / 4) + 4$$

But the A-a gradient has significant limitations in the management of hospital patients. First, the calculation is a bit tedious, although our Pearl (grey box) tells you how to make it easy! But the biggest problem in the hospital is that the "normal" A-a gradient changes as the inspired oxygen changes. We can predict the expected (A-a) gradient for any age group when breathing room air, but "normal values" are not readily available for the expected (A-a) gradient in a hospital patient on a higher level of inspired oxygen concentration.

In the ICU literature, many easy-to-calculate indices of oxygenation are reported. These indices are really modifications of the A-a gradient that simplify the calculation to provide a severity index rather than an indicator of "normal" gas exchange. These measures

Parameter	Description	Sample Values Breathing Room Air (0.21 FiO₂)
P_AO_2	The alveolar partial pressure of oxygen (Big A)	100 mm Hg
P_{ATM}	The atmospheric pressure	760 mm Hg (sea level)
P_{H2O}	The saturated water vapor pressure	47 mm Hg
$PaCO_2$	The partial pressure of carbon dioxide in arterial blood	40 mm Hg
FiO_2	The fraction of inspired oxygen in arterial blood (Little a)	0.21 (room air)
RQ	The respiratory quotient	0.8

Figure 13-1 *Parameters for the alveolar gas equation.*

Note that for most patients at sea level the P_{ATM}, P_{H2O} and RQ are stable. The A-a gradient you calculate is largely determined by 1) the amount of oxygen you are giving the patient (FiO_2), and 2) by the patient's level of alveolar ventilation, The alveolar ventilation is reflected by the $PaCO_2$ level in the arterial blood. If he/she is breathing room air (FiO_2 of .21) and has a normal $PaCO_2$ (40), then

$$P_{A}O_2 = [0.21 \times (760-47) - 40/0.8] \text{ or } 149-50$$

giving a $P_{A}O_2$ = 100. So on a quick evaluation of the patient, if they are on room air and the $PaCO_2$ is normal, you know the $P_{A}O_2$ is ~ 100, from which the arterial PaO_2 can be quickly subtracted for the A-a gradient. The $P_{A}O_2$ can also be quickly adjusted at room air for high or low $PaCO_2$ by subtracting the $PaCO_2$ / 0.8 from 150. Easy so far. The (A-a) gradient gets a little tricky once the patient starts inspiring oxygen concentrations higher than room air. So read a little more for that one.

The severity of ARDS is graded based on the PaO_2/FiO_2 ratio as follows:

- Mild ARDS $300 \geq PaO_2/FiO_2 > 200$
- Moderate ARDS $200 \geq PaO_2/FiO_2 > 100$
- Severe ARDS $100 \leq PaO_2/FiO_2$

In addition to a variable FiO_2, ICU patients are often on elevated levels of positive end-expiratory pressure (PEEP) or continuous positive airway pressure (CPAP). Positive airway pressure applied to the airway will raise the mean airway pressure (MAP) during the respiratory cycle, and this factor can influence the oxygenation independent of the FiO_2. The oxygenation index is another measure of oxygenation used in ICU patients, which incorporates both the FiO_2, PaO_2 and the positive pressure therapy as a measure of the overall gas exchange efficiency. The OI = ($FiO_2 \times$ MAP) / PaO_2. A lower OI is better, meaning the FiO_2 or MAP have reduced or the PaO_2 has improved.

Note that these indices, similar to the (A-a) gradient, show variation with changes in the inspired oxygen concentration and are therefore still limited in the hospital environment.

of hypoxemia are compared to the (A-a) gradient in **Figure 13-2.**

The PaO_2/FiO_2 ratio recognizes that many of the parameters of the alveolar gas equation are relatively constant (P_{ATM}, P_{H2O}, $PaCO_2$) in most patients. The two dominant calculation variables in the (A-a) gradient are therefore the PaO_2 and the FiO_2.

The PaO_2/FiO_2 ratio (sometimes called *the P/F ratio*) is the oxygenation measurement used most frequently in the ICU and for the definition of the adult respiratory distress syndrome (ARDS). We will talk more about ARDS in *Chapter 16 Acute Respiratory Distress Syndrome.*

Because the (A-a) gradient and/or PaO_2/FiO_2 ratio varies across the range of inspired oxygen concentration in critically ill patients, you cannot easily predict the change in FiO_2 required to achieve a reduction or increase in the PaO_2 to a target level. This limitation means that changes in FiO_2 must be titrated to accomplish a given PaO_2, often using non-invasively measured oxygen saturation (pulse oximetry) as a guide. The FiO_2 is titrated to achieve a measured peripheral oxygen saturation of 92-94%.

Parameter	Calculation	Comment
(A-a) gradient	$P_{A}O_2$-PaO_2	• Requires the alveolar gas equation • Normal values are age dependent • Normal values vary with FiO_2 • Does not consider airway pressure in the calculation
P/F ratio	PaO_2/FiO_2	• No alveolar gas calculation required • Varies with the FiO_2 • No accounting for $PaCO_2$ • Does not consider airway pressure in the calculation
Oxygenation Index (OI)	(FiO_2/PaO_2) × Mean Airway Pressure	• No alveolar gas calculation required • Varies with the FiO_2 • No accounting for $PaCO_2$ • Adjusts for airway pressure

Figure 13-2 Oxygenation indices commonly used in the ICU.

13.1.2 Pathophysiology of Hypoxemia

So, how does your patient develop a low PaO_2? Gas exchange in the lung can be described using a schematic with 3 alveolar-capillary units (**Figure 13-3**). Gas exchange in the lung is most optimal when ventilation (V) and perfusion (Q) are matched across all the alveoli (Alveolus A), resulting in a V/Q ratio of 1. The capillary blood leaving this unit has a level of PaO_2 and $PaCO_2$ reflecting equilibration with alveolar gas.

An alveolus with high ventilation relative to perfusion (i.e., pulmonary embolism) has a V/Q ratio approaching infinity (Alveolus B). This alveolus creates a region where capillary blood flow does not equilibrate with alveolar gas. Note the lack of venous return from alveolus B. This region of the lung with ventilation but no perfusion is called *dead space*. The lung contains anatomic dead space regions (conducting airways and pharynx) and physiologic dead space (regions of lung pathology due to vascular occlusion or destruction of the alveolar-capillary interface). The lung typically has a dead space volume (V_D) that equals ~ 20-30% of the overall tidal volume (Vt) or a Vd/Vt = 0.2-0.3. Dead space ventilation increases with lung destruction, reduced blood flow (thromboembolic disease), or overdistention of the alveolus (positive airway pressure). An elevation in dead space (Vd/Vt > 0.3) leads to an elevated $PaCO_2$ and reduced PaO_2. Note that in the regions of physiologic dead space, blood flow must be redistributed to other regions.

An alveolus with no ventilation and retained perfusion (e.g., endobronchial tumor) has a V/Q ratio approaching 0 (Alveolus C). In this case, the blood flow to this region simply passes from the venous to the arterial circulation or "shunts" around the lung. Note the blue blood flowing past alveolus C. The amount of the cardiac output that participates in the intrapulmonary shunt (Q_S), relative to the total cardiac output (Q_T) is termed the *shunt fraction* (Q_S/Q_T) and is normally < 10%. As the shunt fraction increases, the PaO_2 falls progressively. Initially, the $PaCO_2$ is often below normal with an elevated shunt fraction due to hyperventilation. However, as the shunt fraction exceeds 50%, the $PaCO_2$ will also begin to increase.

Individual alveoli with an increase in ventilation relative to perfusion (high V/Q units) or a decrease in ventilation relative to perfusion (low V/Q units) contribute to an overall V/Q imbalance in the lung. Any imbalance in V/Q relationships in the lung contributes to hypoxemia in your patient. Low V/Q units (Alveolus C) produce a reduced oxygen content of post-capillary blood and contribute to the admixture of venous blood with normally oxygenated blood from other V/Q units, leading to hypoxemia. The hypoxemia of low V/Q units can be improved with the administration of supplemental oxygen to increase the P_AO_2 in these low-ventilated units. However, the extreme variant of a low V/Q unit, which is a non-ventilated or "shunt" unit, will not respond to supplemental oxygen. A shunt can occur within the lung parenchyma (atelectasis with failure of hypoxic vasoconstriction) or can occur extrapulmonary in any region where venous blood mixes with post-capillary oxygenated blood (atrial septal defect or patent foramen ovale). Shunt physiology is the type of gas exchange defect often seen in the acute respiratory distress syndrome (ARDS).

The clinical markers of a shunt condition include

1. A very high (A-a) gradient
2. No change in PaO_2 with the administration of 100% inspired oxygen (FiO_2)
3. No improvement in PaO_2 by hyperventilation

Two variables influence the magnitude of hypoxemia in a shunt condition:

1. The actual number of shunt units
2. The venous blood oxygen content (CvO_2)

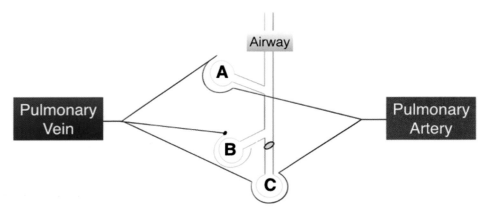

Figure 13-3 *A schematic of 3 different types of alveolar-capillary units. A=normal. B=deadspace. C=shunt.*

In the setting of low V/Q and shunt pathophysiology in an ARDS patient, efforts to increase the venous oxygen content (CvO_2) can increase arterial oxygenation! This can be accomplished by lowering metabolic demand and oxygen consumption (sedation and paralysis) or by increasing oxygen delivery (increasing hemoglobin or cardiac output). In severe cases of ARDS, increasing the oxygen content of venous blood may be life saving when you cannot increase oxygenation with ventilator manipulation.

The venous blood oxygen content (CvO_2) can be an especially important contributor to hypoxemia in the ICU patient with shunt physiology. The venous blood oxygen content in the shunted regions contributes a significant venous "admixture" to post-capillary oxygenated blood from normal regions. High peripheral oxygen extraction from low cardiac output or anemia lowers CvO_2 and will lead to a reduction in PaO_2 due to this contribution of venous admixture.

Logically, low V/Q units and high V/Q units should offset each other and maintain a normal gas exchange. While this does occur for carbon dioxide to a certain degree, this is not the case for oxygen. The difference relates to how O_2 and CO_2 are carried in blood and the role of hemoglobin. Let's now learn a little about the parameters that determine the capacity to carry blood oxygen.

13.1.3 Non-invasive Oxygen Saturation (SpO2)

Maybe you are feeling compassion and do not want to stick your patient for that blood gas. Can you get an assessment of oxygenation non-invasively? One of the most significant technological advances in anesthesia and critical care has been the development of non-invasive SaO_2 monitoring, using pulse oximetry. Quite simply, oximetry involves a light source and a light detector that measure the transmission of the light from a source to a detector. Pulse oximetry relies upon two basic concepts:

1. The light absorption by oxygenated hemoglobin is different than deoxygenated hemoglobin.
2. The light absorption has a pulsatile component that is detected with the change in arterial blood volume.

The blood sample oxygen saturation (SaO_2) is accurately measured by the arterial blood gas analyzer with a co-oximeter using four wavelengths of light to distinguish the four types of hemoglobin. A differential light absorption exists for the four types of hemoglobin: the two major hemoglobin species, oxygenated hemoglobin (O_2Hb) and deoxygenated Hb (Hb); and the two minor hemoglobin species, carboxyhemoglobin (COHb) and methemoglobin (MetHb). In contrast, commercial pulse oximeters are limited to two wavelengths of light and provide a modified pulse oximeter oxygen saturation (SpO_2). HbO_2, COHb, and MetHb are all interpreted as HbO_2 by the pulse oximeter, resulting in false elevations of SpO_2 in the presence of the minor hemoglobins. Other errors associated with pulse oximetry estimates of SaO_2 are listed in **Figure 13-4.**

In addition to the accurate measurement of saturation, the pulse oximeter must distinguish arterial blood from venous and capillary blood to accurately measure arterial saturation. Signal changes in light absorption distinguish the pulsative arterial flow.

The manufacturer establishes a correlation between the ratio of light absorbencies and measured blood SaO_2 during testing in healthy volunteers receiving various levels of inspired oxygen concentration.

Type of Error	Effect of Error	Recognition
Motion artifact or low perfusion	Inaccurate measurement	• Abnormal plethysmograph signal • Poor correlation with heart rate
Nail polish and skin pigmentation	Differential light absorption	• Greater saturation error with darker skin pigmentation • Remove dark (not red) nail polish • Align sideways with nail polish
Ambient light	False low oxygen saturation	• Environmental control with close contact of probe to skin
Hyperbilirubinemia	Falsely high oxygen saturation	• > 4% gradient between ABG oximetry and pulse oximetry
Methemoglobinemia Carboxyhemoglobinemia	Falsely high oxygen saturation	• > 4% gradient between ABG oximetry and pulse oximetry

Figure 13-4 *Potential measurement errors associated with pulse oximetry.*

The calibration curve is stored in the monitor and not altered. The accuracy of pulse oximetry is accepted as $\pm$ 2-3% in comparison to measured blood SaO_2. Translated, measured pulse oximetry of 92% suggests the actual arterial blood saturation should be between 89 to 95%. Based upon the standard oxyhemoglobin dissociation curve, this range of SaO_2 would correspond to a broad range of possible values for PaO_2. While the pulse oximeter can predict a "safe" level of SaO_2 for patient care, the device cannot predict the PaO_2 at any level. Translated into clinical practice, PaO_2 is the best measure to determine how well your lungs are working, but SaO_2, and by association an accurate SpO_2 are a very good measures of systemic oxygen delivery.

Traditional pulse oximetry places the light source and detector on opposite sides, such as seen with a finger probe. Reflectance pulse oximetry (reflecting light off hemoglobin rather than the absorbance of light by hemoglobin-same spectra by mirror images) places the light source and detector on the same surface and allows for the use of forehead probes.

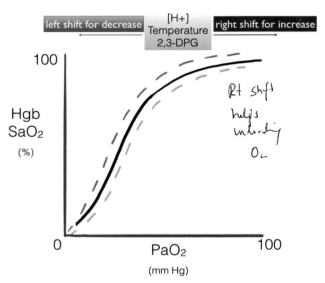

Figure 13-5 *Hemoglobin-oxygen desaturation curve. Hgb SaO_2 = hemoglobin oxygen saturation. PaO_2 = partial pressure of arterial oxygen.*

13.1.4 Assessment of Tissue Oxygen Delivery (DO₂)

After considering the efficiency of oxygen transport across the alveolar-capillary membrane, let's turn to the evaluation of the parameters that influence the transport of oxygen to the tissues. That is, does the patient have adequate blood oxygenation to provide for tissue metabolism?

The relationship between the PaO_2, the SaO_2 and the oxygen content of blood (CaO_2) is determined by

$$CaO_2 = [Hgb \ (gms/dL) \times 10 \ (dL/L) \times SaO_2 \ (fraction) \times 1.34 \ ml \ O_2 \ /gm \ Hgb] + (PaO2 \times 0.0031 \ mL/mmHg)$$

The dissolved oxygen component has a linear relationship between the PaO_2 and CaO_2 but accounts for only a small quantity of the CaO_2 ($PaO_2 \times 0.0031$ mL/mmHg). Most oxygen in blood is transported bound to hemoglobin, and this component is defined by the term [Hgb (gms/dL) $\times$ 10 (dL/L blood) $\times SaO_2$ (%) $\times$ 1.34 ml O_2 /gm Hg]. Simple calculations reveal that when the PaO_2 is 100 mm Hg, there is only 0.31 mL of oxygen dissolved in blood. However, at the same partial pressure of oxygen of 100 mm Hg, the 15 gm/dL hemoglobin is 100% saturated (1.0 fractional saturation), and so there is 200 mL of oxygen bound to hemoglobin per liter of blood)!!! Note the normal value for CaO_2 is ~20 mL/dL of blood or 200 mL /L (multiply by 10 to convert to L).

The CaO_2 is related to the PaO_2 by the hemoglobin-oxygen dissociation curve, which defines the saturation of the hemoglobin molecule for a given PaO_2 (**Figure 13-5**).

On the steep portion of the curve, these two indices show a linear relationship. However, on the upper flat part of the curve, significant changes in the PaO_2 produce relatively small changes in the SaO_2. Thus, PaO_2 values significantly above 60 mm Hg do not increase oxygen binding to hemoglobin (saturation) and therefore do not contribute very much to additional oxygen content in post-capillary blood. The relationship between these two variables is modified in the setting of higher temperature; elevated red blood cell 2,3-diphosphoglycerate (DPG); acidosis; and elevated $PaCO_2$; all of which shift the curve to the right or facilitate unloading of oxygen in the tissues. Note that hemoglobin is already 90% saturated with oxygen at a relatively low PaO_2 of 60 mm Hg.

If we consider the impact of oxygen transport on our schematic lung model (**Figure 13-3**), high V/Q units will have a higher partial pressure of alveolar oxygen, and low V/Q units will have a low partial pressure of alveolar oxygen. Increasing the PaO_2 in post capillary blood from high V/Q units results in a minor increment in oxygen content as they have already maximized their hemoglobin capacity to bind oxygen (flat portion in **Figure 13-5**). High V/Q units therefore do not offset the fall in oxygen content coming from the low V/Q units. Increasing the minute ventilation above normal will increase the P_AO_2 in well-ventilated units (high V/Q), but again will not increase SaO_2 or CaO_2 of blood coming from these units. This principle of oxygen transport explains why V/Q mismatch produces hypoxemia from low V/Q units.

The relationship between $PaCO_2$ and CO_2 blood content ($CaCO_2$) is a bit different. **Figure 13-6** compares the relationship between PaO_2 or $PaCO_2$ on the X-axis, and blood O_2 or CO_2 content on the Y-axis. Note that CO_2 content has a more linear relationship over the physiologic range of $PaCO_2$ in blood. CO_2 does not saturate the blood carriers, so there is no flat portion of the CO_2 dissociation curve, and CO_2 is much more diffusible than oxygen.

The importance of these differences in oxygen and carbon dioxide transport from a gas exchange perspective is that a well-ventilated lung region (high V/Q) can compensate for a poorly ventilated region (low V/Q) with respect to CO_2 content—but not the O_2 content.

What does this all this information mean for the patient with respiratory distress?

First, the target PaO_2 for resuscitation is a value ≥ 60 mm Hg. When the PaO_2 is on the flat upper portion of the oxyhemoglobin dissociation curve ($PaO_2 > 60$ in **Figure 13-5**), minimal changes in saturation (SaO_2) and arterial oxygen content are realized with further increases in PaO_2. Since oxygen content of the blood is the critical variable that determines oxygen delivery (content × flow) to the tissues, clinicians target a SaO_2 of > 90% or a $PaO_2 > 60$mmg Hg when they provide supplemental oxygen.

Second, these unique transport mechanisms of oxygen and carbon dioxide in human blood explain gas exchange abnormalities in the patient with respiratory failure. Hyperventilation can compensate for V/Q units that would normally lead to hypercapnia. Hyperventilation cannot compensate for low V/Q units that would normally lead to hypoxemia. As a

result of these physiologic concepts, the most common presentation in sick patients with parenchymal lung disease will be hypoxemia, hyperventilation, and relative hypocapnia.

13.2 Supplemental Oxygen and Hypoxemic Respiratory Failure

Supplemental oxygen is administered to immediately address hypoxemia. Patients unresponsive to the administration of supplemental oxygen via low- or high-flow oxygen delivery systems most likely have shunt physiology. Shunt physiology in a patient may require alternative strategies, such as positive end-expiratory airway pressure (PEEP) or other airway pressure maneuvers to recruit new alveolar units and thus improve V/Q matching and reduce shunt physiology.

Non-invasive oxygen systems are divided into low-flow and high-flow systems, reflecting the total device flow to the patient. The distinction is somewhat arbitrary, however, as the patient's inspiratory flow rate – rather than the device flow rate – actually determines whether the device delivers all the inspired gas (patient inspiratory flow < device flow) or leads to mixing with ambient air (patient inspiratory flow > device flow).

13.2.1 Low-Flow Oxygen Systems

Low-flow systems provide a total device flow lower than the patient's inspiratory flow rate. The expected peak inspiratory flow rate for a patient breathing comfortably at rest is approximately 35 L/min. Low-flow systems allow the patient to inspire (entrain) ambient air to make up the difference between the device flow rate and the patient's inspiratory flow rate. The exact inspired oxygen concentration is a mix of the device FiO_2 and the amount of the room air entrained As a result of this room air entrainment, an increase in the patient's inspiratory flow rate (i.e., tachypnea) with low-flow systems increases the inspired room air entrained and lowers the inspired oxygen concentration.

The most frequently used low-flow oxygen system is the *nasal cannula* **(Figure 13-7).** With a low-flow oxygen delivery system, an oxygen regulator is connected to the wall oxygen outlet, and the nasal cannula tubing is connected to the regulator. A specific flow rate is selected on the regulator, typically in the range of 1-5 L per minute of 100% oxygen flow for a nasal cannula. No premixing of oxygen and room air occurs before the patient. The 1-5 L delivered flow rate of the nasal cannula is expected to be significantly below the patient's inspiratory flow requirement. Between breaths, the oxygen fills the nasopharynx, creating a reservoir of oxygen for inspiration, but this is still quite limited.

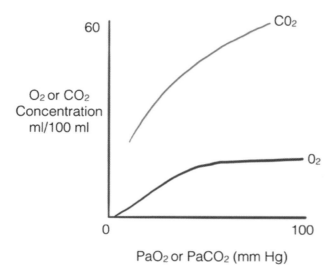

Figure 13-6 Relationship between arterial partial pressure and arterial concentration of oxygen or carbon dioxide.

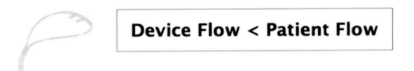

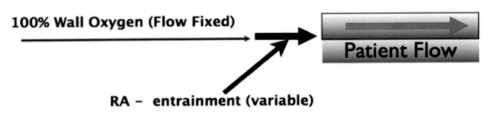

Figure 13-7 Schematic illustrates the components of a low-flow oxygen delivery system.

The patient's inspired oxygen concentration will vary based on the patient's inspiratory flow rate and the delivered flow rate of the device. A very rough rule of thumb is that every 1 L flow increase from the cannula increases the FiO_2 by 4%. If the patient's minute ventilation increases, then the inspiratory flow rate will usually increase. The cannula flow rate, however, remains fixed, and the inspired oxygen concentration will decrease due to a greater mix (called *entrainment*) of room air by the patient.

Low-flow oxygen systems can be modified with the incorporation of a reservoir **(Figure 13-8)**. The reservoir is part of the oxygen delivery system and fills with oxygen during the expiratory phase. The reservoir then supplements the inspiratory flow of oxygen to minimize the room air entrainment required to meet the inspiratory flow demand. By enhancing the inspiratory flow, reservoirs achieve an increase in the effective inspired oxygen concentration. The reservoir system with a nasal cannula can be located near the nose (nasal reservoir) or along the tubing (pendant reservoir). A downside of reservoir cannula systems is that they frequently do not allow humidification.

Consider a reservoir nasal cannula when the patient requires a higher flow rate of continuous oxygen (i.e., 3-10 L), but the higher flow rate is uncomfortable or creates local complications (e.g., nasal irritation).

A summary of low-flow oxygen delivery systems is outlined in **Figure 13-9**.

13.2.2 High-Flow Oxygen Systems

In contrast, high-flow systems are targeted to exceed the patient's inspiratory flow rate. A high-flow system theoretically meets the patient's total respiratory demand without any mixing of ambient air.

High-flow oxygen systems usually deliver supplemental oxygen via a face mask, although more recently, high-flow (and humidified) nasal cannula systems have been developed and are widely available in ICUs. High-flow systems, in theory, provide all the inspiratory flow required by the patient at a consistent FiO_2 **(Figure 13-10)**. The figure illustrates a high-flow bottle system. The inspired gas is premixed before delivery to the patient at the bottle by changing the size of the opening. The premixing of oxygen is accomplished based upon an air entrainment effect, which mixes oxygen and room air at a constant ratio. This ratio achieves the desired inspired oxygen concentration in the gas delivered to the patient. The key to high-flow systems is that they are blasting the flow at a rate higher than the patient's inspiratory rate, so that if the patient takes a fast breath, the air is all coming from the high-flow, fixed FiO_2 system, with no room air entrainment.

A Venturi mask incorporates a simple face mask with a special jet device that attaches to the traditional face mask and can be changed to accomplish a set inspired oxygen concentration **(Figure 13-11,** left panel). The jets are usually color coded for the desired FiO_2 and labeled for the particular flow of 100% oxygen, which is connected to the device. The jet devices are designed to entrain a specific ratio of room air to modify the delivered 100% oxygen.

This system really consists of an oxygen flow rate combined with an ambient air flow rate to give you a total flow rate **(Figure 13-11)**. By controlling the flow rate of ambient air and oxygen, a high total flow rate is delivered to the patient with a relatively constant inspired oxygen concentration. Alternatively, a Venturi mask may have a rotating device that is used to select the desired FiO_2 in place of the jet device. A summary of the airflow settings for a traditional Venturi mask and jets are included in **Figure 13-12.**

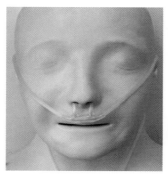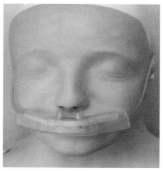

Figure 13-8 *Nasal cannula (left) and a nasal cannula with a reservoir (right).*

Device	Liter Flow (LPM)	FiO$_2$	Advantages	Disadvantages	Comments
Nasal cannula	1-6	22-45% (estimate of 4% per L flow)	Patient comfort Easy speaking and eating Effective for low FiO$_2$	Limited to FiO$_2$ < 40% Dry mucous membranes at high flow without humidification	Maximum flow 5-6 L/min Humidity for flow > 4 L/min Use restricted to patients with adequate tidal volume
Simple face mask	5-12	35-60%	Delivers FiO$_2$ up to 60%	Can be hot and confining Impractical for long-term use	Minimum 6L flow to flush mask of carbon dioxide No humidification
Partial rebreather mask	8-15	35-60%	Delivers FiO$_2$ up to 60%	Can be hot and confining Impractical for long-term use	Must have flow to maintain bag 1/3 to 1/2 inflated
Non-rebreather mask	8-15	60-90%	Delivers FiO$_2$ up to 100% One-way valve does not allow exhaled gas in reservoir One-way valve on expiratory ports does not allow room air entrainment	Can be hot and confining Impractical for long-term use	Must have flow to maintain bag 1/3 to 1/2 inflated

Figure 13-9 *Summary of low-flow oxygen systems.*

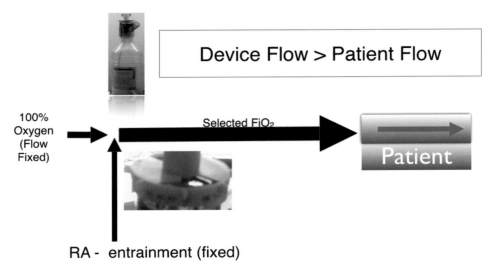

Figure 13-10 *Schematic illustrates the components of a high-flow oxygen delivery system.*

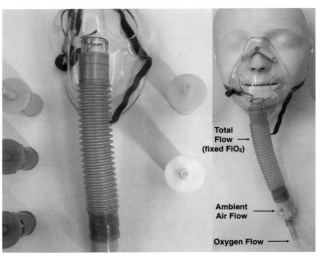

Figure 13-11 *Basic components of a Venturi mask (left panel) assenbled into an oxygen delivery system (right panel).*

Venturi Jet FiO$_2$	Oxygen Flow (100% O$_2$ L/min)	Ambient Air Flow (L/min)	Total Flow to Patient (L/min)
24%	2	51	53
28%	4	41	45
31%	6	41	47
35%	8	37	45
40%	10	32	42
60%	15	15	30

Figure 13-12 *FiO$_2$, oxygen flow, and total airflow with Venturi oxygen delivery system.*

While the oxygen flow connected to a Venturi Jet would be considered low flow ($\leq$ 15 L), the combined flow of oxygen and ambient air to the patient is $\geq$ 30 L/min. Because the total flow is high, a Venturi mask is considered a high-flow device. Also, note that the total flow declines as the target FiO$_2$ increases.

A different high-flow system may achieve the air:oxygen ratio at the regulator using a *nebulizer and bottle system*. Gas flow of 100% oxygen from the regulator is passed through a humidification bottle. A wheel attachment on the humidification bottle adjusts an opening that regulates the mix of room air with the 100% oxygen gas flow to provide a continuous oxygen:room air ratio (**Figure 13-13**).

At 100% oxygen, the entrainment opening is closed, and only gas from the regulator is provided to the patient. As the inspired oxygen concentration is lowered, the entrainment opening becomes larger, and flow from the regulator (100% oxygen) is mixed with increasing quantities of ambient air flow to achieve the desired FiO$_2$. You will notice the device gets louder as the selected FiO$_2$ gets lower. The noise is the ambient air rushing through the opening. Similar to the Venturi mask, as the FiO$_2$ is increased, the total flow rate (oxygen + room air) from the device is decreased. Sample settings with airflows for a bottle system are outlined in **Figure 13-14.**

Although the Venturi mask and bottle systems are considered high-flow in concept, that principle only holds if the total device flow to the patient exceeds the patient's inspiratory flow rate.

Consider a patient you are treating with 40% oxygen and a normal inspiratory flow rate on a bottle system. The patient would have the following settings on a bottle system (**Figure 13-14**):

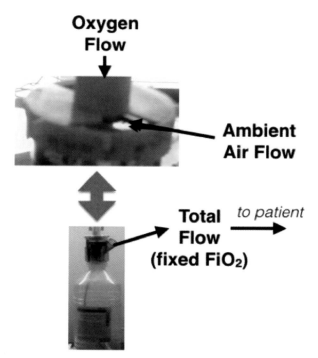

Figure 13-13 *Components of a nebulizer and bottle system.*

FiO$_2$ (%)	Oxygen Flow (100% O$_2$ L/min)	Ambient Air Flow (L/min)	Total Flow to Patient (L/min)
36	14	60	74
40	15	47	62
50	15	26	41
60	15	15	30
80	Flush	Minimal	54
95	Flush	Minimal	43

Figure 13-14 *Sample FiO$_2$, oxygen flow, and total airflow for a nebulizer and bottle delivery system.*

- FiO$_2$ = 40%
- Oxygen Flow = 15 L / min of 100% Oxygen
- Total Device Flow to Patient = 62 L / min
- Patient's Resting Inspiratory Flow = 30 L / min

Because the device flow > patient's inspiratory flow, the patient will receive gas at close to an FiO$_2$ of 40%.

The nurse reports the patient is suddenly having desaturation (SaO$_2$ = 85%) with marked tachypnea. You elect to increase the FiO$_2$ to 60% to address the desaturation. Your patient's tachypnea will be associated with an increase in inspiratory flow rate. The new settings for the patient are:

- FiO$_2$ = 60%
- Oxygen Flow = 15 L / min of 100% Oxygen

A patient with marked tachypnea and a high respiratory rate, such as a patient with an acute exacerbation of idiopathic pulmonary fibrosis, may have a very high inspiratory flow rate that exceeds most high -flow oxygen systems (i.e., > 60 L/min). Hypoxemia in this patient may actually deteriorate by increasing the aerosol nebulizer FiO2. As the FiO2 increases in these systems, the flow rate falls, which requires the patient to entrain more room air. Correction of hypoxemia in these patients often requires attention to very high gas flows using reservoir systems, dual flow circuits, or specialized high- flow delivery devices.

- Total Device Flow to Patient = 30 L / min
- Patient's Resting Inspiratory Flow = 60 L / min

Now the device flow < patient's inspiratory flow by 30 L/min. The 30 L/min device flow at FiO$_2$ of 60% will be mixed with 30 L/min of ambient air to match the patient's inspiratory flow rate. Under these conditions, the high-flow system has converted to a low-flow system!!

If the flow rate from a high-flow system is less than the patient's inspiratory flow demand, the patient must meet that flow demand through another source, which could include

- Additional room air is entrained to compensate for the low-flow rate of the delivery system. This would lead to a reduction in the inspired oxygen concentration.
- Adding a reservoir device would serve to help maintain the inspired oxygen concentration.
- Adding a second oxygen delivery system by connecting two high-flow systems together would also serve to help maintain the inspired oxygen concentration.

13.2.3 High-Flow Nasal Cannula

A newer high-flow system is a *high-flow nasal cannula* (*HFNC*). HFNC refers to a nasal oxygen delivery system that can deliver up to 100% heated/humidified oxygen at a maximum flow rate of ~ 60 L per minute. Based on bench models, the HFNC systems may also generate an element of positive pressure in the posterior pharynx, estimated at ~ 1 cm/H$_2$0 per 10 L/min flow. A HFNC system requires three components (**Figure 13-15**):

1. A high-flow nasal cannula interface device
2. A gas delivery device to control the oxygen and air flow mix, called a *blender*
3. A gas heater/humidifier

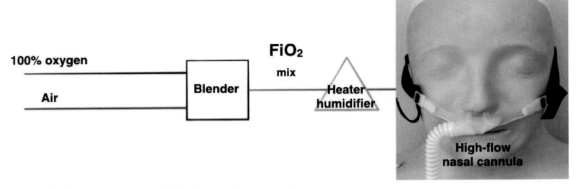

Figure 13-15 *Components of a high-flow nasal oxygen setup.*

The gas delivery system provides the precise FiO_2 delivery.

More recently, HFNC has been promoted as an alternative to oxygen delivered via a face mask or via non-invasive ventilation. HFNC systems have been examined in a variety of patient care areas, including pre-intubation (apneic oxygenation), post-extubation, and for non-invasive support of patients with severe hypoxemic respiratory failure. Proponents have argued that HFNC is more comfortable for the patient and may reduce the work of breathing. However, randomized trials comparing the efficacy of these various modalities have been limited and present conflicting results.

HFNC use prior to and during intubation may achieve better oxygenation throughout the procedure, although these results are controversial.[99,100] In patients with severe hypoxemic respiratory failure secondary to pneumonia, HFNC may be favored over standard face mask therapy or non-invasive positive pressure ventilation.[101]

Pending further clinical trials, we can probably come to two conclusions regarding HFNC:

1. HFNC is not inferior to other methods of support for patients with severe hypoxemic respiratory failure and appears to provide favorable comfort to the patient.
2. HFNC for apneic oxygenation is likely beneficial to patients during intubation, but multiple variables influence the rate of desaturation during intubation and require careful consideration as to modality.

13.2.4 Fixing Hypoxemia

The correction of hypoxemia in the non-mechanically ventilated ICU patient involves consideration of three variables:

1. Device oxygen concentration setting
2. Device flow rate
3. Patient's inspiratory flow rate

Once these variables are appreciated, a few general guidelines apply:

- Target oxygen therapy to achieve a peripheral capillary oxygen saturation (SpO_2) of 90-94%. A slightly reduced target of 88-92% is appropriate for patients with hypercapnic respiratory failure.
- Patients with V/Q mismatch as the etiology for hypoxemia usually have modest FiO_2 requirements, i.e., < 40% oxygen. Manage these patients with low-flow delivery systems, including a nasal cannula or a simple face mask. This category of patient would include patients with COPD exacerbations, status asthmaticus, or pulmonary embolism.
- Patients with V/Q mismatch who require higher oxygen flows from a nasal cannula (> 5 L/min) or a simple face mask may benefit from a reservoir nasal cannula to reduce oxygen flow rate requirements.
- Patients with hypercapnia may be at risk for further hypoventilation with over-oxygenation. Treat these patients with high-flow delivery systems with a controlled inspiratory oxygen concentration, such as a Venturi mask. This category of patient would include patients with hypercapnic COPD and obesity hypoventilation syndrome.
- Patients with shunt physiology as the cause of hypoxemia (very low V/Q) typically have high FiO_2 requirements, i.e., > 40% oxygen. These patients require high-flow delivery systems to regulate the FiO_2. This category of patients could include patients with acute lung injury, pneumonia, pulmonary edema, or atelectasis.
- Patients with shunt physiology and high inspiratory flow demand who remain hypoxemic on high-flow systems may require the addition of a second reservoir or second high-flow system.
- Patients with shunt physiology who stay hypoxemic on high-flow systems may need the

addition of positive end-expiratory pressure (PEEP) to resolve alveolar collapse and lessen shunt physiology. This is typically the case in patients with the adult respiratory distress syndrome and cardiogenic pulmonary edema.

13.3 Assessment of Ventilation (PaCO$_2$)

For the bedside clinician, the most basic assessment of ventilation comes from the measurement of respiratory frequency (f) and tidal volume (Vt). A normal respiratory rate is typically in the range of 12-18 breaths/min, and an average tidal volume in the range of 4-5 ml/kg of ideal body weight. Clinical features of ventilation failure can occur with changes in respiratory frequency or tidal volume in either direction. A reduction in rate or tidal volume, in association with hypercapnia, is characteristic of patients with primary ventilatory failure of a central or neuromuscular basis. Alternatively, a rapid respiratory rate (> 35 breaths/min), often in association with a reduction in tidal volume (< 300 ml), can be a sign of respiratory muscle fatigue with actual or impending respiratory failure (rapid shallow breathing = bad).

Further, the efficiency of that ventilation in clearing carbon dioxide cannot be known from an assessment of tidal breathing and frequency alone. For these reasons, the "right" level of ventilation for a given patient is determined by a combination of physical examination and assessment of arterial blood gases. A discussion of ventilation will introduce several new terms and symbols outlined in **Figure 13-16**.

The blood PaCO$_2$ is determined by the relationship between CO$_2$ production (VCO$_2$) and elimination through alveolar ventilation (V$_A$) as shown in

$$PaCO_2 = VCO_2 \times 0.863 / V_A$$

Breathing pattern has been explored extensively in the assessment of the patient during weaning from mechanical ventilation. The frequency/tidal volume (f/Vt) ratio has been used as a measure of respiratory muscle fatigue during weaning. A value < 105 has both a high positive predictive value (0.78) and a negative predictive value (0.95) for the ability to maintain unassisted breathing after extubation.[4] The f/Vt correlates well with markers of mechanical work and capacity. The efficacy of the f/Vt ratio may obviate the need to routinely measure other weaning variables.

Under normal conditions, the respiratory control center adjusts the level of minute ventilation to achieve clearance of the carbon dioxide generated from tissue metabolism. During exercise, when tissue carbon dioxide production (VCO$_2$) increases significantly, the level of alveolar ventilation (V$_A$) is adjusted proportionally to maintain a relatively constant PaCO$_2$.

In this equation, 0.863 is a constant, which converts fractional concentrations to pressures and corrects volume to standard conditions, so don't worry too much about that number. Note the inverse relationship between the PaCO$_2$ and the V$_A$. You can use this relationship when adjusting ventilators to fix hypercapnia. If the CO$_2$ production and the dead space remain constant, the blood PaCO$_2$ and minute ventilation should have an inverse relationship. If you want to reduce the PaCO$_2$ by ½, you best double the minute ventilation.

To refine this relationship a little further, we know that two additional clinically relevant variables must be incorporated into the relationship as:

$$PaCO_2 \propto K \left[VCO_2 / (V_E - V_{DS}) \right]$$

Anatomic Dead Space	Symbol	Description
Anatomic dead space		Inhaled gas that does not reach gas exchange units
Physiologic dead space		Inhaled gas that reaches gas exchange units with no perfusion and no carbon dioxide exchange
Dead space volume	Vd	Sum of anatomic and physiologic dead space tidal volume
Dead space ventilation	V$_{DS}$	Vd × frequency (f)
Tidal volume	Vt	Exhaled gas volume
Minute ventilation	V$_E$	Vt × frequency (f)
Alveolar ventilation	V$_A$	V$_E$ − V$_{DS}$
Carbon dioxide production	VCO$_2$	Total carbon dioxide production from metabolism

Figure 13-16 Definition of terms used in the analysis of ventilation.

The measured f and Vt do not define the alveolar ventilation, but rather the total minute ventilation (V_E). The total minute ventilation includes a component of alveolar ventilation (V_A), which participates in gas exchange, and dead space ventilation (V_{DS}), which does not participate in the exchange of carbon dioxide. Dead space includes both anatomic dead space (conducting airways) and alveolar dead space (V/Q = infinity). The physiologic dead space can be estimated by the Bohr Equation, which defines the fraction of each tidal breath that is "wasted," i.e., does not clear carbon dioxide. The parameters to define this relationship are

$$V_d /Vt = [P_ACO_2 - P_ECO_2]/P_ACO_2$$

Vd/Vt is the ratio of tidal physiological dead space to tidal volume. In this calculation, alveolar carbon dioxide (P_ACO_2) is assumed to be equivalent to blood $PaCO_2$ (since CO_2 diffuses so fast in the alveolus), and P_ECO_2 is the partial pressure of mixed expired CO_2. A sample of expired gas is collected, and the P_ECO_2 is measured as the "average" partial pressure of carbon dioxide in the sample. In an entirely efficient lung, the P_ECO_2 would equal the P_ACO_2, meaning all the breath volume is devoted to clearing carbon dioxide. However, some volume of the tidal breath must be dedicated to dead space regions, and this gas with 0% CO_2 mixes with alveolar gas to dilute the mixed (alveolar plus dead space) CO_2 concentration. The Bohr equation tells us that the larger the gradient between blood $PaCO_2$ and the expired P_ECO_2, the larger the fraction of the tidal breath that did not participate in gas exchange.

A good way to remember this relationship is to say three times:

P_ACO_2 minus P_ECO_2 over P_ACO_2,
P_ACO_2 minus P_ECO_2 over P_ACO_2,
P_ACO_2 minus P_ECO_2 over P_ACO_2!!!

In the critically ill, the dead space fraction can increase due to disease factors (such as pulmonary thromboembolism) or due to anatomic factors (such as extra ventilator tubing). As the dead space fraction increases, the total minute ventilation must increase to maintain the same alveolar ventilation (carbon dioxide clearance), or the blood carbon dioxide will rise. A critically ill patient can have a very high minute ventilation (f $\times$ Vt) but a low or normal alveolar ventilation (V_A). Because only V_A participates in the removal of carbon dioxide, an ICU patient with a high minute ventilation can be hypocapnic, normocapnic, or even hypercapnic depending on the magnitude of the dead space ventilation. When considering the efficiency of CO_2 removal in the critically ill, the $PaCO_2$ must be considered in comparison to the level of total minute ventilation (frequency $\times$ tidal volume). The variability in the minute ventilation / $PaCO_2$ relationship can be illustrated by considering three different clinical examples:

Example #1. A patient with a centrally mediated reduction in respiratory drive or neuromuscular weakness will have reduced minute ventilation leading to hypercapnia. No contribution of altered V/Q relationships is required to explain the hypercapnia, as minute ventilation is merely inadequate to match the normal CO_2 production (VCO_2).

Example #2. The patient with pulmonary embolism (PE) illustrates the effect of changing V/Q relationships in the normal lung. Total dead space ventilation increases in PE because lung units continue to be ventilated despite diminished or absent perfusion. However, medullary chemoreceptors respond to an increase in the blood arterial $PaCO_2$ and function to increase total minute ventilation, often lowering the arterial $PaCO_2$ to normal or below normal values. So most patients with PE present with a lower than normal arterial $PaCO_2$ and respiratory alkalosis but a high total minute ventilation. If measured correctly, an elevated dead space fraction of ventilation is very characteristic of the PE patient population and is the most sensitive gas exchange parameter for the diagnosis of PE. But the measurement is time-consuming and requires careful gas collection to measure accurately. Analysis of Vd/Vt is rarely done in clinical practice. Evidence suggests the increased total minute ventilation may also occur because of reflex stimulation of irritant and juxtacapillary (J) receptors in the lung, leading to increased total ventilation. This additional stimulus may explain the tendency for PE patients to overventilate. Hypercapnia in acute PE occurs only in association with large pulmonary emboli or in the setting of advanced lung disease.

The vascular obstruction of PE can also cause redistribution of blood flow to low V/Q units, whereas other lung units have excessively high ratios of ventilation to perfusion. Arterial hypoxemia results from the redistribution of flow to these low V/Q units. In addition, atelectasis (caused by loss of surfactant) and alveolar hemorrhage can also contribute to reduced ratios of ventilation to perfusion and produce further arterial hypoxemia. In acute PE, intracardiac shunting may also occur through a patent foramen ovale, since right atrial pressure exceeds left atrial pressure. The use of positive end-expiratory pressure (PEEP) could worsen intracardiac shunting by increasing pulmonary vascular resistance and/or compressing pulmonary vessels. A low pressure of oxygen in venous blood secondary to a reduced cardiac output also may contribute to arterial hypoxemia when PE causes right ventricular failure. Hypoxemia in PE can be a contribution of increased perfusion of low V/Q units, R to L shunting, and low mixed venous oxygen saturation. Not surprisingly, the measured PaO_2 in PE patients can be very hard to predict, and this has been confirmed by numerous clinical studies. In fact, a low percentage (~5-10%) of patients with PE can have a normal PaO_2.

Example #3. The patient with ARDS presents with non-cardiogenic pulmonary edema with flooding of the alveolar space and significant disturbances in gas exchange. The classic gas exchange defect in ARDS is the right-to-left intrapulmonary shunt, leading to marked arterial hypoxemia. However, numerous clinical studies have confirmed that a marked increase in dead space also characterizes ARDS. Anatomic dead space can be increased by components of the ventilator circuit and by low tidal volume ventilation. In lower tidal volume ventilation, the normal anatomic dead space of 150 mL in the trachea and airways starts to represent a large contribution of the small tidal volume. Physiologic dead space can be attributed to injury of pulmonary capillaries by thrombotic and inflammatory mechanisms, leading to obstruction of pulmonary blood flow. In shunt units, venous blood passes through the lung without exchanging carbon dioxide and then mixes with arterial blood. Venous blood has a higher carbon dioxide content than does arterial blood from ventilated and perfused lung units, and a shunt thereby leads to an increase in arterial $PaCO_2$. Shunt physiology thus contributes to the classical concept of physiological dead space. In ARDS, the shunt component may reach .50% of cardiac output, significantly increasing the VE needed to maintain a normal $PaCO_2$. An increased Vd/Vt in early ARDS is an important gas exchange predictor of mortality.

How do we accurately measure the Vd/Vt? Vd/Vt can be measured by collecting exhaled gas into a 30-60L Douglas bag. An arterial blood gas is obtained during the midpoint of the collection. Vd/Vt is calculated using a modification of the Bohr equation, where P_ACO_2 is assumed to equal the blood $PaCO_2$, and the expired CO_2 (P_ECO_2) is obtained from the Douglas bag collection. P_ACO_2 minus P_ECO_2 over P_ACO_2! The normal Vd/Vt

A patient is reported to have "apnea" during a weaning trial. Before you decide the patient has suffered a devastating neurologic event, the first parameter to assess is the blood $PaCO_2$. If low, the apnea is "normal" and the patient has not ventilated due to the lack of an appropriate metabolic stimulus. If observed for an appropriate period of time (blood $PaCO_2$ increases appropriately 3 mm Hg per minute), the patient will develop a normal spontaneous ventilation as the $PaCO_2$ rises. The patient has likely been overventilated prior to the weaning trial.

is within the range of 0.15-0.35 and is influenced by such variables as age, tidal volume, and body position. This value can rise significantly in critical illness and usually accounts for the high minute ventilation with hypercapnia seen in patients with advanced lung disease. An increase in physiologic dead space can occur in the setting of hypovolemia (no Q), or lung overdistention in air-trapping, due to the conversion of very high V/Q units to physiologic dead space. Your friend "P_ACO_2 minus P_ECO_2 over $PACO_2$" can tell you how bad your lung disease is in a variety of disorders.

In the early phases of most parenchymal lung disorders, increasing V_E compensates for abnormalities in V/Q relationships that can produce hypercapnia. Commonly, patients initially present with hypoxemia, hyperventilation, and normal to low blood $PaCO_2$ levels. As the disease advances, however, a combination of increasing dead space ventilation or mechanical fatigue from the increased workload of ventilation leads to progressive hypercapnia.

13.3.1 Non-Invasive Assessment of Carbon Dioxide

The non-invasive assessment of $PaCO_2$ is most commonly approached using the technique of capnometry. Capnometry involves the measurement of expired carbon dioxide at the airway opening (P_ECO_2). A continuous real-time measurement is displayed as a capnogram and shows the measured P_ECO_2 continuously in a gas sample from near the mouth over the entire respiratory cycle (Figure 13-17). Capnometry typically uses infrared light transmission through the sample of gas to measure carbon dioxide partial pressure.

The capnograph rises from 0% during the inspiratory phase to a flattened height or plateau termed the end-tidal CO_2 ($P_{ET}CO_2$). $P_{ET}CO_2$ differs slightly from P_ECO_2), which is a sample from a collected volume of gas. The capnography uses real-time monitoring and does not collect the gas sample.

The $P_{ET}CO_2$ should reflect the partial pressure of carbon dioxide in the alveolar space and therefore the blood $PaCO_2$. As the patient exhales, a CO_2 sensor at the airway will detect no CO_2, since this initial portion of exhaled air is all dead space from the conducting airways (Phase I in Figure 13-17). As exhalation continues, the CO_2 concentration will gradually rise as the CO_2 is emptied from the alveoli. Phase II will reflect a mixture of anatomical and physiologic dead space with alveolar gas. The tracing will reach a relative plateau, which indicates the concentration of CO_2 from alveolar gas (Phase III). Once the patient begins inhalation of air (CO_2 free), the CO_2 concentration returns to zero.

The slope of the curve between the inspiratory value and the $P_{ET}CO_2$ provides a rough indicator of the variable

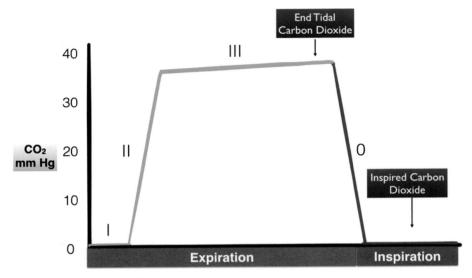

Figure 13-17 Capnograph tracing.

emptying of dead space volume and alveolar volume. Although the $P_{ET}CO_2$ can be used as a surrogate for blood $PaCO_2$ in the patient on mechanical ventilation, the values are not necessarily equivalent. The blood $PaCO_2$ rapidly equilibrates with alveolar P_ACO_2, but this is not necessarily equivalent to the $P_{ET}CO_2$. During expiration, lung regions with high V/Q ratios or physiologic dead space dilute the expired CO_2 from more normal V/Q units, so a gradient exists between blood $PaCO_2$ and $P_{ET}CO_2$. Remember P_ACO_2 minus P_ECO_2? This dilution creates a ($PaCO_2$ - $P_{ET}CO_2$) gradient. The normal gradient is 4-5 mm Hg, attributable to normal physiologic dead space. A more significant gradient is seen in clinical conditions associated with an increase in physiologic dead space (i.e., age, emphysema, low cardiac output, pulmonary or air embolism). Higher tidal volumes or more prolonged expiratory times would limit the dilution component and narrow the gradient. Controlling for all these variables is difficult in the interpretation of capnography results, and $\Delta P_{ET}CO_2$ cannot reliably predict $\Delta PaCO_2$ in critically ill adult patients. This makes arterial blood gas analysis still an important component in the assessment of ventilation for these patients.

Despite these limitations, capnography can be used effectively in several important clinical situations, including the following:

- $P_{ET}CO_2$ is a reliable method for evaluating the effectiveness of cardiopulmonary resuscitation correlating with cardiac output during chest compressions in humans. As cardiac output drops, CO_2 is not delivered from the body to the alveolus, and the detection of $P_{ET}CO_2$ is no longer present.

Measurement of a low end-tidal CO_2 (< 10 mm Hg) during CPR in an intubated patient would suggest that the quality of chest compressions needs improvement. When the patient has the return of spontaneous circulation (ROSC), there will be a significant increase in the $P_{ET}CO_2$ (35-45 mm Hg).

- The ($PaCO_2$-$P_{ET}CO_2$) gradient correlates strongly with dead space ventilation and therefore is an indicator of dead space volume (P_ACO_2 minus P_ECO_2). During therapeutic maneuvers that might alter dead space, such as the application of positive end-expiratory pressure or lung recruitment strategies, the monitoring of the gradient can provide an indicator of therapeutic success. Positive end-expiratory pressure can improve gas exchange through recruitment of collapsed V/Q units. However, overdistention of high V/Q units can increase physiologic dead space, making the use of the monitoring tool very helpful.

13.4 Hypercapnic Respiratory Failure

The treatment for hypercapnic respiratory failure is to improve the $PaCO_2$ to a value that achieves a pH > 7.30. Improvement in hypercapnia can be achieved by maneuvers that reduce metabolism (CO_2 production), limit dead space, or, most commonly, augment minute ventilation (V_E). The augmentation of V_E can be achieved through either invasive (endotracheal tube) or non-invasive mechanical ventilation (NIV).

A major component in the assessment of ventilation is determining whether the hypercapnia is acute or chronic. This assessment generally involves the interpretation of arterial blood gases and the analysis of blood pH. *Acidemia* is defined as a pH < 7.35 and *alkalemia* as a pH > 7.45. An acid-base disorder can be suspected when the $PaCO_2$ is outside the normal range of 35-45 mm Hg, the plasma bicarbonate concentration is outside the normal range of 22-26 mEq/L, or the arterial base excess is more than 3 or less than −3 meq/L. The body responds to an acid-base disorder by making compensatory changes in either the $PaCO_2$ (respiratory compensation) or HCO_3^- (renal compensation). A trick to remember is that the compensation serves to protect the $HCO_3/PaCO_2$ ratio, and therefore the pH requires a compensatory response that varies in the same direction as the primary disorder (low $PaCO_2$ leads to low bicarbonate and high $PaCO_2$ to a high bicarbonate). The relationship between the pH and $PaCO_2$ provides a starting point for the assessment of acid-base disorders. Hypocapnia with alkalemia defines respiratory alkalosis, while hypercapnia with acidemia defines a respiratory acidosis.

The relationship between pH, $PaCO_2$, and the plasma bicarbonate concentration can be conceptualized as:

$$[H+] = [PaCO_2] / [HCO_3^-]$$

A normal proton concentration is maintained by a $PaCO_2$ of about 40 mm Hg and by a HCO_3^- of 24-26 mEq/L. For acidosis, increasing $PaCO_2$ increases hydrogen ion, and decreasing bicarbonate increases hydrogen ion. For alkalosis, decreasing $PaCO_2$ decreases hydrogen ion, and increasing bicarbonate decreases hydrogen ion.

Easy!!!

13.4.1 Primary and Secondary Compensation

When you have a primary disturbance that changes the hydrogen ion concentration, the body will attempt to compensate to keep the pH normal. The lung defends (compensates) the hydrogen ion concentration (and pH) by changing $PaCO_2$, and the kidney defends (compensates) the hydrogen ion concentration by changing HCO_3^-. The lung can do this by hyperventilating or hypoventilating. The kidney can do this by retaining HCO_3^- at the proximal tubule or by increasing fixed acid excretion at the distal tubule. The proximal tubule reabsorption of bicarbonate is massive, with up to 4,500 mEq per day reabsorbed! However, other tricks are needed to clear the acid being generated from metabolism. The kidney has two tricks to do this. The first is a high-capacity ATP-dependent proton pump

that pumps out a proton and recovers bicarbonate. One proton removed, *AND* one bicarbonate saved! The second trick is to hydrolyze glutamine and generate NH_4+ ions, which are excreted in the urine; this removes $H+$ and saves a HCO_3^-. The relationship between these variables is summarized as

$$[H+] + [HCO_3^-] \leftrightarrow [H_2CO_3] \leftrightarrow [H_2O] + [CO_2]$$

So, let's consider a few examples in our brain......

Respiratory acidosis. Your patient is not ventilating well and does not blow off enough $PaCO_2$. Hypoventilation increases the $PaCO_2$, which reacts with water to increase carbonic acid, which increases protons, causing an acidosis. Note that bicarbonate will also increase as you drive the full balanced equation to the left and your kidneys begin to compensate to excrete proton and retain bicarbonate.

Respiratory alkalosis. Your patient is hyperventilating (from pain, sepsis, liver failure), and you are removing too much CO_2. This "pulls" the balance equation to the right, so the proton is removed, bicarbonate is removed, carbonic acid is down, and the patient develops an alkalosis. The kidney responds by reducing proton/bicarbonate exchange and letting go the bicarbonate.

To determine if the kidney has developed the appropriate compensation for a respiratory change in $PaCO_2$, we have many fascinating compensation rules to guide us.

The expected compensatory changes of HCO_3^- and $H+$ for *acute* respiratory acidosis are

$$\Delta[H+] = 0.8 \; \Delta \, P_ACO_2 \; OR \; 10 \; \Delta \, [HCO_3^-] = \Delta \, P_ACO_2$$

This means that for every 10-point increase in $PaCO_2$, the pH will decrease by 8 units. *This is the easiest to memorize: 10 changes pH by 0.08.* If $PaCO_2$ increases from 40 to 50, we expect the pH to drop from 7.40 to 7.32. For the same patient, the HCO_3^- would increase from 24 to 25.

For *chronic* respiratory acidosis, the parameters are modified to

$$\Delta \, [H^+] = 0.3 \; 10 \; \Delta P_ACO_2 \; OR \; 10 \; 10 \; \Delta \, [HCO_3^-] = 3.5 \; 10 \; \Delta P_ACO_2$$

This means that for every 10-point increase in $PaCO_2$, the pH will decrease by 3 units. If $PaCO_2$ increases from 40 to 50, we expect the pH to drop from 7.40 to 7.37. For the same patient, the HCO_3^- would increase from 24 to 27.5. Note that with chronic compensation, the kidney has time to retain more HCO_3^- and this limits the pH decrease.

If the measured values of compensation do not correlate with the predicted values, this suggests a superimposed metabolic acid-base disorder or a "mixed" disorder. It is important to note that the pH improves but never normalizes even with sufficient compensation for respiratory acidosis. A complete normalization or over-shoot in pH suggests another disorder.

The compensation rules for respiratory acidosis and hypercapnia can be used to help you determine whether the ventilation failure is acute or chronic.

13.4.2 Etiology of Ventilation Disorders in the ICU

Respiratory alkalosis in the ICU patient can be secondary to a broad range of disorders summarized in **Figure 13-18**.

Alkalemia is usually associated with an adverse outcome when the pH > 7.60. This level of pH change is associated with electrolyte abnormalities (i.e., hypokalemia), pulmonary vasoconstriction, decreased cardiac contractility, and seizures.

In contrast, *respiratory acidosis* in the ICU patient is usually secondary to some type of mechanical respiratory failure. The causes are classified by etiology and listed in **Figure 13-19**.

Etiology of Respiratory Alkalosis	Examples
Central disorder	Meningitis, fever, anxiety
Peripheral disorder	Pain, hypoxemia
System disorder	Hepatic disease, pregnancy
Drug induced	Salicylate overdose
Iatrogenic disorder	Mechanical ventilation-induced hyperventilation

Figure 13-18 Classification of respiratory alkalosis by cause with clinical examples.

Etiology of Respiratory Acidosis	Examples
Upper airway obstruction	Laryngospasm, tracheal tumor
Lower airway obstruction	COPD, status asthmaticus
Parenchymal lung disease	ARDS, pneumonia, interstitial lung disease
Central disorders of ventilation	Drug overdose
Neuromuscular disorders	Guillain-Barre, critical illness polyneuropathy
Chest wall disorders	Kyphoscoliosis, obesity

Figure 13-19 Classification of respiratory acidosis by cause with clinical examples.

If the required minute ventilation for CO_2 clearance exceeds the capacity of the ventilatory muscles, the patient develops hypercapnia and often requires ventilatory assistance. While mechanical ventilation can usually "normalize" the hypercapnia, this may come at the cost of a high tidal volume or respiratory frequency, which can have risks for the patient. In the ICU patient some degree of hypercapnia may be tolerated, termed "permissive hypercapnia," until the dead space ventilation improves with treatment of the underlying disease process. Permissive hypercapnia is commonly employed in severe obstructive pulmonary disease or advanced ARDS to prevent complications of mechanical ventilation related to high tidal volumes. Current data suggests this produces little adverse effect and that hypercapnia and respiratory acidosis may actually be protective in these settings. Permissive hypercapnia is contraindicated in the setting of disordered cerebral blood flow (i.e., cerebral edema) due to the recognized cerebral vasodilating effects of hypercapnia.

The patient's clinical symptoms of ventilatory failure and respiratory acidosis may range from confusion, lethargy, and agitation to more advanced signs and symptoms, including seizures, cardiac arrhythmias, and pulmonary hypertension. The patient may also be asymptomatic.

Because the patient may present with variable levels of compensation for hypercapnia, the target for correction is not based upon the $PaCO_2$. The target for correction in hypercapnic respiratory failure is based upon the pH with a goal to achieve a pH > 7.30. Although this can be achieved by maneuvers that reduce metabolism (CO_2 production), limit dead space, or augment minute ventilation (V_E), most commonly we approach the patient with severe hypercapnia with the use of positive pressure ventilation. The augmentation of V_E can be achieved through either invasive (endotracheal tube) or non-invasive mechanical ventilation (NIV). Let's move to a discussion of mechanical ventilation. But first, we better talk about *a little basic respiratory mechanics, so you can understand that ventilator.*

Suggested Reading

- Dantzger DR. Pulmonary Gas Exchange. In: Dantzger DR, ed. Cardiopulmonary critical care. 2nd Edition. Phladelphia: WB Saunders, 1991:25–43.
- Nuckton TJ, Alonso JA, Kallet RH, et al. Pulmonary dead-space fraction as a risk factor for death in

the acute respiratory distress syndrome. NEJM 2002;346(17):1281–6.

- Siddiki H, Kojicic M, Li G, et al. Bedside quantification of dead-space fraction using routine clinical data in patients with acute lung injury: secondary analysis of two prospective trials. Critical Care 2010;14(4):1–8.
- Girardis, M., Busani, S., Damiani, E., Donati, A., Rinaldi, L., Marudi, A., et al. Effect of conservative vs conventional oxygen therapy on mortality among patients in an intensive care unit: The Oxygen-ICU Randomized Clinical Trial. JAMA 2016: 316(15), 1583–1589.
- Siemienium RA, Chu DK, Kim LH, et al. Oxygen therapy for acutely ill medical patients: a clinical practice guideline. BMJ 2018:363:k4169

14

Mechanics of Respiratory Failure

14.1 Simple Mechanics of Lung Inflation – the EOM

Understanding the mechanics of lung inflation and deflation can be a little intimidating and even downright annoying. Pressures, flows, volumes, elastance, resistance, compliance, etc., etc. can give you a headache. Relax—it is easiest to learn the mechanics of breathing in the hospital setting. Not only do you have patients to help you, but you also get a fancy machine with bells, whistles, curves, and all sorts of buttons to change. When you watch how the ventilator and patient interact as you change the parameters or as the patient's condition varies, the whole thing starts to make a little sense. And you now remember why it is so important to learn it all in the first place!

The mechanical ventilator can provide total assistance to breathing (such as in the operating room under anesthesia), no assistance (a spontaneous breathing trial), or partial assistance (a pressure support trial). So, where to start? Most discussions of lung mechanics begin with the spontaneously breathing patient. But let's be radical and approach this a little differently. Let's start with an ICU or operating room patient who is sedated and paralyzed, on mechanical ventilation. In this example, the patient is on total assistance or is a *passive patient* during lung inflation. Remember, our *passive* patient is providing no muscular effort. We will need to define some terms, using **Figure 14-1** to help us.

In a passively ventilated patient, the pressure required to deliver the tidal breath and inflate the respiratory system (Prs) is equivalent to the airway pressure applied by the ventilator (Pao). The simplified *Equation of Motion*

Mechanics Parameter	Definition
Pao	Positive pressure located at the airway opening. This would be the pressure generated by the ventilator to inflate the lung and chest in a paralyzed patient.
Pmus	Negative pressure generated by the respiratory muscles
Prs	Pressure required to inflate the respiratory system
Vt	Tidal volume (the amount of air exchanged per breath)
Vt/Ti	Inspiratory flow (tidal volume/inspiratory time)
Rrs	Resistance of the respiratory system
Crs	Compliance of the respiratory system
PEEPtotal	The total alveolar pressure at end expiration (includes extrinsic or applied PEEP and intrinsic PEEP)

Figure 14-1 Terms used to define respiratory mechanics.

(EOM) of the respiratory system defines the pressure requirement for lung inflation.

$$Prs = Pao = (Vt/Crs) + (Vt/Ti \times Rrs) + PEEPtotal$$

Remember this equation! We are going to keep coming back to this over and over when we think about the ventilator. Look closely at the terms of this equation and **Figure 14-2**. Essentially, this equation consists of three components:

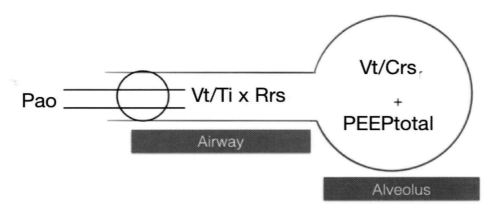

Figure 14-2 *Graphic illustrating components of lung mechanics. See Figure 14-1 for definition of terms.*

1. *Flow × resistance* (Vt/Ti × Rrs). The pressure required to inflate the lungs and chest wall (respiratory system) to a new volume has a resistive component originating primarily within the conducting airways. The higher the flow and the resistance, the greater the pressure needed to move a constant tidal volume of air. Thus, the magnitude of the pressure change is determined by the speed of gas flow (Vt/Ti) and the respiratory system resistance to airflow (Rrs).

2. *Compliance* (Vt/Crs). The pressure required to inflate the lungs and chest wall (respiratory system) to a new volume has an elastic component related to lung and chest wall inflation. The magnitude of the pressure change is determined by the size of the tidal volume (Vt) and is inversely related to the respiratory system compliance (Crs). Since Crs is in the denominator, low lung compliance (*stiff lung* in an ARDS patient) results in higher Vt/Crs and higher-pressure requirement. Note this is a volume-dependent elastic parameter.

3. Basal end-expiratory pressure (PEEPtotal). One additional component is best characterized as an elastic component. Under normal breathing conditions, alveolar pressure is 0 at the end of a breath. When the ventilator increases airway pressure above 0, inspiratory airflow occurs along an airway to alveolar pressure gradient. In the ICU, alveolar pressure is often maintained above 0 at end expiration. This positive end-expiratory pressure (PEEP) must be figured in the total pressure requirement for a tidal breath. PEEP can be produced externally by the ventilator or internally by the mechanics of the lung (often called *intrinsic* or *auto-PEEP*). The airway pressure required to inflate the lung to a new volume must include the positive end-expiratory pressure used to maintain alveolar volume including both intrinsic (auto-PEEP) and extrinsic PEEP.

The Equation of Motion shows you that changing a parameter alters the pressure required to deliver a breath. At a constant tidal volume, any decrease in the respiratory system compliance, increase in flow, increase in resistance, or increase in total PEEP, will augment the pressure requirement for the ventilator to deliver a given tidal volume.

So, the mechanics of each ventilator breath are determined by 4 × 3 components:

4 Set Ventilator Parameters → Pressure, Flow, Volume, Extrinsic PEEP
3 Patient Parameters → Compliance, Resistance, Intrinsic PEEP

A model that illustrates the respiratory system might be a tube connected to a balloon (**Figure 14-3**). Inflation of the balloon requires adequate pressure at the tube

> The Equation of Motion (EOM) is great to remember when the nurse calls to say the airway pressures on the ventilator are too high in a patient on volume-controlled ventilation. The Equation of Motion tells you how to organize the types of problems to look for in your patient (i.e., resistance problems, compliance problems, or anything that increases total PEEP). In a later pearl, we will tell you how to tell resistance from compliance problems. The EOM also tells you what you can do to fix high airway pressures, including lowering the tidal volume, reducing flow, or decreasing PEEP.

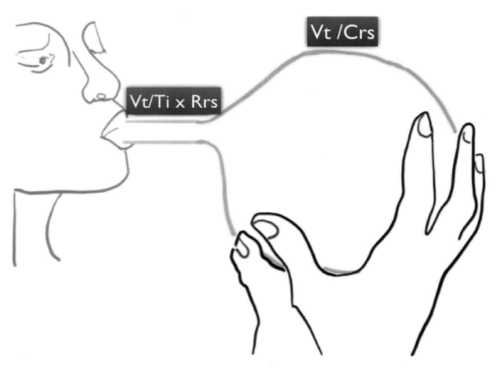

Figure 14-3 *A model to illustrate lung inflation. See Figure 14-1 for definition of terms.*

opening to overcome the resistance of the tube and then enough pressure to overcome the elastic recoil of the balloon. In the interest of accuracy, however, the respiratory system has two elastic components: the lungs and the chest wall/diaphragm. The first component (the lungs) lives inside the other component (chest wall and diaphragm), and both of these are connected to the same tube. The balloon represents the elastic elements of the lung, while the tube represents the resistive elements of the conducting airways. Think of a pair of hands around the balloon representing the chest wall. At lower lung volumes, the chest wall recoils (hands pull) to assist the lung opening. At higher lung volumes, the chest wall recoils (hands squeeze) to add to the elastic recoil of the lungs. In certain conditions, such as obesity, the chest wall is less compliant (hands squeeze), and a greater airway pressure is needed to inflate the lungs. In other conditions, the lung (balloon) is less compliant and higher airway pressures are needed. To accomplish ventilation, the respiratory pump (muscles) or a mechanical ventilator must overcome these elastic properties of the lung and chest wall and the resistive properties of the conducting airways.

How do we think about the PEEP term in the Equation of Motion? Let's suppose someone else (hopefully a very close friend) first partially inflated the balloon, pinched the tube (PEEP), and handed it to you. To finish the inflation, you would first need to blow hard enough and

generate enough pressure to overcome the elastic recoil from the partially expanded first breath (overcome the higher pressure already in the balloon or the PEEP). Then, if you continued to increase the airway pressure, you could further increase the balloon volume above the first breath. Do not try this at home!

Let's move from a passive breath to an assisted breath. An excellent clinical example here might be a pressure support weaning trial where the patient provides some effort and the ventilator provides some assistance. The Equation of Motion still applies to an assisted breath, but we need to make a little change. The patient's respiratory muscles now contribute to the pressure generated to achieve the tidal volume. We need to rewrite the Equation of Motion as shown

$$Prs = Pao + (-Pmus) = (Vt/Crs) + (Vt/Ti \times Rrs) + PEEPtotal$$

Whoa! What is that -Pmus term, after a positive sign?? Very confusing? No, not really. The pressure to inflate the respiratory system can include a positive pressure at the airway (Pao) or a negative pressure produced by the respiratory muscles (Pmus). The pressure generated by the respiratory muscles is measured as a negative intrathoracic pressure. A negative intrathoracic pressure creates a vacuum around the lung and drops alveolar pressure, effectively pulling air in from the airway (high

A patient is being supported on mechanical ventilation with set parameters of a tidal volume of 400ml, RR 14, PEEP 10, FiO_2 0.60. The patient is breathing at 40 breaths per minute, and you elect to paralyze the patient. The respiratory rate falls to 20 bpm, but you note his airway pressures have risen by 20 cm H_2O. What happened? Prior to paralysis, you were only seeing the Pao of the ventilator and not the Pmus of the patient. Once the patient was paralyzed, the Pao now must increase to make up for the loss of the Pmus. The transpulmonary pressure is really unchanged – if tidal volume and flow remain constant. We just shifted all the pressure requirement to the ventilator and rested the respiratory muscles.

pressure) into the alveoli (low pressure). Thus, the actual lung inflation pressure is the sum of the airway pressure (+) and the negative respiratory muscle pressure (−). The equation can get confusing with the positive and negative terms. Keep it simple. Add the airway pressure from the ventilator to the respiratory muscle pressure (ignore the negative), creating a delta which is the sum of the positive and the negative value. So for the EOM, we are going to convert all the negative muscle pressures (Pmus) to a positive value so we get the sum of the two inflation pressures.

The airway pressure (Pao) generated by the ventilator and the negative intrathoracic pressure produced by the inspiratory muscles (Pmus) combine to create the total respiratory system inflation pressure Prs. As the patient shifts to spontaneous ventilation, the respiratory muscles will need to generate the total pressure required to inflate the respiratory system. Whether it is the ventilator, the respiratory muscles, or a little bit of both, the pressure required for a given tidal volume is determined by the elastic and resistive components of the respiratory system. Let's take a little closer look at those parameters on the right side of the EOM.

14.2 Compliance/Elastance and Pleural Pressure

We can break the pressure required to inflate the lungs into static and dynamic components. The static components are measured in the absence of airflow and reflect the pressure required to create a volume change in the lung and chest wall (functionally the chest wall and abdomen). Under conditions of zero airflow and relaxed respiratory muscles, the pressure required to inflate the

respiratory system (Prs) (both lung and chest wall) will be equivalent to the airway pressure (Pa_o) measured on the ventilator. From the EOM, in this clinical condition, the Pmus is 0 and our equation simplifies to

$$Prs = Pao = (Vt/Crs) + PEEPtotal$$

If we increase the airway pressure (Pao) with the ventilator to a new value, what tidal volume change can we expect? This gets a little more complicated because we are actually changing the volume of both the lung and the chest wall.

The pressure required to distend the respiratory system to a given volume is dependent on the recoil pressure of the lung and chest wall. The unique feature of the lung and chest wall is that the recoil pressure of each structure changes based upon the state of their inflation. The lung recoil is directed inwards at all lung volumes. The chest wall has different mechanical characteristics dependent on the state of inflation. At low lung volumes (residual volume), the chest wall tends to recoil outwards, favoring lung inflation. At the higher lung volumes, the chest wall recoil pressure is directed inward and favors lung collapse. In the transition from residual volume to total lung capacity, the chest wall assists lung inflation to about 60% of total lung capacity, where it transitions to favor lung collapse with progressive lung inflation.

The pressure gradient required to change the lung volume is called the *transpulmonary pressure (Ptp)*, and the pressure gradient needed to change the chest wall volume is called the *transthoracic pressure (Pw)*.

The transpulmonary pressure (Ptp) is equivalent to the difference between airway pressure (Pao) and pleural pressure (Ppl) as:

$$Ptp = Pao − Ppl$$

The transthoracic pressure (Pw), or pressure across the chest wall, is the difference between pleural pressure and atmospheric pressure as:

$$Pw = Ppl − Patm$$

Interesting, but is any of this information relevant to treating patients? Understanding the relationship between airway pressure and inflation of the respiratory system is very important when considering mechanical ventilation. Let's consider two different alveoli as shown by the schematic of an alveolus (large red circle) within the chest wall (blue box) as outlined in **Figure 14-4.** The ventilator delivers a breath to a specific level of airway pressure (Pao). In alveolus A, the Pao will be 25; in alveolus B, the Pao will be 50. Under conditions of no airflow, the airway pressure (Pao)

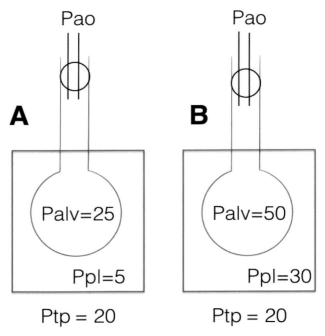

Figure 14-4 *Comparison of transpulmonary (Ptp), airway opening (Pao), alveolar (Palv), and pleural (Ppl) pressures under conditions of normal (A) and high (B) pleural pressures.*

will be approximately equal to the alveolar pressure (Palv). The transpulmonary pressure (pressure across the lung) determines the actual change in lung volume. Transpulmonary pressure (Ptp) is the difference between airway (Pao) = alveolar pressure (Palv) and pleural pressure (Ppl). In alveolus A, the Ptp is equal to 25 − 5, or 20, leading to a change in alveolus volume, which is determined by the compliance of the alveolus. In alveolus B, the Ptp is equal to 50 − 30, or 20. In the case of alveolus B, the Pao is markedly elevated in comparison to alveolus A, BUT the transpulmonary pressure is identical. The change in alveolar volume between alveolus A and B would also be equal because of the higher pleural pressure in alveolus B.

Clinical examples that can lead to higher than normal pleural pressures include morbid obesity, abdominal distention from abdominal compartment syndrome, or pleural effusions. In all these conditions, airway pressures may read high, but the change in lung volume can be small.

We will use airway pressure measurements frequently in the ICU patient with respiratory failure to estimate lung mechanics. In doing this, we will "assume" that with zero airflow, Pao = Palv. We will use Pao, measured on the ventilator, to estimate lung compliance and guide us in efforts to minimize the risk of lung overinflation. We will also apply positive end-expiratory pressure (PEEP) to maintain lung volume. We will assume that

Ppl is low in most patients and that Pao predicts lung volume. But we need to remember that Pao reflects the components of both lung and chest wall mechanics. Pao may be markedly elevated, but this only indicates a significant change in lung volume if Ppl is "normal."

If you wanted to measure Ppl, you would need to place an esophageal balloon manometer. We will talk more about this issue when we consider the use of positive end-expiratory pressure (PEEP) in patients with hypoxemia.

A static respiratory system pressure-volume curve can be measured in intubated patients by inflating and deflating the respiratory system to sequential lung volumes and measuring the static (zero flow) airway pressure (**Figure 14-5**). On the X-axis, we have the change in pressure across the respiratory system. On the Y-axis we have the change in lung volume above baseline. The pressure measured at the airway opening (Pao) at each lung volume, during a period of interrupted airflow with relaxed (paralyzed) respiratory muscles, will be equal to the elastic recoil pressure of the lung and chest wall. The inflation curve is slightly different than the deflation curve, a feature termed hysteresis, resulting in an inspiratory-expiratory pressure-volume loop. Hysteresis is produced by surface tension at the gas-liquid interface of the alveoli and collapse of small airways at small lung volumes, both of which must be overcome to inflate the lung. Remember this curve only accurately reflects the respiratory system elastic recoil characteristics in a patient without respiratory *muscle activity (no Pmus)*.

During normal tidal volume breathing (30% to 70% vital capacity), the relationship between pressure and volume is linear, and the system's elastic properties can

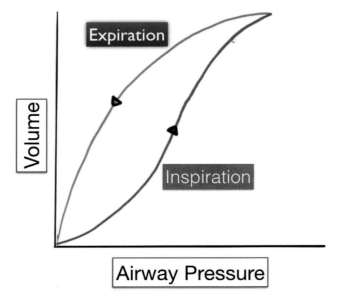

Figure 14-5 *Pressure – volume replationship of the respiratory system during the respiratory cycle.*

be defined by a constant, namely *elastance*. Elastance measures the change in pressure required for a given change in volume. The term *compliance* is most frequently used in the ICU setting and is simply the inverse of elastance, defined as the change in volume per unit change in applied pressure ($C_{rs} = V_t/\Delta P_{ao}$). The normal respiratory system compliance is 80-100 mL/cm H_2O. The slope of the curve in **Figure 14-5** is a measure of compliance, since this reflects the rise over the run or the volume generated with increasing pressure ($V_t/\Delta P_{ao}$).

Note that at high lung volumes, the compliance of the respiratory system declines (curve flattens). This flattening of the pressure-volume relationship is primarily due to a limitation of lung compliance at total lung capacity. At low lung volumes, again the respiratory system compliance declines, but in this case the change is primarily due to a change in chest wall compliance and collapsing alveoli that stick together.

The lung recoil is a collapsing force that is offset by the transpulmonary pressure distending force created by the inspiratory muscles and chest wall. This lung recoil component is composed of tissue components and surface tension components. Surface tension is generated from the interaction of liquid and air molecules along the alveolar surface. Surface tension accounts for about 50% of the elastic recoil component associated with lung inflation. Surfactant's role in the lung is to lower surface tension. Depletion of surfactant during lung injury will further increase the elastic recoil properties of the lung and promote alveolar instability and collapse, especially at lower lung volumes. This results in a requirement for higher transpulmonary pressures to maintain inflation of the surfactant-depleted lung. This physiology is characteristic of the patient with the adult respiratory distress syndrome (ARDS). Common causes of decreased respiratory system compliance in an ICU patient are listed in **Figure 14-6**.

14.2.1 Measurement of Compliance

Respiratory system compliance can be measured in the ICU patient using the mechanical ventilator (**Figure 14-7**). The airway pressure is shown in this figure on the Y-axis, and time is the variable on the X-axis. The breath is divided into phases consisting of inspiration, an inspiratory hold, and expiration. The measurement requires the delivery of a tidal breath (V_t) with a constant rate of gas flow during the breath delivery (termed *square wave flow*). Airway pressures are measured before the breath starts (end-expiration) and at the end of the breath (end-inspiration). Immediately following the delivery of the target tidal volume, an inspiratory hold is produced on the ventilator so that no additional flow of gas occurs as either inspiration or expiration – a brief "inspiratory hold" maneuver. The patient's respiratory muscles must be either relaxed or paralyzed so they do not contribute to changes in pleural pressure. When the breath hold maneuver is performed, the pressure components of the Equation of Motion determined by flow and airway resistance ($V_t/T_i \times R_{rs}$) are zero. Under these conditions, the pressure measured at the airway (Pao) is equivalent to the alveolar pressure (Palv). The airway pressure (Pao) that you measure during the breath hold maneuver is called the *plateau pressure* (Pplat). We can calculate the change in alveolar pressure during the tidal breath as [Pplat- end-expiratory pressure (PEEP)]. This pressure gradient is called the *driving pressure*. We can also measure the change in tidal volume. From these two variables, we can calculate the respiratory system compliance as the change in tidal volume/change in alveolar pressure.

This pressure-time curve in **Figure 14-7** is a critical measurement that you will use regularly in your ICU practice. The Pplat is most closely related to the risk of ventilator-induced injury from barotrauma or volutrauma (provided the pleural pressure is not elevated). The Pplat gives you a physiologic indicator of the "stiffness" of the lung and chest wall.

As mentioned, for Pplat to accurately reflect Palv, the patient cannot have respiratory muscle activity. Active expiratory muscle contraction can falsely elevate the Pplat. Active inspiratory muscle contraction can falsely lower the Pplat. If your patient is paralyzed – no worries. If your patient is not paralyzed, look carefully at your Pplat tracing. You would want to see a very flat Pplat measurement tracing. Upward or downward drift would strongly suggest respiratory muscle activity.

Compliance is calculated as:

tidal volume/(end-inspiratory pressure [Pplat] - end-expiratory pressure [PEEPtotal])

The calculation of total PEEP is the additive level of ventilator set PEEP and intrinsic PEEP. A couple of examples for the compliance calculation are outlined in **Figure 14-8**.

Causes of Decreased Lung/Thorax Compliance	Causes of Decreased Chest Wall Compliance
Pulmonary edema	Obesity
Pulmonary fibrosis	Ascites or increased abdominal pressure
Adult respiratory distress syndrome	Flail chest
Mainstem intubation (only ventilating one lung)	Kyphoscoliosis
Dynamic hyperinflation (intrinsic PEEP to overcome)	Neuromuscular weakness
	Pleural disease (e.g., fibrothorax, tension pneumothorax)

Figure 14-6 Conditions which impact respiratory system compliance.

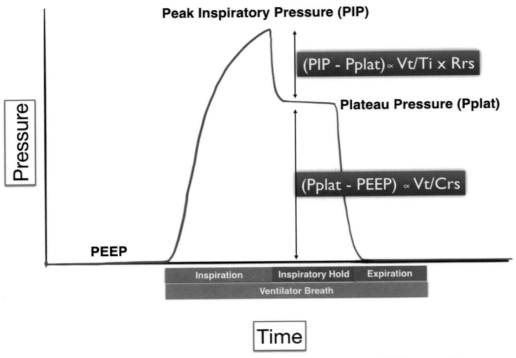

Figure 14-7 *A pressure-time curve showing an inspiratory hold maneuver which illustrates the components for the measurement of respiratory system compliance. See Figure 14-1 and text for definition of terms.*

Parameter	Clinical Example 1	Clinical Example 2	Clinical Example 3	Clinical Example 4
Tidal volume (mL)	500	500	500	500
Peak inspiratory pressure (PIP) cm H_2O	25	30	35	40
Plateau pressure (Pplat) cm H_2O	20	20	25	15
Set PEEP cm H_2O	5	5	5	5
Intrinsic (auto) PEEP cm H_2O	0	10	5	10
Compliance calculation mL/ cm H_2O	500/20-5	500/20-15	500/25-10	500/15-15

Figure 14-8 *Example calculations of respiratory system compliance based upon variable input measurements.*

The compliance term, if appropriately measured, provides an indicator for the Vt/Crs term in the Equation of Motion. The normal compliance on mechanical ventilation should be in the range of 50-100 mL/cm H_2O. Notice that the PIP does not accurately reflect the compliance of the lung and chest wall because it includes the effects of flow and airflow resistance (Vt/Ti × Rrs). We need to dig a little deeper.

14.3 Resistance and Time Constants

The transpulmonary pressure generated by the respiratory pump, in addition to the static forces associated with volume change (Vt/C_{RS}), must also overcome the resistive forces (Vt/Ti × R_{RS}) related to gas flow (i.e., the tube and airways). The resistance to flow in the airways depends on the dimensions of the airway, the viscosity of the gas, and whether the flow is laminar or turbulent.

The resistance to gas flow is not uniform across the lung, and we can take advantage of this in treating patients. Peripheral airways are characterized by low gas velocity, favoring laminar flow. Resistance during laminar flow is calculated based upon Poiseuille's Law, which states that R=8ln/πr⁴, where l=length of the tube, n=gas viscosity, and r=radius of the tube. As this equation illustrates, minimal changes in airway radius create large changes in airway resistance. In patients with asthma or COPD, airway inflammation can compromise airway patency, leading to a marked reduction in expiratory airflow. The resistance to flow in the airways is also influenced by the lung volume, as the airways are tethered to the entire connective tissue network and pulled open with larger inflation volumes.

> This density dependence of turbulent flow is occasionally exploited in the use of heliox, a low-density helium-oxygen mixture given to patients with central airway lesions or asthma to assist their breathing.

14.3.1 Measurement of Airways Resistance

Let's return to the pressure-time curve with the inspiratory hold maneuver on the ventilator (**Figure 14-7**). The highest pressure on the curve that occurs just before airflow is stopped is called the *Peak Inspiratory Pressure (PIP)*. The PIP happens with airflow, so it is a measure of the pressure needed to offset both the compliance and resistance of the lung. If you see a big drop in pressure from the Peak Inspiratory Pressure (PIP) to the plateau pressure (Pplat), this indicates that you have a significant flow-related parameter that disappears when airflow stops. This gradient means you have either a very high rate of airflow or high airways resistance. This can occur with high inspiratory flow settings on the ventilator and with obstruction of the endotracheal tube or intrinsic obstructive airways disease, such as asthma and COPD.

In the ICU, we can simply monitor the difference between the PIP and Pplat. As the gradient between these two parameters increases, the greater likelihood your patient has a resistance problem. The common causes of airway resistance problems in patients on mechanical ventilation are summarized in **Figure 14-9**.

Causes of Increased Airway Resistance
Bronchospasm
Fixed airflow obstruction in OLD
Biting of the endotracheal tube
Small endotracheal tube
Mucous plug in airway or endotracheal tube
Kink in ventilator circuit or endotracheal tube

Figure 14-9 *Common clinical causes of increase airway resistance in ventilator patients.*

In patients on mechanical ventilation, the time required to fill and empty the lung becomes critical because you (the clinician!) will often determine the time parameters for your patient. The respiratory time constant (τ) reflects the time required to fill or passively discharge the lung volume. This time constant is a product of the respiratory system resistance (Rrs) and compliance (Crs):

$$\tau = Rrs \times Crs$$

Patients with a high respiratory system resistance or a high compliance (or low elastance) have an increased time constant for alveolar filling and emptying. Think of this simply: The time required to exhale is slowest (long time constant) if the airway resistance is high (breathing through small tubes) and the lung compliance is high (less elastic squeeze to push air out of alveoli). If the resistance is low and the compliance is low, then air rushes out and the time constant is short. Increased Rrs can result from internal factors (tissue and airways resistance) or from external factors such as the resistance of the respiratory tubing in mechanical ventilation, leading to increased τ. The respiratory time constant will be an important variable to consider in mechanical ventilation.

As τ increases, a higher fraction of each breath cycle length (time between breaths) must be allocated to expiratory time for the lungs to return to their relaxation volume. Failure to meet these expiratory time requirements will result in trapping of inhaled volume in the lung, a process termed *dynamic hyperinflation of the lung*, leading to intrinsic PEEP.

Patients with advanced COPD can have a very long time constant because of an increase in airways resistance and increased lung compliance (decreased elastance). If the Vt is not completely exhaled by the end of the breath, then a certain amount of air is "trapped" in the alveoli. This breath stacking will occur until a new end-expiratory lung volume (functional residual capacity) is achieved. At a higher lung volume, the elastance will increase (or the compliance will decrease) and the time constant will become shorter in duration. The patient with dynamic hyperinflation will reach a new plateau where expiratory time is once again adequate to allow expiration of the tidal breath. But to accomplish this improvement in the time constant, a patient must enable hyperinflation to the point of decreased lung compliance.

14.4 Let's Put it Together

Now that we have reviewed static and dynamic factors affecting lung mechanics, let's turn to the most common problem you will face: the patient on a mechanical ventilator who is sucking in air while at the same time you are pushing in air (*Patients suck and ventilators blow!*). The ventilator introduces an increase in pressure that directly relates to an increase in volume and inspiratory flow. Note that ventilators can be set to target a change in airway pressure or lung volume. The change applied (pressure or volume) then results in a net change in the non-targeted or dependent variable (volume or pressure). The magnitude of the non-targeted change results from the interaction of both the static (lung and chest wall mechanics) and dynamic components (time constant) of the respiratory system. This assumes the patient is paralyzed and makes no respiratory muscle contribution to the transpulmonary pressure. When the patient actively assists the breathing effort, the combined ventilator-induced positive airway pressure and respiratory muscle pressure generates the necessary flow and tidal volume to create lung inflation. *Keep reading!*

Suggested Reading

- Lucangelo U, Bernabè F, Blanch L. Lung mechanics at the bedside: make it simple. Current Opinion in Critical Care 2007;13(1):64–72.
- Grinnan DC, Truwit JD. Clinical review: Respiratory mechanics in spontaneous and assisted ventilation. Critical Care 2005;9(5):472.
- Tobin MJ. Physiologic basis of mechanical ventilation. Ann Am Thorac Soc 2018;15(Supplement_1):S49–S52.

15

Mechanical Ventilation

Your patient presents acutely ill, and you move rapidly to intubation. You manage the airway during endotracheal intubation, and now you are ready to connect your patient to the ventilator. *What is all this mode stuff and those crazy letters all combined? Does it really need to be this confusing? Are the respiratory therapists that much smarter than the rest of us?* Mechanical ventilation is pretty simple once you break it down to a couple of fundamental components.

The *modes* of positive pressure ventilation (PPV) are descriptions of how the ventilator controls the breath delivery to the patient. The terms used (usually reduced to letter acronyms such as SIMV, AC, or PRVC) are assigned by the ventilator manufacturer without strict industry standards, leading to an alphabet soup of confusing terminology (**Figure 15-1**). Unfortunately, these terms don't always clearly describe the characteristics of breath delivery. To add to the confusion, different manufacturers use different names for virtually the same type of breath delivery. As a result, the presentation of the modes of ventilation can be very confusing for the new practitioner in the ICU. Let's try to simplify.

15.1 Ventilator Components

Figure 15-2 illustrates the necessary components of a hospital ventilator. The gas delivery begins at the hospital gas outlets, which bring air and oxygen under high pressure to a *blender*, typically inside the ventilator. The blender mixes the two gases to achieve the inspired

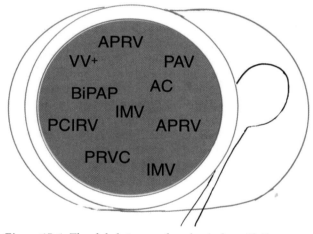

Figure 15-1 The alphabet soup of mechanical ventilation.

oxygen concentration selected by the physician or therapist. The mechanical ventilator has a flow controller to drive gas flow, based upon input from the mode control unit. After all, a ventilator is just a very expensive air blower!! The mode control unit regulates the type of breaths, based on the variables you select and feedback data it receives from the ventilator circuit. The ventilator is connected to the patient via a Y circuit, which includes an inspiratory limb (air to the patient) and an expiratory limb (air back to the ventilator). Sensors (S) in either the inspiratory or expiratory limb recognize pressure or flow-based changes in the airway circuit and provide feedback information to the mode control.

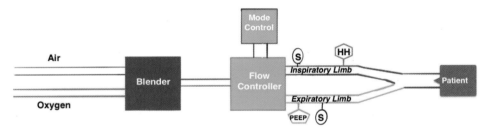

Figure 15-2 *The basic components of a ventilator circuit.*

A humidifier (HH) adds heat and moisture to the blended gas on the inspiratory limb to approximate body conditions. A valve or gas flow in the expiratory limb regulates end-expiratory pressure (PEEP). The tubing of this Y circuit will expand while the airway is pressurized. As a result, the ventilator circuit will take up some of the delivered gas during the inspiratory phase of the ventilator. The expansion of the tubing can be predicted based on the tubing compliance (normal 3-5 ml/cm H_2O). Modern ventilators will adjust the volume of breath delivery to account for this volume loss in the ventilator circuit.

15.2 Setting the Breath Rate (Triggering)

The blender delivers the right gas mixture to the flow controller. The flow controller regulates the airflow to the patient based on input from the mode control unit, which has the requested breath parameters and frequency. The interaction of the set ventilator rate and the patient's respiratory rate determines the breath frequency.

Let's talk about how the patient starts or triggers a breath. *Triggering* refers to the method of initiating a breath or most simply considered, how do we get this whole thing started? A breath can be initiated by the machine or by the patient. A breath triggered by the patient is called an *assisted breath*, meaning the patient started the breath. Once the patient triggers the breath lots of changes can happen. Keep reading!

The most straightforward triggering mechanism is a *time-based trigger*, which initiates ventilator breaths based upon a set respiratory rate or frequency per minute (i.e., a respiratory rate of 10 triggers a breath every 6 seconds). With this mechanism, the ventilator controls each breath. The obvious limitation of a time-based trigger mechanism is that it does not allow for patient interaction with the ventilator. If the patient's metabolism (CO_2 production) changes, the respiratory controller of the patient would be unable to effect a change in the set minute ventilation of the machine without a patient-based trigger. To allow patient adjustment of the respiratory rate, one of two patient-initiated breath triggering methods is used by modern ventilators: pressure triggering or flow triggering.

15.2.1 Pressure-Based Triggering

Pressure-based triggering results when the patient's inspiratory effort creates a negative airway pressure (**Figure 15-3**) below the end-expiratory pressure. The user sets the amount airway pressure must be reduced to initiate the ventilator breath. This setting on the ventilator is called the *sensitivity* and is typically set in the range of 1-2 cm H_2O below the end-expiratory pressure. The negative airway pressure produced by the patient's inspiratory effort then triggers the ventilator to deliver the set breath characteristics. In **Figure 15-3**, the sensitivity is set at -2 cm H_2O. If the PEEP level was 5 cm H_2O, the breath would trigger if the airway pressure was reduced to 3 cm H_2O. The patient makes an initial negative respiratory effort to the target baseline, which triggers the ventilator breath (labeled P in the diagram). If the patient's effort fails to achieve the required pressure reduction, no inspiration is triggered (F in the diagram). A breath triggered by the ventilator based upon time does not require an airway pressure reduction (T in the diagram).

A significant limitation of pressure-based triggering is a potential phase lag between the patient's neural onset of inspiration (brain trigger) and the flow response of the ventilator (ventilator trigger). The negative alveolar pressure generated by the patient must be transmitted to the airway, appropriately sensed by the airway pressure sensor of the ventilator, and the ventilator must then create an immediate flow response. The traditional phase lag is measured in milliseconds but can be more prolonged. The greater the phase lag, the longer the patient pulls against an inspiratory system with restricted airflow. Patients with unusually high respiratory drive can experience significant post-triggering work of breathing if the phase lag is prolonged.

The reduction in pressure required for triggering the ventilator should be set low enough to allow minimum patient effort to initiate a breath. However, a setting too low can cause an event call *auto-triggering*. During auto-triggering, small fluctuations in the tubing airway pressure "simulate" a patient effort, causing the ventilator to cycle as if the patient triggered it. So, the sensitivity setting is adjusted – not too high – not too low – just right.

15.2.2 Flow-Based Triggering

The alternative to pressure-based triggering is flow-based triggering (**Figure 15-4**). *Flow-based triggering* attempts to eliminate the phase lag associated with pressure-based triggering. Flow-based triggering is restricted to modern ventilators, which can deliver a constant low flow through the respiratory circuit during the respiratory cycle (termed *flow-by* or *bias*

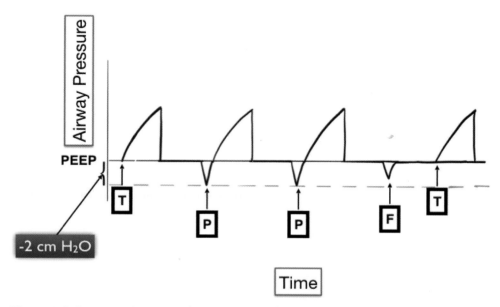

Figure 15-3 Pressure – time curve shows patient breaths triggered by the ventilator based upon time (T) and breaths triggered by the patient (P). The patient triggered breaths require the patient to lower the airway pressure – 2 cm H20. If the patient effort does not meet this threshold the breath will fail (F) to trigger.

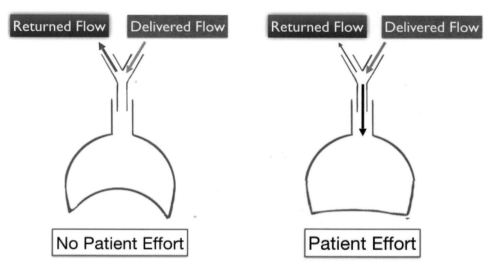

Figure 15-4 Illustration of changing flow in the inspiratory and expiratory limb of the ventilator in relation to patient effort.

flow). The delivered flow provided on the inspiratory limb is compared to the returned flow in the expiratory limb (left image). A reduction in the flow on the expiratory limb of the circuit, below the delivered bias flow, is sensed by the ventilator when the patient begins an inspiratory effort (right image). This triggers the ventilator to deliver the breath. In theory, the continuous delivered flow is immediately available to the patient and would minimize any phase lag characteristic of pressure-based triggering. An initial setting of 2 L/min for flow-based triggering is appropriate. This level sets the ventilator to deliver the control breath once the patient generates 2L/min of inspiratory flow An even more advanced method of triggering is based upon reading the patient's neural output via a diaphragm EMG signal. If clinically perfected, this method would allow triggering based upon the patient's respiratory control signal rather than airway pressure or flow signals. This form of breath triggering is limited to only a few currently available ventilators.

A summary of the triggering methods for mechanical ventilation breaths is outlined in **Figure 15-5.**

15.3 Setting the Breath Type

Simply stated, the goal of positive-pressure mechanical ventilation is to maintain appropriate levels of oxygen and carbon dioxide in arterial blood while replacing the workload of the respiratory muscles. The ventilator "pushes" oxygen and nitrogen mixtures down an endotracheal tube at specific flows, volumes and pressures and, for many modes, synchronizing this with a patient's respiratory effort. The workload replacement of the respiratory muscles can be either total or partial. This section will make a lot more sense if you read *Chapter 14, Mechanics of Respiratory Failure* first. You need a little foundation before you build! Let's break this down into two fundamental control breaths. *Control breaths* can be delivered by the ventilator without any

Method	Description	Limitation/Benefits
Time	Ventilator breath initiated every 60 sec/frequency	Unable to adjust for metabolic changes
Pressure	Ventilator breath initiated in response to a minimum pressure decline below end-expiratory pressure, generated by the patient's negative inspiratory effort. Set as sensitivity on the ventilator and traditionally set in the range of 1-2 cm H_2O.	Phase delay between patient's neural onset of inspiration and machine flow delivery
Flow-by	Ventilator breath is triggered when a continuous bias flow in the ventilator circuit is redirected to the patient during inspiration.	Restricted to modern ventilators with rapid microprocessors. May minimize phase delay
Neural	Ventilator breath is initiated based upon recognition of esophageal pressure or diaphragm EMG signal.	Minimize phase delay and triggering limitation associated with a threshold load. Very limited availability

Figure 15-5 *Methods used to initiate or trigger a breath in mechanical ventilation.*

Both pressure-and flow-based triggering depend on the transmission of a negative pressure or negative flow signal to the mechanical ventilator sensor. This process assumes an equilibration of the patient's alveolar pressure with the circuit pressure of the ventilator at end expiration. However, some patients, particularly those with airflow obstruction, suffer from a condition in which the alveolar and circuit pressures do not reach equal values. These patients suffer from dynamic hyperinflation (or intrinsic-PEEP). During inspiration, alveolar pressure must first be lowered by the respiratory muscles to equal the circuit pressure and then further reduced to trigger the inspiratory sensor of the ventilator. Clinically, you can see the patient make an effort (starts a breath), but it looks like the ventilator did not respond. So if your patient is on an external PEEP of 5 cm H_2O, with a sensitivity of -2 cm H_2O, the patient needs to lower the airway circuit pressure to 3 cm H_2O to trigger the ventilator. The patient does this by generating a net negative 2 cm H_2O. However, if the patient's breath ends with an alveolar intrinsic-PEEP pressure of 10 due to hyperinflation, the patient must lower the alveolar pressure from 10 to 3 to effect the circuit pressure. So the triggering threshold is now 7 cm H_2O. However, this high triggering threshold is not readily apparent to the bedside clinician.

patient participation. In other words, all the necessary breath parameters are set to allow the breath to be given to a completely passive patient – such as a patient under sedation/paralysis in the ICU or a patient in the operating room.

The first positive pressure ventilators were designed to provide a breath that inflated the lungs until a preset pressure was achieved. This type of *pressure control* breath was limited by changing lung mechanics (compliance and resistance), which led to a variable tidal volume. Now the more commonly employed breaths provide a specific tidal volume, termed a *volume control* breath. Volume control breaths are favored in adult ICUs because they deliver a consistent tidal volume independent of changes in lung mechanics.

If you take a second to think about this – mechanical ventilation control breaths are extremely simple. To make a ventilator breath, you have four input variables to consider, and *you can only CONTROL two at one time:*

- Pressure and inspiratory time
- Tidal volume and flow

Think of your four major ventilator variables as playing cards, and you can only play two at a time: airway pressure, inspiratory time, tidal volume, and inspiratory flow (**Figure 15-6**). A simple way of summarizing your breaths is:

- The *volume control breath* plays with two cards: volume and flow. These volume control breaths cannot use the pressure card.
- The *pressure control breath* plays with two cards: pressure and inspiratory time. The pressure control breath cannot play the volume or flow cards.

Now that time card is a little sneaky. Modern ventilators provide many different options to set the duration of inspiration.

1. In a volume control breath, if you set volume and flow, then inspiration ends when the tidal volume is delivered at the set flow rate. So, you did set the inspiratory time!
2. In a volume control breath, you could alternatively set the tidal volume and inspiratory time. Remember that FLOW = Volume/time, so in essence, you have set flow. *Sneaky – huh?*
3. In a pressure control breath, you can set the inspiratory time.

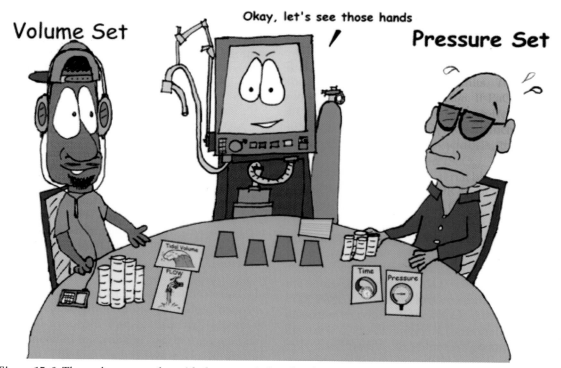

Figure 15-6 *The cards you can play with the two main breaths of mechanical ventilation.*

209

4. In a pressure control breath, you can also set the respiratory rate and the ratio of inspiratory time to expiratory time (called the I:E ratio). If you think about that for a minute, you will realize that this is the same thing as setting the inspiratory time.

So maybe that time card is a bit of a wild card! In both volume control and pressure control breaths the inspiratory time is set – we use slightly different ways of getting to it. The machines vary a bit in how you set the parameters – *that is to keep you guessing and provide job security for your respiratory therapists!*

PEEP is also set on the ventilator but is not part of the breath construction so should be considered as an added variable, like the respiratory rate.

15.3.1 Control Breaths

Let's compare these two very basic types of ventilator control breaths by going back to the Equation of Motion (EOM) from *Chapter 14.*

$$Prs = Pao + (-Pmus) = (Vt/Crs) + (Vt/Ti \times Rrs) + PEEPtotal$$

As a reminder, the total pressure required to inflate the respiratory system (Prs) to a new lung volume can be contributed by either positive ventilator pressure at the airway (Pao) or negative intrathoracic pressure generated by the respiratory muscles (Pmus), i.e., patient effort.

The Prs requirement is influenced by the size of the tidal volume (Vt), the compliance of the lung and chest wall (Crs), the inspiratory flow rate (Vt/Ti), and the airways resistance (Rrs). Finally, we need to add in the total value of PEEP (PEEPtotal) to control for the baseline alveolar pressure at the start of the breath.

We can break the EOM down into two components:

1. *Patient-controlled variables.* Patient characteristics determine these breath parameters, which are not set by the ventilator.
2. *Ventilator-set variables.* Ventilator settings control these breath parameters, which do not change with patient (disease) fluctuations in effort or lung mechanics (disease).

The patient-controlled variables in the EOM include:

- (-Pmus)—the patient's negative inspiratory muscle effort
- (Crs)—the compliance of the patient's lung and chest wall (respiratory system)
- (Rrs)—the resistance of the patient's airways
- PEEPtotal—the end-expiratory pressure in the alveolus, ordinarily atmospheric but could be

elevated at end expiration due to an abnormal patient time constant (τ) leading to intrinsic PEEP

In the equation below, we indicate the potential patient-determined variables in bold.

$$Prs = Pao + (-\mathbf{Pmus}) = (Vt/\mathbf{Crs}) + (Vt/Ti \times \mathbf{Rrs}) + \mathbf{PEEPtotal}$$

The ventilator-set variables might include:

- Pao – positive pressure at the airway opening
- (Vt) – the tidal volume in mL or size of the breath delivered
- (Vt/Ti) – tidal volume divided by time or the inspiratory flow rate of the breath delivered
- PEEPtotal – the end-expiratory pressure in the alveolus, ordinarily atmospheric but could be maintained at a positive pressure level by the ventilator setting

Note that PEEPtotal is listed as both a patient-controlled and a ventilator-set variable. This one is a little tricky because it can be controlled by the patient (intrinsic PEEP) or the machine (extrinsic PEEP).

Let's compare the parameters between *pressure control* and *volume control* breaths in **Figure 15-7.**

15.3.1.1 Pressure Control Breath

$$Prs = \mathbf{Pao} + (-Pmus) = (Vt/Crs) + (Vt/Ti \times Rrs) + PEEPtotal$$

The inspiratory airway pressure (Pao) is the control variable in pressure control breaths (bold). Pao can provide the total respiratory system inflation pressure, as Pmus would be 0 in a paralyzed patient. In a patient with spontaneous respiratory muscle effort, Pao interacts with the patient effort (-Pmus) to determine the tidal volume and flow rate for a constant respiratory system compliance (Crs) and resistance (Rrs). If Pao and (-Pmus) remain constant, the tidal volume is only constant if lung mechanics (Crs and Rrs) remain constant. Otherwise, pressure control breaths result in a variable tidal volume based upon the interaction of the set ventilator inflation pressure (Pao), the patient's respiratory muscle effort (-Pmus), and the lung mechanics (Crs and Rrs). *Remember that Equation of Motion!*

Pressure control breaths allow more precise control over airway pressures, including peak airway and mean airway pressure. As we will soon review, mean airway pressure can directly relate to oxygenation in patients with hypoxemic respiratory failure. Our ability to specifically regulate mean airway pressure in these conditions can be a significant advantage of the pressure control breath. There is also some evidence that pressure control breaths provide for a more even distribution of

Parameter	EOM	Volume Control	Pressure Control
Tidal volume	Vt	Ventilator-set	Variable parameter
Flow	Vt/Ti	Ventilator-set	Variable parameter
Airway pressure	Pao	Variable parameter	Ventilator-set
Inspiratory time	Ti	Ventilator-set	Ventilator-set
Respiratory system complicance	Crs	Patient-controlled	Patient-controlled
Respiratory system resistance	Rrs	Patient-controlled	Patient-controlled
Respiratory muscle parameter	Pmus	Patient-controlled	Patient-controlled
PEEP (extrinsic)	PEEP	Ventilator-set	Ventilator-set
PEEP (intrinsic)	PEEP	Patient-controlled	Patient-controlled

Figure 15-7 *Comparison of respiratory mechanics between volume control and pressure control breaths.*

lung ventilation. Because we do not control tidal volume or flow, patients can influence those two variables, making this type of breath more responsive to patient inspiratory demands.

15.3.1.2 Volume Control Breath

The tidal volume and inspiratory flow rate are the set variables in volume control breaths. We focus on the right side of the EOM by setting a target tidal volume (Vt) and inspiratory flow (Vt/Ti) (bold), leaving the left side of the equation variable.

$$Prs = Pao + (-Pmus) = (\mathbf{Vt/Crs}) + (\mathbf{Vt/Ti} \times Rrs) + PEEPtotal$$

If the patient is paralyzed, the Pao measured at the airway reflects the interaction of the set tidal volume (Vt) and inspiratory flow (Vt/Ti) and the respiratory system mechanics (Crs and Rrs). *Note from the EOM:* If V_T and Vt/Ti remain constant, the Pao is only constant if lung mechanics (Crs and Rrs) and patient effort (Pmus) remain constant. Otherwise, volume control breaths result in a variable airway pressure based upon the interaction of the set ventilator parameters (Vt and Vt/Ti), the patient's respiratory muscle effort (-Pmus), and the lung mechanics (Crs and Rrs). *Remember that Equation of Motion!!*

With *volume control* breaths, the ventilator provides an inspiratory flow based upon a user set flow rate and pattern. The flow is maintained until the tidal volume is delivered, and then the breath terminates. If patient effort increases, the flow pattern would be kept constant by the flow controller of the machine. As a result, the patient pulls against a restricted flow, and the measured airway pressure is reduced, resulting in "dyssynchrony" between the patient and the machine. The patient wants a specific flow rate and tidal volume, and the machine is set to deliver a different flow rate and tidal volume. The patient will look uncomfortable. The nurse will call you and say the patient is "agitated." To be more precise, the nurse should probably call and tell you the patient is "suffocating," but that does not sound so good. In reality, the patient wants to breathe one way, and the ventilator happens to think it has a better idea.

Either the ventilator will need to be adjusted to match the patient's desired parameters, or the patient will need to be sedated to match the ventilator's desired parameters. The main advantage of *volume control ventilation* is that tidal volume remains constant when the respiratory system mechanics change. The main disadvantage can be the patient's comfort (synchrony), especially if the set breath parameters do not match the awake patient's respiratory drive.

In contrast, for *pressure control* breaths, the ventilator adjusts inspiratory flow to achieve a user-determined pressure target. If patient effort increases, the effect is to drop airway pressure, which is immediately offset by the flow controller to increase inspiratory flow to maintain the target Pao. If the patient wants a bigger flow rate and tidal volume, they just need to make a greater inspiratory effort (Pmus), and the machine will generally respond proportional to the patient effort. The patient is less likely to have dyssynchrony with pressure control breaths. However, the patient will be subject to a variable tidal volume as previously outlined.

The advantages and limitations of these two main types of ventilator breaths are summarized in **Figure 15-8**.

15.3.1.3 Respiratory Cycle Length

The time between breaths, or the sum of the inspiratory time (Ti) and expiratory time (Te), is called the *respiratory cycle length*. The cycle length duration is inversely related to the breath frequency. Tachypnea shortens the cycle length and requires inspiration and expiration to

	Volume Control	**Pressure Control**
Advantages	Set tidal volume and inspiratory flow independent of changing lung mechanics. The breath ends when the tidal volume is delivered.	Set airway pressure and inspiratory time with variable tidal volume and inspiratory flow. The breath ends when the inspiratory time is expired. Favorable for patient comfort; does not deliver dangerously high pressures if lung mechanics change
Disadvantages	Patient-ventilator dyssynchrony if a mismatch between the set inspiratory flow and tidal volume and the patient's respiratory drive	Variable tidal volume if lung mechanics change
Common use	Initial support in an adult patient with respiratory failure	Alternative support in a patient with elevated airway pressures or marked dyssynchrony

Figure 15-8 Comparison of volume control and pressure control breaths.

be completed in a shorter span to avoid stacking breaths or the more proper term, *dynamic hyperinflation.*

A volume control breath is easy to understand – the breath ends when the specified tidal volume is delivered. The inspiratory duration of the breath comes from the interaction of the set volume and flow parameters.

Let's look at this type of breath graphically as the ventilator might show it to you in **Figure 15-9**. Here we illustrate the three components (volume, flow, pressure in that order) over the time of a single volume control breath. At the end of inspiration, we have introduced a brief pause, before allowing the onset of expiration. This pause helps with the illustration but is not usually present for this type of breath.

For our volume control breath, the breath could be time-triggered or patient-triggered. The ventilator initiates a flow of gas immediately to the target level and pattern set for the volume control breath (**Figure 15-9**, middle graphic). The ventilator maintains the flow target until the tidal volume is delivered (**Figure 15-9**, top graphic). Expiration begins after the tidal volume delivery – or in our example, after a brief end-inspiratory pause.

For the volume control breath, we will need to set the flow parameters (remember the two cards we can play). Flow represents the rate of gas delivery to the patient or essentially *volume delivery/time*. The highest rate of gas flow during the inspiration cycle is termed the *peak flow*. We can set the peak flow, and we can also establish a pattern for the flow delivery. The inspiratory flow pattern could be a square wave pattern (most common pattern with flow rising fast and staying constant until the tidal volume target is achieved). Alternatively, a ramp pattern (accelerating or decelerating), or sinusoidal pattern can be set. The middle graphic in **Figure 15-9** illustrates the square wave flow pattern. The flow pattern you select in volume control breaths will influence the shape of the pressure waveform (**Figure 15-9,** bottom graphic). The pressure, in this case,

rises to a peak value based upon patient airways resistance and compliance and then falls back with expiration to the baseline or end-expiration value.

Remember in a volume control breath, the airway pressure is really a passive result from the elastic (Crs) and resistive forces (Rrs) of the lung, the patient effort (Pmus), and the initial system pressure at the start of flow delivery (PEEPtotal). (Remember that EOM!).

At end inspiration in our example, the pause interval is associated with a drop in airway pressure until it reaches a new plateau pressure value *(Remember Pplat from Chapter 14)*. The Pplat occurs due to the lack of continued airflow, so resistance is no longer an active component. This Pplat reflects only the elastic recoil pressure (or compliance) of the respiratory system.

Ventilators can get a little confusing when it comes to setting the flow parameter. Any of the following parameters could be involved in setting the flow characteristics for a volume control breath based upon how the different manufacturers choose to construct their ventilator.

- *Peak inspiratory flow* – the highest rate of flow during the inspiratory phase
- *Flow pattern* – square, descending ramp, sinusoidal
- *Inspiratory time* – duration of inspiration
- *Inspiratory:Expiratory time ratio* – defines the relationship between the inspiratory and expiratory time by setting a timing relationship

Although ventilators differ slightly in the required set elements related to this flow parameter, some combination of volume and time *(Remember, flow = volume/time)* creates the actual flow rate and pattern for the *volume control* breath delivery.

Now let's look at the graphics for a pressure control breath (**Figure 15-10**). For a pressure control breath, the breath could also be time triggered or patient triggered. The ventilator will immediately deliver

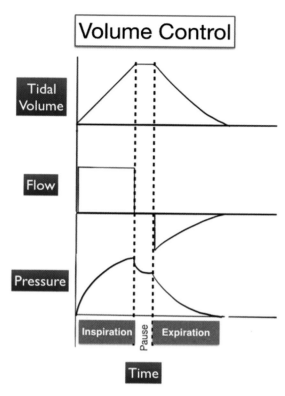

Figure 15-9 *Volume control breath parameters during the respiratory cycle interval.*

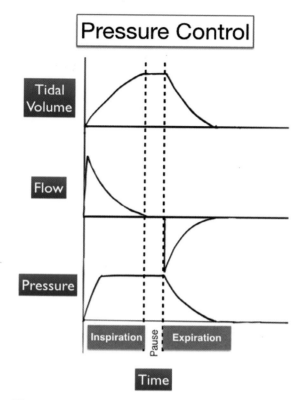

Figure 15-10 *Pressure control breath parameters during the respiratory cycle interval.*

flow to achieve a set target inspiratory pressure (**Figure 15-10**, bottom graphic). Flow is initially rapid to accomplish the set pressure target (**Figure 15-10**, middle graphic). Some manufacturers allow you to set the rise time for the pressure waveform, which will modify the rate of gas flow from the ventilator. Setting the rise time can allow you to minimize that rapid, sudden increase in airway pressure.

For the pressure control breath, the breath ends based upon a time duration. In pressure control breaths, the user sets either an inspiratory time (most common) or an inspiratory:expiratory time ratio with a respiratory rate, which, of course, equals the same thing as setting the inspiratory time! The flow is initially high reflecting a gradient between airway pressure and alveolar pressure. However, as the lung continues to inflate, this gradient will gradually decline, and the flow rate will decelerate over the inspiratory cycle. The flow level will be maintained at a level necessary to achieve the inspiratory pressure target. For a pressure control breath, the pressure wave is constant (square wave) (**Figure 15-10**, bottom graphic), while the flow wave is decelerating (**Figure 15-10**, middle graphic). The peak inspiratory pressure will never exceed the set pressure target by design. If the inspiratory

flow reaches zero, this means the alveolar pressure has reached the target airway pressure. The airway pressure with zero flow would then equal the Pplat.

During expiration, the lung is emptied, based upon the recoil forces of the lung and chest wall, until the airway pressure returns to the end-expiratory pressure (typically the PEEP level of the ventilator). If the expiratory time is long enough to reach zero flow, the alveolar pressure and external PEEP pressure will be equal.

A critical variable in a pressure control breath is the change in pressure from end-expiration (PEEP) to end-inspiration (PIP). This difference in pressure or driving pressure is a primary determinant of tidal volume. The tidal volume (**Figure 15-10**, top panel) is dependent on this driving pressure, the inspiratory time, and the compliance and resistance of the respiratory system.

Note that in patients with dynamic hyperinflation and significant intrinsic PEEP, the end-expiratory alveolar pressure may be higher than the set external PEEP. In this case, the driving pressure will be the difference between the PIP and the intrinsic PEEP.

As we move along, we will also learn about pressure target breaths that are not cycled through a time setting but by the flow signal. These breaths (termed *pressure*

For volume control breaths, respiratory rate and tidal volume are always uncoupled, so that changing one parameter does not change the other. In contrast, for pressure control breaths, the target pressure and respiratory rate may not always be independent. If we increase the respiratory rate, we shorten the time available for expiration. If the reduction in expiratory time leads to incomplete lung emptying, the end alveolar pressure rises (intrinsic PEEP). Under these conditions, the driving pressure (PIP-intrinsic PEEP) falls and the tidal volume is reduced. So, the use of pressure target breaths in the right clinical setting (typically a patient with airflow obstruction) can result in a situation where increasing the respiratory rate can be associated with a reduction in tidal volume and, therefore, minute ventilation.

support) cycle off when the flow curve decline achieves a certain value. We will discuss this later in our chapter.

Timing (cycling) refers to the mechanism by which the ventilator switches between inspiration and expiration. The duration of inspiration relative to the entire breath duration is termed the *duty cycle.*

The duty cycle in volume control breaths is determined by the interaction of the set tidal volume and flow. A time parameter sets the duty cycle in pressure control breaths.

15.3.1.4 Pressure-Regulated Volume Control Breath

Now that we understand volume and pressure control breaths, we come to a crucial question: *Hey, can't we have a little of both?* We want a breath that provides a consistent tidal volume but does not promote patient-ventilator dyssynchrony and sudden surges in airway pressure.

Newer ventilators attempt to incorporate the favorable components from both a volume control breath and a pressure control breath into a mixed breath. A hybrid of ventilator breaths! To make it even a little more confusing the ventilator manufacturers use crazy terms to describe this one breath, including pressure-regulated volume control (PRVC), volume ventilation plus (VV$^+$), pressure control adaptive support ventilation, and volume-assured pressure control (VAPC). We will use the term *pressure-regulated volume control* or *PRVC* to describe how this hybrid of volume and pressure control breaths works.

The hybrid breaths rely on a feedback loop from the airway sensors to the mode control to allow continuous adjustments in the breath parameters, based upon breath-by-breath analysis. Modes which incorporate PRVC breaths deliver a breath with pressure control characteristics (set pressure and inspiratory time) but maintain a relatively fixed tidal volume. *How is that possible? You are not allowed to play three cards!*

The PRVC breath does this by cheating and adjusting the inspiratory pressure target on a breath-to-breath basis to maintain a relatively constant tidal volume. The algorithm uses a step-wise increase or decrease in pressure with each breath to hit the tidal volume with the lowest pressure possible (thus the name *Pressure Regulated Volume Control).*

The algorithm for a PRVC breath is illustrated in **Figure 15-11**. The ventilator first delivers a volume "test" breath along with an inspiratory "hold" maneuver. The measured Pplat then becomes the pressure target for the next breath to presumably give the required target tidal volume. The ventilator then measures the exhaled tidal volume and compares it to the set tidal volume. The ventilator adjusts the pressure level on each subsequent breath to achieve the target tidal volume. The breath $\times$ breath pressure target change is often limited (i.e., $+/- 3$ cm H_2O per breath). Most manufacturers also limit the inspiratory pressure increase as a safety mechanism (i.e., < 5 cm H_2O below the set high-pressure alarm limit).

Note that some ventilators take a different approach to the test breath. The alternative approach is to deliver a pressure control test breath and measure the tidal volume that results. This test breath allows calculation of compliance, and the ventilator can then adjust the target pressure for the next breath. Regardless of the method, a test breath is needed to start the PRVC cycle, and then the ventilator adjusts the pressure control target breath by breath to achieve the goal tidal volume.

After the initial test breath, a PRVC breath will look similar to the pressure control breath in **Figure 15-10**, with the caveat that the pressure target will vary on a breath-by-breath basis based upon the tidal volume delivered on the previous breath.

This combination of pressure control and volume control breaths could provide potential advantages over a pure volume control or pressure control breath. Tidal volume remains relatively constant in PRVC breaths. The relatively constant tidal volume is the primary advantage of PRVC over a pressure control breath. Airway pressure is limited to the minimum value needed to deliver the required tidal volume, which may provide better distribution of ventilation and improved oxygenation. The mode allows some flow and volume

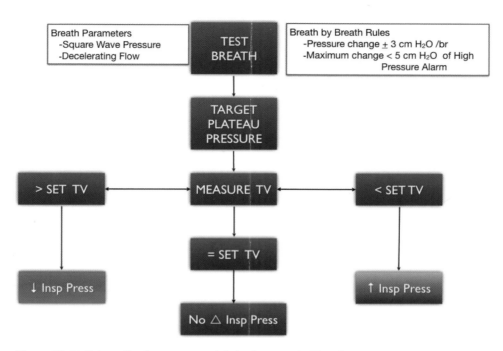

Breath Parameters
- Square Wave Pressure
- Decelerating Flow

TEST BREATH

Breath by Breath Rules
- Pressure change ± 3 cm H_2O /br
- Maximum change < 5 cm H_2O of High Pressure Alarm

TARGET PLATEAU PRESSURE

> SET TV ← MEASURE TV → < SET TV

= SET TV

↓ Insp Press

↑ Insp Press

No △ Insp Press

Figure 15-11 Schematic of pressure-regulated volume control breaths.

variability for the patient, which may improve patient synchrony.

A primary disadvantage is that tidal volume and airway inflation pressures are not explicitly regulated. This might be important in clinical situations where strict tidal volume regulation has been shown to be beneficial (e.g., ARDS).

In practice, PRVC is used clinically like traditional volume control breaths. These hybrid modes of ventilation may be favored for patients with very high ventilatory drives when patient-ventilator dyssynchrony is common.

15.3.2 Support Breaths

In contrast to control breaths, a *support breath* is designed to follow or respond to the patient's inspiratory efforts. A support breath achieves this close physiological response by providing inspiratory flow support to a specific volume or pressure target. In the case of pressure support, this means the patient initiates the breath, and the ventilator assists the patient with a flow to achieve a target positive airway pressure above

the end-expiratory baseline. So far this sounds like pressure control. *What's the diff, dude?*

The key differences between a pressure control and pressure support breath are:

1. The patient must be spontaneously breathing for a pressure support breath, so all breaths are patient-triggered. In pressure control breaths, the trigger can be the patient or machine.
2. The mechanism for ending inspiratory flow is different between pressure support and pressure control.

Figure 15-12 illustrates a *pressure control breath*. The breath can be time-triggered by the machine. The flow duration during inspiration is time limited, based on setting an inspiratory time or I:E ratio (+ respiratory rate). The tidal volume delivery is completed at the end of the set inspiratory time duration. A pressure control breath could alternatively be patient-triggered but would have the same pressure limit and time cycle characteristics.

In contrast, **Figure 15-13** illustrates a pressure support breath. A pressure support breath is always

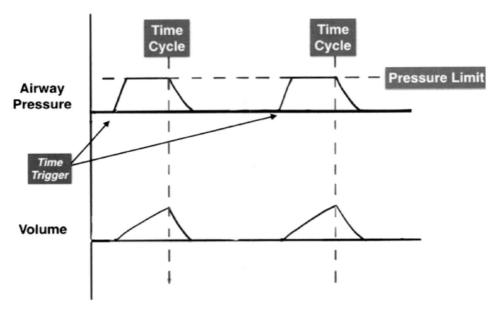

Figure 15-12 Graphic illustration of airway pressure and tidal volume changes during a pressure control breath. Note the breath termination (red dotted line) based upon a time cycle.

patient-triggered. Again, airflow is generated to achieve a specific airway pressure target. In contrast to a pressure control breath, the inspiratory duration is determined by the characteristics of the inspiratory flow curve. Remember, a pressure target breath is characterized by a decelerating ramp flow curve to keep the pressure right at the target even as the lung fills up and becomes less compliant. When the decelerating flow achieves a specific reduction in flow (flow limit), the pressure support breath cycles off to allow exhalation. A specific decelerating flow limit tells the pressure support breath when to end. This is typically an inspiratory flow reduction to 25-33% of the peak flow, as shown by the yellow dotted lines in the bottom panel Figure 15-13. The ventilator may allow the user to set the flow level, which causes the breath to cycle off from inspiration to expiration.

During a pressure control breath, the flow may decelerate to zero, essentially an inspiratory breath hold, waiting for the inspiratory time cycle to allow exhalation. An inspiratory breath hold will never happen with a pressure support breath, as it cycles off when the flow drops to 25-33% of peak flow, so this mode is more physiologically linked to the patient's inspiratory and expiratory effort, while still providing a positive pressure to augment the inspiratory effort.

We like to think of pressure support as the completely patient-sculpted breath. Let's try to summarize the pressure support breath:

- *Patient trigger* - a characteristic of all support breaths
- *Pressure target* - supports the patient's inspiratory effort, compliance, and airways resistance
- *Flow cycle* - turns off when the patient has had enough!

The primary advantage of the pressure support breath is that you can provide partial patient support for each breath to allow a more gradual transition from ventilator support to spontaneous breathing. The breath is not designed for a patient with an irregular breathing pattern or reduced respiratory drive.

You will not be surprised to learn that a few ventilators also include a volume support breath. Again, these breaths are all spontaneous. For volume support breaths, a target tidal volume is maintained by the ventilator by adjusting the pressure support level on a breath-by-breath basis. SO, quite simply, volume support is really a pressure support breath that changes the pressure target breath by breath to maintain a target tidal volume.

Since pressure support is the most common support breath used in weaning, we will focus on it here.

So, with all these options, which breath to pick?? Let's compare the variables we spoke about earlier and contrast the two control breaths and a pressure support breath in **Figure 15-14**.

Let's summarize. Volume control breaths are machine (time) or patient-triggered (pressure or flow). Volume control breaths provide the benefit of a guaranteed tidal

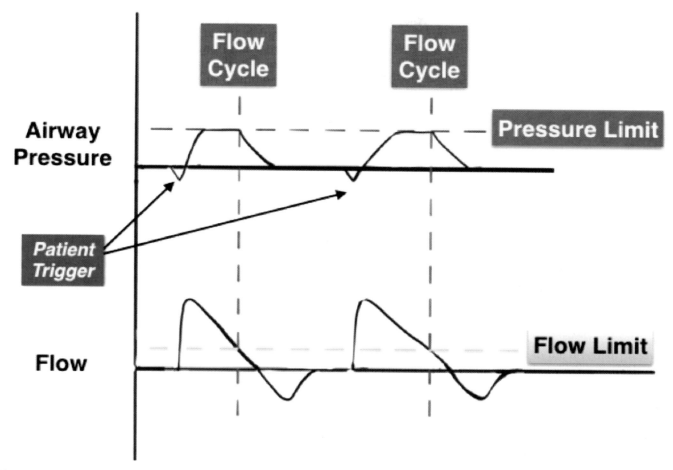

Figure 15-13 *Graphic illustration of airway pressure and flow changes during a pressure support breath. Note the breath termination (red dotted line) based upon a reduction from the peak flow (yellow dotted line).*

Parameter	EOM	Volume Control	Pressure Control	Pressure Support
Tidal volume	Vt	Set Parameter	Variable Parameter	Variable Parameter
Flow	Vt/Ti	Set Parameter	Variable Parameter	Variable Parameter
Airway pressure	Pao	Variable Parameter	Set Parameter	Set Parameter
Inspiratory time	Ti	Set Parameter	Set Parameter	Variable Parameter
Respiratory system complicance	Crs	Patient Parameter	Patient Parameter	Patient Parameter
Respiratory system resistance	Rrs	Patient Parameter	Patient Parameter	Patient Parameter
Respiratory muscle parameter	Pmus	Patient Parameter	Patient Parameter	Patient Parameter
PEEP (extrinsic)	PEEP	Set Parameter	Set Parameter	Set Parameter
PEEP (intrinsic)	PEEP	Patient Parameter	Patient Parameter	Patient Parameter

Figure 15-14 *Comparison of respiratory breath mechanics between volume control, pressure control, and pressure support breaths.*

volume. If the patient's lung mechanics change, the measured airway pressure will vary, but the ventilator will deliver the set tidal volume and flow. Because of this feature, volume control breaths are the most frequent breath used for acute respiratory failure. However, volume control breaths provide a fixed breath pattern with a set flow, volume, and inspiratory duration. If the set parameters fail to match the patient's desire for volume or flow, a condition called *dyssynchrony* develops.

Pressure control breaths are machine (time) or patient-triggered (pressure or flow). Pressure control breaths provide the advantage of flow and volume variability. For the patient with a high respiratory drive to breathe, there is no ventilator limit to tidal volume or flow. So, generally speaking, patients are more comfortable on pressure control breaths. But two problems exist. The tidal volume is not regulated, so conditions where a smaller tidal volume is preferred (such as ARDS) are treated with no control of tidal volume using these breaths. Secondly, if the patient's lung mechanics change, the tidal volume will vary.

Pressure support breaths are all spontaneous. Pressure support breaths have the benefits of a pressure-regulated breath with the addition that inspiratory time is patient determined. Most patients breathe very comfortably in this mode. Tidal volume will vary, however, as the patient changes effort (Pmus) or the lung mechanics change. Also, any leak in the ventilator - patient circuit (e.g., endotracheal tube cuff leak or bronchopleural fistula) can confuse this mode as the flow pattern does not cycle and the mode gets confused about when to turn off.

15.4 Modes of Mechanical Ventilation—The Full Monty

Now that we understand the components of the basic ventilator breaths, let's review the names and properties of the modes. *Modes* of mechanical ventilation refer to all the components that come together to define the full inspiratory support. *The full monty so to speak!*

Don't let this scare you. The modes are just formed with the same basic building blocks we have already discussed. The modes of ventilation are often divided into control and support modes. In a control mode, the ventilator delivers control breaths. A control mode can be entirely passive, with no participation by the patient. A patient in the operating room under anesthesia would require a control mode of ventilation.

In contrast, a support mode provides support breaths in response to a patient trigger only. The level of inspiratory support can be varied but always occurs in response to a patient effort. Support modes are commonly used when weaning the patient from mechanical ventilation.

15.4.1 Control (Assist Control) Ventilation

In a "pure" *control mode*, all breaths are triggered on a time basis. The breath type can be either a volume control, a pressure control, or hybrid (PRVC) breath. This leads to the mode terms of *Volume Control (VC)*, *Pressure Control (PC)*, or *Pressure Regulated Volume Control (PRVC)*. A simple modification to the Control Mode incorporates patient-based triggering, leading to the term *Assist Control (AC) Mode*. The Assist Control Mode is the most common form of ventilation used initially in adult respiratory failure.

The AC mode includes a combination of ventilator-triggered control breaths and patient-triggered control breaths (**Figure 15-15**). The machine set respiratory rate (RRset) establishes a maximum respiratory cycle time between breaths. If the RR = 10, then the maximum cycle time is 6 seconds. Using **Figure 15-15**, let's start with a time-triggered breath (A) from the ventilator, which resets the respiratory cycle duration to 6 seconds. If the patient triggers a breath before the end of the cycle length (B and C), the ventilator responds with the prescribed control breath. Each breath resets the timing for the maximum cycle length. If the ventilator reaches the end of the cycle length before a patient-initiated breath (D), the ventilator triggers the control breath on the basis of time.

The Assist Control Mode really involves two respiratory rates:

- RRset = the value set on the ventilator, which determines the maximum cycle length between breaths
- RRpatient = the value specified by the patient, which determines the minimum cycle length between breaths

To put it simply, faster rate wins. If the patient breathes at a RR of 20 breaths/min with a set rate of 10, the ventilator triggers at a rate of 20 breaths/min. If the patient breathes at a rate of 8, with a set rate of 10, the ventilator wins. The patient may "assist" to a higher frequency, but the breath characteristics (volume vs. pressure control) are identical for all breaths regardless of whether the patient initiated, or the ventilator began the breath in the *Assist Control Mode*.

The distinction between the terms *Control Mode* and *Assist Control (AC) Mode* is nothing to worry about. All modern ICU ventilators provide patients the option of triggering breaths if they have a respiratory drive and muscle capacity to accomplish the trigger. Assist control implies patient triggering. However, if the patient-triggering rate is less than the ventilator rate, then the ventilator sets the rate. Hence, assist control becomes "control" only if the patient rate is < set rate. Therefore, clinicians and ventilator companies use *control* and *assist*

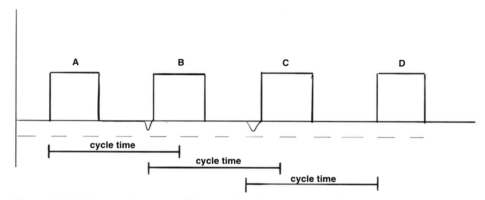

Figure 15-15 *Pressure-time curve illustrates breath triggering in the assist control mode. Breaths can be patient triggered (B and C) or time triggered (D) based upon the timing of the breath in the cycle interval.*

control interchangeably to refer to the same mode with both ventilator and patient-triggering capacity.

15.4.1.1 Setting the Ventilator—Control (Assist Control) Ventilation

Let's start with Volume Assist Control. Patients with acute respiratory failure and unstable lung mechanics are most frequently placed on the volume assist control mode initially. Pressure control modes in the adult population are traditionally reserved for the management of patients with high airway pressures such as advanced ARDS. So, AC should be your first go-to mode, and you should memorize your parameters. *Right after you intubate your patient and the therapist asks, "What settings doc?," you are ready to go.*

This is a volume control breath mode, so you know you have two choices:

1. *Tidal volume.* The selected tidal volume is adjusted for body size (proportional to lung size) with a target equal to ~ 6-8 ml/kg of ideal body weight. Usually 350-500 mL tidal volume.
2. *Inspiratory flow.* The rate of inspiratory flow is set initially in the range of 60-80 L/min. The flow rate is adjusted to be fast enough to shorten inspiration time and allow adequate time for expiration (maintain an I:E ratio > 1:2). The inspiratory flow is set low enough to keep peak airway pressures < 30 cm H_2O.

Next set your rate. The respiratory rate is adjusted to provide an appropriate backup rate from the ventilator, usually at about 2/3 of the spontaneous rate. The respiratory rate is adjusted to assure the necessary minute ventilation (checking pH and CO_2 levels after stabilization).

If you have just intubated a patient and your heart is racing and your mind is boggled and the therapist asks you what settings you want, just say: Assist Control, Rate 12, Tidal Volume 400, PEEP 5 and FiO2 of 100. This is a safe bet while you make sure the patient is stable, get a blood gas and a post intubation chest X-ray. Then you can check your plateau pressures, blood gas and chest X-ray to make sure everything is good and think harder about specific ventilator adjustments based on the data and disease. You will learn more about refinements as we move forward.

If you chose Pressure Assist Control, you would have two different settings:

1. You would need to set the target inspiratory airway pressure. Usually this would be set to achieve either a desired tidal volume or to maintain an airway pressure below a specific value.
2. You would need to set the duration of the inspiratory phase.

The key features of the Assist Control Mode are

- The clinician sets a minimum mandatory breath rate.
- The total breath rate may be ventilator- or patient-triggered.
- For a Pressure Control – AC breath, the clinician sets

  o Inspiratory pressure
  o Inspiratory time or fraction (I:E ratio)

- For a Volume Control - AC breath, the clinician sets

    o Tidal volume
    o Inspiratory flow pattern
    o Inspiratory time or fraction (I:E ratio)

- For both modes, the clinician sets the inspired oxygen concentration (FiO_2) and the level of positive end-expiratory pressure (PEEP) to regulate oxygenation.
- For both modes, the mandatory and spontaneous breaths are identical and determined by the set parameters of the machine (Control ventilation).

15.4.2 Intermittent Mandatory Ventilation (IMV)

A modification of the Control mode is the *Intermittent Mode of Ventilation (IMV)*. This mode provides a mix of control breaths and spontaneous breaths. The control breaths can be volume or pressure control. The spontaneous breaths can be unassisted (just breathing all alone through the tubing like using a snorkel) or assisted by the ventilator (pressure support modes— easier than the snorkel).

The switching between control breaths and spontaneous breaths can only be on the basis of time or can be adjusted to assure that a control breath and a spontaneous breath do not overlap. This latter modification of IMV is called the *Synchronized Intermittent Mode of Ventilation (SIMV)*. SIMV sets a cycle interval based upon the set respiratory rate (**Figure 15-16**). During the first portion of that interval, either a patient or time trigger will result in a control breath (labeled C). Subsequent breaths in the cycling interval will be spontaneous breaths (S). Then the cycle repeats itself. The control breaths can be volume control, pressure control, or a hybrid (PRVC) breath. These control breaths are mixed with the spontaneous breaths.

If you remember the Assist Control (AC) mode, we had a RRset and a RRpatient. In the AC mode, regardless of whether the patient or machine triggered the breath, the actual breath delivered was a control breath (determined by the ventilator settings).

In the SIMV mode, we also have a RRset and a RRpatient. In this case, RRset determines the control breath rate. If the RRpatient exceeds the RRset, the additional breaths are spontaneous. We can assist the spontaneous breaths with additional support. The combination of control breaths and spontaneous breaths can lead to confusing terminology such as *Volume Control IMV with Pressure Support.* **Figure 15-17** outlines the possible breath combinations that can occur with the Intermittent Mode of Ventilation.

15.4.2.1 Setting the Ventilator—Intermittent Mandatory Ventilation (IMV)

Although we have many possible combinations, IMV is most commonly delivered as volume control breaths. The volume control settings are similar to the description for the Assist Control Mode of ventilation above. The primary difference in the IMV mode is that any breath above the set respiratory frequency will be a spontaneous breath. A level of pressure support may be set for these breaths to assist or maintain a desired tidal volume.

The key features of the (S)IMV Mode are

- The clinician sets a minimum mandatory breath rate.
- The mandatory breaths may be machine- or patient-triggered.
- The clinician sets the control breath characteristics for the mandatory breaths.
- The clinician sets the inspired oxygen concentration and the level of positive end-expiratory pressure.
- The patient may trigger additional breaths above the set rate (spontaneous breaths).

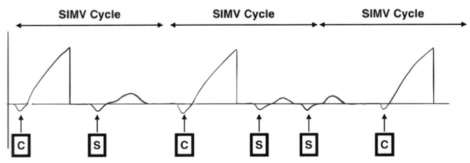

Figure 15-16 *A volume-time tracing indicates the SIMV mode with spontaneous (S) and control (C) breaths depending on their timing in the SIMV cycle interval.*

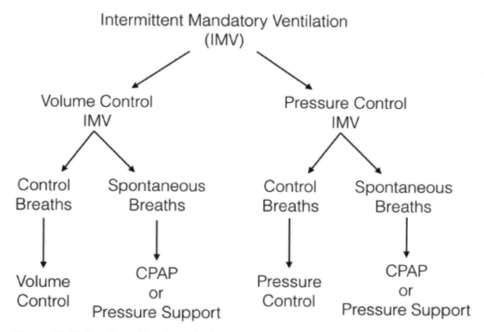

Figure 15-17 *Breath combinations which are possible with the SIMV mode.*

- The mandatory and spontaneous breaths are different and determined by the set parameters of the machine for the mandatory breaths (Control ventilation) and either spontaneous or support settings for the spontaneous breaths.

15.4.3 Spontaneous Mode of Ventilation

The spontaneous mode of ventilation provides no mandatory breaths. The patient triggers each breath. True spontaneous ventilation can occur through the endotracheal tube without a connection to the ventilator. The respiratory circuit used for this is called a *T-piece*. If the spontaneous mode is delivered to a tracheostomy tube, the respiratory circuit is called a *trach mask.*

Alternatively, the spontaneous mode can be "adjusted" to maintain a continuous low-level positive airway pressure. This mode of spontaneous ventilation is called *CPAP (continuous positive airway pressure)*. The spontaneous breaths can also be supported on the inspiratory phase by a support breath—typically pressure support.

So, the key features of the Spontaneous Mode are

- The clinician sets no mandatory breath rate as all breaths are spontaneous.
- The clinician can set a minimal level of airway pressure during the entire respiratory cycle, termed *continuous positive airway pressure (CPAP)*.

- The clinician can also set an inspiratory level of breath assistance or support based upon either a pressure target or a volume target.
- The clinician sets the inspired oxygen concentration and the level of positive end-expiratory pressure.

15.4.3.1 Setting the Ventilator—Spontaneous Ventilation

When the spontaneous mode of ventilation is provided either as a T-piece (connected to an endotracheal tube) or a trach mask (attached to a tracheostomy), the clinician only sets the inspired oxygen concentration.

Alternatively, a spontaneous mode can be provided with a fixed level of expiratory pressure, typically 5 cm of H_2O. When positive end-expiratory pressure is set in the AC or SIMV mode, we call the term *PEEP*. When end-expiratory pressure is set in a spontaneous mode, we term this *continuous positive airway pressure (CPAP)*. No control breath characteristics are set in this mode as all breaths are spontaneous.

We can assist the patient's spontaneous breaths with a support breath. These support breaths employ one variable as the set parameter (pressure or volume) and the opposite parameter as the goal variable.

In the case of pressure support, the pressure target is titrated to achieve a target tidal volume. A common tidal volume target is ~ 4 ml/kg IBW.

Less commonly on some machines, a volume support breath is accomplished by setting the tidal volume target.

The mode will adjust the pressure level on a breath-by-breath basis to maintain the desired tidal volume.

15.4.4 APRV and BiLevel Ventilation

BiLevel ventilation refers to pressure control intermittent ventilation that allows unrestricted spontaneous breathing during the respiratory cycle. A very confusing list of terms are used by the ventilator manufacturers to describe their own versions of BiLevel ventilation including BiLevel, BIPAP, Bi Vent, BiPhasic, PCV+, and DuoPAP. A variant of the BiLevel mode of ventilation is termed *airway pressure release ventilation* and is used primarily for patients with ARDS. This mode of ventilation, which is available on newer ventilators, cycles the patient between a high and low level of pressure. The high level is termed high $PEEP_H$ and the low level is termed low $PEEP_L$. The clinician sets the relationship between the high and low PEEP level ($PEEP_H$/ $PEEP_L$). Spontaneous breaths may occur at either the high or low PEEP level. Ventilation occurs in the transitions from low to high levels in addition to the spontaneous breaths. We will talk more about this very specialized mode in *Chapter 16* on the *Acute Respiratory Distress Syndrome.*

15.5 Mode summary

We can start to organize this soup of ventilator terms. We have four modes of ventilation:

1. Assist-Control (AC)
2. Synchronized Intermittant Mandatory Ventilation (SIMV)
3. Spontaneous Ventilation (SV)
4. Bilevel Ventilation (BiLevel)

And we have five different breath types that we can provide in these modes:

1. Volume Control (VC)
2. Pressure Control (PC)
3. Pressure Regulated Volume Control (PRVC)
4. Pressure Support (PS)
5. Volume Support (VS)

We start putting the mode and breath combinations together, and this starts to get a little crazy!!

1. Control/AC mode with either VC, PC, or PRVC mandatory breaths
2. SIMV mode with

   a. VC or PC mandatory breaths determined by the set rate
   b. Spontaneous, PS, or VS breaths determined by the spontaneous rate

3. Spontaneous Ventilation (or CPAP) with PS or VS spontaneous breaths
4. BiLevel Ventilation

Hey – not so bad when we organize it a little!
Always ask yourself (or that therapist) two basic questions:

1. Is the breath delivery based on a pressure or volume goal?
   Once you learn this, you always know to monitor the opposite variable, i.e., volume goal means monitor pressure.
2. Is the breath triggering based upon timing, the patient, or both?

Once you learn this, you can align the breath types with the triggering mechanism.

Pressure control breaths occur in modes labeled as

- Pressure Control Mechanical Ventilation (PC-CMV)
- Pressure Control Intermittent Mandatory Ventilation (PC-IMV)
- Pressure Regulated Volume Control Ventilation (PRVC)
- Pressure Control Inverse Ratio Ventilation (PC-IRV)
- BiLevel Pressure Ventilation (BiLevel)

Volume control breaths occur in modes labeled as

- Volume Control Mechanical Ventilation (VC-CMV)
- Volume Control Intermittent Mandatory Ventilation (VC-IMV)
- Volume Control Inverse Ratio Ventilation (VC-IRV)

Basic initial ventilator settings for the three common breath types are summarized in **Figure 15-18.**

Refinement of the initial breath and rate settings are then based on the following goals:

- Minute ventilation (RR × Tidal volume) is adjusted to control hypercapnia and maintain pH > 7.30.
- Tidal volume is adjusted to achieve the target minute ventilation while maintaining the plateau (end-inspiratory) airway pressure less than 30 cm H_2O and tidal volume in the range of 6-8 ml/kg ideal body weight.
- Inspiratory flow is adjusted to maintain plateau pressures less than 30 cm H_2O but still allow a ratio of inspiratory:expiratory time of 1:2 or greater.
- Sensitivity is adjusted to minimize triggering related workload for the patient but avoid auto triggering.
- PEEP and FiO_2 combinations are adjusted to achieve an oxygen saturation of 92-94% or a measured oxygen partial pressure of >_60-65 mm Hg.

Don't let those nasty respiratory therapists confuse you!! You got this!! The majority of patients with respiratory

Parameter	EOM	Volume Control	Pressure Control	Pressure Support
Tidal Volume	Vt	6-8 ml / kg ideal body weight	Variable Parameter	Variable Parameter
Flow	Vt/Ti	~ 60-80 L/min adjusted to keep I:E > 1:2 (standard ratio) and peak airway pressure < 30 cm H_2O Can also set flow delivery pattern as a square wave, descending ramp, or sinusoidal pattern	Variable Parameter	Variable Parameter
Airway Pressure	Pao	Variable Parameter	Set to achieve a goal tidal volume and/or maintain peak airway pressures < 30 cm H_2O	Set to achieve a goal tidal volume of ~ 4-6 ml/kg ideal body weight
Inspiratory Time	Ti	Determined by set flow rate or set to meet flow rate targets	Set to keep I:E > 1:2 (standard ratio)	Variable Parameter
PEEP (extrinsic)	PEEP	5 cm H_2O and titrated to target oxygenation	5 cm H_2O and titrated to target oxygenation	5 cm H_2O (if receiving with CPAP mode)

Figure 15-18 Initial ventilator settings for three common breath types.

failure will do well with your basic settings in the AC volume assist mode while you treat their underlying pulmonary condition. Two of the toughest ventilator problems are severe hypoxemia and severe airflow obstruction. We are going to talk more about these specialized ventilation concepts in the chapters on ARDS and COPD. ARDS is the classic disease to learn about managing severe hypoxemia. Obstructive lung disease is the clinical disease to learn about mechanical ventilation with severe airflow obstruction. *So, keep reading!!* But first, let's talk a little about end-expiratory pressure.

15.6 Positive End-Expiratory Pressure—PEEP, CPAP, and EPAP

In addition to supporting the inspiratory muscles for the work of breathing, positive pressure ventilation must correct gas exchange abnormalities. Advanced hypoxemia due to physiologic shunting and V/Q mismatch is often present in hospital patients due to alveolar edema, loss of surfactant, or collapsed alveoli. In this situation, manipulation of airway pressures can be used to recruit these collapsed alveoli and increase alveolar ventilation (thus improving V/Q matching). The most common method to recruit these alveoli is through the use of positive end-expiratory pressure. End-expiratory airway pressure is usually equivalent to ambient atmospheric pressure. Under these conditions, the balance of inward lung and outward chest wall elastic recoil forces determines the lung volume at end-expiration, sometimes called the *lung equilibration volume*

(or *functional residual capacity—FRC*). Positive pressure applied to the airway at end expiration (PEEP) increases the transpulmonary pressure (alveolar pressure - pleural pressure) above ambient pressure and increases the lung volume at end-expiration (higher than FRC).

Positive end-expiratory pressure can occur due to patient factors (e.g., air is trapped at end-expiration) or can be due to external factors, such as a face mask or ventilator used to increase end-expiratory pressure. Confusing terminology is used for the many variations of positive end-expiratory pressure. The term used for the same physiologic end-expiratory pressure is different based on the mode of ventilation (**Figure 15-19**). For example, during pressure control or volume control breaths, we refer to positive end-expiratory pressure as *PEEP*. During spontaneous ventilation, we call positive end-expiratory pressure *continuous positive airway pressure (CPAP)*. With a non-invasive BiPhasic (BiPAP) system, we call it *expiratory positive airway pressure (EPAP)*. In essence, these are many terms for the same physiologic equivalent, positive end-expiratory airway pressure. For the remainder of this discussion, we will use the single term *PEEP*.

There are numerous potential benefits to the application of PEEP, including

- Recruitment of collapsed lung units to improve ventilation and V/Q matching, reduce shunt physiology, and correct significant hypoxemia poorly responsive to augmentation of F_iO_2
- Stabilization of "recruitable" alveoli during inspiratory/expiratory cycles to prevent opening and closing cycles that may extend lung injury

Mode of Ventilation	Inspiratory Pressure	Expiratory Positive Pressure Term
Volume or Pressure Control Ventilation	Determined by a Volume or Pressure Goal	Positive End-Expiratory Pressure (PEEP)
Spontaneous Ventilation	Inspiratory Pressure = Expiratory Pressure	Continuous Positive Airway Pressure (CPAP)
Non-Invasive BiPhasic Ventilation	Inspiratory Pressure > Expiratory Pressure	Expiratory Positive Airway Pressure (EPAP)

Figure 15-19 *Terms for end-expiratory pressure settings with mechanical ventilation based upon the mode of ventilation.*

(called *open lung ventilation*)
- Improving lung volumes in the setting of chest or abdominal wall restriction that limits lung expansion
- Reducing preload and afterload on the heart in a patient with congestive heart failure
- Improving ventilator triggering and reducing work of breathing in the setting of a COPD patient with intrinsic PEEP and dynamic hyperinflation

The most common reason for the use of positive end-expiratory pressure is to recruit collapsed alveolar units and improve oxygenation in the setting of alveolar collapse.

15.6.1 Adverse Effects of End-Expiratory Pressure

In addition to the benefits, there are a few potentially adverse consequences from the application of PEEP including

- Increase in anatomical shunting
- Decline in cardiac output
- Alveolar distention and barotrauma

Let's first take a look at these adverse effects of PEEP.

15.6.1.1 PEEP and Anatomical Shunting

The ideal application of PEEP results in recruitment of collapsed alveoli while maintaining the blood flow to those alveoli (thus improving V/Q matching). We assume, however, that the increase in end-expiratory pressure is uniformly distributed across all the alveoli. In fact, an injured lung is a heterogeneous group of alveolar units with widely variable V/Q relationships. The heterogeneous nature of ICU lung disease can make the physiologic response to PEEP quite variable, with some alveoli over-distending and some not distending at all.

Let's consider a two-alveolus lung model shown in **Figure 15-20**. Alveolus B is characterized by loss of surfactant, poor compliance, and collapse. The absence of ventilation would lead to characterization of alveolus

B as a low V/Q unit. The local hypoxemia leads to vasoconstriction and a decrease in blood flow to alveolus B as a method of compensation for the low V/Q unit. In contrast, alveolus A has a normal compliance and blood flow or essentially a more normal V/Q unit. These baseline conditions are illustrated in **Figure 15-20**, left panel.

Application of airway or extrinsic PEEP is uniform at the trachea, but the effects could be variably distributed between the alveoli. Ideally, the application of PEEP to the airway "recruits" alveolus B and improves the V/Q match in alveolus B, reducing the overall shunt (middle panel). However, PEEP could create a volume change most significantly in alveolus A (right panel), given the better compliance. This volume change could lead to over-distention of alveolus A, with the alveolus pressing against the capillaries and increasing local vascular resistance and reducing blood flow. The redistributed blood would be directed to alveolus B despite the lack of recruitment in this alveolus. In essence, the application of end-expiratory pressure has moved alveolus A to a higher V/Q unit (dead space) and alveolus B to a lower V/Q unit (shunt). The lower V/Q unit worsens hypoxemia, and the higher V/Q unit contributes to dead space and hypercapnia.

This example illustrates that the application of PEEP has the potential to both improve and worsen gas exchange parameters, depending on the overall effect on V/Q relationships in the lung. Optimizing PEEP is a balance of opening recruitable alveoli without over-distending normal alveoli. Fortunately, PEEP is more likely to increase alveolar recruitment, improve V/Q matching, and relieve hypoxemia than to alter V/Q relationships unfavorably. It is important to assess the response to incremental PEEP on oxygenation with each change of the ventilator settings. So as a rule, titrate PEEP with careful monitoring of gas exchange parameters.

In patients with intracardiac shunts, like an atrial septal defect or a patent foramen ovale, increasing intrathoracic pressure with PEEP can also produce paradoxical effects. If PEEP increases pulmonary vascular resistance, right atrial pressure rises, and an intracardiac right-to-left shunt is favored. This increase in intracardiac shunt could offset any beneficial effects

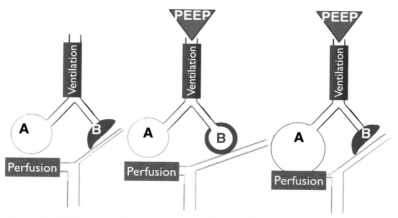

Figure 15-20 *Two alveolus lung model with variable V / Q relationships (see text).*

of PEEP on improving lung gas exchange.

15.6.1.2 PEEP and Cardiac Output

A second significant impact of increasing end-expiratory pressure is the effect on cardiovascular hemodynamics. As positive end-expiratory pressure increases, mean intrathoracic pressure must increase. PEEP therefore augments the effects of positive airway pressure on cardiac function. In a review from *Chapter 9 Acute Decompensated Heart Failure*, positive airway pressure accomplishes important hemodynamic changes through heart-lung interactions. Positive airway pressure

1. *Reduces right ventricular preload* by increasing intrathoracic pressure and reducing venous blood flow to the right atrium
2. *Increases right ventricular afterload* by potentially increasing lung volume, leading to compression of alveolar vasculature, raising pulmonary vascular resistance
3. *Decreases left ventricular preload* through reduced pulmonary venous return resulting from decreased RV preload and increased RV afterload with a possible additional contribution from a shift of the septum to compromise LV filling
4. *Reduces left ventricular afterload* by creating a favorable gradient between increased intrathoracic pressure and the lower atmospheric pressure in the extrathoracic cavities. The systemic vasculature is at a lower pressure than the left ventricular and intrathoracic aorta.

The hemodynamic effect of PEEP will be dependent on the interaction of these variables and the patient's hemodynamic parameters before the application of PEEP.

A 60 yo previously healthy male presents to the ED with rapidly progressive fever, dyspnea, and confusion. On arrival, the patient has tachycardia, tachypnea, and severe oxygen desaturation (SaO$_2$ 75%). The patient undergoes rapid intubation and is placed on 100% oxygen. The radiograph on presentation reveals a dense right lung consolidation. The oxygen saturation improves slightly to 82%. PEEP is added to the ventilatory circuit at 10 cm H$_2$O. The saturation improves minimally. Gradual titration of PEEP leads to no improvement in the patient's measured saturation and is associated with hypotension. In this case, the patient has unilateral lung disease (pneumonia); PEEP is not beneficial and may worsen gas exchange if it overdistends the normal lung. Positional therapy, which involves placing the patient L lung down, may be the most effective approach to improve V/Q match and reduce the physiologic shunt.

15.6.1.3 PEEP and Alveolar Distention

Alveolar overdistention can occur with PEEP, as illustrated in **Figure 15-20**, particularly in compliant alveoli, often in nondependent lung regions, which remain open at end-expiration. Overdistention can lead to alveolar injury (popped lungs!). Alveolar over-distention may manifest as pneumothorax, pneumomediastinum, or subcutaneous emphysema.

In all ventilator modes except CPAP, the inspiratory phase is associated with an augmentation of airway pressure, which is provided on top of the end-expiratory pressure. An increase in PEEP therefore leads to an associated increase in end-inspiratory pressure as well. The latter increase may be adversely associated with overdistention of compliant alveolar units. This overdistention would place this region of the lung at risk for ventilator-related lung injury.

OK – now that we know the bad parts, let's set the ventilator.

15.7 How to Set Your Best PEEP on the Ventilator

Clinical investigators have described many models for selecting the "best" PEEP value for your patient. However, the most common clinical approach is based on simple titration and observation. PEEP is applied in increments of 2.5 cm H_2O progressively to a maximum value usually in the range of 15-20 cm H_2O. Selection of the "best" PEEP level for a patient is clinically determined by monitoring four variables:

1. Oxygenation (PaO_2 or SaO_2)
2. Cardiac output or systemic perfusion
3. Dead space fraction (minute ventilation and $PaCO_2$)
4. Airway pressures (target plateau pressure < 30 cm H_2O)

Only a single variable, the PEEP level, is adjusted during each incremental PEEP titration, while other variables such as tidal volume, body position, and F_iO_2 are kept constant. At each PEEP level, assessment of the benefit (PaO_2) and possible detriment (cardiac output, $PaCO_2$, and airway pressure) must be assessed.

You increase the PEEP from 10 to 15 cm H_2O in a patient with severe ARDS, and his PaO_2 increases from 60 to 194 mm Hg, and his cardiac output changes from 5 to 4 L/min (or mixed venous saturation drops from 74% to 60%). Which is the "best PEEP, 10 or 15? The answer is not straightforward:

Because the PaO_2 increases dramatically, this might lead you to think that 15 cm H_2O of PEEP might be the best choice. However, if you review your hemoglobin-oxygen dissociation curve, you will remember that a PaO_2 of 60 mm Hg results in a hemoglobin oxygen saturation of 89%, and a PaO_2 of 194 increases it to 100% saturation, so the oxygen delivery would increase by 11%. However, your cardiac output decreased by 20% from 5 to 4 L/min. Therefore, your net oxygen delivery DECREASED by 9%, so your best PEEP was paradoxically 10 cm H_2O!

Impairment of cardiac output is most commonly seen in the setting of relative volume depletion and PEEP levels > 15 cm H_2O. While cardiac output changes occur quickly after each PEEP titration, gas exchange parameters usually change more slowly over 15-30-minute intervals. So, your PEEP titration usually occurs over 30-60-minute intervals if your patient allows.

The effect of PEEP titration is assessed using arterial oxygenation from a blood gas and assessing cardiac output either non-invasively by clinical exam or monitoring $ScvO_2$ (mixed central venous oxygen saturation). Alternatively, an invasive approach can be chosen by shooting a thermodilution cardiac output from your PA catheter. This allows you to determine the best PEEP that improves oxygen delivery. Remember that oxygen delivery depends on both the hemoglobin oxygen saturation (dictated by PaO_2 and the hemoglobin-oxygen dissociation curve) AND the cardiac output (which you can estimate by the mixed venous saturation).

Weaning of PEEP, as the patient clinically improves, is also conducted in a stepwise fashion. Premature reduction in PEEP can be associated with alveolar collapse, oxygen desaturation, and a requirement for levels of end-expiratory pressure above the former baseline to re-recruit the lung.

We will further review more complex options for PEEP titration including PEEP tables and lung mechanics in Chapter 16, our chapter on *ARDS*.

15.8 Extrinsic vs. Intrinsic PEEP

The application of end-expiratory pressure through the use of expiratory circuit valves is termed *applied* or *extrinsic PEEP*. The clinician, through the specific ventilator setting, always knows the level of extrinsic PEEP. The alveolar pressure at end expiration is equal to the airway pressure or set PEEP – *easy!*

PEEP can also occur, however, from the interaction of the mechanical ventilator and the patient's lung mechanics. This type of PEEP is termed *intrinsic PEEP (PEEPi)* or *auto-PEEP* and is not evident to the clinician unless accurately measured. Intrinsic PEEP is the alveolar pressure when the alveolar units do not empty to FRC at end-expiration. At end-expiration, the alveolar pressure remains greater than the airway pressure or extrinsic PEEP setting. PEEPi occurs in the setting of a prolonged expiratory time constant (high resistance × high compliance). Any combination of four variables can interact to elevate intrinsic PEEP:

1. *Elevated respiratory rate*, which shortens the available time for expiration (i.e., tachypnea)
2. *Increased inspiratory time* due to increased tidal volume or reduction in inspiratory flow

A patient with severe emphysema is admitted to the ICU with respiratory failure. The patient is placed on mechanical ventilation with settings of TV=450, RR$_{set}$ 20, FiO$_2$ 5 0.50, PEEP 5. You note the patient is breathing at a rate of 30 bpm. The patient is also hypotensive and has required norepinephrine to support his blood pressure.

You carefully assess the patient for intrinsic PEEP and note persistent end-expiratory airflow. You sedate the patient to reduce the respiratory rate and prolong the cycle time. With sedation the patient's blood pressure improves. What happened?

The high RR provides a short cycle length in a patient with a fixed long expiratory time (airflow obstruction and reduced elastic recoil), leading to intrinsic PEEP. The intrinsic PEEP compromises venous return and reduces cardiac output, leading to hypotension.

Sedation reduces the RR to the set ventilator rate, prolongs the cycle length, allows greater expiration, reduces intrinsic PEEP, and improves blood pressure.

3. *Increased expiratory time* due to airflow obstruction (e.g.,. asthma or COPD)
4. Increased expiratory time due to a reduced respiratory system elastic recoil (e.g., high lung compliance with emphysema)

Given the characteristics that are associated with intrinsic PEEP, you can expect this condition will be most common in patients with severe airflow obstruction.

The adverse effects of intrinsic and extrinsic PEEP are similar on gas exchange and cardiovascular hemodynamics, although the distribution of PEEPi across the lung may not be equivalent. The primary difference between extrinsic and intrinsic PEEP is the lack of easy recognition and measurement for PEEPi. Even though the patient's ventilator says PEEP = 5, the intrinsic PEEP may be much higher. Since the pressure is related to air trapped in the lung, it is harder for us to get inside the lung and measure the pressure. We need to be vigilant, especially in any patient with obstructive lung disease and hemodynamic instability, and think about PEEPi.

Because of the strong association of PEEPi with obstructive lung disease, we will review the techniques for the measurement of intrinsic PEEP in detail in Chapter 19 on *Obstructive Lung Disease and Respiratory Failure.*

15.9 Mean Airway Pressure and Oxygenation

Recruitment of alveoli and stabilization of alveolar volume is most closely linked to the average airway pressure during the entire respiratory cycle, termed the *mean airway pressure* (MAP). PEEP augments mean airway pressure by increasing the baseline pressure during both inspiration and expiration. An alternative approach to increase airway pressure would be to change the characteristics of the breath delivery.

Figure 15-21 A is a conventional control breath with inspiratory time much shorter than expiratory time. For these breaths, if we increase PEEP, we would also increase peak inspiratory pressure and mean airway pressure (MAP). In **Figure 15-21 B,** we have extended the inspiratory time of the conventional breath rather than increasing the PEEP. Both the PEEP level and peak inspiratory pressure values are the same for both breaths A and B. However, the more prolonged inspiratory phase in Breath B leads to a greater mean airway pressure. If we assume that the risk of overdistention and barotrauma links best to the peak inspiratory pressure, and recruitment to the mean airway pressure, you can appreciate the possible benefit to this alternative method for raising mean airway pressure. This approach offers the potential advantage of recruitment without further distending normal alveolar units.

Many methods are used in mechanical ventilation to increase the mean airway pressure without increasing PEEP. These might include

- Lengthening the inspiratory time cycle of pressure control breaths
- Adding an end-inspiratory pause to volume control breaths
- Reducing the inspiratory flow rate of volume control breaths

These concepts are the basis for specialized modes most frequently applied in the patient with severe hypoxemic respiratory failure. The modes manipulate the normal inspiratory:expiratory timing ratio away from the traditional 1:2 relationship. The modes include the following:

- Pressure Control Inverse Ratio Ventilation (PC-IRV)
- BiLevel Pressure Ventilation (BiLevel) including Airway Pressure Release Ventilation (APRV)

These modes of ventilation have been most commonly employed in the patient with ARDS and will be discussed further in *Chapter 16 Acute Respiratory Distress Syndrome.*

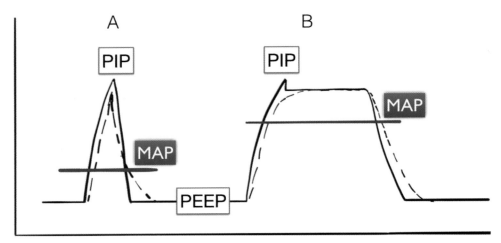

Figure 15-21 *Pressure-time tracing showing a conventional pressure control breath (A) and a breath with an extended inspiratory time (B).*

A little caution here. Any maneuver that lengthens the inspiratory time can compromise expiratory time and may lead to an increase in intrinsic PEEP. Your extrinsic PEEP setting may be the same, but your intrinsic PEEP level may be increased with all the associated risks. A primary effect of prolonging the inspiratory phase on improving your oxygenation when you lengthen the inspiratory phase may be through the development of intrinsic PEEP.

Alveolar recruitment maneuvers can also be used to recruit collapsed alveoli and again are based on the principle of increasing *(briefly)* the airway pressure. The procedure involves temporary inflation of the lung during positive pressure ventilation to total lung capacity. A variety of protocols has been described for these maneuvers but generally involve sustained inflation of the lung to 30-40 cm H_2O for a prolonged interval (i.e., 1-2 min). These "maximal" recruitment maneuvers are only temporarily effective in recruiting collapsed alveoli and require changes with modification in PEEP or inspiratory time to sustain the recruitment effect. While they are often beneficial on a temporary basis, controversy exists about whether the routine application of recruitment maneuvers is advantageous to the patient with lung injury.

Oxygenation made simple: Just increase the MAP!!!

You will notice that most of our mechanical methods used to improve oxygenation on the ventilator involve adding more pressure in one way or the other. These maneuvers all distend alveoli and increase the number of alveoli that are in contact with capillaries for gas exchange.

Suggested Reading

- Rittayamai N, Katsios CM, Beloncle F, Friedrich JO, Mancebo J, Brochard L. Pressure-controlled vs volume-controlled ventilation in acute respiratory pailure: A physiology-based narrative and systematic review. Chest 2015;148(2):340–55.
- Pontoppidan H, Geffin B, Lowenstein E: Acute respiratory failure in the adult (parts I-III). NEJM 1972;287:690–698, 743–752, 799–806
- Loring, S. H., Topulos, G. P., & Hubmayr, R. D. (2016). Transpulmonary pressure: The importance of precise definitions and limiting assumptions. *Am J Resp Crit Care*, 194(12), 1452–1457.

16

Acute Respiratory Distress Syndrome (ARDS)

Acute Respiratory Distress Syndrome (ARDS) is one of the most common diseases requiring mechanical ventilation due to severe hypoxemic respiratory failure. ARDS is not a specific disease entity, but rather a clinical syndrome. We will use the ARDS condition for a discussion of interventions to treat acute hypoxemic respiratory failure.

The justification for classifying ARDS as a syndrome is a clinical observation that a specific trigger initiates a characteristic pattern of disease pathophysiology in the lung (**Figure 16-1**). The host response to the insult begins alveolar capillary injury that includes a neutrophilic inflammatory process within the lung parenchyma. Complications of patient care, including ventilator-induced lung injury (VILI) and nosocomial infections, can extend the alveolar capillary injury beyond the initial insult. The damage to the lung parenchyma is associated with permeability lung edema, loss of normal surfactant in the airspace of the lung, and capillary thrombi formation. The pathophysiologic process leads to marked hypoxemia secondary to shunt physiology (alveolar edema), loss of lung compliance with restrictive lung mechanics (loss of surfactant), and the development of pulmonary hypertension (capillary microthrombi). The justification for grouping diverse etiologies into the single ARDS syndrome is that the pathophysiologic process appears to have a common clinical and pathologic progression, regardless of the trigger.

Other terms, often used interchangeably with ARDS, include acute lung injury (ALI), permeability pulmonary edema, and/or non-cardiogenic pulmonary edema.

16.1 ARDS Ridiculously Simple Overview

ARDS is a *lung injury syndrome triggered by many kinds of severe "hits" that cause lung inflammation and leak.* These hits can be a systemic infection (sepsis and septic shock) or a lung infection (pneumonia). The hit can be massive trauma, systemic inflammation from pancreatitis, burns, near-drowning, or aspiration. *Think of an inflammatory or traumatic hit to the lung!*

The syndrome ARDS is defined by specific clinical criteria which include

1. *Infiltrates on the radiograph.* When the lung fills up with water and pus (inflammatory neutrophils, fibrin and collagen), it whites out.
2. *A leaky lung, causing non-cardiogenic edema.* This is *NOT* cardiac, pulmonary edema. The diagnosis of normal heart function can be confirmed based on clinical evidence (history, examination, plasma BNP, echocardiogram) rather than using an invasive pulmonary artery catheter, so long as there is an accepted risk factor (a bad hit) for developing ARDS and no history of heart failure.

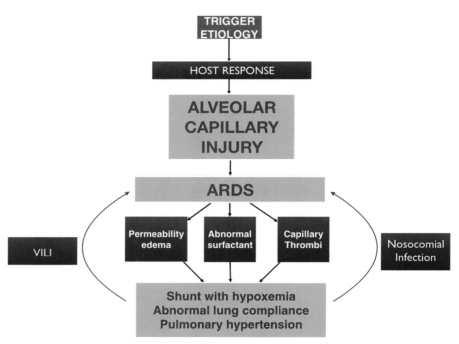

Figure 16-1 *Summary of the progression from an ARDS trigger etiology to lung injury.*

3. *Low oxygen.* How low can you go? The ratio of the PaO_2/FiO_2 is referred to as the *P/F ratio,* and as the lung V/Q worsens, the PaO_2 drops and we dial up the FiO_2. So, a low PaO_2/FiO_2 level is bad. The P/F ratio has to be less than 300 mm Hg to meet ARDS criteria. Think of a PaO_2 of 100 mm Hg (which is normal) but on a FiO_2 of 0.35 (normal air is 0.21). This gives us a value of 285.7. It does not take much hypoxia to meet the definition of mild ARDS. Severe ARDS is less than 100, so this would be a PaO_2 of 60 mm Hg with an FiO_2 of 0.6 or higher. As you will see below, the lower the P/F ratio, the lower the survival.

Pharmacological therapy. There are no drugs for ARDS. What? In the modern age of medicine and science, we have no drugs for one of our most common diseases in the ICU? Many drugs have been tested for ARDS, including high- and low-dose steroids, β-agonists, statins, ketoconazole, lisofylline, and omega-3 feedings. To date, none has proven efficacious. The only drug that seems to work is the non-steroidal paralytic drug *cisatracurium,* which is thought to protect the lung from injury, but may have direct effects on lung injury or repair that we do not yet understand. We use inhaled nitric oxide and inhaled prostacyclin as salvage therapy in severely hypoxemic patients, but these have not been proven to change outcomes and are not FDA-approved for ARDS. But we will keep trying to find new drugs.

Non-drug therapy. But the good news is that we seem to be getting better at treating ARDS, and this may all be due to better non-drug therapy. This therapy includes

1. *First and foremost, put out the fire!* What we mean is, "Stop the first hit that caused ARDS." Infection causes 70% of ARDS with sepsis or pneumonia, common "hits." You must kill the buggers. Hit the patient with broad-spectrum antibiotics, and narrow your coverage once you have positive identification. Find the source and clear it. Sometimes this requires a surgical solution, for example with gallstone pancreatitis or cholangitis or an abscess. Draining or operating on an infectious source is called *source control.*

2. *Resuscitate, ventilate and oxygenate:* fluid resuscitation, intubation, and mechanical ventilation. Good old-fashioned *ABCs* to limit multi-organ injury. The more organs you lose, the less likelihood of survival.

3. *Do no harm and dial it down! DO NOT DEEP SIX YOUR PATIENT.* As you will see below, a major problem with ARDS is that our primary therapy to save the patient is mechanical ventilation, and this can hurt the patient by causing barotrauma and volutrauma. Turn down the tidal volume to 6 ml/kg of ideal body weight. If you do not do this, you may *DEEP SIX (>6 cc/Kg) YOUR PATIENT.*

4. *Know how to oxygenate a rock.* When the lung fills with pus, fibrin and fluid, it becomes a rock with severe V/Q mismatch (shunt), leading to hypoxemia and low compliance, leading to high airway pressures. ARDS will teach you how to manage severe hypoxemic respiratory failure. There are seven primary strategies to improve oxygenation, which are reviewed in the context of ARDS management in this chapter and outlined in **Figure 16-2:**

a. *Oxygenate! FiO$_2$.* Turn up the oxygen. This is a simple adjustment based upon the alveolar gas equation.

b. *Turn up the pressure!* Improve V/Q by recruiting alveoli with high mean airway pressure (MAP). Mean airway pressure recruits collapsed alveoli to increase the number of alveoli that are in contact with capillaries for gas exchange and health V/Q matching. You can increase MAP by increasing peak inspiratory pressure, positive end-expiratory pressure, or changing the I:E ratio (more time with higher inspiratory pressure) (*See Chapter 15 Mechanical Ventilation.*)

c. *Squeeze out the sponge. Diuresis.* After resuscitation, you should run your ARDS patient dry, often with active daily diuresis when the patient is hemodynamically stable. Diuresis improves oxygenation (V/Q matching again) and allows for earlier extubation.

d. *Flip the burger. Prone positioning* improves V/Q matching, oxygenation, and mortality in the sickest patients.

e. *Paralyze and suspend animation. Cisatracurium* will improve ventilation efficiency and reduce oxygen consumption.

f. *Inhaled vasodilators.* As a rescue therapy for the sickest patients, you can try and mprove V/Q by inhaling drugs (typically, inhaled NO or prostacyclin) that recruit blood flow to ventilated regions.

g. *When all else fails, add more boxcars to the train. Transfuse and maintain cardiac output.* When you really are facing hypoxemic respiratory failure, you can always improve oxygen delivery by blood transfusion and ensuring cardiac function is normal. At any given

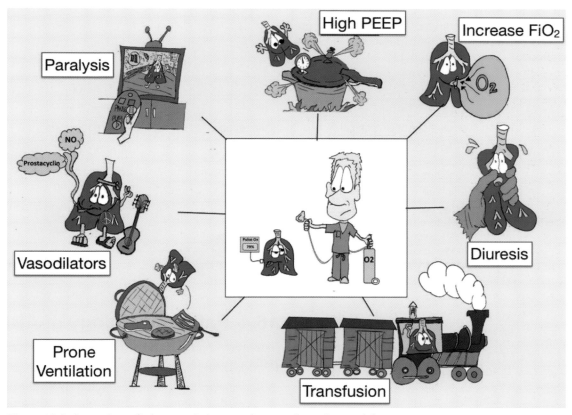

Figure 16-2 Strategies to fix hypoxemia in severe hypoxemic respiratory failure.

PaO$_2$, you will have more oxygen delivery with a higher hemoglobin level.

5. *Wake up and breathe!* As we describe in our weaning chapter, daily interruption of sedation, daily trials of spontaneous breathing/weaning, and early mobilization will allow for earlier extubation, improved survival, and better post-ICU functional recovery.

6. *Tender loving care.* Your patient will be in the ICU for more than a week, and you have to avoid second hits, drug and therapy complications, and secondary infections. Be vigilant every day.

And now let's dive in deep!

16.2 Berlin Definition

The current parameters used to define ARDS, often called the *Berlin definition,* are based upon the specific parameters outlined in **Figure 16-3**.[102]

Why does the Berlin classification define the severity of ARDS based on PaO$_2$/FiO$_2$ as mild (200-300), moderate (100-200), or severe ($\leq$ 100)? The Berlin definition stages of mild, moderate, and severe ARDS were associated with increased mortality from 27% to 32% to 45%, respectively, and increased median duration of mechanical ventilation in survivors from 5 days to 7 days to 9 days, respectively. The term acute lung injury (ALI) from earlier definitions of ARDS has been eliminated.

Clinical Feature	Description
Timing	Within 1 week of a known clinical insult or new or worsening respiratory symptoms
Chest imaging	Bilateral opacities – not fully explained by effusions, lobar/lung collapse or nodules
Origin of edema	Respiratory failure not fully explained by cardiac failure or fluid overload. Need objective assessment (e.g., echocardiography) to exclude hydrostatic edema if no risk factor is present
Oxygenation:	
Mild	200 mm Hg< PaO$_2$/FiO$_2$ $\leq$ 300 mm Hg with PEEP $\geq$ 5 cm H$_2$0
Moderate	100 mm Hg< PaO$_2$/FiO$_2$ $\leq$ 200 mm Hg with PEEP $\geq$ 5 cm H$_2$0
Severe	PaO$_2$/FiO$_2$ $\leq$ 100 mm Hg with PEEP $\geq$ 5 cm H$_2$0

Figure 16-3 *Cinical features that define ARDS based upon the Berlin criteria.*

16.3 Causes of ARDS

The most common etiology for ARDS is an infection, whether intrapulmonary (pneumonia) or systemic. Additional etiologies are outlined in **Figure 16-4**. It is worth noting that the majority of ARDS cases are associated with infection, either sepsis or pneumonia.

ARDS is characterized by a typical "evolution" with time. The early phase of ARDS, termed the *exudative phase,* is dominated by the rapid onset of an alveolar-capillary leak syndrome and alveolar damage with airspace edema and radiographic alveolar infiltrates, marked hypoxemia secondary to physiologic shunting, and markedly increased work of breathing. Other clinical features are dominated by the associated inciting condition (i.e., sepsis or trauma). The lung pathology in this phase is dominated by neutrophilic inflammation, interstitial and alveolar edema, and atelectasis.

Along the pathway to healing, the disease will often progress through a recognizable *fibro-proliferative phase* characterized by alveolar Type II cell proliferation, interstitial infiltration by myofibroblasts, collagen formation and deposition, a transition to more interstitial than alveolar radiographic changes. These changes during the fibroproliferative phase are typically associated with an improved oxygenation (but with a persistent high ventilatory workload and need for mechanical ventilation).

ARDS Etiology	
Sepsis	Drugs and alcohol
Aspiration	Pneumonectomy
Pneumonia	Near drowning
Severe trauma	Lung and stem cell transplantation
Lung contusion	
Massive transfusion	Fat embolization syndrome
Pancreatitis	Sickle cell acute chest syndrome

Figure 16-4 *List of potential trigger etiologies for ARDS.*

16.4 Pathophysiology of ARDS

Three components dominate the pulmonary pathophysiology of ARDS:

1. *Impaired gas exchange*—ruled by shunt physiology with advanced hypoxemia and increased physiologic dead space ventilation with high total ventilatory requirements

2. *Decreased pulmonary compliance*—secondary to stiff and nonaerated lungs, leading to high inflation pressures and limited tolerance for higher tidal volumes

3. *Pulmonary hypertension*—secondary to hypoxic vasoconstriction, vascular compression from lung overdistention, parenchymal destruction, pulmonary microthrombi, and therapy with vasoconstrictors

A traditional time course of ARDS is a 14-day ICU hospitalization and a 3-month recovery. Patients typically show an improvement in the severe hypoxemia between days 3-5 of the hospitalization. The time course is widely variable, however, especially if complications intervene in the routine care of these patients.

16.4.1 ARDS as a Heterogeneous Lung Disease

The management of severe hypoxemia dominates the early phase of ARDS. Although ARDS occurs in the setting of a multi-system disease, a primary focus of management is to support the respiratory system during the evolution of the ARDS syndrome.

Patients with ALI/ARDS are characterized by heterogeneous lung injury so that there is normal lung interspersed with inflammatory cells and edema fluid within the lung parenchyma. As shown in the CT Scan from a representative ARDS patient, the lung infiltrates are often worse in gravitationally dependent regions where the alveoli are likely to collapse (atelectasis) **(Figure 16-5)**.

The injured ARDS lung potentially produces three variants of alveoli units:

1. *Normal lung* with alveoli ventilated throughout the respiratory cycle, but prone to overdistention and stretch-related lung injury during lung inflation.

2. *Recruitable lung* characterized by fluid-filled or collapsed alveoli that are inflated during the inspiratory portion of the respiratory cycle only to collapse again at end-expiration. These latter units may be returned to normal ventilation throughout the respiratory cycle, with the use of specific ventilatory techniques. These units are called *recruitable* as we can bring them back into gas exchange function with the application of positive pressure on the ventilator.

3. *Consolidated lung* characterized by fluid-filled or collapsed alveoli that are never inflated during the respiratory cycle (*non-recruitable*).

Variable local airway resistance, compliance, and residual capacity characterize each alveolar unit. In pressure- and volume-control breath delivery, the delivered tidal volume is preferentially distributed to alveolar units with low airway resistance, high compliance, or both (i.e., more normal lung units). This heterogeneity of alveolar unit physiology and tidal volume distribution leads to a potential risk for overdistention of normal lung units, which can cause ventilator-induced lung injury (VILI) superimposed on the underlying disease process. In ARDS, the disease process can injure the lung, but the lung can also be injured by the therapy we use to treat the disease process. So in the case of mechanical ventilation we must – *DO NO HARM!*

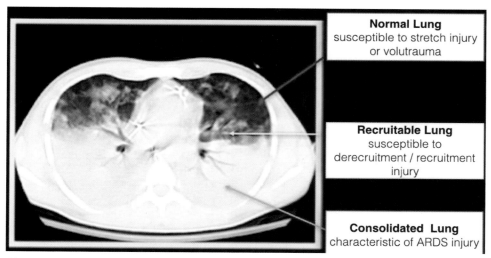

Normal Lung
susceptible to stretch injury or volutrauma

Recruitable Lung
susceptible to derecruitment / recruitment injury

Consolidated Lung
characteristic of ARDS injury

Figure 16-5 CT image of ARDS patient showing the heterogeneous injured lung in ARDS.

16.5 Airway Management in ARDS

ARDS patients typically manifest tachypnea, severe hypoxemia, and hypo- to normocapnia on presentation. A significant work of breathing to maintain hyperventilation often leads to a requirement for intubation and support with mechanical ventilation. Endotracheal tube size in ARDS should be selected to allow for bronchoscopy, if possible, which requires a tube $\geq$ 7 mm. Many of the respiratory conditions, which are ARDS "look-alikes," can be assessed with the technique of bronchoalveolar lavage, including alveolar hemorrhage and eosinophilic pneumonia. Hemodynamic issues to consider during the process of intubation relate primarily to the underlying condition that precipitated the ARDS.

23 yo with AAF and modest obesity presents with upper respiratory tract congestion for 72 hours prior to admission, which has now progressed to SOB, fevers, and chills. On initial presentation, she is noted to have tachypnea (RR 28), tachycardia (HR 115), and normal blood pressure (BP 130/70). She is febrile at 39.°C. She is speaking in short sentences. The initial assessment reveals a pulse oximetry value of 75%. Her lungs have diffuse rales anterior in the lung bases. She has tachycardia, but no gallop or murmur is appreciated. Her abdomen is soft and non-tender with normal bowel sounds. Her extremities are very cool, with a delayed capillary refill, and peripheral pulses are hard to palpate. Her WBC is elevated at 15.5 cells/mm³ with a shift to immature forms. The patient is initially resuscitated with 500 mL normal saline and high-flow oxygen. Her peripheral saturation improved to 85% with a 100% non-rebreather mask. She continues to have tachypnea. Her mental status is confused and disoriented.

Our patient presents with clinical findings of severe community-acquired pneumonia. She has persistent hypoxemia despite high-flow oxygen and her mental status is confused. The use of non-invasive ventilation (NIV) could be considered for this patient, but her mental status and severe hypoxemic respiratory failure suggest early endotracheal intubation is indicated. In contrast to patients with a COPD exacerbation or cardiogenic edema, the beneficial effects of non-invasive ventilation (BiPAP) in ARDS are not as clearly established.

16.6 ARDS and the Ventilator – First Do No Harm

16.6.1 Oxygen Toxicity: Hyperoxic Lung Injury

Both normal human and animal investigations suggest a spectrum of airway and parenchymal injury occurs in association with the administration of supplemental oxygen at high inspired oxygen concentrations. Lung injury has been attributed to the generation of reactive oxygen species. Excess oxygen administration is associated with an early, mild inflammatory response in the normal human lung, and a more severe pathologic picture consistent with diffuse alveolar damage in animal models. From these investigations, it is inferred that supplemental oxygen is potentially injurious in the setting of hypoxemic respiratory failure. However, the specific role oxygen toxicity plays in the diseased human lung, such as ARDS, has been most problematic to determine because of the presence of confounding variables (i.e., the more severe the lung injury, the more oxygen we give, *so guilty by association!*).

16.6.2 Barotrauma—No Pressure!

Early in the everyday use of ventilator support for respiratory failure, clinicians recognized that lungs inflated with high inspiratory pressures had a propensity to develop extra-alveolar air leaks attributed to high inflation pressures. This form of ventilator-induced lung injury was termed *barotrauma*. Barotrauma includes ventilator-associated pneumothorax, pneumomediastinum, subcutaneous emphysema, and pneumoperitoneum. Barotrauma is attributed to the extension of alveolar air into the interstitial space. The air then dissects along tissue planes, and the manifestations of barotrauma depend upon the path of dissection.

Additional clinical manifestations of barotrauma include bronchopleural fistula, tension pneumothorax, tension lung cysts, systemic gas embolism, and subpleural air cysts. Although generally accepted that higher inflation pressure contributes to the development of barotrauma, the evidence to support this association has been inconsistent. Barotrauma as a complication of ARDS management is less common in the current era, where we restrict tidal volumes and plateau pressures. The first manifestation of barotrauma can be pneumothorax or pneumomediastinum. Either can be associated with subcutaneous emphysema **(Figure 16-6)**. In subcutaneous emphysema, blebs of black air can be seen under the skin. On physical examination, if you push down on the skin, it feels like pushing a Rice Krispies treat (called *crepitations*). If you hold the stethoscope down and push on the skin, you can hear the snap, crackle, and pop of your Rice Krispies hitting the milk! Patients can also develop pneumomediastinum and pneumoperitoneum. Pneumomediastinum and pneumoperitoneum can occur without a pneumothorax, but the patient remains at very high risk for this complication.

Barotrauma can be a life-threatening complication of mechanical ventilation, primarily related to pneumothorax. Pneumothorax should be considered in any mechanically ventilated patient with ALI/ARDS who

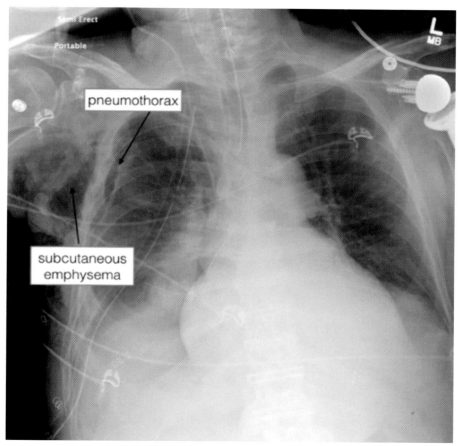

Figure 16-6 Radiograph showing evidence for pneumothorax and subcutaneous emphysema.

develops sudden, unexplained worsening of hypoxemia, respiratory distress, or hemodynamic instability. A chest radiograph (preferably upright) is usually sufficient to make the diagnosis, but in many cases there may not be time to obtain one. Bedside point of care ultrasound offers a more immediate option to assist in the diagnosis (*See Chapter 3, Point of Care Ultrasound*). Pneumomediastinum and subcutaneous emphysema can be painful but, other than analgesia, do not require specific therapy. Air embolus is a rare and potentially fatal complication of positive-pressure mechanical ventilation, which has been occasionally reported in patients with ALI/ARDS and usually occurs in conjunction with other evidence of pulmonary barotrauma.

16.6.3 Volutrauma—Turn Down the Volume!

More recent investigations have identified an additional form of ventilator-induced lung injury termed *volutrauma*. Volutrauma results from overexpansion of alveolar units in association with increased tidal volume.

Alveolar units with normal compliance and low airway resistance would be particularly prone to this form of injury.

An extensive experimental dataset gathered in animal models of ALI-ARDS has confirmed histologic changes characterized by permeability edema in previously uninjured lungs, and exacerbated injury in the diseased lung during mechanical ventilation with high tidal volumes. Comparison of high airway pressure ventilation with restricted chest expansion (performed by placing bands around the chest) compared with low airway pressures with high tidal volumes (performed by surgically opening the chest) has suggested that overdistention, rather than pressure-related injury, is most injurious to the lung (volutrauma).

The strongest evidence for ventilator-associated lung injury in humans was demonstrated by the ARDS Network (ARDSNet) tidal volume trial.[103] Patients in this trial who received a tidal volume of 6 mL/kg predicted ideal body weight (IBW) with a plateau pressure maintained at ≤ 30 cm H_2O had a reduced ICU mortality compared to a higher (~ 12ml / kg IBW) tidal volume group. The ARDSNet tidal volume trial clearly established a negative effect of high tidal volume and high plateau airway pressures on patient outcome in ARDS. From this landmark study, lung protective strategies have evolved as a standard of care for patients with ALI-ARDS on mechanical ventilation, although clinicians often modify the specifics of the ARDSNet protocol in their practice.

Based upon the available information, a tidal volume goal of 6 mL/kg predicted IBW with a plateau pressure maintained at ≤ 30 cm H_2O should be a standard of care for patients with ARDS **(Figure 16-7)**.

16.6.4 Atelectrauma—The Elusive Best Peep!

While the issue of optimal tidal volume has been addressed in ARDS, the selection of the optimal PEEP to support these patients has been more elusive. While excessive tidal volume has been associated with the lung injury we call *volutrauma*, PEEP has been associated with an additional form of ventilator-induced lung injury (VILI) termed *atelectrauma*.

Animal models have suggested that a form of lung injury occurs in response to the shear stress caused by unstable alveoli recruiting (opening) and derecruiting (closing) with each tidal breath. In the heterogeneously injured lung, the strain of alveolar unit inflation is also heterogeneously distributed. The principle of alveolar interdependence can produce increased and potentially harmful stress at the interface between collapsed and expanded lung units, extending the lung injury. In theory, the correct application of PEEP could minimize the risk of this form of damage. The combination of low tidal volume (no volutrauma) *AND* higher PEEP to maintain alveolar recruitment (no atelectrauma) is often termed the *open-lung approach*.

Theoretically, an optimal PEEP setting would minimize this form of lung injury. But setting the optimal PEEP in the ARDS patients has been difficult to define for the bedside clinician. We will outline the existing data on setting the "best PEEP" below.

These three ventilator-related forms of lung injury (barotrauma, volutrauma, and atelectrauma) are collectively referred to clinically as *ventilator-induced lung injury* or VILI.

Don't VILIfy the ventilator in ARDS. As you are playing your cards for ventilator parameters, remember the complications of mechanical ventilation. Pick those cards to keep the pressure and tidal volume low and the lung alveoli open **(Figure 16-8)!**

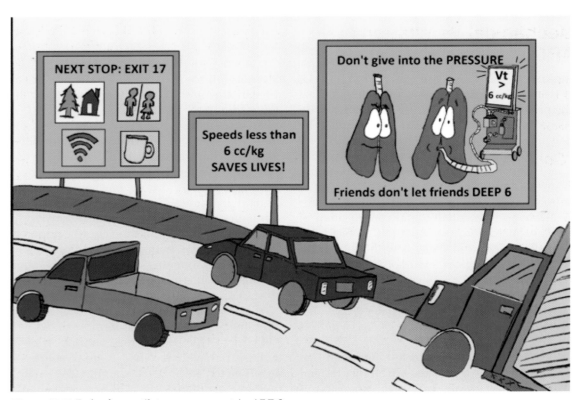

Figure 16-7 *Rules for ventilator management in ARDS.*

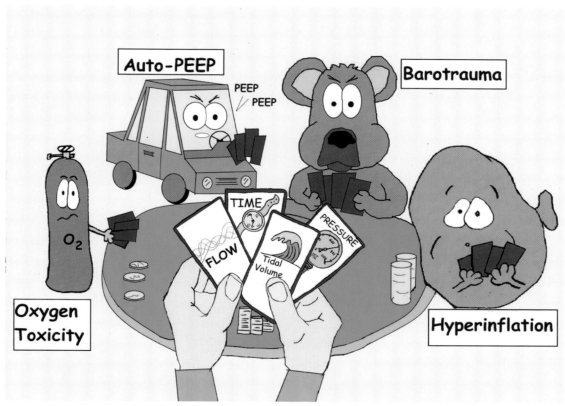

Figure 16-8 *Risk of playing the wrong cards in ARDS ventilator management.*

16.7 Mechanical Ventilation in ARDS

Recognizing the complex lung injury pattern and associated risks of mechanical ventilation, how do we manage the ventilator support for patients with ARDS and respiratory failure?

16.7.1 Control Breaths

Patients with ARDS-ALI can be supported with either pressure control or volume control breaths, most commonly with the assist mode of ventilation, with the provision that appropriate focus is placed on the specific goals of mechanical ventilation. Volume control ventilation offers a predictable tidal volume, which can be limited to 6 ml per kg ideal body weight, and predictable minute ventilation with variable airway pressures based on changing lung mechanics. Pressure control breaths offer predictable airway pressures, which can be limited to plateau airway pressures < 30 cm H_2O yet provide variable lung volumes with changing lung mechanics. The attention of the clinician to these distinct differences and prompt recognition and explanation of changing physiologic variables is most important. In general, full-support modes are favored over partial-support modes early in the disease course because of variable lung mechanics and patient comfort. The majority of ARDS clinical studies have used volume control modes of ventilation. This focus towards volume control modes is appropriate given the clear relationship between tidal volume and disease mortality

The key information to remember includes:

- The proper physiologic targets for ventilator management in ARDS/ALI include a tidal volume in the range of ~6 mL/kg ideal body weight and a plateau pressure < 30 cm H_2O. Hypercapnia experienced with low tidal volume ventilation seems to be modest and well tolerated.
- The current clinical data suggest that tidal volume restriction be a focus for the clinician as a primary treatment goal *RATHER* than achieving normocapnia or avoiding oxygen toxicity.

Emphasis is placed on the use of ideal body weight to determine an appropriate tidal volume, as the use of actual body weight can overestimate the target tidal volume by a value of 10-15% or more. If the tidal volume selected is associated with end-inspiratory (plateau) pressures > 30 cm H_2O, the tidal volume is gradually reduced to lesser values (as low as 4ml/kg predicted IBW). The exception to this plateau pressure target is a clinical situation where pleural pressures might be elevated (e.g., obesity).

The use of low tidal volumes (actually normal size for a spontaneously breathing patient) may cause two potential changes for the ARDS patient:

1. The patient may demonstrate patient-ventilator dyssynchrony with breath stacking and double triggering of breaths. Patient-ventilator dyssynchrony can be addressed by increasing the inspiratory flow rate, sedation of the patient, or, as the patient improves, gradual titration of the tidal volume to ~ 8 ml/kg if the plateau pressures remain < 30 cm H_2O. Neuromuscular blockade should probably be restricted if possible beyond the initial 48-72 hours to avoid the complication of critical illness polyneuropathy and myopathy.

2. Desaturation may occur since the reduction in tidal volume leads to a reduction in inspiratory pressure and mean airway pressure (remember your area under the breathing curve contributes to your mean airway pressure!). Desaturation is compensated for by raising PEEP to maintain mean airway pressure as the cycling pressure is lowered.

16.7.2 PEEP Management

In general, oxygenation is addressed by titrating FiO_2 and PEEP, based upon monitoring of oxygen saturation and cardiac output. Higher PEEP / lower FiO_2 strategies are favored for patients with the more advanced disease.

So how do you set the correct PEEP level? PEEP is applied in increments of 2.5-5 cm H_2O to a maximum value usually in the range of 15-20 cm H_2O. Selection of the "best" PEEP level for a patient is usually determined by the interaction of four goals:

1. Improve oxygenation
2. Maintain cardiac output
3. Limit any elevation of dead space fraction

4. Limit airway pressures (plateau pressure < 30 cm H_2O)

The PEEP level is adjusted during an incremental PEEP titration while other variables such as tidal volume, body position, and F_iO_2 are kept constant. At each PEEP level, the benefit (PaO_2) and possible detriment (cardiac output and $PaCO_2$) must be assessed. Impairment of cardiac output is most commonly seen in the setting of relative volume depletion and PEEP levels > 15 cm H_2O. The risk is also greater in patients with underlying cardiac disease. While cardiac output changes occur quickly after each PEEP titration, gas exchange parameters usually change more slowly over 15-30-minute intervals.

Because ARDS is the prototype disease for severe hypoxemic respiratory failure, many alternative strategies have been employed to suggest the optimal PEEP level for the patient.

16.7.2.1 PEEP Tables

Investigators have described $PEEP/FiO_2$ combinations to guide PEEP therapy, primarily for the design of ARDS clinical trials. The ALVEOLI clinical trial treated all ARDS patients with low tidal volume ventilation (~ 6 ml/kg IBW), but then randomized patients to one of two different $PEEP/FiO_2$ table combinations (**Figure 16-9**).[104] The $PEEP/FiO_2$ combination is adjusted to achieve a PaO_2 55-80 mm Hg or SpO_2 88-95%. When patients fall outside the range for the target oxygenation, the ventilator settings are changed up or down the blocks, based on the $PEEP/FiO_2$ table selected. Managing a patient with the low PEEP table might have ventilator settings with a FiO_2 of 0.70 and PEEP 10 cm H_2O. When the measured PaO_2 is > 80 mm Hg or SpO_2 > 95%, the patient would move one block down to a FiO_2 of 0.60 and PEEP 10 cm H_2O. These changes would occur a minimum of every 4 hours.

No specific difference was noted in patient mortality or ventilator-free days in the ALVEOLI trial. Comparing patients managed with the low vs. high PEEP table in the ALVEOLI trials showed no difference in patient outcome.

Low PEEP													
FiO_2	0.30	0.40	0.40	0.50	0.50	0.60	0.70	0.70	0.70	0.80	0.90	0.90	0.90	1.0
PEEP	5	5	8	8	10	10	10	12	14	14	14	16	18	18-24

High PEEP													
FiO_2	0.30	0.30	0.30	0.30	0.30	0.40	0.40	0.50	0.50	0.50-.80	0.80	0.90	1.0	1.0
PEEP	5	8	10	12	14	14	16	16	18	20	22	22	22	24

Figure 16-9 Outline of low and high PEEP tables used for titration in ARDSNet ventilation protocols.

A meta-analysis examining set PEEP levels confirmed that treatment with higher vs. lower levels of PEEP is not associated with improved hospital survival when all patients (ALI and ARDS) in these trials are combined.[105] However, when subphenotypes from the combined patient population are isolated, the patients with more severe ARDS (PaO_2/FiO_2 ratio < 200) demonstrated an improved overall patient survival with the higher PEEP strategy.

Further attempts to subphenotype the ARDS population have incorporated biomarkers. Calfee and colleagues have described two unique subphenotypes of ARDS.[106] They describe a hyperinflammatory subphenotype (phenotype 2) characterized by high plasma concentrations of inflammatory biomarkers, greater prevalence of vasopressor use, lower serum bicarbonate concentrations, and a high prevalence of sepsis. Phenotype 2 patients appeared to benefit from a high PEEP management strategy. The work of Calfee et al, hopefully, begins an era of precision medicine in ARDS where therapies are individualized to an optimal patient outcome. But much work remains to confirm these findings before they can provide a standard for clinical care.

Considering these clinical trials together, we have data to suggest a favorable outcome for the use of a higher PEEP strategy in the more severe ARDS patients. For milder patients, we have no clinical evidence to favor a higher PEEP strategy. Unfortunately, the trials use slightly different protocols, so our ability to outline a simple approach to PEEP titration from the trials is limited. The ARDSNet PEEP/FiO_2 tables have been extensively used in U.S. clinical trials and can be readily adopted by all clinicians as an acceptable high PEEP strategy in patients with moderate to severe ARDS (http://www.ardsnet.org/files/ventilator_protocol_2008-07.pdf).

16.7.2.2 Transpulmonary Pressures

Alternative approaches to defining "best PEEP" rely upon more detailed physiologic assessment, which might not be as widely applicable to all clinicians. One measurement that has been advocated to set optimal PEEP is the measurement of transpulmonary pressure.

Remember that our airway pressure measurements reflect the compliance of *both* the lung and chest wall. When we apply PEEP, our traditional goal is to recruit the lung to a new lung volume. We want to recruit, but not overdistend, the lung to limit lung injury. To limit lung overdistention at end-inspiration, we set a traditional upper limit for airway plateau pressures of 30 cm H_2O, based upon studies of the alveolus from animal models. So the ARDSNet ventilation model for ARDS targets a tidal volume of 6 ml/kg IBW and a plateau pressure (Pplat) of ≤ 30 cm H_2O.

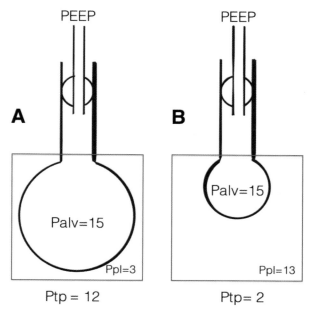

Figure 16-10 Illustration of the impact of low (A) and high (2) pleural pressures (Ppl) on transpulmonary pressure (Ptp) and alveolar volume changes with a constant PEEP level

We measure Pplat during an end-inspiratory hold maneuver, and this measurement provides an indicator of the end-inspiratory alveolar pressure (Palv). The Palv at end-inspiration should determine the end-inspiratory lung volume based upon the lung compliance. We assume the pleural pressure (Ppl) is a low and constant value, and Palv primarily determines the change in lung volume. We illustrate this condition in **Figure 16-10, A.** Likewise, we measure PEEP at end-expiration and assume this provides the primary indicator of end-expiratory lung volume.

Transpulmonary pressure is the difference between airway pressure (Pao) and pleural pressure (Ppl), both at the end of inspiration (transpulmonary plateau pressure) and expiration (transpulmonary PEEP).

In patients with high pleural pressure (e.g., obesity or abdominal distention), external PEEP may overestimate transpulmonary PEEP due to a high Ppl, leading to poor lung recruitment and underinflation with hypoxemia **(Figure 16-10, B).** In contrast, patients with low Ppl may be at risk for overdistention if PEEP leads to underestimated high transpulmonary pressures. Simply stated, for a given alveolar pressure, the lung recruitment decreases when Ppl increases and the chest wall becomes stiffer.

Ideally, transpulmonary pressure (Pplat- Ppl) would provide the optimal method to titrate PEEP to achieve optimal lung recruitment and avoid lung overinflation. The primary limitation to the widespread use of this technique is the measurement of Ppl. Esophageal pressure is traditionally used as a surrogate for pleural pressure, and this requires placement of an esophageal balloon catheter, correct placement, and correct interpretation of the pressure waveforms. Widely variable values for Ppl can be obtained, based upon variable positioning of the balloon catheter in the esophagus. The technical limitations are the main reason transpulmonary pressures are *NOT* frequently used clinically to titrate PEEP in ARDS.

A randomized trial compared PEEP settings based upon the ARDSNet PEEP/FiO$_2$ table vs. PEEP set by transpulmonary pressure measurements.[107] The use of transpulmonary pressure measurements to titrate PEEP demonstrated improved oxygenation and lung compliance. The investigation did not include enough patients to reach a definite conclusion regarding mortality. Despite the physiologic appeal of this technique, the measurement of esophageal pressures requires specialized expertise and is unlikely to be widely employed.

16.7.2.3 Stress Index

Airway pressure measurements, other than transpulmonary pressures, may be more readily available to clinicians. Both the lower inflection point of maximum curvature on the pressure-volume curve and the stress index have been studied in the ARDS population. The stress index has been advocated as a measurement to more optimally set PEEP and avoid potential hyperinflation in patients with a heterogeneous ARDS distribution. The stress index requires measurement of the airway pressure (Pao) during the inspiratory phase measured under conditions of constant flow (square wave) with volume-controlled ventilation. The stress index describes the slope of the Pao over the breath duration. A stress index > or < 1 suggests changing lung compliance during the inflation period.

The optimal pressure-time curve shows a linear pattern over the inspiratory cycle (see yellow line in **Figure 16-11**, top Pao graphic) during constant flow ventilation with no patient effort. If the curve shows an upward concavity over the inspiratory cycle, the stress index is > 1, suggesting a decrease in compliance over time (**Figure 16-11**, middle Pao graphic). If the curve shows a downward concavity, this represents a stress index < 1 and suggests a continuous increase in compliance during lung inflation **Figure 16-11,** bottom Pao graphic).

For PEEP titration, the stress index target is 0.9-1.1. If the stress index is greater than 1.1, the PEEP level is titrated down to avoid overdistention. If the stress index is < 0.9, the PEEP level is increased to promote recruitment.

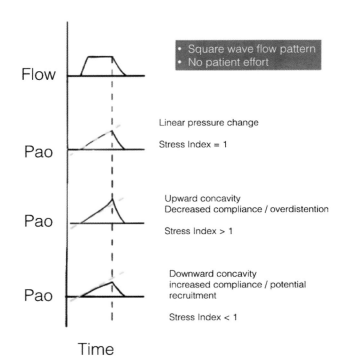

Figure 16-11 *Airway pressure (Pao)-time curves illustrating the patterns associated with the stress index.*

In contrast to the PEEP/FiO$_2$ titration tables mentioned above, titration of PEEP based on the stress index leads to a consistent reduction in the prescribed PEEP level.[108] Titration of PEEP to the stress index also has led to reductions in plasma inflammatory mediators, including interleukin-6, interleukin-8, and soluble tumor necrosis factor receptor, suggesting a reduction in overall lung injury.

The value of the stress index in critical patient outcome parameters, such as ventilator-free days or mortality, remains to be determined in larger populations. However, modern ventilators now incorporate the stress index as a measurement parameter to guide PEEP titration. Remember, the stress index requires constant flow ventilation with no patient effort!

16.7.2.4 Imaging Techniques

Radiographic studies using serial CT imaging have been used to look at the success of lung recruitment under conditions of increasing PEEP.[109] These studies have suggested that alveolar recruitment with PEEP is quite variable among patients with ARDS. A poor correlation between radiographic recruitment of lung parenchyma and changes in gas exchange indices (PaO$_2$/FiO$_2$ or PaCO$_2$) has been found. The use of quantitative CT in ARDS to measure recruitment, while appealing, has generally not been accepted as a clinical tool. This may be related to perceived disadvantages for patient care, including risk of patient transfer, radiation exposure, cost, and processing limitations.

16.7.2.5 Driving Pressure

Driving pressure (DP) is calculated as the difference between the airway inspiratory plateau pressure (Pplat) and the PEEP level. Driving pressure results from the relationship between tidal volume (Vt) and the compliance of the respiratory system (Crs) where DP = Vt/Crs. DP adjusts for the patient's real physiologic parameters and does not attempt to assume lung "size," which is inherent when Vt is based upon ideal body weight. Driving pressure is a dynamic indicator of lung physiology unlike the static parameters of Pplat, PEEP, or Vt. A retrospective analysis of patients receiving lung protective ventilation suggested that DP may be the strongest ventilator parameter predictive of mortality in ARDS patients.[110] The following limitations of DP in clinical management are multiple and require further exploration in clinical trials:

- DP is an accurate physiologic measure only in a patient without spontaneous respiratory effort. Patients with active inspiratory or expiratory muscle effort will alter the relationship between DP and lung distention.
- DP is determined by respiratory system compliance and therefore is influenced by the chest wall mechanics. Patients with identical DP, may have very different transulmonary pressures and therefore a different risk of VILI.
- A focus on manipulation of DP rather than Vt or PEEP has not been shown to be beneficial in prospective ARDS clinical trials.

At the current time, DP is an important physiologic parameter for monitoring the interaction of PEEP and Vt in the ARDS patient population, but specific guidelines for the bedside clinician to adjust this parameter are lacking.

16.7.2.6 PEEP Conclusion

To date, no specific technique has been widely adopted to select the optimal PEEP setting for the patient with ARDS. Ideally, PEEP should be selected to provide optimal lung recruitment (diseased regions) without overdistention (normal regions). PEEP should prevent injury to the lung resulting from recurrent cycles of alveoli opening and closing (atelectrauma).

Meta-analyses suggest higher PEEP strategies may be favorable for patients with more advanced disease. The use of PEEP tables to select higher PEEP strategies for patients with more advanced disease is an approach that is easily implemented in most ICUs and requires no specialized training. In comparison to other methods, PEEP tables provided better correlation to radiographically measured lung recruitability in a small patient sample with ARDS.[111]

16.7.3 Alveolar Recruitment Maneuvers

Briefly raising the transpulmonary pressures to higher levels than are associated with tidal ventilation is intended to promote alveolar recruitment. These brief changes in inflation pressures are termed *recruitment maneuvers*. Recruitment maneuvers are used to establish initial alveolar patency, which is then maintained at lower tidal pressures and PEEP levels than are needed to open the same collapsed units. Numerous methods for recruitment have been explored in the literature, including intermittent sighs, episodic increases in PEEP, and sustained application of pressure to achieve total lung capacity. Alternatively, alterations in the timing of breath delivery may be used to produce a more sustained inspiratory elevation in mean airway pressure (prolonged inspiratory time) or intrinsic PEEP (inverse inspiratory/expiratory ratio).

Two methods of alveolar recruitment have been commonly advocated. The first uses a sustained elevation in airway pressure using a continuous positive airway pressure of 35 to 40 cm H_2O for 40 seconds before reinstituting the previous level of PEEP. Alternatively, a high level of pressure-controlled ventilation (PEEP of 15–20 cm H_2O, driving pressure of 30 cm H_2O, plateau pressure of 50 cm H_2O) is provided for 1 to 2 minutes as tolerated. These pressures may be titrated upward for patients with a markedly reduced extrathoracic compliance. Patients who demonstrate an improvement in oxygenation during these maneuvers are labeled *PEEP responsive* and likely to benefit from upward titration of the PEEP settings. The benefit to gas exchange from recruitment maneuvers is that maneuvers are limited in duration and may depend on pre-existing PEEP levels. The routine application of recruitment maneuvers seems to offer little benefit over appropriate PEEP titration and remains controversial in the ARDS population.

These recruitment maneuvers can be highly effective for the patient on high levels of PEEP that has the ventilator accidentally or purposefully disconnected. The patient may "de-recruit" open alveoli and desaturate. Prior to putting the patient back on the high PEEP settings, a recruitment maneuver may be helpful to bring the oxygenation up to the prior baseline.

16.8 Fluid Management in ARDS—Wet or dry?

Often the first, and most difficult, step in managing the patient with ARDS is excluding cardiogenic pulmonary edema. The combination of clinical history and non-invasive assessment parameters (such as clinical examination, chest film radiography, brain natriuretic peptide levels (< 100 pg/ml), and bedside echocardiography) can be combined to give an accurate assessment. An accurate diagnosis of cardiac function is especially important because many of the conditions that precipitate ARDS, such as sepsis or trauma, require volume resuscitation. In the setting of ARDS, the potential adverse effect of volume resuscitation on oxygenation must be carefully considered in relation to the beneficial impact resuscitation may have on organ perfusion. Although intuitively it would seem that right heart catheterization might resolve much of the debate over cardiogenic vs. non-cardiogenic edema, the current data do not suggest this measurement tool offers any advantage over central venous catheter measurements.

A common clinical condition associated with ARDS is sepsis. From a cardiac standpoint, sepsis is characteristically associated with a rightward shift in the Starling curve (**Figure 16-12,** top). Under these conditions, volume loading is required to increase left ventricular end-diastolic volume (LVEDV) to maintain stroke volume (SV) (blue line). Patients may respond to volume resuscitation with improved cardiac output and tissue perfusion. However, increased LVEDV will lead to increased left ventricular end-diastolic pressure with an associated increase in pulmonary capillary hydrostatic pressure.

Under normal conditions, pulmonary capillary hydrostatic pressure (PCHP in **Figure 16-12,** bottom) must exceed a critical value before we see an increase in lung water due to capillary leak from elevated hydrostatic vascular pressures in the lung capillaries. However, ARDS is associated with a leftward shift in the relationship between PCHP and lung water because the capillaries are injured and leak at lower hydrostatic pressures.

So ARDS patients classically benefit from volume resuscitation for cardiac output and tissue perfusion but suffer adversely from volume resuscitation due to lung water and adverse effects on oxygenation. *What to do???* Further complicating fluid management is the association of ARDS and acute kidney injury. Do we want more or less fluid to maintain cardiac output to the kidneys? This brings the world-famous wet (*give me fluid*) vs. dry (*give me Lasix*) question to the bedside. Excessive fluid administration leads to worsening edema and a prolonged time on mechanical ventilation. Excessive diuretics could lead to intravascular volume contraction and impaired organ perfusion, especially the kidney.

Start wet and resuscitate. The early phase of patient management is focused on the treatment of the underlying disease process. The patient may require volume resuscitation to resolve hypotension or stabilize organ perfusion. But the clinician must carefully provide an ongoing assessment at the bedside to assure that volume resuscitation is beneficial. As described in *Chapter 4* on *Sepsis Resuscitation*, bolus fluid administration, monitoring mean arterial pressure, urine output, and gas exchange are essential. The bedside exam can be supplemented by a range of non-invasive tools to guide fluid resuscitation (See *Chapter 7 Hemodynamic Monitoring*).

Stabilize and then keep the deck of the ship dry. After the initial 48 hours, the patient often enters a more stable hemodynamic phase. The average patient with medical ARDS might gain 6-7 liters of fluid over the initial 7 days of patient management due to antibiotics, sedatives, and enteral feeding in addition to scheduled fluid administration. Is this harmful or beneficial?

The Fluids and Catheter Therapy Trial (FACTT) randomized ARDS patients to two fluid management strategies.[112] The basic principles of resuscitation were

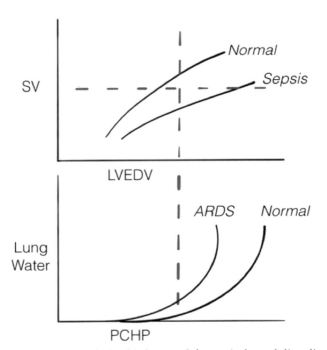

Figure 16-12 Relationship between left ventricular end-diastolic stroke volume (LVEDV) and stroke volume (SV) in top graphic. Relationship between pulmonary capillary hydrostatic pressure (PCHP) and lung water in bottom graphic. Fluid loading in the ARDS patient can elevate the LVEDV and PCHP.

maintained (i.e., vasopressors for resistant hypotension), but in the setting of hemodynamic stability, one patient group was randomized to a "dry" fluid status and the second to a "wet" fluid status. The FACTT clinical protocols created an ARDS "wet" group managed to ~ 7 liters positive over the first seven days post randomization, while the "dry" group was managed to an even fluid balance. The "dry" strategy did not produce a statistical impact on mortality but did achieve an improvement in ventilator-free days. Ventilator-free days is a measure of weaning time in patients with ARDS – a bigger number is better – meaning more time off mechanical ventilation.

The FACTT algorithm is based upon the assessment of four variables (mean arterial pressure, urine output, markers of perfusion [capillary refill or cardiac output], and central venous pressure or pulmonary capillary wedge pressure). The measurements occur every 4 hours and lead to a decision. The algorithms are complex and require an experienced bedside nurse to implement (http://www.ardsnet.org/files/factt_algorithm_v2.pdf). The complexity of the algorithms has limited their widespread application in clinical ICUs, but the outcome data strongly support maintaining a dry fluid balance in the setting of hemodynamic stability in ARDS patients.

You cannot diurese a hypotensive patient, but you can set a goal for a more optimal fluid balance of "even" for the initial week of ARDS management. To put this more directly, so long as 1) the blood pressure is good, 2) the patient has a good estimated cardiac output and systemic perfusion, and 3) urine output and kidney function are normal, you should try to dry the patient out and maintain a daily negative 0.5 to 1 L fluid balance. Try to get your patient's total fluid balance as even by the 6-7th ARDS day.

As in patients with sepsis and cardiac dysfunction, the $ScvO_2$ can provide an important global measurement of the relationship between tissue oxygen consumption and oxygen delivery. This variable can also be helpful to monitor in ARDS patients in order to further manage their hypoxemia. A reduced $ScvO_2$ contributes to the venous admixture, with hypoxic blood shunting through the injured lung, and can thus worsen arterial oxygenation. Attention to transfusion and inotropic therapy in the acute phase of ARDS management can be beneficial. Indiscriminate transfusion in the absence of impaired tissue oxygenation is not indicated. A transfusion threshold for stable ARDS patients without evidence of tissue anoxia would be 7.0 gms / dL. Inotropes are *NOT* beneficial in ARDS if cardiac function is normal.

The topic of fluid balance and hemodynamics cannot be considered without appreciating that the selection of mechanical ventilation variables in ALI-ARDS will impact cardiac function. Positive pressure ventilation is frequently associated with the development of hypotension and reduced cardiac output. The increase in mean intrathoracic pressure associated with mechanical ventilation can reduce the gradient for systemic venous return. Further elevations in mean intrathoracic pressure with extrinsic or intrinsic PEEP can additionally compromise venous return, and this effect is most evident in patients with intravascular volume contraction. PEEP-related increases in alveolar volume could increase pulmonary vascular resistance, leading to increased right ventricular afterload. Increased right ventricular afterload can shift the intraventricular septum, leading to impaired left ventricular filling. If not titrated carefully, beneficial outcomes of PEEP on oxygenation indices (PaO_2/FiO_2 ratios) can be significantly offset by marked reductions in cardiac output and tissue oxygenation.

Volume loading can overcome the adverse effects of positive pressure ventilation on venous return. But this fluid accumulates and can delay weaning from mechanical ventilation

16.9 Approach to Intractable Hypoxemia in ARDS

ARDS is the most common respiratory disease leading to intractable hypoxemia. As a result, a variety of alternative therapies and ventilation strategies have been employed in ARDS patients to address the management of severe hypoxemia. While these therapies may not apply to all causes of severe hypoxemic lung disease, they have been most extensively investigated in the ARDS patient population.

The patient with hypoxemia can be approached using the following treatment algorithm in order of increasing aggressiveness:

1. Increase FiO_2 concentration (Major way 1)
2. *Increase mean airway pressure* (Major way 2)
   a. Positive end-expiratory pressure
   b. Increase inspiratory time duration
3. *Pharmacologic paralysis*
4. *Prone ventilation*
5. *High-frequency oscillation*
6. *Extracorporeal circuits*
7. Correct SvO_2

16.9.1 Pharmacologic Paralysis

Pharmacologic paralysis has been extensively used in the management of severe hypoxemic respiratory failure for many years, primarily to improve the gas exchange defect. Muscle relaxation has two effects:

1. Reduced ventilator-breathing dysynchrony that may limit the efficiency of gas exchange
2. Reduced oxygen consumption, thus improving $ScvO_2$

The ARDS clinical trials studying PEEP application showed a range of patients on paralytics between 30-55% at enrollment. Pharmacologic paralysis is commonly used by clinicians to promote patient-ventilator synchrony, improve gas exchange, and reduce oxygen consumption. However, the potential adverse effects of paralytics, particularly on neuromuscular function, have raised concerns for clinicians regarding their more widespread application.

A single randomized trial had suggested a favorable risk:benefit ratio for routine paralytic use during the first 48 hours of care in ARDS patients with moderate to severe ARDS ($PaO_2/FiO_2 \geqslant 150$ with PEEP $\geqslant$ 5 cm H_2O).[113] However, a subsequent multi-center randomized trial was unable to confirm a mortality benefit to early routine use of paralytic agents in ARDS management. These patients were all treated with a high PEEP strategy and no significant difference in mortality was seen at 90 days between patients who received an early, continuous cisatracurium infusion and those who were treated with a usual-care approach with as needed use of paralytic agents.

The mechanism by which neuromuscular blocking agents might improve mortality in ARDS is not defined. These drugs might reduce metabolism (VCO_2 production) and therefore ventilatory demand. Alternatively, they may simply promote patient-ventilator synchrony. Patients on low tidal volume ventilation are recognized to have variable breathing patterns and a significant risk of breath stacking. Breath stacking can lead to larger tidal volumes that could be injurious to the patient (volutrauma) and would be eliminated by neuromuscular blockade. Finally, a non-identified effect, specific to the drug cisatracurium, might be at play, which would make the mortality benefit specific to a single paralytic agent. Additional research will be required to resolve these issues.

The combination of low tidal volume ventilation with paralysis can predispose your patient to hypercapnia. In the patient with ARDS, we accept this outcome and allow the hypercapnia. Acceptance of the hypercapnia while maintaining the low tidal volume ventilation strategy is called *permissive hypercapnia*. An abundance of data suggests permissive hypercapnia is not only safe but may be protective in patients with advanced respiratory failure. The primary contraindication to permissive hypercapnia would be neurologic conditions at risk for increased intracranial pressure.

There is some debate among clinical investigators whether the acidosis that accompanies permissive hypercapnia requires metabolic correction. The majority of clinical trials that have explored permissive hypercapnia have provided supplementation of sodium bicarbonate to maintain a pH > 7.15-7.20.

16.9.2 Prone Ventilation

With the ready availability of chest CT for evaluating ARDS, investigators have appreciated the heterogeneous distribution of the ARDS infiltrates, despite the homogeneous appearance by plain film radiography. As shown in **Figure 16-5**, the lungs tend to collapse in the gravitational-dependent (down) regions, or posteriorly when patients are lying supine on their backs. Prone ventilation refers to the delivery of mechanical ventilation in the prone position. Moving the patient from the supine to the prone position can immediately improve oxygenation.

The precise mechanism that allows prone ventilation to have a favorable effect in patients with severe ARDS is likely multifactorial but almost certainly relates to improved V/Q matching:

1. *Increases in ventilation (V).* Several mechanisms improve the ventilation of the collapsed areas of the lung by moving the heart off the collapsed left lower lobe, applying gravitational traction to the previously collapsed dorsal lung, and diverting positive pressure ventilation to the now previously collapsed dorsal lung.
2. *Improved blood flow (Q).* Improved blood flow to the lower gravitationally dependent lung zones which, after prone positioning, are the open (more "normal") ventilated alveoli

Some of the proposed effector mechanisms for Prone Ventilation are outlined in **Figure 16-13**.

Some clinical trials using prone position were conducted in ARDS patients between 2001 and 2011. Although investigators were consistently able to show an improvement in oxygenation in ~80% of patients using prone ventilation, no mortality effect was demonstrated. These studies were limited by a mix of ventilator management strategies, variable duration of the prone position, and patients with widely variable disease severity.

The PROSEVA trial examined prone ventilation for 16 hours in moderate to severe ARDS patient (PaO_2/FiO_2 ratio < 150 mm Hg on a PEEP $\geqslant$ 5 cm H_2O).[114] This

Description	Physiologic Effect
Change in distribution of ventral (back) compared to dorsal (chest) pleural pressure with more even distribution in prone position	Transpulmonary pressure is more evenly distributed, leading to more uniform ventilation of ventral and dorsal alveoli compared to supine position.
Change in lung and thorax configuration, making heart dependent and smaller volume of lung dependent	Improves ventilation distribution and increases the functional residual capacity (decreased shunt)
Reduced lung compression from the heart and diaphragm	Reduction in medial posterior lung compression and decreased compression of the posterior-caudal lung
Redistribution of blood flow	Blood flow redistributes to better-ventilated alveoli that are not collapsed, with improved cardiac output due to reduced hypoxic vasoconstriction.

Figure 16-13 Proposed mechanisms for prone ventilation to improve gas exchange.

investigation demonstrated a marked reduction in 28- and 90-day mortality in the prone ventilation group. The risk of adverse events was not statistically different in the two study populations. When all prior prone positioning trials are considered, three parameters may be important for the management of patients with prone ventilation to be effective:

1. The patients must be managed with a protective ventilation strategy (~ 6 ml/kg ideal body weight).
2. The prone cycle must be a minimum of 12-16 hours in duration.
3. The patient must have moderate to severe hypoxemia (PaO_2/FiO_2 ratio $\leqslant$ 150 mm Hg).

Under these restrictions, meta-analysis has suggested a consistent beneficial effect of prone positioning in the ARDS patient population.[115]

How do you accomplish prone ventilation? Gather up your ICU team, including nurses, your respiratory therapist, and a few generally strong people hanging out in the ICU. *Plan this out!* You need to pay attention to your lines and tubes as you plan the turning process and how they will be situated after you finish. Protect areas of your patient that will be pressure points. You will need to support the head and endotracheal tube. A number of helpful videos are available to train your team (https://www.youtube.com/watch?v=E_6jT9R7WJs).

Contraindications to the prone position based upon the Guerin protocol are outlined in **Figure 16-14**.

16.9.3 Inhaled Vasodilators

An additional option for the patient with severe hypoxemia is the use of inhaled vasodilators (IVD) to produce selective pulmonary vasodilation. The appeal of inhaled selective vasodilators is their distribution to well-ventilated lung regions, leading to reduction of vascular resistance in these regions and improved blood flow to these well-ventilated areas. The overall result is

an improvement in ventilation-perfusion matching in the lung. As illustrated in **Figure 16-15, alveolus A,** in a heterogeneous lung, the inhaled vasodilator (green triangles) is preferentially distributed to the well-ventilated alveolus A.

The local effect on the pulmonary vasculature promotes redistribution of flow to alveolus A. Note: This effect would *NOT* be characteristic of systemically administered vasodilators, which are delivered to all lung blood vessels and vasodilate all areas, even those with poor ventilation. For this reason, in contrast to inhaled vasodilators, systemically administered vasodilators can worsen hypoxemia in patients with advanced pulmonary disease or ARDS. The adverse effect of systemic vasodilators on gas exchange has been attributed to the reversal of hypoxic vasoconstriction in poorly ventilated lung regions **(Figure 16-15, alveolus B)**, thus worsening V/Q matching.

Selective pulmonary vasodilators are characterized by a short half-life, which minimizes any systemic effect. The two most common inhaled selective pulmonary vasodilators used in the ARDS patient population have been inhaled nitric oxide (iNO) and inhaled prostacyclin (epoprostenol).

iNO and epoprostenol appear to have similar effects on pulmonary vascular resistance, cardiac output, and

If nitric oxide is a highly diffusible gas molecule, why does it only act on the pulmonary vessels (a selective pulmonary vasodilator). Why is nitric oxide not carried in the blood to vasodilate the systemic circulation? The answer is that any NO that diffuses into the blood reacts with hemoglobin and is inactivated. This reaction with hemoglobin is so fast that the half-life of NO in whole blood is less than 2 milliseconds!

Contraindications to Prone Ventilation
• Increased intracranial pressure > 30 mm Hg or cerebral perfusion pressure < 60 mm Hg
• Massive hemoptysis with the need for immediate surgical or interventional radiology procedure
• Tracheal surgery or sternotomy during the previous 15 days
• Serious facial trauma or facial surgery during the previous 15 days
• Deep venous thrombosis treated for less than 2 days
• Cardiac pacemaker inserted in the last 2 days
• Unstable spine, femur, or pelvic fractures
• Mean arterial pressure lower than 65 mm Hg
• Pregnancy
• Single anterior chest tube with air leaks
• Burns on more than 20 % of the body surface

Figure 16-14 Contraindications to prone ventilation.

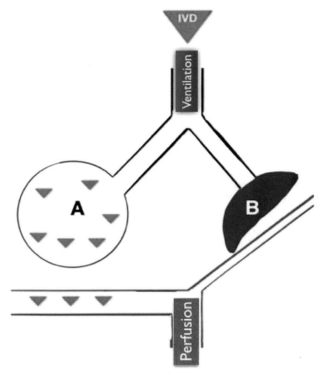

Figure 16-15 Inhaled vasodilator (IVD) preferentially distributes to well-ventilated alveolus (A) causing local vasodilation and improved V/Q match.

right ventricular function. iNO was the initial pulmonary selective vasodilator explored in human ARDS studies. NO is a highly diffusible gas molecule that binds to its receptor, soluble guanylate cyclase, in the pulmonary arteriolar smooth muscle. Activation of soluble guanylate cyclase coverts GTP to cGMP, which is a downstream signaling molecule that relaxes the smooth muscle to produce selective pulmonary vasodilation. Clinical trials of iNO in ARDS patients have characteristically shown improvements in gas exchange for up to three days. The iNO is typically delivered at a starting concentration of 40 parts per million, while monitoring nitrogen dioxide (formed when NO reacts with oxygen) concentrations to limit exposure to this toxic gas. The concentration can be reduced to as low as 5 parts per million and still exert efficacy. While oxygenation improves on iNO, no trial has demonstrated an improvement in patient mortality, and some analysts have suggested a potential adverse effect on renal function. The lack of efficacy on patient mortality, high cost, unique delivery system, and potential toxicity has led clinicians to look for other options.

Epoprostenol, while having similar physiologic effects to iNO, has very few comparative clinical trials to assess outcome other than improvements in the PaO_2/FiO_2 ratio. The medication is delivered over a dose range of 10-40 ng/kg/min. The dosing is based upon ideal body weight. The drug requires a specific diluent (glycine buffer) and is both photosensitive and stable for only about 8 hours at room temperature. A specific nebulizer protocol is required, and the expiratory filter of the ventilator must be monitored for partial occlusion and changed daily. The nebulizer is placed on the wet side of the ventilator humidifier. Other nebulized medications are discontinued, and heat and moisture exchangers are removed from the ventilator circuit.

Selective pulmonary vasodilators are used for salvage therapy in patients with intractable hypoxemia and/or pulmonary hypertension. The lack of benefit on patient mortality and ventilator weaning has limited their use appropriately to patients with intractable hypoxemia.

We tend to use these medications most commonly in the patient with both severe ARDS (PaO_2/FiO_2 ratio > 150 mm Hg) *AND* with pulmonary arterial hypertension (which can develop in some patients with ARDS), where one would expect to improve both V/Q matching and right heart cardiac output.

16.9.4 High-frequency Oscillation

High-frequency ventilation is a unique form of ventilation that uses respiratory rates > 150 breaths per minute. There are many types of high-frequency ventilation, but the two most studied have been high-frequency jet ventilation (HFJV) and high-frequency oscillatory ventilation (HFOV).

In adult critical care, high-frequency ventilation is most commonly used when conventional ventilation has failed, for the treatment of bronchopleural fistulas or for management of difficult airways.

The general principle of high-frequency oscillatory ventilation (HFOV) is to achieve ventilation using very small tidal volumes (generally smaller than physiologic dead space) at a baseline high mean airway pressure (**Figure 16-16,** top graphic). Respiratory rates (f) are in the range of 1-50 Hz, with 1 Hz equal to one cycle per second, or 60 breaths per minute. The small tidal breaths "oscillate" around a high mean airway pressure.

The baseline mean airway pressure is set as the CPAP or PEEP level, and then the breaths oscillate around the MAP (**Figure 16-16**, bottom graphic).

The goal is to minimize volutrauma from the overdistention of alveoli associated with traditional larger tidal volumes and to minimize alveolar collapse due to reduced mean airway pressures. Theoretically, this mode of ventilation should provide the optimal "open-lung" approach. The adverse hemodynamic effects on the cardiovascular system should also be minimized in this mode.

Clinical trials have suggested that HFOV is frequently associated with improved parameters of oxygenation in the ALI/ARDS population, but have not shown a reduction in mortality in comparison to more standard lung protective ventilation. The technique for HFOV is not familiar to many clinicians and should remain a rescue therapy for consideration after other options have proven ineffective.

16.9.5 APRV and BiLevel Ventilation

Novel pressure-oriented modes of ventilation have been explored for the patient with advanced ARDS and hypoxemia. If you understand the basic concepts from our discussion in *Chapter 15, Mechanical Ventilation,* you will recognize that all these "fancy" modes are just

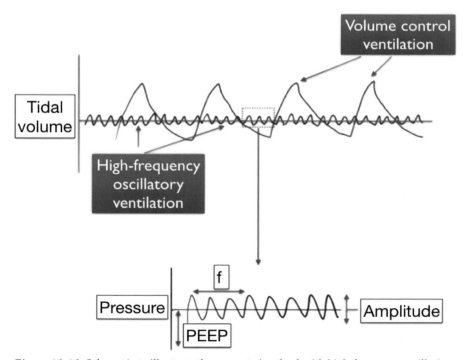

Figure 16-16 Schematic to illustrate the concepts involved with high-frequency oscillation.

modifications of the original principles we outlined. We will use variations of the pressure control breath to achieve high mean airway pressures.

Airway pressure release ventilation (APRV) is a form of pressure-controlled breaths operating in the intermittent mandatory ventilation mode. Mandatory breaths are machine triggered, pressure targeted, and time cycled. With APRV the inspiratory time is very long, with only brief exhalation.

These specialized pressure-oriented modes involve cycling between a high pressure (P_H) and a low airway pressure (P_L). In addition, the duration of each cycle is set, giving a high and low pressure time duration (T_H and T_L). The duration of T_L is often called the *release time*. **Figure 16-17,** top diagram, illustrates the pressure cycling curves for a patient without spontaneous breaths. Note that the high-pressure cycles are longer than the low-pressure cycles ($T_H > T_L$). The mean airway pressure is determined by the combination of the P_H and T_H and the P_L and T_L variables. The transition from P_H to P_L deflates the lungs and allows CO_2 elimination.

The unique feature of APRV is that throughout these pressure cycles, the patient is also allowed spontaneous ventilation. **Figure 16-17,** bottom graphic, illustrates the pressure cycles with superimposed spontaneous breathing. On some ventilators, an additional setting for pressure support is available for these spontaneous breaths. Note that the majority of spontaneous breaths will occur during the P_H cycles as more time is spent in this phase.

What distinguishes APRV from pressure control inverse ratio ventilation is that the patient is allowed spontaneous breaths during the high and low pressure cycles (similar to breathing during a very high pressure CPAP setting).

The outcome of APRV mode is to achieve high mean airway pressures with smaller tidal volumes in patients with low lung compliance and poor oxygenation. Often the patients also are managed with permissive hypercapnia.

Confusion occurs because the ventilator manufacturers have used a variety of terms for similar methods of breath delivery that employ two levels of positive airway pressure, including APRV, BiLevel, and BiVent. APRV characteristically uses extreme inverse ratios of ventilation, whereas other forms of BiLevel pressure ventilation do not.

The literature does not clearly outline protocols for the APRV form of mechanical ventilation. *This is not a mode for the novice at mechanical ventilation* because the patient can incur significant risk if the ventilator is managed improperly. **Figure 16-18** compares the main parameters for three different pressure-targeted modes of ventilation: conventional pressure control breaths, inverse ratio pressure control breaths, and APRV ventilation.

The theoretical advantages to APRV include the following:

- Ease of manipulating airway pressures and inspiratory:expiratory ratios to accomplish higher mean airway pressures
- Provides a form of lung-protective ventilation, which controls the high airway pressures to a maximum target
- May improve overall gas exchange with better lung recruitment with the superimposed spontaneous breaths

The patient may feel uncomfortable with this mode of ventilation and require heavy sedation and paralysis.

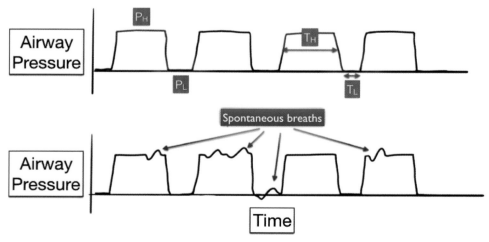

Figure 16-17 *Airway pressure – time tracing of airway pressure release ventilation (APRV).*

Parameter	Pressure Control Breaths	Inverse Ratio Ventilation	APRV
I:E ratio	1:4 to 1:1	> 1:1	> 2:1
Mean Airway Pressure	Less	Increased	Increased
Spontaneous Breaths	No	No	Yes
Auto-PEEP	Less common	Common	Common
Sedation/Paralytics	Maybe	Required	Uncommon

Figure 16-18 A comparison of three pressure-targeted modes of ventilation.

This removes the spontaneous ventilation component and transitions the mode to a form of pressure control inverse ratio ventilation.

Small studies have suggested a possible advantage in oxygenation parameters in patients using these alternative pressure-regulated modes of ventilation. However, no single trial has shown a benefit to patient mortality. Just remember, > 3000 patients have been studied on the ARDSNet protective ventilation strategy, which uses only volume-assist control ventilation. These patients have been managed with the lowest reported mortality rates for the ARDS patient population. These specialized forms of pressure control ventilation must be considered a rescue strategy for patients with advanced hypoxemia.

16.9.6 Extracorporeal Support

Extracorporeal membrane oxygenation (ECMO) circuits have logical appeal for the management of ARDS patients with severe hypoxemia. An ECMO circuit consists of the access cannula, heparin-coated tubing, an oxygenator, a pump, and a heat exchanger. The ECMO circuit oxygenator must accept a high volume of blood flow, similar to the patient's cardiac output, to adequately oxygenate the blood. Within the oxygenator, hemoglobin is fully saturated with oxygen, and carbon dioxide is removed. The heat exchanger limits excessive cooling of the blood outside the body. The type of ECMO is based upon the location of the access cannula.

For respiratory support, a conventional access method is a catheter placed into the inferior vena cava via the femoral vein and a catheter placed through the internal jugular into the superior vena cava. This arrangement is called *veno-venous ECMO (VV-ECMO)* and is the most common type of ECMO used for support of the respiratory system. Exchange of the femoral catheter for an arterial access (femoral artery) is *veno-arterial ECMO (VA-ECMO)*, which is most commonly used for both respiratory and cardiovascular support. Newer ECMO systems can use a single cannula placed through the internal jugular vein into the intrahepatic portion of the inferior vena cava. These single cannula systems offer the significant advantage of mobility for patients on ECMO. The management of patients on ECMO requires specialized training, so we will limit our discussion to general concepts.

The primary limitation to widespread acceptance of ECMO for support of the ARDS population is the complication rate, with bleeding complications being most common. Activation of clotting factors within the bypass circuit can lead to a consumptive coagulopathy and thrombocytopenia. This process can be limited by the administration of heparin and the use of biocompatible materials; however, this modification does not eliminate the risk of bleeding complications. Platelet transfusions may be required to maintain the platelet count > 50,000 per microliter. Additional circuit complications include air embolization, intravascular hemolysis, and nosocomial infection.

Because of the significant risk profile, ECMO is a salvage regimen for patients with advanced hypoxemic respiratory failure resistant to all other strategies to improve oxygenation. **Figure 16-19** summarizes the indications and contraindications for ECMO (https://www.elso.org/default.aspx).

Indications for ECMO	Contraindications for ECMO
✓ Refractory hypoxemia ($PaO_2/FiO_2 < 70$ mmHg) or hypercarbia (pH < 7.20) in acute/reversible pulmonary conditions	✓ Advanced age (> 65 yo) / premorbid clinical status
✓ Failure of alternative rescue strategies like paralysis, inhaled vasodilators, and prone positioning	✓ Contraindication to anticoagulation
✓ Refractory cardiovascular shock	✓ Non-recoverable neurologic injury
✓ Massive pulmonary embolism	✓ > 7- 10 days on mechanical ventilation
✓ Cardiac arrest	✓ Advanced malignancy
✓ As a bridge to lung or cardiac transplantation or device	

Figure 16-19 ECMO indications and contraindications.

While on the ECMO circuit, the lungs are rested, with the ventilator settings adjusted to minimize oxygen toxicity ($FiO_2 < 0.50$), barotrauma (plateau pressures < 30 cm H_2O), and volutrauma with a low minute ventilation (tidal volume 200-400 ml and a respiratory rate of 4-6). The PEEP level is set at 10-15 cm H_2O to maintain recruitment.

Early studies of ECMO therapy in ARDS were unable to achieve a favorable outcome. However, advances in circuit design and careful patient selection have suggested improvements in patient outcome. During the H1N1 influenza outbreak, a number of centers reported very favorable outcomes in patients with severe hypoxemic respiratory failure in comparison to historical controls.[116]

16.9.7 Hypoxemia Overview

For the patient with ARDS, the management of severe hypoxemia is often the most significant clinical challenge for the intensivist. A large number of clinical trials have been conducted in the population to provide guidance on how to organize the approach to intractable hypoxemia, as illustrated in **Figure 16-20**. The graphic is based upon entry criteria for the successful clinical trials in ARDS and forms the building blocks for ARDS gas exchange management.

Think of the management as a series of steps that increase based on ARDS severity. The foundation of all management is lung protective ventilation with a target tidal volume of ~ 6ml / kg IBW. This principle extends across the full spectrum of ARDS management. Patients with mild ARDS may be managed successfully with non-invasive mechanical ventilation, although clear outcome data for this mild ARDS group are lacking. Both low PEEP and high PEEP strategies outlined in clinical trials appear to be equivalent when all ARDS patients are considered. However, subgroup analysis suggests a higher PEEP strategy may be advantageous in the more severe population ($PaO_2/FiO_2 \leq 200$). As the severity advances, our most recent trials indicate favorable outcomes for patients using prone ventilation in advanced disease ($PaO_2/ FiO_2 \leq 150$ with $FiO_2 > 0.60$ and PEEP ≥ 5 cm H_2O). Neuromuscular paralysis can also be considered in advanced ARDS with intractable hypoxemia and/ or ventilator dyssynchrony. Patients who fail these regimens may be candidates for inhaled selective pulmonary vasodilator therapy. Since this form of treatment remains unproven, it must be considered a salvage regimen at this time. Finally, patients with very severe hypoxemia ($PaO_2 /FiO_2 < 70$ mmHg) who fail our initial step therapies, with a reversible disease process, may be candidates for consideration of ECMO.

The principles outlined for the management of severe hypoxemia in ARDS may also apply to other disease populations with severe hypoxemic respiratory failure. However, the clinical guidelines have been most extensively studied in the ARDS population.

16.10 The Little Things

Successful mechanical ventilation in the ARDS patient frequently requires sedative administration due to the combination of increased patient ventilatory drive and the clinician's desire to restrict tidal breath size. Effective sedation can decrease the work output for ventilation and reduce total body metabolism.

Ventilation can be completely synchronized with the mechanical ventilator by the use of paralytic agents. These agents should never be administered without an accompanying sedative to the point of full anesthesia. *The patient may look asleep but is just paralyzed with these medications.* If paralytic medications are needed, remember to adjust the set ventilator rate to match the total ventilator rate, because the patient will lose all spontaneous breaths.

Early bronchoscopy, if gas exchange parameters allow, is helpful to exclude ARDS "look-alikes" in patients without a clear precipitating factor for the development of ARDS. These would include opportunistic pneumonia (pneumocystis pneumonia for example), idiopathic eosinophilic pneumonia (elevated BAL eosinophils),

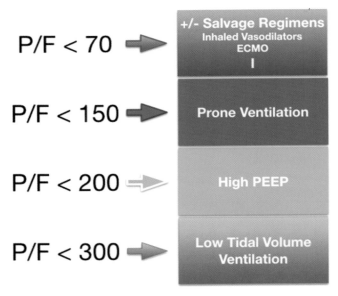

Figure 16-20 Management strategy for severe hypoxemia based upon severity.

diffuse alveolar hemorrhage (hemosiderin-laden macrophages), and disseminated cancer (positive cytology).

During the acute phase management of ARDS, the clinician must always be aware of the risk for complicating barotrauma in the ARDS patient. Barotrauma is estimated to occur in roughly 10-15% of ARDS patients and can include the clinical manifestations of pneumothorax, pneumomediastinum, subcutaneous emphysema, and pneumoperitoneum. The best predictor of risk for the development of barotrauma may be higher levels of PEEP.

Patients with ARDS spend longer intervals in the ICU. Attention to prophylaxis for complications associated with a more prolonged ICU stay—such as deep vein thrombosis (heparin prophylaxis) and stress gastritis (H2 receptor antagonist)—is essential. Catheters will be needed for fluid management and monitoring. Attention to infection prevention of these catheters both during the insertion process and with daily care is critical to minimizing infection risk.

As ARDS is often considered a disorder of an unregulated inflammatory response, the appeal of corticosteroids as a therapeutic agent is always present. To date, a mortality benefit for corticosteroid therapy in early or late ARDS has not been demonstrated.

16.11 Prognosis

On day 1 in the ICU, the spouse of your patient with severe community-acquired pneumonia and ARDS asks you whether the patient is going to live. What to say? You can provide some general guidelines based upon many years of published outcome studies in the population.

The initial days of ARDS management are focused on managing severe hypoxemia and FiO_2/PEEP levels, although these may not be the most important determinants of outcome. Lung-specific injury scores have shown poor prediction for outcome, while more global scores of overall organ function, including the *Acute Physiology and Chronic Health Evaluation (APACHE) score*, are more reflective.[117] The overall mortality rate from ARDS has decreased dramatically over the past 20 years. **Figure 16-21** illustrates the mortality rates from the control populations of large clinical trials in ARDS over approximately 25 years. Because this data reports the control group, which received no experimental therapy, the mortality rate reflects the "usual care" mortality during that era. The year each trial was reported is included adjacent to the trial. Note the marked decline in mortality rate from the late 1980s to the current period, with declines from almost 60% mortality to close to 20%!!! This change has occurred

ARDS Mortality

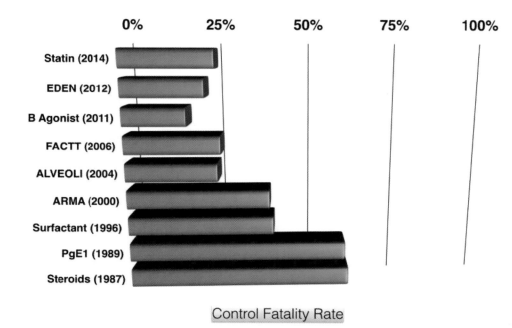

Figure 16-21 ARDS mortality from control populations in clinical trials from 1987 to 2014

despite the lack of new specific drug therapy to treat the disorder. Much of this change has been attributed to our improvements in patient support, particularly the use of lung protective ventilation. Other factors contribute, such as improved resuscitation, early antibiotics, and coordinated highly trained multidisciplinary care. Similar improvements in outcomes have occurred for patients with septic shock in ICUs. Patients with limited additional organ dysfunction with proper management can be expected to have a mortality rate < 25% in the current era. ARDS is a prolonged illness, with more severe cases typically spending ~ 2 weeks in the ICU and ~ 3 months in recovery. Obviously, these numbers will vary from patient to patient, but this data helps the clinician to give the family some perspective regarding the duration of the illness on admission. For many days, the patient will look unchanged to family members, with ventilator support, sedation, and paralysis. Help your patient's family to appreciate the small changes in hemodynamics and gas exchange parameters during these early days that reflect clinical improvement. These changes can help control surrogate anxiety during the early days of ARDS management.

Do patients with ARDS die of hypoxemia? Despite the fact that we work so hard keeping the oxygen up with all our therapies, most patients with ARDS die of multiorgan failure. Being critically ill on the ventilator for weeks wears down the body, and patients often suffer from second hits, like ventilator-associated pneumonia, line infections, acute kidney injury from dye or drugs or shock, and many other causes.

With a greater population of the ARDS patient population surviving, what can we expect in terms of longer term outcomes? The majority of patients appear to recover their lung function by the 3-6-month time frame post ARDS. However, a significant fraction of patients show evidence for persistent functional disability at one year and five years post follow-up.[118] Important psychiatric disorders, including post-traumatic stress disorder (PTSD), have been recognized, but current studies suffer from methodological limitations to determine the true incidence. The "late" physical and psychological limitations of ARDS survivors have contributed to a renewed focus on the possible role that ICU sedation practice and mobility management contributes to this delayed outcome in the population. Ongoing studies in these areas hope to evolve a best practice management for the future of ARDS patients. We discuss how to improve outcomes with rapid weaning and rehabilitation *(Wake up, breathe!* protocols) in the next few chapters.

A summary for ARDS management is outlined in **Figure 16-22.**

Suggested Reading

- Donahoe M. Acute respiratory distress syndrome: A clinical review. Pulmonary Circulation 2011;1(2):192–211.
- Fan E, Del Sorbo L, Goligher EC, et al. An Official American Thoracic Society/European Society of Intensive Care Medicine/Society of Critical Care Medicine Clinical Practice Guideline: Mechanical ventilation in adult patients with Acute Respiratory Distress Syndrome. Am J Respir Crit Care Med. 2017;195(9):1253–63.
- Scholten EL, Beitler JR, Prisk GK, Malhotra A. Treatment of ARDS with prone positioning. Chest 2017;151(1):215–24.
- Hess DR. Recruitment maneuvers and PEEP titration. Respiratory Care. 2015;60:1688-1704
- Walkey AJ, Goligher EC, Del Sorbo L, et al. Low tidal volume versus non-volume-limited strategies for patients with acute respiratory distress syndrome. A systematic review and meta-Analysis. Ann Am Thorac Soc 2017;14(Supplement_4):S271–9.

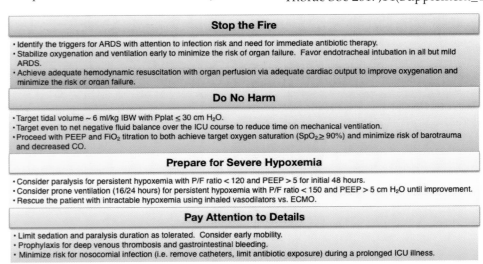

Figure 16-22 Summary of key concepts for management of the ARDS patient.

17

Obstructive Lung Disease (OLD) and Respiratory Failure

The management of patients with *obstructive lung disease (OLD)* is a frequent challenge for the critical care practitioner. While we will focus our discussion on the COPD patient, note that many of the acute management issues are similar for the patient with severe asthma, advanced bronchiectasis (cystic fibrosis), and bronchiolitis. Important clinical variations will exist in these diagnostic groups, but common management strategies exist in the hospital setting. Asthma patients, for example, rarely have pulmonary hypertension and may be younger, with fewer co-morbidities. But the lung mechanics, presence of dynamic hyperinflation / intrinsic-PEEP, drug therapy, and approach to mechanical ventilation are very similar in these populations.

For COPD patients, we must remember that some disease "exacerbations" will be precipitated by ischemic heart disease, pneumonia, or pulmonary thromboembolic disease. A high clinical suspicion must be maintained for complicating factors.

Patients with severe obstructive lung disease may require mechanical ventilation for a broad range of indications:

- Following cardiac or general surgery
- In connection with thoracic surgery such as lobectomy, wedge resection, lung reduction or bullectomy

- During an episode of acute respiratory failure secondary to a disease other than obstructive lung disease, such as sepsis, drug overdose, or trauma
- For acute-on-chronic respiratory failure (the classic "COPD exacerbation") where acute illness, usually presumed to be infectious in nature, destabilizes the characteristically compensated state

While this chapter will focus on mechanical ventilation of the patient with OLD, it should be stressed that the primary goal is to *avoid intubation whenever possible*. There are two principal reasons for this:

1. In most exacerbations of OLD, intubation is unnecessary if appropriate management is undertaken early.
2. Intubation is fraught with iatrogenic, infectious, and ventilator-associated complications. It is clear the intubated COPD patient has a high mortality rate, which probably reflects not only the severity of illness leading to intubation but also the complications inherent in the intubated and mechanically ventilated state. Consequently, there is a growing body of literature that supports the use of non-invasive positive pressure ventilation, in place of intubation, in COPD patients with acute ventilatory failure.

For these reasons, the initial management of this population favors the use of non-invasive positive pressure ventilation for patients with respiratory failure.[119] For patients intolerant or unsuccessful with this form of therapy, invasive mechanical ventilation is necessary.

17.1 Pathophysiology of Airflow Obstruction

Respiratory failure in the OLD patient is specifically defined by the presence of hypoxemia and often hypercapnia. However, respiratory failure is most frequently identified clinically by a marked increase in the work of breathing.

Hypoxemia in OLD results from a mismatch of alveolar unit ventilation (V) and perfusion (Q). Both high and low V/Q units are recognized in OLD patients. The severity of gas exchange derangement in any patient is defined by multiple variables, including the level of total alveolar ventilation, total pulmonary vascular perfusion, and the match of these variables within individual alveolar units. Shunt physiology plays an insignificant role in this population. While patients will often require supplemental oxygen, they will rarely require advanced methodologies for hypoxemia (i.e., PEEP or prone ventilation). If your OLD patient is markedly hypoxemic, you should be looking for complicating factors such as pneumonia or atelectasis.

Let's examine how these gas exchange parameters might interact to increase the demand (minute ventilation) on the respiratory system in the patient with OLD. Returning to *Chapter 13 Acute Respiratory Failure*, we remember the metabolic parameters that interact to determine the blood $PaCO_2$.

$$PaCO_2 = K \times \frac{VCO_2}{V_E(1 - Vd/Vt)}$$

The blood $PaCO_2$ is determined by the relationship between CO_2 production (VCO_2) and CO_2 clearance (alveolar ventilation [V_A]). In respiratory medicine, we measure the minute ventilation based upon the expired gas volume (V_E). We frequently use the ratio of dead space to tidal volume (Vd/Vt) as a marker of the efficiency of ventilation. As the Vd/Vt increases, the effective alveolar ventilation (V_A) declines. Conversely, as the ratio declines, the effective alveolar ventilation increases. Unlike V_A, we can directly measure V_E and the Vd/Vt. This equation shows us important relationships that are especially relevant in the OLD patient population. Any variable that raises carbon dioxide production (VCO_2) will require an increase in V_E to maintain a constant $PaCO_2$. Any variable that raises the Vd/Vt will again require an increase in V_E to maintain a constant $PaCO_2$. Any desire to lower the $PaCO_2$ must also be associated with an increase in minute ventilation.

Now think about these relationships in your OLD patient with a disease exacerbation. As illustrated in **Figure 17-1**, the combination of hypoxemia, dyspnea, altered V/Q relationships, and fever can all combine to increase the ventilation demand on the respiratory system. *What's the big deal – just raise your minute ventilation, and everyone stays happy?*

Increasing your minute ventilation to meet metabolic demand solves the issue in healthy lungs. After all, this is what happens when you exercise. But (hopefully) you

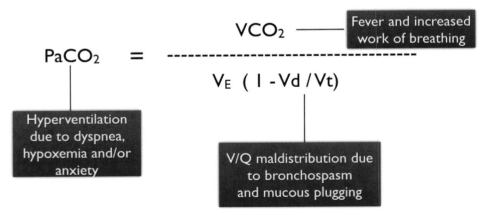

Figure 17-1 *Relationship between arterial blood carbon dioxide ($PaCO_2$), CO_2 production (VCO_2), minute ventilation (V_E), and deadspace ventilation (Vd/Vt).*

have healthy lungs, so you can increase your minute ventilation to very high levels with limited metabolic cost. Not so for the OLD patient. In OLD patients, small changes in minute ventilation come at a very high metabolic cost due to an increased work of breathing. A lot of seemingly minor variables, such as controlling fever, managing anxiety, resolving airway secretions and bronchospasm, can all add up to a significant impact when weaning OLD patients from mechanical ventilation. To understand the source for this high metabolic cost of breathing in the OLD patient, we need to shift our focus to the abnormal mechanics of chest inflation/deflation in these patients.

Expiratory airflow obstruction is the cardinal feature of OLD exacerbations. The morphologic basis of reduced expiratory airflow involves obstructive changes in the peripheral conducting airways (e.g., bronchitis and/or mucous hypersecretion), leading to expiratory airflow resistance. In certain conditions, such as emphysema, destructive changes in the terminal respiratory bronchioles lead to reduced lung elastic recoil. This combination of airflow obstruction and reduced elastic recoil leads to a *marked prolongation of the expiratory time constant.*

The OLD patient's ability to increase the rate of expiratory airflow is limited. Any attempt to voluntarily increase expiratory effort leads to more positive pleural pressure during expiration and serves only to promote further airway collapse. Despite the inefficiency of this expiratory effort, your patient will keep trying! You will notice your OLD patient often contracts the abdominal muscles to "force" expiration during a disease exacerbation. Ineffective, but a frequent sign of advanced airflow obstruction. Dynamic airway collapse in the OLD patient promotes air trapping in the lung at end-expiration, often called *dynamic hyperinflation.*

Figure 17-2 illustrates the timing components of a single tidal breath with tidal volume (Vt) on the Y-axis and time on the X-axis. The respiratory rate determines the total time between breaths (T_{TOT}). We divide T_{TOT} into inspiratory (T_i) and expiratory (T_e) time components. If the respiratory rate increases (blue compared to red figure), then T_{TOT} is shorter. Either T_i, T_e or some combination must also shorten to allow full expiration before the next breath occurs. T_e is a passive event determined by the elastic recoil pressure of the lung and chest wall and airway resistance. In the patient with OLD, expiratory time is prolonged. Any increase in respiratory frequency (to meet a metabolic demand) shortens the total breath duration, while expiratory time remains persistently prolonged.

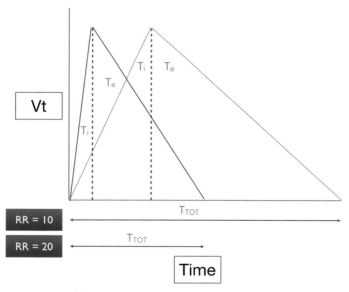

Figure 17-2 Tidal volume – time graph showing relationships between inspiratory time (Ti), expiratory time (Te), and total breath time (TTOT) at two different respiratory rates (RR).

With tachypnea, inspiratory time must shorten in the OLD patient to avoid hyperinflation. To shorten T_i either the ventilator or the patient's respiratory muscles must generate a faster inspiratory flow rate. If you follow the concept, you realize that OLD is an expiratory obstructive lung disease that places a significant burden on the inspiratory muscles to accelerate inspiratory flow, maintain a short inspiratory time, and avoid hyperinflation.

As an alternative to shortening the inspiratory time, OLD patients can just accept hyperinflation. Breathing at a lung volume closer to total lung capacity allows expiratory airflow to increase, as elastic recoil pressures increase and airway resistance decreases at the higher lung volume. The hyperinflated patient can reach a new equilibrium that allows both inspiration and expiration to occur within the allotted T_{TOT}. But hyperinflation comes as a price, whether the patient is breathing spontaneously or is on the ventilator.

The elastic work of tidal ventilation increases at the higher lung volumes, so taking the same size tidal breath at a higher resting lung volume is a greater burden on the inspiratory muscles. Again, expiratory airflow limitation places a work burden on the inspiratory muscles. Further, hyperinflation in the setting of dynamic airway collapse increases the end-expiratory elastic recoil pressure of the respiratory system. This positive end-expiratory pressure has been variously termed *auto* or *intrinsic PEEP (PEEPi)*.

Intrinsic PEEP, in effect, places an additional "threshold" load on the process of inspiration, which contributes to a high respiratory muscle workload, respiratory distress, and at times a failure to cycle mechanical ventilation. The residual positive alveolar pressure at end-expiration must be overcome, either by the respiratory muscles (spontaneous ventilation) or ventilator for inspiratory airflow to begin.

To summarize, the mechanics of OLD are primarily related to expiratory airflow obstruction. The prolonged expiratory phase complicates spontaneous breaths or mechanical ventilation, especially in a setting that increases the respiratory frequency. Compensation by either increasing the inspiratory flow rates to shorten inspiratory time or hyperinflation to allow an increased expiratory flow rate both come at a significant metabolic cost.

We can summarize the relationship between minute ventilation (V_E) and the metabolic work associated with breathing in **Figure 17-3**. The metabolic work for breathing alone is represented by the oxygen consumption of the respiratory muscles (VO_{2resp}). For the healthy individual, the metabolic cost associated with increasing minute ventilation is minimal and only grows significantly at very high levels of minute ventilation ($\sim 60\text{-}80\ L/min$). For the OLD patient, limited changes in minute ventilation create a marked workload for the respiratory and cardiovascular systems. We will focus our management in OLD on controlling minute ventilation and relieving airflow obstruction.

Cardiovascular changes also occur in OLD, especially the COPD patient with acute respiratory failure, and are dominated by the presence of pulmonary hypertension and the associated right heart dysfunction. Some patients

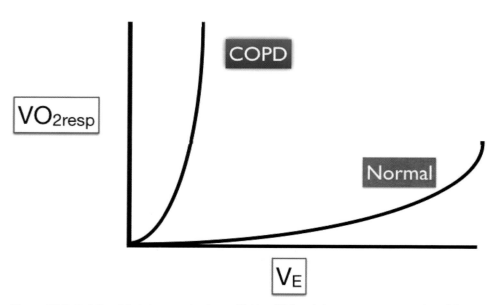

Figure 17-3 Relationship between minute ventilation (V_E) and the oxygen consumption of the respiratory muscles (VO_{2resp}).

may have underlying chronic pulmonary hypertension, which can be worsened during acute exacerbations. The change in mean pulmonary artery pressure is often related to the degree of hypoxemia and may return to baseline values once the exacerbation subsides. Secondary changes in right ventricular function include a reduced ejection fraction. Positive pleural pressure, seen with dynamic hyperinflation, can limit systemic venous return and raise right ventricular afterload, further limiting right ventricular function.

17.2 Intrinsic PEEP (PEEPi) in OLD

The application of end-expiratory pressure through the use of expiratory circuit valves is termed *applied* or *extrinsic PEEP* and was reviewed in *Chapter 15 Mechanical Ventilation*. The clinician, through the specific ventilator setting, always knows the level of extrinsic PEEP. PEEP can also occur, however, from the interaction of the mechanical ventilator and the patient's lung mechanics, most commonly in the setting of severe OLD. This type of PEEP, which is called *intrinsic PEEP (PEEPi)*, is not evident to the clinician unless measured. Any combination of four variables can interact to elevate intrinsic PEEP:

1. Increased minute ventilation with a reduced expiratory time

2. Longer inspiratory time due to increased tidal volume or reduction in inspiratory flow
3. Longer expiratory time due to airflow obstruction
4. Longer expiratory time due to a reduced respiratory system elastic recoil

The adverse effects of intrinsic and extrinsic PEEP on cardiovascular hemodynamics are similar. The primary difference is the lack of easy recognition and measurement for intrinsic PEEP. Even though the patient's ventilator says PEEP=5, the patient's internal expiratory pressure may be much higher.

17.2.1 Intrinsic PEEP Assessment

How do you recognize the presence of intrinsic PEEP in your ICU patient? A few simple steps make this easy.

1. *Examination and smarts.* The first trick is to have a high index of suspicion. Does your patient have known COPD or asthma that leads to airflow obstruction? Is the patient wheezing? Wheezing on physical exam that lasts right up to the start of the next breath can be a good clinical indicator of dynamic hyperinflation and intrinsic PEEP.
2. *Flow-Time profiles.* A qualitative assessment of intrinsic PEEP can be made from the flow-time curve on the ventilator screen as illustrated in **Figure 17-4**. Examine the flow-time curve for the pattern of persistent expiratory flow at end expiration (red arrow). The normal expiratory

Flow - Time Waveform

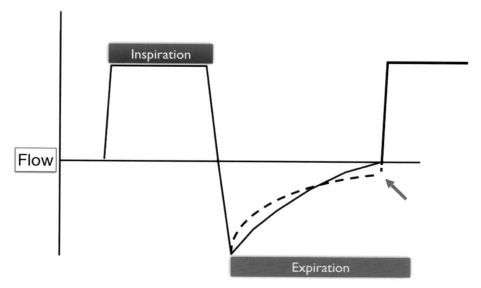

Figure 17-4 *Flow-time waveform in a patient with airflow obstruction and evidence for persistent end-expiratory airflow (red arrow).*

time curve returns to zero flow prior to the onset of inspiration (solid line). In the setting of PEEPi, alveolar pressure remains > airway pressure at end-expiration, so expiratory flow continues right up to the onset of the next ventilator inspiratory cycle (dotted line). In the setting of intrinsic PEEP (PEEPi), the following breath starts from the point of continuous expiratory airflow. If you disconnect a paralyzed patient from the endotracheal tube during expiration, a patient with PEEPi will show a prolonged period of continued expiration, often with an audible wheeze. During this period, intrathoracic airway pressures will fall, and venous return may increase to resolve hypotension. On reconnection to the ventilator, a reduction in the plateau airway pressures will be noted.

Some modern ventilators will show you a digital readout of airflow at end-expiration, which should fall to 0. This approach is a qualitative measure of the presence of intrinsic PEEP but does not give you a pressure or measured volume of intrinsic PEEP or trapped air, respectively.

3. *End-expiratory occlusion pressure.* This more *quantitative* occlusion technique requires cessation of airflow at exactly end-expiration and closure of both the inspiratory and expiratory limbs of the ventilator. The patient must be relaxed,

and the timing must assure that the patient has reached end-expiration. The maneuver is difficult to accomplish in the absence of paralysis and a regular breathing pattern.

To understand this technique for measurement of PEEPi, let's consider a basic respiratory circuit as illustrated in **Figure 17-5**. The inspiratory limb of the ventilator consists of an inspiratory airway pressure monitor and a valve to occlude the inspiratory limb. The expiratory limb consists of an airway pressure monitor with an expiratory occlusion valve. During inspiration, the expiratory occlusion valve is closed, and the delivered airflow from the inspiratory limb goes down the ETT to the patient's lungs. During expiration, the inspiratory occlusion valve is shut, and the expiratory occlusion valve is open. The lung and chest wall elastic recoil drives airflow down the expiratory limb. If at any point in the respiratory cycle, both the inspiratory and expiratory valves are closed, airflow stops and pressure equilibrates throughout the system. In that situation, the alveolar pressure = expiratory airway pressure = inspiratory airway pressure. If we time the expiratory valve occlusion to precisely the point of end expiration, the measured ventilator airway pressure is equivalent to the alveolar pressure. Modern ventilators have a button to help time the expiratory port occlusion to end-expiration. Older ventilators required the clinician

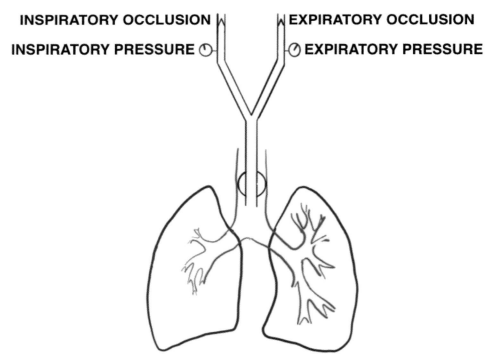

INSPIRATORY OCCLUSION

INSPIRATORY PRESSURE

EXPIRATORY OCCLUSION

EXPIRATORY PRESSURE

Figure 17-5 *A respiratory circuit graphic illustrating the position of pressure manometers and occlusion valves.*

to time the occlusion of the expiratory limb, often using your hand to do it. The specific timing of expiratory valve occlusion could be a challenge, as premature occlusion will measure alveolar pressure before end-expiration and will show elevated alveolar pressures mid-expiration, which could be normal.

During the expiratory hold, you can monitor the pressure-time curve on the ventilator. You will see a rise in the measured pressure above the set extrinsic PEEP value to the intrinsic PEEP value, as illustrated in **Figure 17-6**. Note the period of the end-expiratory hold.

Both of the techniques for the assessment of PEEPi are limited by the presence of expiratory muscle contraction, which can raise end-expiratory airway pressure in the absence of dynamic hyperinflation.

4. *Trigger failure.* Failure to trigger a breath during inspiratory efforts can be another sign of intrinsic PEEP. This one is easy to recognize but not so easy to explain. Your patient with OLD makes recurrent efforts to inspire, but you notice the effort does not trigger a ventilator control breath. This patient effort to trigger a breath can sometimes look like hiccups and can be misdiagnosed as hiccups. Don't be fooled by this presentation of intrinsic PEEP! The patient is pulling hard enough, but nothing is happening – *what gives?*

The triggering dysfunction produced by PEEPi results from the disequilibrium between the ventilator circuit pressure and alveolar pressure. An inspiratory threshold exists for the respiratory muscles, which must lower alveolar pressure to the equivalent of circuit pressure before the initiation of end-expiration.

Figure 17-7, Example A shows the alveolus at end expiration in a patient with PEEPi equal to 10 cm H_2O. The alveolar pressure (10) is higher than the external PEEP (5). In the absence of respiratory muscle effort, the intrapleural pressure (10) is equivalent to the alveolar pressure (10). The limitation to further expiratory airflow is dynamic airway collapse, which limits flow independent of the external PEEP setting.

To achieve inspiratory airflow, the respiratory muscles in the patient with Example A must first lower the alveolar pressure below the external PEEP. So, our patient has an external PEEP setting of 5 cm H_2O and a trigger sensitivity of -1 cm H_2O. This means that the airway pressure would need to fall to 4 cm H_2O to initiate inspiratory airflow.

In Example B, the alveolar pressure would need to decrease from 10 to 4 to achieve inspiratory flow if the triggering pressure was set at -1. So, the patient has a threshold load equal to the PEEPi value above the external PEEP (5) plus the set triggering value (-1) for a total triggering value of 6. The ventilator may show a sensitivity value of -1 cm H_2O, but in this case, the real triggering value for this patient with PEEPi is - 6 cm H_2O.

In Example C, note the external PEEP has been increased to match the end-expiratory alveolar pressure or the PEEPi. At this level, note that no change in alveolar volume occurs because the alveolar pressure and PEEP are equivalent. However, the threshold for lowering the pleural pressure has been reduced from 10 to 9. At this

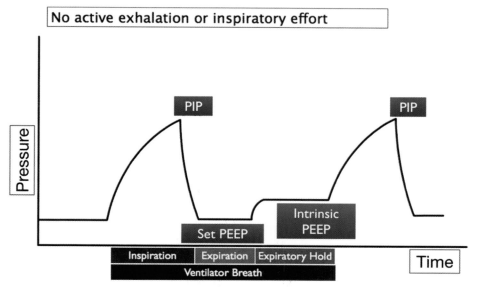

Figure 17-6 Pressure – time graphic that illustrates the measurement of intrinsic PEEP during an inspiratory hold maneuver.

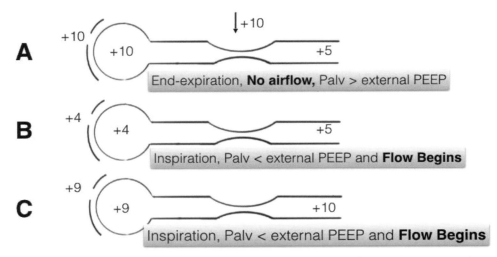

Figure 17-7 *Trigger failure results when alveolar pressure (Palv) at end expiration is greater than airway pressure or external PEEP (A). Ventilator trigger requires alveolar pressure to be lowered to a value less than airway pressure (B). Increasing external PEEP to match end-expiratory alveolar pressure allows triggering with less patient effort (C).*

level, alveolar pressure is lower than circuit pressure, and airflow begins.

Application of extrinsic PEEP to match PEEPi can serve to equilibrate circuit and alveolar pressure without additional hyperinflation if applied correctly. Extrinsic PEEP is generally applied at approximately 85% of the PEEPi value if this approach is used. The correct application of extrinsic PEEP can reduce the mechanical work of patient-triggered breaths. However, the application of extrinsic PEEP in this setting must be undertaken with some caution. Extrinsic PEEP applied in the absence of expiratory airflow limitation may increase alveolar pressure and end-expiratory lung volume, and further reduce expiratory airflow.

You will often see a patient with severe COPD or asthma on the ventilator take one or more breath attempts, without reversing flow or pressure enough to trigger a ventilator breath. This concept is further illustrated in **Figure 17-8**. This figure shows a comparison of the airway (Paw) and esophageal pressures (Pes) in the same patient. The patient makes intermittent efforts to decrease esophageal (pleural) pressure but does not achieve the necessary threshold to overcome intrinsic PEEP. So for the breaths above the threshold (red), no airway pressure change occurs and no inspiratory breath is triggered. For those breaths at or below the threshold (green), airway pressure change occurs, and the breath is triggered. The effort is reflected in the *pleural pressure change* (~ 10 cm H$_2$) and not the airway pressure change (~ 1-2 cm H$_2$O).

Figure 17-9 shows you a ventilator screen with the characteristic features of severe airflow obstruction and intrinsic PEEP. The top yellow curve is a pressure-time curve. The middle green curve is a flow-time curve. The bottom curve is a volume-time curve.

Note that the patient is receiving a volume control breath (Arrow 1) with a constant (square) rate of flow during the breath delivery (green curve). The pressure-time curve (yellow) rises to the highest value (peak inspiratory pressure) and then falls to a new value we call the plateau pressure (Pplat) (Arrow 2). This fall in airway pressure occurs during a short inspiratory hold we introduced on the ventilator—meaning a short period with no further inspiratory or expiratory airflow.

The flow-time curve (green) shows a prolonged expiratory phase consistent with significant airflow obstruction (Arrow 3). Although the scaling on the flow-time curve does not easily allow you to determine if the patient has persistent flow at end-expiration, the ventilator lists the end-expiratory flow (Vee) as positive at 2 L/min (Arrow 4). *Don't be afraid of that ventilator screen!* You can learn a lot about your patient's physiology by looking at the curves and recordings. If you don't look and ask questions of your therapist, you will never learn.

17.2.2 Complications of Intrinsic PEEP

So why do we care about intrinsic PEEP in the patient with severe airflow obstruction? *Complications and more complications!*

Potential complications of intrinsic-PEEP and dynamic hyperinflation are threefold and can be remembered by thinking of your COPD patient with extremely labored breathing needing to be intubated. The patient has a very high W*ork* O*f* B*reathing*

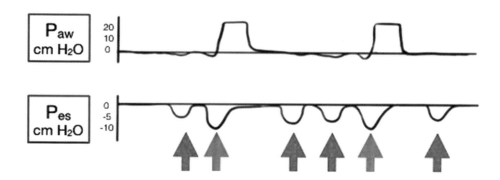

Figure 17-8 Comparison of the airway (Paw) and esophageal (Pes) pressure – time tracing. The patient makes an effort to inspire (red arrows) but does not meet the triggering threshold due to intrinsic PEEP. Only with significant effort (green arrows) are ventilator breaths triggered. This will appear clinically as a patient making ventilatory effort without an associated ventilator response.

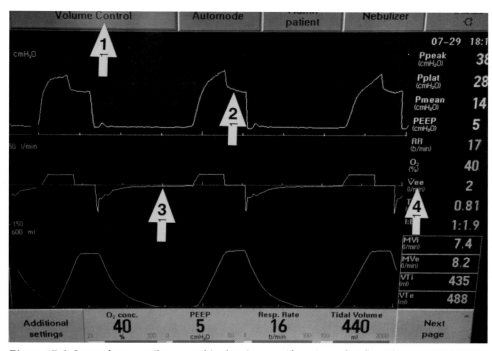

Figure 17-9 Image from ventilator graphic showing manifestations of airflow obstruction. See text.

1. **W: Work** of breathing. Increased work of breathing during spontaneous breathing and patient cycled mechanical ventilation
2. **O: Output.** Elevated intrathoracic pressures reduce heart preload and drop Cardiac Output, resulting in cardiovascular compromise and hypotension
3. **B: Barotrauma.** Increased risk for barotrauma

17.2.2.1 W: Work of Breathing

The impact of intrinsic PEEP and dynamic hyperinflation on the patient's WOB, both on and off the ventilator, are significant. With dynamic hyperinflation a significant effort can be expended just to trigger the ventilator breath. PEEPi represents an inspiratory threshold load that must be overcome if the patient is to breathe spontaneously or trigger the ventilator. Furthermore, this must occur at higher lung volumes, such that inspiration occurs on a less compliant portion of the pressure-volume curve, where there is a greater inward elastic recoil of the overexpanded chest wall.

How to reduce this work of breathing? Carefully applying extrinsic PEEP to the COPD patient with high PEEPi increases the proximal airway pressure and reduces the pressure gradient required to reverse flow on inspiration. Theoretically, the application of extrinsic PEEP to the level of PEEPi should serve to prevent early dynamic airway closure by maintaining a positive airway pressure that counterbalances the positive extramural pressure that surrounds the airways during forced exhalation. Unfortunately, the concept that applied PEEP thus "stents" open airways and facilitates lung emptying is not supported by clinical studies. The application of external PEEP rarely leads to actual reductions in lung volume.

But you want to be careful. As the level of applied external PEEP approaches that of PEEPi, the lung volume increases. Think of the classic waterfall analogy when setting applied PEEP. As the downstream water of the waterfall or a dam rises, the water backs up behind the dam. In fact, the most significant risk of applied PEEP in the COPD patient is inducing further hyperinflation with cardiovascular compromise. A rule of thumb is extrinsic PEEP induces hemodynamic impairment when the levels of applied PEEP exceed 85% of the measured PEEPi. It is therefore reasonable to apply PEEP to about 80% of the measured PEEPi level, to reduce WOB associated with patient-initiated mechanical ventilation. However, there is *NO RATIONALE* for its use during controlled mechanical ventilation when there is no patient inspiratory effort, such as in a deeply sedated or paralyzed patient, or to "stent" open airways to reduce lung volume

17.2.2.2 O: Output—Hemodynamic Instability

With dynamic hyperinflation, lung volume and intrathoracic pressure increase, venous return is impaired, and the right ventricle and pulmonary veins are mechanically compressed. Increased intrathoracic pressure reduces left ventricular preload and cardiac output. Central venous and pulmonary artery occlusion pressures are elevated, reflecting increased intrathoracic pressure rather than increased intravascular volume. The combination of high filling pressures, reduced cardiac output, and hypotension may be mistakenly diagnosed as left ventricular failure. Progressive severe dynamic hyperinflation when extreme may result in pulseless electrical activity (PEA) and cardiac arrest.

The patient with COPD may be at greatest risk for this complication immediately following intubation. The urgency of the situation often leads to overzealous manual bag-mask ventilation. The resultant large tidal volumes and rapid respiratory rates increase lung volume and shorten expiratory time, preventing adequate exhalation and potentiating dynamic hyperinflation. In the setting of non-elective emergency intubation, the reduction in cardiac output associated with dynamic hyperinflation is often compounded by

volume depletion and sedation. In fact, hypotension may occur in up to 25 % of all emergency intubations of COPD patients.

17.2.2.3 B: Barotrauma

Barotrauma is a recognized complication of mechanical ventilatory support in OLD patients. The incidence of this complication relates at least in part to the level of ventilator cycling pressures. Dynamic hyperinflation results in overdistention of lung parenchyma, which may lead to alveolar disruption and extra-alveolar air.

Remember that peak inspiratory pressure (PIP) reflects both lung compliance and flow-resistive properties (airway and endotracheal tube resistance and peak inspiratory flow) of the lung and chest wall. The plateau pressure (P_{PLAT}) more directly relates to alveolar pressure and overdistention forces. As long as plateau pressure remains low, increasing peak inspiratory flow to reduce inspiratory time is a reasonable strategy to prevent dynamic hyperinflation. This is a bit of a paradox unique to the patient with OLD:

- Increased inspiratory flow will raise PIP, as measured at the airway opening.
- By shortening the inspiratory time, the patient has a long time to expire, which reduces dynamic hyperinflation and PEEPi.
- The reduction in PEEPi lowers plateau airway pressures.

Normally, changes in PIP and P_{PLAT} will move in the same direction. The patient with OLD is one exception where this may not occur.

A slightly reduced tidal volume (6-8 ml/kg ideal body weight) and therapy directed at reducing minute ventilation and airway resistance are also helpful to control P_{PLAT} in OLD patients. For patients with severe dynamic hyperinflation, we often need to accept hypercapnia until the airflow obstruction improves.

17.2.3 Limiting Intrinsic PEEP in OLD

Focus medical treatment for dynamic hyperinflation on reducing expiratory airflow obstruction, using bronchodilators and anti-inflammatory agents. Because these therapies take hours to days to work, you must limit the intrinsic PEEP with your ventilator management to stabilize the patient and prevent complications of dynamic hyperinflation while you wait for your other treatments to take hold.

Avoid the complications of dynamic hyperinflation through suspicion, detection, and therapy. Control of dynamic hyperinflation is primarily achieved by facilitating adequate lung emptying by *prolonging expiratory time* on the ventilator.

How to prolong expiratory time?

1. *Reduce overall minute ventilation (respiratory rate and tidal volume).* Use tidal volumes of 5-8 ml/kg ideal body weight and rates of 8-10 breaths/min. You should also control fever and manage anxiety to help minimize any increase in ventilatory demand. In severe OLD you will need to accept hypercapnia until airflow obstruction is relieved.

2. *Reduce inspiratory time by increasing the inspiratory flow rate,* which, as we discussed above, will increase peak inspiratory pressure. However, alveolar or plateau pressures will be unaffected or paradoxically drop as dynamic hyperinflation is reduced. The use of non-compressible ventilator tubing will also increase inspiratory flow rate and reduce inspiratory time by lowering the volume the ventilator must deliver to reach the set tidal volume. Depending on your ventilator, you can reduce inspiratory time by setting a specific flow rate, a specific inspiratory time duration, or setting the inspiratory:expiratory time ratio. All produce the same effect, but the key outcome is to reduce inspiratory time.

3. *Increase expiratory time with bronchodilator therapy.* Beta-adrenergic and anticholinergic bronchodilators can be effectively delivered to the mechanically ventilated patient via small volume nebulizers or metered-dose inhalers (MDI). These medications, when dosed and delivered effectively, will reduce airway resistance.

With these maneuvers, you may be able to reduce dynamic hyperinflation and manage your patient. But often, several patient factors will interfere with your plan:

- Despite your goal to reduce minute ventilation, your patient has a fever, elevated dead space fraction from bronchoconstriction and airway secretions, and a high work of breathing from the mechanical workload associated with severe airflow obstruction. These factors will drive the need for a higher, not lower, minute ventilation.
- Despite your goal to reduce minute ventilation, your patient has extreme dyspnea and hypoxemia. You can correct the hypoxemia with supplemental oxygen, but the marked dyspnea will be associated with a high ventilatory drive and tendency to hyperventilate on mechanical ventilation.
- Bronchodilators will provide temporary relief, but sustained improvement usually requires antibiotics and corticosteroid therapy, and the timing for improvement will be delayed.

So, your OLD patient will not always be cooperative with your plan to lower minute ventilation! You will be faced with a decision to either maintain an appropriate level of ventilation and $PaCO_2$ (accepting high airway pressures and dynamic hyperinflation) <u>OR</u> control high airway pressures and dynamic hyperinflation (accepting a reduced minute ventilation with the associated hypercapnia). In OLD patients with respiratory failure, *dynamic hyperinflation is considered a much greater risk to the patient than hypercapnia.* So, in severe OLD disease, we hypoventilate the patient on purpose – called *controlled hypoventilation or permissive hypercapnia.*

Sedation and occasionally paralysis may be required to control the minute ventilation. The use of neuromuscular blocking agents should be limited, to avoid precipitating the necrotizing myopathy associated with these agents and the administration of corticosteroids. Short-acting agents such as propofol, fentanyl, or dexmedetomidine may allow for more rapid weaning, but little evidence exists to support one agent over the other. Cisatracurium (trade name Nimbex) is a non-depolarizing neuromuscular blocking drug that is rapidly degraded by Hofmann elimination and ester hydrolysis, so it has a very short half-life. Interestingly, this drug is associated with lower rates of myopathy and can be used in cases of severe dyssynchrony and dynamic hyperinflation until things are under control. Remember to deeply sedate and provide analgesia prior to paralysis.

17.3 Mechanical Ventilation in OLD

Now that you have a good understanding of obstructive physiology in your OLD patient, let's get down to management issues. Although the physiology principles we have learned apply to both forms of ventilation, we need to consider both non-invasive and invasive mechanical ventilation.

17.3.1 Non-Invasive Mechanical Ventilation in OLD

Non-invasive mechanical ventilation refers to the delivery of positive pressure ventilation via a nasal mask, nasal prongs, or face mask. COPD patients with respiratory failure who receive NIV have a reduced rate of intubation, ICU stay, and possibly nosocomial infections. For other forms of OLD, clinical trials of sufficient patient numbers do not exist to confirm equal efficacy, but there is no reason to believe NIV would be less beneficial.

NIV is the preferred ventilation method in any COPD patient with marked dyspnea, increased work of breathing, and evidence of hypercapnia. Many factors predict limited success with NIV in the COPD patient population including a higher APACHE II score ($>$ 29), a lower Glasgow Coma Score ($<$ 11), a PH $<$7.25, a respiratory rate $>$ 35/min, mask air leakage, and copious secretions.[120] One additional variable predicting success is improved gas exchange and heart rate within two hours of NIV application.

Contraindications to the use of NIV include unstable cardiovascular status (including respiratory arrest), inability to protect the airway, agitated or uncooperative patient, recent upper tract surgery (GI or ENT), excessive secretions, or failure to fit a mask.

Ventilators that provide a separate inspiratory and expiratory positive pressure settings for pressure regulated breath delivery are used to provide NIV. This mode is frequently called BPAP for bilevel positive airway pressure. Specific "NIV modes" in modern ventilators attempt to compensate for mask leaks and the unique monitoring needs of non-invasive ventilation to improve the overall patient tolerance. However, any ICU ventilator can be adapted for delivery via a face mask, and no specific ventilator has been shown superior for this mode.

An interface is selected to provide a comfortable fit with minimal air leaks. For acute respiratory failure, a full-face mask may be preferred over a nasal mask, but this preference is very patient-dependent.

NIV settings are individualized to reduce the work of breathing, relieve dyspnea, and hopefully to correct abnormal pH secondary to acute hypercapnia. For the BPAP, an inspiratory positive airway pressure (IPAP) is selected to reduce the work of breathing, usually initiating in the range of 8-10 cm H_2O. The level of inspiratory positive airway pressure is adjusted based upon a target tidal volume to relieve dyspnea and the work of breathing, balanced against the discomfort and leaks from positive pressure applied to the mask. A level of positive expiratory pressure is also selected in the BPAP mode. In NIV, this is often called *EPAP* for *expiratory positive airway pressure* but essentially is identical to PEEP. This value is usually set in the range of 5-7 cm H_2O and helps to maintain airway patency and limit the threshold load on inspiration that characterizes the OLD patient with dynamic hyperinflation. Both the IPAP and EPAP are titrated to achieve patient comfort and control hypercapnia. The tidal volume is not regulated in the simple BPAP mode of NIV. Think of effective ventilation using BPAP in a two-compartment respiratory model, in which EPAP achieves the upper airway patency needed to allow the effective delivery of IPAP to the lower airways. BPAP devices can operate in a spontaneous (S) or timed (T) mode. Most commonly the spontaneous and timed mode are combined (ST). In the S mode, the patient initiates all the breaths, while in the ST mode

a backup machine triggered rate exists if the patient's spontaneous rate falls below the set value.

A modification of BPAP allows for the setting of a fixed tidal volume. In this form of NIV, the system output adjusts automatically with variations in the inspiratory pressure to assure a predetermined target tidal volume. This modification of BPAP has been termed AVAPS (average volume assured pressure support ventilation). AVAPS may offer a more favorable form of NIV to rescue acute COPD exacerbations with hypercapnic encephalopathy.

Complications of NIV include mask leaks, mask discomfort, eye irritation, sinus congestion, and skin breakdown over the bridge of the nose. More severe complications include patient-ventilator dysynchrony, gastric insuflation, and hemodynamic compromise. For these reasons, in the patient with acute respiratory failure NIV warrants very close monitoring especially during the initial phase. NIV in acute respiratory failure is not the same as NIV for home therapy or palliative care. The patient with acute respiratory failure treated with NIV must be cautiously monitored to assure a good mask fit, comfort, appropriate triggering of spontaneous breaths, and appropriate cycling off with breath termination. Patients who are "dependent" on NIV and unable to survive without continued therapy should be in a closely monitored environment. NIV is weaned no differently than invasive mechanical ventilation – regular spontaneous breathing trials of progressively increasing duration.

Based upon a numerous clinical trials, NIV is strongly advised as the initial ventilatory support mode for two clinical scenarios in patients with COPD exacerbation:

1. Use NIV on initial assessment in COPD exacerbation patients with acute or acute on chronic respiratory acidosis (pH $\leq$7.35).
2. Use NIV as a clinical trial in COPD patients with exacerbation that meet your clinical consideration for endotracheal intubation.

17.3.2. Invasive Mechanical Ventilation in OLD

Base your decision to initiate invasive mechanical ventilation in COPD on a complete evaluation of the patient rather than any specific level of pH or $PaCO_2$. Assessment of the patient's hemodynamic stability, mental status, and response to initial therapy are used as factors to determine the need for mecanical support. As soon as you intubate a patient with OLD, you are likely to land yourself in hot water. You may face two immediate problems: 1) acid-base disturbances and 2) hypotension (shock!).

17.3.2.1 Acid-base Issues

In the face of increased dead space ventilation (Vd/Vt) and work of breathing, patients with severe COPD frequently develop a stable, compensated respiratory acidosis. Arterial $PaCO_2$ rises to allow adequate steady-state elimination of CO_2 at a reduced level of alveolar ventilation (V_A). The kidneys retain HCO_3^- until a compensated state is achieved, characterized by a high $PaCO_2$, high HCO_3^-, and normal or near-normal arterial pH. If this pre-existing state is not appreciated by the clinician when such patients are first intubated and ventilated, acute overventilation and potentially life-threatening alkalemia can result. Furthermore, if a "normal" minute ventilation (e.g., to $PaCO_2$ 40 mmHg) is pursued in a patient with chronic hypercapnia, the patient's kidneys will progressively excrete the previously retained HCO_3^- until the overall acid-base balance returns to "normal." The patient loses the buffering capacity for hypercapnia, and is unable to maintain the ventilation necessary to keep $PaCO_2$ normal during weaning. This causes the patient to develop acute respiratory acidosis during weaning or post extubation.

There is no $PaCO_2$ target for ventilation. The real goal for ventilation is the pH. Mechanical ventilation is adjusted to achieve a pH target in the range of 7.25 to 7.40. In the acute OLD exacerbation, a lower pH is often accepted to allow controlled hypoventilation. Controlled hypoventilation and permissive hypercapnia are well tolerated even at pH levels as low as 7.15-7.20, and this strategy buys time for the primary pharmacologic interventions, corticosteroids, bronchodilators, and antibiotics, to take effect.

17.3.2.2 Hypotension Post Intubation

Dynamic hyperinflation reduces left ventricular preload and cardiac output. This hemodynamic risk is greatest immediately after intubation, because the patient is often aggressively diuresed to improve hypoxemia and prevent intubation, and sedatives used to intubate the patient can venodilate the circulation, further reducing preload to the heart. Finally, in an emergency after intubation, most of us can't help but bag a patient as hard as we can (big bagged tidal volumes!) and at a respiratory rate equal to our heart rate! This severely reduces expiratory times and increases dynamic hyperinflation and PEEPi. There are a few tricks to prevent this from happening:

1. *Prehydrate.* As you prepare for your intubation, start a liter of normal saline wide open. Get some fluid on board to increase preload.
2. Have a push dose vasopressor (PDP) on the ready. Have diluted epinephrine or phenylephrine

available for immediate use as outlined in *Chapter 12 on Basic Airway Management.*

3. *Bag the patient very slowly!* This is the most important and simple step. A severe COPD patient after intubation has little problem with oxygenation and just needs about 6-10 breaths per minute. Think for a minute how slow this is… You can give a single bag breath, let go of the bag, have a sip of coffee, say hi to your neighbor, and then give the next breath (6-10 seconds between breaths!).

17.3.3 Ventilator Management in OLD

We can divide ventilator management in the OLD population to the acute phase and more chronic ventilator dependent phase for discussion.

17.3.3.1 Acute Phase

Set your ventilation parameters early in the resuscitation period to adequately "unload" the work of the respiratory muscles. For most patients, the mode will be a form of volume control ventilation. Pressure control breaths provide variable levels of minute ventilation, depending on the patient's effort and respiratory impedance, and therefore are less desirable. Variable mechanics are especially true for the acute management of the OLD patient, where variable degrees of bronchospasm, airway secretion, and response to therapeutic intervention exist.

Utilize a tidal volume of approximately 6-8 ml/kg of ideal body weight in the early management period. Further adjustments are based upon patient response and additional arterial blood gas monitoring. A rough rule of thumb is that the machine-supported minute ventilation should be adjusted to approximately 2/3 of the patient's spontaneous minute ventilation in the acute phase. This setting assures the ventilator will provide an adequate level of minute ventilation if there is a sudden decline in the output of the respiratory system. Normalization of the $PaCO_2$ is not the target of ventilatory assistance, but rather a level of minute ventilation that appears to "rest" the neuromuscular system and slowly correct acidosis. Overventilation can lead to complications of respiratory alkalosis with cardiac arrhythmias and seizures. Overventilation can complicate weaning as previously outlined. The inspired oxygen concentration is usually guided by arterial blood gas data or pulse oximetry.

Attention to timing parameters, specifically inspiratory time is essential. Different ventilators will adjust inspiratory time, based upon a flow setting, a time setting, or an I:E ratio setting. But the impact of all three is to set the duration of the inspiratory phase. An inspiratory flow rate that is 5-6 times the resting minute ventilation will meet inspiratory flow demands without causing excessively high peak cycling pressures. Mechanically ventilated patients with COPD typically have a high respiratory drive, which requires a high inspiratory flow rate. If the inspiratory flow rate is insufficient, the patient workload to overcome pulmonary and ventilator impedance is markedly increased. An increased inspiratory flow rate also prolongs expiratory time.

The increased airway resistance and reduced elastic recoil characteristic of COPD patients, particularly those patients with emphysema, provides a requirement for a prolonged expiratory duration. An elevated dead space ventilation increases ventilatory requirements, which are most frequently met through tachypnea, leading to a short cycle time between breaths. The combination of short cycle length and prolonged expiratory phase places the patient at high risk for dynamic hyperinflation. Inappropriate settings for triggering, inspiratory flow, and tidal volume can lead to marked patient-ventilator dyssynchrony in the population. Under these circumstances, the patient's work of breathing on mechanical ventilation may equal or exceed the work of breathing for spontaneous ventilation. Adjustment of ventilator support settings is preferred for patient-ventilator dyssynchrony, but if not successful, the patient may require sedation for the initial period of ventilator support to rest the ventilatory muscles.

Treatment for dynamic hyperinflation, if present, is focused on reducing expiratory airflow obstruction, using bronchodilators and anti-inflammatory agents. In passive patients, reductions in minute ventilation will produce an increase in expiratory time and decrease PEEPi. Increasing the inspiratory flow rate will also extend expiratory time, provided the flow change is not associated with any change in respiratory frequency.

As previously mentioned, the relationship between augmented ventilation and energy consumption is hyperbolic in these patients. Small increments in ventilation require disproportionate increases in resting oxygen consumption. Hypermetabolism secondary to fever or agitation must be reduced. Treatable causes of high dead space ventilation (e.g., volume depletion or lung overdistension) should also be identified and reversed, if possible.

17.3.3.2 Chronic Phase

Mechanical support is usually continued for a minimum of 24-48 hours while therapy directed at the underlying pathophysiologic processes is instituted. The focus for COPD patients on more long-term ventilation must be to minimize the risk of complications associated with this support.

For the more alert COPD patient on mechanical ventilation, the management of anxiety becomes a significant issue. Anxiety can provoke periods of panic during the weaning phase, leading to hyperventilation, dynamic hyperinflation, and worsening dyspnea. While sedation is often necessary early in the treatment phase to minimize ventilatory requirements, regular sedation can interfere with the normal weaning process. Patients with more chronic ventilatory support appear to benefit from a regular daily schedule. Nighttime intervals are best conducted with full ventilatory support to allow adequate rest periods. The addition of regular physical therapy, including ambulation on mechanical ventilation, appears also to be helpful. If patients understand the goals for the weaning process and actively participate in the daily program, anxiety can often be minimized and the need for pharmacologic intervention eliminated. The use of specific biofeedback techniques in the weaning process has been reported and may be beneficial.

Particular attention to the "external" workload associated with the ventilator system is warranted, especially in the COPD patient, as small changes in minute ventilation or mechanical work produce significant changes in respiratory muscle energy requirements. The resistance of the endotracheal tube increases in an exponential relationship with reductions in tube size. The use of smaller endotracheal tubes (< 8 mm) in the COPD patient can limit secretion clearance and significantly increase the work of breathing. The use of low levels of pressure support (3-5 cm H_2O) during spontaneous breaths on mechanical ventilation can limit the effects of endotracheal tube resistance.

Demand valves associated with breath-triggering or synchronized intermittent mandatory ventilation (IMV) circuits can require a significant reduction in airway pressure by the patient to initiate airflow. This factor, combined with the lack of immediate delivery of gas flow, can cause a significant increase in the mechanical workload of ventilation. Ventilator circuits that incorporate a continuous flow design may serve to minimize this workload. Finally, the importance of matching ventilator sensitivity and flow rates to patient inspiratory flow demands should be emphasized. Significant amounts of respiratory work can be performed by the patient, even in the assist mode of ventilation if these variables are adjusted incorrectly.

17.4 Drug Therapy in OLD

While you are avoiding problems and limiting PEEPi to the best of your ability, you are buying time for your pharmacologic therapy to work. Easy to remember medical therapy for OLD – you need to know your *ABC*'s. Many of the treatment principles are similar for the two most common forms of OLD: asthma and chronic obstructive pulmonary disease. We will highlight the differences when they exist.

17.4.1 Antibiotics

Antibiotic therapy is advised for hospitalized patients with moderate to severe COPD exacerbations and may provide a mortality benefit in patients who require mechanical ventilation.[121] The initial selection of antibiotic therapy is guided by the patient's history and local antibiotic resistance patterns. The most common bacterial pathogens include Streptococcus pneumoniae, Haemophilus influenzae, and Moraxella catarrhalis. Patients with risk factors for Pseudomonas and more resistant gram-negative infections include COPD patients with frequent disease exacerbations (> 3 per year), a recent hospitalization, a prior isolate of Pseudomonas, or severe disease ($FEV_1 < 50\%$ predicted). Therapy for these patients should include an anti-Pseudomonas agent such as cefepime, ceftazidime, or piperacillin-tazobactam. Duration of antibiotic therapy is typically limited to 3-7 days. Anti-viral treatment is recommended for patients with confirmed influenza infection.

In contrast to the COPD patient, antibiotics are not beneficial for the patient with an asthma exacerbation.

17.4.2 Bronchodilators

Standard bronchodilator therapy in OLD exacerbations would be short-acting beta-agonists including albuterol and levalbuterol. These medications are favored due to their rapid onset in producing bronchodilation. Administer the medications via a nebulizer or metered dose inhaler with a spacer. Although clinical studies suggest these two delivery methods are therapeutically equivalent, patients and clinicians seem to prefer the nebulized method of drug delivery in acute disease exacerbations. We prefer albuterol administered at doses of 2.5 mg (in 3mL) or 4 puffs of an MDI q 1-4 hours. On initial presentation, the patient may benefit from "stacked" treatments, meaning 2-3 treatments repeated every 20 minutes to provide initial symptomatic relief.

The inhaled beta-agonists can be delivered with additional dosing of an inhaled cholinergic agent such as ipratropium bromide (500 mcg) at similar dosing frequency. The inhaled anticholinergic medications work on unique receptors, but the added benefit of anticholinergic therapy to frequent beta-agonist administration is controversial.

Bronchodilators via nebulizer should be delivered by high-flow room air rather than oxygen to avoid the risk of hyperoxia in COPD patients with hypercapnia.

17.4.3 Corticosteroids

Clinical trials have convincingly demonstrated that hospitalized patients with COPD exacerbations benefit from the administration of systemic corticosteroids.[122–124] But controversies remain. Clinical studies suggest that oral corticosteroids are equivalent to the intravenous administration for COPD exacerbations, although many clinicians continue to use IV corticosteroids in hospitalized patients. The optimal dose of corticosteroids remains unknown. The Global Initiative for Chronic Obstructive Pulmonary Disease (GOLD) guidelines advise a dose equivalent to 40 mg of prednisone per day, but clinicians frequently choose higher dosing for patients with respiratory failure.[121] A final controversy in corticosteroid therapy for COPD exacerbations is the duration of therapy. More recent trials suggest the maximum therapy duration recommended for corticosteroid therapy is 14 days, and shorter courses may be equally valid.

For patients with acute asthma exacerbations, the guidelines for corticosteroid therapy are oddly like the patient with a COPD exacerbation. The administration is indicated for any hospitalized disease exacerbation, oral equal to intravenous drug delivery, dosing not defined, and duration at ≤ 14 days. *Easy to remember!*

17.4.4 Miscellaneous Interventions

Helium is a non-toxic gas that is lower in density than nitrogen and oxygen. By adding helium to oxygen (replacing nitrogen), the density of the inspired gas is reduced. Airflow resistance is impacted by the density of the inspired gas, especially in areas of turbulent flow. The major region of airflow resistance in the lung occurs in the larger airways, where turbulent flow is more common. These physiologic principles have prompted clinicians to employ helium:oxygen mixtures (called *heliox*) in the management of patients with significant airway obstruction. Heliox is a therapeutic option in upper airway obstruction and OLD exacerbations – both COPD and asthma.

For the patient presenting with an acute asthma exacerbation, the routine use of heliox has not been shown to alter outcome.[125] The application may offer a form of rescue therapy when applied individually to patients with status asthmaticus. Similar data define the experience in the COPD patient population presenting with acute respiratory failure.

The administration of intravenous magnesium (2 g IV over 20 min) has been advocated for patients not responsive to initial bronchodilator therapy. Magnesium does have bronchodilator properties and has been used primarily in the emergency room setting for patients who fail to respond to initial therapy. Current data suggests that the agent may offer an additional form of rescue therapy in asthma patients not responsive to beta-agonists and corticosteroid therapy.

17.5 Patient Outcome

Hospitalization for a bout of respiratory failure identifies a COPD patient with a higher risk for short-term (~ 3 month) mortality. The risk is exacerbated by advanced age, disease comorbidity, a requirement for long-term oxygen therapy, and Pseudomonas colonization. The ability to confidently predict which patients will survive the acute hospitalization is limited, however.[126] We would advise caution in physician judgment regarding which patient may or may not recover from a bout of acute respiratory failure. Attention to the pre-morbid patient condition may be the most important prognostic variable.

Like the COPD patient population, patients with status asthmaticus who require mechanical ventilation have both an increased in-hospital and post-discharge mortality. Labeled as having "near fatal" asthma, these patients warrant intensive monitoring and follow-up post discharge.

A summary for COPD management is outlined in **Figure 17-10**.

Suggested Reading

- Gladwin MT, Pierson DJ. Mechanical ventilation of the patient with severe chronic obstructive pulmonary disease. Intensive Care Med. 1998 Sep;24(9):898–910.
- Pepe PE, Marini JJ. Occult positive end-expiratory pressure in mechanically ventilated patients with airflow obstruction. Am Rev Respir Dis 1982; 126:166–170.
- Rochwerg, B. *et al.* Official ERS/ATS clinical practice guidelines: noninvasive ventilation for acute respiratory failure. *Eur. Respir. J.* 50, (2017).
- Selim BJ, Wolfe L, Coleman JM, et al. Initiation of noninvasive ventilation for sleep related hypoventilation disorders. Chest 2018;153:251–265

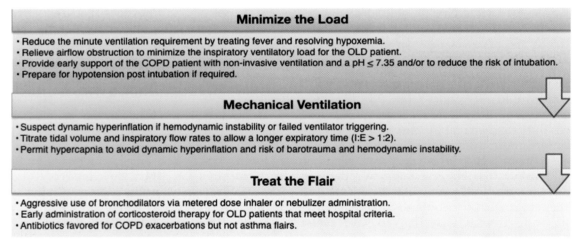

Figure 17-10 *Summary of key concepts for management of the OLD patient.*

18

Weaning from Mechanical Ventilation

You expertly managed your patient with respiratory failure, with careful correction of the abnormal gas exchange physiology, regulation of airway pressures, and a period of rest for the respiratory muscles. Now how do you get that tube out?

18.1 Control That SOB

We present an approach to weaning in this chapter that *FIRST* includes an assessment of whether the patient is truly ready to wean and *SECOND* the specific weaning trials that can be performed to see if the endotracheal tube can be removed. A series of questions can be answered to prepare a patient for liberation from the mechanical ventilator. One way to remember the approach is that to wean a patient, we must *Control That SOB* (**Figure 18-1**)!

Control the offense: Is the primary problem that resulted in mechanical ventilation resolved or controlled? If the patient had septic shock, the patient's fevers should be resolved, minute ventilation reduced, and vasopressors weaned off. If the reason was congestive heart failure, the cardiac output should be improved. If the reason was pneumonia, the oxygenation and compliance should be improved. If the problem was a stroke, the patient should be able to cough and gag and protect his/her airway. If the problem was renal failure and volume overload the patient should have undergone diuresis or be well-controlled on hemodialysis.

Control the defense: Are we protected from any unexpected left hooks? Keep an eye on total fluid volume. After massive resuscitation from septic shock or surgery, the fluid could begin to mobilize into the vasculature and cause flash pulmonary edema during the weaning process.

T for Tracheal tube: Does the patient need an endotracheal tube? Patients should be able to protect their airways, with a good strong cough and gag reflex with minimal secretions.

S for Sedation: Is the patient off sedation or on minimal sedation? Your patient should be alert and able to follow commands. A transition from longer- to shorter-acting sedatives may help, as will daily trials of sedation interruption to keep total sedation at a minimal level.

O for Oxygen: Is the oxygen requirement minimal? The patient should be on a FiO_2 of 0.40 and PEEP of 5. Remember, 40 and 5 and your patient is ready to come alive!

B for Breathing Trial: Can the patient breathe spontaneously? Now that you are controlling the offense and the defense and the patient has lower oxygen requirements and is off vasopressors, you are ready to think about weaning from the ventilator. The single most important test will be the *spontaneous breathing trial (SBT)*, but let us first review the general principles of weaning.

The physical process of removing a patient from mechanical ventilation is called *weaning*. Weaning involves a two-component patient assessment by the treating physician:

1. Is the patient ready to fully accept the burden of gas exchange and the work of breathing?
2. Is the patient able to maintain airway patency to allow successful ventilation?

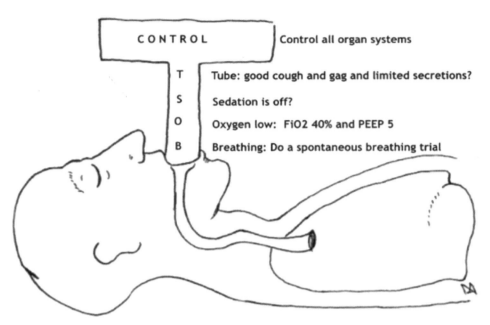

CONTROL — Control all organ systems

T — Tube: good cough and gag and limited secretions?

S — Sedation is off?

O — Oxygen low: FiO2 40% and PEEP 5

B — Breathing: Do a spontaneous breathing trial

Figure 18-1 *A summary of the key steps to weaning a patient from mechanical ventilation.*

In other words, does the patient need the machine, and does the patient need the tube? The two assessments are not always in agreement. A patient may have adequate gas exchange parameters during spontaneous ventilation to liberate from positive pressure ventilation yet have a poor mental status to protect the airway and tolerate extubation. The patient may also be producing too many airway secretions or have an insufficient cough and gag response to clear the secretions once the tube is removed.

After controlling the offense and the defense, and removing sedation, the assessment of the patient's tolerance for removal of positive pressure ventilation begins with an evaluation of the general support parameters. As a general guideline, the patient should achieve a level of inspired oxygen concentration ≤ a FiO_2 of 40% and a PEEP level ≤ 5 cm H_2O to be confident he/she can tolerate non-invasive oxygenation post-extubation. Likewise, a global assessment of the patient's ventilatory demand would include a review of resting minute ventilation on mechanical support (target < 8-10 L/min), airway pressures (< 30 cm H_2O plateau pressure), and the presence or absence of dynamic hyperinflation (PEEPi). As the level of these indices rises above the targeted norms, the patient's ability to assume the full range of mechanical ventilation declines. Despite knowledge of these parameters, no single variable appears to predict the success of weaning with a high positive and negative predictive value.

The most common approach to assess the patient's tolerance for extubation is the weaning trial. The weaning

trial transitions the patient from a controlled mode of ventilation to a full or partial spontaneous mode of ventilation. The most straightforward weaning trial is the *spontaneous breathing trial* or *SBT*. For ICU management of patients, *this is the one you all HAVE TO KNOW…*

18.2 Spontaneous Breathing Trial (SBT)

Numerous clinical trials have been conducted to compare breathing trials with or without partial ventilatory support. These trials strongly suggest that the most efficient method of weaning patients involves a spontaneous breathing trial (SBT) – also referred to as the *"Sink or Swim" method of weaning.*

Proceed with your spontaneous breathing trial in one of three ways:

1. *CPAP 5 SBT.* Place the patient on continuous positive airway pressure (CPAP) with or without pressure support (≤ 5 cm H_2O). Pressure support may be more essential if the endotracheal tube is less than 7 mm internal diameter, to overcome the resistance of the tube.
2. *T-piece trial.* Place the patient on a flow-by oxygen breathing circuit attached to the endotracheal tube.
3. *Aerosol trach mask.* This circuit refers to a spontaneous breathing circuit used when your patient has a tracheostomy tube.

During an SBT, the patient's response to the complete absence of support from the mechanical ventilator is carefully observed over a defined interval (30 minutes to 2 hours). The patient is placed on an aerosol T piece (endotracheal tube) or trach mask (tracheostomy) or on the ventilator with a continuous positive airway pressure (CPAP) of 5 cm H_2O and allowed to breathe spontaneously. In addition to the simple clinical observation, indices gathered during the SBT have been explored in order to successfully predict the success for removing positive pressure ventilation. In larger intensive care units, these spontaneous weaning trials proceed most efficiently if directed by the respiratory therapy team operating under a specific protocol. A combined sedation interruption and spontaneous breathing trial protocol is outlined in **Figure 18-2**.[127,129]

The best weaning predictor is the Rapid Shallow Breathing Index (RSBI). Clinical experiments that stress the respiratory muscles of normal individuals to fatigue demonstrate a consistent evolution of signs and symptoms in the study subject. Early signs of respiratory muscle fatigue include tachycardia and tachypnea. The tachypnea appears in tandem with a progressive decline in tidal volume. Not surprisingly, then, a simple measure of the respiratory rate (f) and the tidal volume (Vt) appears to best predict the patient who is ready to breathe without the mechanical ventilator. A person who is not fatiguing will breathe at a respiratory rate of less than about 30 breaths per minute and at a tidal volume of greater than 0.3 Liters mL (300 mL or > 4 mL per kg). Dividing the respiratory frequency (f) by the tidal volume (value in Liters) gives us a number that is called the *rapid, shallow breathing index or RSBI (f/Vt).* It is easy to remember that it is good to breathe less than 30 per minute and have a tidal volume greater than 0.3 Liters. This RR and Vt relationship gives a number for RSBI of less than 100, which is good, while more than 100 is bad.

Clinical studies have examined the operating characteristics of many weaning modalities and have found that an RSBI value < 105 has an approximately 80% positive predictive value for successful extubation and a 95% negative predictive value for unsuccessful extubation.[130] This simple test outperformed other tests, like fancy measures of compliance and the measured maximal inspiratory pressure. Plus, it is straightforward to measure!! While the utility of this parameter over simple, careful observation of the patient has been challenged, this measure is simple to do and can be incorporated into a protocol for nurses or respiratory therapists to perform.

In addition to changes in rate and tidal volume, progressive respiratory muscle fatigue can be recognized by atypical breathing patterns, including paradoxical respirations, use of accessory muscles,

tachycardia, hypertension, and confusion. Of particular note, all these signs and symptoms of respiratory muscle fatigue appear before the development of hypercapnia, measured by blood gas analysis. So, in the case of an SBT, careful clinical observation is more important to detect early signs of respiratory muscle fatigue than serial blood gas measurements.

A spontaneous breathing trial is typically continued for 30-120 minutes or until failure (tidal volumes < 0.250-0.300 Liters and respiratory rates >35-40, hypoxemia, agitation, etc.). A successful trial occurs when a patient maintains an RSBI <105 for 30-120 minutes with stable oxygenation, stable vital signs, and apparent low work of breathing.

OK. Let's put it all together in **Figure 18-3**.

18.2.1 *Spontaneous Breathing Trial Intolerance*

What happens if your patient fails the SBT? Think of this from an economic perspective, and focus on supply and demand. Supply refers to the capacity of the respiratory muscles to sustain the workload needed for spontaneous ventilation. Demand refers to the load placed upon the ventilatory muscles. Consider factors on both sides of the imbalance to advance the patient to a successful SBT.

Simple parameters to assess ventilatory demand are the minute ventilation and airway pressures (with volume cycled ventilation). A high resting minute ventilation or high airway pressures during full ventilator support suggest a high demand is placed on the respiratory muscles. Keep it simple. Ventilatory demand is produced by any factor that increases the total number or size of individual breaths required (minute ventilation) or increases the workload per individual breaths. Possible contributors to increased ventilatory demand are highlighted in **Figure 18-4**.

Ventilatory capacity, on the other hand, refers to the potential work output by the entire respiratory and cardiovascular system in response to the ventilatory demand. Many potential problems can occur in the critically ill patient that compromise the capacity for spontaneous ventilation. Examples are highlighted in **Figure 18-5**.

Particular attention should be given to the relationship between the cardiovascular and respiratory systems during the weaning process. Positive pressure ventilation can reduce the metabolic demand on the cardiovascular system by 10-15% in the patient with respiratory failure. Weaning returns the metabolic demand to the cardiovascular system. Positive pressure ventilation also acts to unload the heart by regulating venous return and reducing left ventricular afterload. The weaning process can increase myocardial filling

Sample Weaning Protocol

1. Screen patient for sedation interruption (SI) if on continuous sedative infusion:

    a. Exclusion criteria for sedation interruption protocol might include:

        i. Active seizures or alcohol withdrawal

        ii. Paralytic administration

        iii. Myocardial ischemia

        iv. Vasopressor requirement (norepinephrine > .03 mcg/kg/min or dopamine infusion > 5 mcg/kg/min, vasopressin or milrinone at any dose)

    b. If the patient has no exclusion criteria, turn off sedative and evaluate the patient for signs of intolerance to sedation interruption. These include:

        i. Increased HR, RR, or BP more than 20% over baseline vital signs; or a RR greater than 30, SpO2 less than 90% for up to 5 minutes, elevated airway pressures, hemodynamic instability, or cardiac arrhythmias.

        ii. If intolerance noted, restart sedation infusion(s) at 50% of dose utilized before interruption and up-titrate as needed.

    c. If the patient is not on a continuous infusion, proceed directly to a spontaneous breathing trial.

2. If no signs of intolerance to sedation interruption are present, evaluate for the safety of a spontaneous breathing trial.

    a. Exclusion criteria from spontaneous breathing trial might include:

        i. FiO2 $\geq$ 0.60 and/or PEEP $\geq$ 8 cm H_2O

        ii. SaO_2 < 88 %

        iii. The patient is not able to trigger the ventilator in a 5 min observation.

        iv. Myocardial ischemia in the past 24 hours

        v. Elevated intracranial pressure

        vi. Vasopressor requirement (norepinephrine > 2mcg/min or dopamine infusion > 5 mcg/kg/min, vasopressin or milrinone at any dose)

        vii. Agitated patient

    b. If the patient passes the SBT safety screening, the respiratory therapist may proceed with a SBT trial.

3. If the patient passes safety criteria for sedation interruption and SBT, proceed to SBT trial.

    a. Place the patient on one of three ventilator circuits, using a constant FiO_2 and PEEP.

        i. T tube circuit

        ii. Ventilator circuit with

            1. CPAP $\leq$ 5

            2. CPAP 5 and PS $\leq$ 5

    b. Assess patient for SBT trial failure with

        i. a respiratory rate > 35 or < 8 breaths per min for 5 min or longer

        ii. hypoxemia (SpO2 <88% for $\geq$5 min)

        iii. abrupt changes in mental status

        iv. an acute cardiac arrhythmia

        v. two or more signs of respiratory distress

            1. tachycardia (>130 bpm) or bradycardia (<60 bpm)

            2. use of accessory muscles including abdominal muscles

            3. diaphoresis or marked dyspnea

    c. Patients who show no signs of SBT trial failure within 120 min are candidates for extubation.

    d. Patients who fail the SBT trial are returned to the original ventilator settings.

Figure 18-2 *An example protocol for weaning patients from invasive mechanical ventllation.*

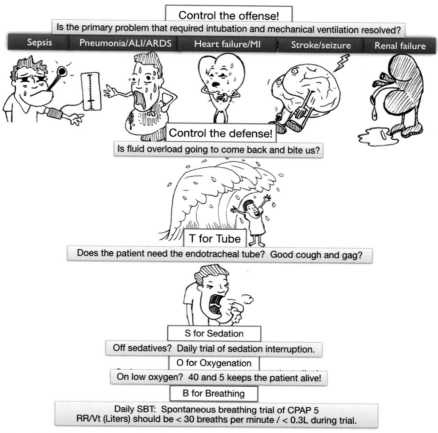

Figure 18-3 *Prepare your patient for extubation using the steps outlined by Control That SOB.*

Mechanism	Clinical Examples	Possible Solutions
High minute ventilation (V_E) secondary to increased CO_2 production	Fever, overfeeding, anxiety, pain	Resolve infections Reassess nutritional intake Mild sedative use
High V_E secondary to increased dead space ventilation	Pulmonary thromboembolism, volume contraction	Anticoagulation Volume repletion
Abnormal respiratory system compliance	CHF / Fluid overload, abdominal distention, dynamic hyperinflation	Diuresis Decompress or drain ascites Adjust ventilator parameters
Abnormal respiratory system resistance	Bronchospasm, excess secretions	Bronchodilators Treat tracheobronchitis

Figure 18-4 *Factors to consider as increasing to respiratory demand during weaning.*

Mechanism	Clinical Examples	Possible Solutions
Reduced central respiratory drive	Sedatives/narcotics, CNS depressants	Remove nonessential meds Treat underlying disorder
Reduced neuromuscular transmission	Phrenic nerve dysfunction Critical illness neuropathy	Anticoagulation Volume repletion
Neuromuscular failure	Corticosteroid-induced myopathy Electrolyte disorders	Wean medications to limit exposure Correct deficiencies
Cardiovascular dysfunction	CHF, CAD	Inotropic support

Figure 18-5 *Factors to consider as limiting to respiratory system capacity during weaning.*

pressures, leading to pulmonary edema in patients with poor ventricular function. Pulmonary edema leads to a further increase in ventilatory demand, and a cycle of failed spontaneous ventilation persists. The combination of increased left ventricular preload and heightened metabolic demand can lead to myocardial ischemia. Prior work has suggested that maintenance or elevation of cardiac output with sustained mixed venous oxygen content is an important parameter of weaning success.

18.2.2 Removing the Tube

The decision to extubate an intubated patient or move the patient to a spontaneous trach mask trial is based upon the patient's clinical response to the SBT. In addition to an RSBI < 105, clinical signs to follow include the oxygen saturation, heart rate, respiratory rate, tidal volume, accessory muscle use, and general distress prior to and during the spontaneous trial.

In addition to tolerance of the SBT, an assessment of the patient's airway is needed. The two most important parameters for the clinician to assess are the presence of a spontaneous cough and gag reflex and the need for endotracheal suctioning. No clean measurement exists for the airway assessment, and objective thresholds for the extubation decision do not exist to guide the clinician.

The duration of the SBT trial is controversial. Not surprisingly, shorter SBT trials lead to higher rates of successful extubation but also higher rates of reintubation. Studies suggest that a duration of 30 minutes is adequate, but the original studies were conducted for 120 minutes. A role for non-invasive ventilation to facilitate early extubation in COPD patients is favored. The balance between early, successful extubation and rates of reintubation remains a thorny issue to consider. If your reintubation rate is too low, you are likely delaying extubation too long, increasing the risk of ventilator-associated pneumonia, and moving too many patients to tracheotomy procedures. On the other hand, patients who require reintubation appear to have a much worse outcome than patients who did not progress to extubation.[131] Achieving a 7-10% reintubation rate is probably about right, as this balances the risk of waiting too long to extubate and limiting the downside of unsuccessful extubation. Careful clinical assessment remains the most critical parameter to guide the clinician, and the period of observation on the SBT should be sufficient to provide confidence of successful extubation.

18.3 Non-invasive Ventilation (NIV) and Weaning

Mechanical ventilation delivered via a face mask, rather than the endotracheal tube (non-invasive ventilation), may have a role during the weaning process. Potential clinical situations where non-invasive ventilation (NIV) could be employed include:

- Patients who pass the initial SBT and are extubated but require reintubation due to recurrent respiratory failure could use NIV for *rescue* to prevent the need for reintubation.
- Patients who fail SBT trials could be directly extubated to NIV as a *supportive* mode to facilitate earlier extubation.
- Patients who pass an SBT trial but are at high risk for extubation failure could receive *preventative* therapy with immediate application of NIV post extubation.

The literature here is a little mixed and can be confusing to interpret because of the variable conditions.

The *rescue* application of NIV has not been favored, based upon a large randomized clinical trial.[132] Patients with mixed etiologies for respiratory failure rescued within 48 hours post extubation demonstrated an increased patient mortality. The investigators hypothesized that delayed decisions to reinstitute mechanical ventilation may have explained the mortality effect.

The *supportive* use of NIV to accelerate extubation in patients who fail traditional weaning trials is most favored in the COPD patient population.[133] Meta-analyses have suggested that early extubation to NIV in the COPD patient population can reduce ventilator days, ICU time, and ventilator-associated pneumonias, all without increasing the risk of recurrent respiratory failure and reintubation.

The *preventative* use of NIV refers to extubating high-risk patients immediately to NIV. The strategy of immediate application of NIV post-extubation is favorable, particularly in high-risk patients with hypercapnia. The approach appears to lower the risk of reintubation in this population.[134] It gets a little tricky deciding who the high-risk population is, but older patients with underlying hypercapnia or COPD appear to be a good target for this intervention.

In summary, the immediate application of NIV post-extubation is an important tool to facilitate weaning in high-risk COPD patients and patients with hypercapnia (suggesting more ventilator failure than hypoxia). The delayed application of NIV in patients post-extubation is not helpful and may be harmful to rescue the patient from a failed extubation. Before you decide whether the supportive or preventative approach is right for your ventilator-dependent patient, think about how this might go. Is your patient likely to adapt to NIV post-extubation? Does the patient have COPD and hypercapnia that could benefit? Is the patient's mental status adequate to cooperate with NIV and protect the airway? Does the patient have experience with NIV to suggest that the patient will be compliant? Consider these factors prior to planning extubations in your weaning protocol.

18.4 Alternatives to the SBT Trial

For the patient who initially fails an SBT, the clinician will focus on interventions to reset the balance of ventilatory demand and ventilatory capacity. The patient should continue to be assessed daily for successful spontaneous breathing capacity. Current evidence strongly suggests that daily or twice daily SBTs, directed by respiratory therapists under protocol guidance, reduce weaning time and shorten ICU stay.

The clinician may choose from additional modes of ventilation to progress in the weaning process. We don't have any good evidence to support these alternative strategies, but that will not stop clinicians from trying them!!

Pressure support weaning. The alternative mode to a wholly spontaneous breathing trial is a support mode of ventilation. A *support mode* is always patient-triggered and attempts to assist the patient's normal spontaneous ventilation with support breaths only (See *Chapter 15 Mechanical Ventilation*). The most common support mode for weaning is pressure support.

The pressure support level is traditionally targeted to a level that supports patient comfort and a respiratory rate in the range of 25-30 breaths per minute. To wean, the pressure level is gradually reduced in 2-4 cm H_2O decrements until a level of 5-8 cm H_2O exists. This level of support is generally felt to reflect the airway pressure support required to overcome the resistance of the endotracheal tube. This mode of weaning is a common approach after using daily trials of spontaneous breathing (SBT).

Not surprisingly, some modern ventilators also provide a volume support mode for weaning. In the *volume support mode,* sufficient gas flow is provided to accomplish a target tidal volume. The airway pressure required to achieve the target tidal volume is adjusted on a breath-by-breath basis to reach the target. If the patient's inspiratory effort increases, the ventilator progressively reduces the airway pressure during the breath delivery to support only the minimum target volume.

The theoretical advantage of support modes is a more gradual transition to spontaneous breathing. The mode retains all ventilator monitoring and alarms. However, clinical trials have not shown an advantage to pressure support titration over a simple daily spontaneous breathing trial, even in patients with prolonged mechanical ventilation.[128]

Synchronized intermittent mandatory ventilation (SIMV) is another weaning mode that has fallen into disfavor. SIMV provides both controlled breaths and spontaneous breaths. Controlled breaths can be volume-assisted or pressure-assisted. Weaning is accomplished by reducing the set rate of the mechanical ventilator (controlled breaths) and allowing the patient to assume progressively additional spontaneous breaths. Prospective, randomized clinical trials have confirmed that the SIMV method of weaning is much less effective than other modes of weaning. For this reason, SIMV has not been considered a favored mode for weaning the patient.

18.5 Beyond the SBT Trial – Pain, Sedation, and Delirium

Weaning is not just the brilliant lung physician deciding which mode to use. Weaning is a multidisciplinary attack. In addition to the focus on respiratory care issues, coordination of general medical care is also essential in the weaning process. The timing of rehabilitation services and intervention procedures must be adjusted to assure the patient has uninterrupted time to participate in weaning. Rehabilitation efforts, including mobilization, often need to be conducted with full ventilator support until the patient has regained neuromuscular function to allow weaning from mechanical ventilation.

Pain, sedation, and delirium management in the ventilator-dependent patient deserve particular attention. Many patients on mechanical ventilation are also receiving continuous or intermittent sedation. Do not underestimate the interaction between sedative management and weaning. Your success at getting the patient awake, comfortable, and cooperative with your SBT trials will have a *MAJOR* impact on his time on that ventilator.

18.5.1 Sedation Management: Less Is More

Many observational and randomized studies have shown the benefit of limiting sedative administration to the minimal amount possible. Three approaches to sedative administration have a significant impact on weaning time. These include

1. Sedation Interruption
2. Sedation protocols
3. No sedation

The initial benchmark study for sedation management in the ventilator-dependent patient was the *sedation interruption.*[135] In this landmark trial, patients received an infusion for both pain (morphine) and a sedative (propofol or midazolam). The sedative was titrated to a standard scale. In the intervention group, an investigator not directly involved in the patients' care interrupted the sedative and narcotic infusion on a daily basis until either the patients were awake and could follow instructions or until they became uncomfortable or agitated. The sedative infusion was not interrupted if the patient was receiving a paralytic drug. A research nurse stopped the infusions until the patients were either awake or uncomfortable and in need of resumed sedation. The sedative infusions were started again if agitation prevented successful waking, at half the previous rate and were adjusted according to the need for sedation. This systematic approach to sedation reduced the median time on mechanical ventilation by 2.4 days!!

A key component of effective sedation management is the use of a measurement tool to describe the patient's level of alertness. An objective measurement tool allows effective communication between the members of the treatment team. Two commonly used tools are outlined in **Figure 18-6** (*Richmond Agitation and Sedation Scale = RASS*) and **Figure 18-7** (*Riker Sedation Agitation Scale = RSAS*). Which scale you elect to use in your ICU is less critical than a standardized approach all caregivers can

Riker Sedation Agitation Scale		
Score	Scale	Description
1	Unarousable	Minimal to no response to noxious stimuli
2	Very sedated	Arouses to physical stimuli. Doesn't communicate or follow commands. May move spontaneously
3	Sedated	Difficult to arouse. Awakens to verbal stimuli or gently shaking, but drifts off again. Follows simple commands
4	Calm/cooperative	Calm, awakens easily, follows commands
5	Agitated	Anxious or mildly agitated. Attempts to sit up. Calms with verbal instruction
6	Very agitated	Doesn't calm despite frequent verbal reminding of limits. Requires physical restraints. Bites ET tube
7	Dangerous agitation	Pulling at ET tube. Tries to remove catheters, climb over bedrail, strike at staff and/or thrashing side-to-side.

Figure 18-7 Riker Sedation Agitation Scale.

Richmond Agitation and Sedation Scale		
Score	Scale	Description
+4	Combative	Violent, combative, immediate danger
+3	Very agitated	Pulls or removes tubes/lines, aggressive
+2	Agitated	Non-purposeful movements, fights ventilator
+1	Restless	Anxious, not aggressive
0	Alert and calm	
−1	Drowsy	Not alert, opens eyes and makes eye contact to VERBAL for 10+ secs
−2	Light sedation	Not alert, opens eyes and makes eye contact to VERBAL for < 10 secs
−3	Moderate sedation	Not alert, briefly opens eyes but NO eye contact to VERBAL
−4	Deep sedation	Not alert, opens eyes to PHYSICAL stimulation
−5	Unarousable	No response to VERBAL or PHYSICAL

Figure 18.6 Richmond Agitation and Sedation Scale.

use to communicate. These scoring systems provide an excellent target for rounds discussion. Your severe ARDS patient on paralysis may be a Riker target of 1 early in his course when paralytic agents may be required. Later in his course, that target may shift to a Riker of 4 when you are weaning the patient. By incorporating these scoring systems into your rounds discussion, all members on the treatment teach are working toward the same goal. These scoring systems are very similar, with slightly different value assignments to the specific clinical states. A multidisciplinary goal is to get your ventilator-dependent patient ready for weaning to a target of 0 to −1 on the RASS or 3 to 4 or the Riker = awake and cooperative. Both scores have good reliability and are in everyday use.

As previously mentioned, the sedation interruption method combines with a spontaneous breathing trial to provide a *Wake Up and Breathe* method for weaning patients from mechanical ventilation.[127]

An alternative strategy to sedation interruption is the strict use of a sedation protocol. The Canadian Critical Care Trials group compared the use of a sedation protocol with sedation interruption.[136] The bedside nurse titrated analgesic and sedative administration using a target RSAS of 3 or 4 or a RASS of −3 to 0. This approach was equivalent to the sedation interruption approach.

The third and most dramatic approach is the use of *NO SEDATION!* Not possible, you say? A group of Danish investigators compared no sedation (n=70) patients to sedation patients (20 mg/mL propofol for 48 h, 1 mg/mL midazolam thereafter).[137] The group that received sedation had a daily interruption until awake. The no sedation group had more ventilator-free days and shorter ICU stays. No difference was recorded in the occurrence of accidental extubations. Agitated delirium was more frequent in the intervention group than in the control group.

How should we interpret these studies? You must strive to minimize sedation to the minimum required to keep your patient safe on mechanical ventilation. Exactly how the doctors and nurses accomplish this goal is probably not specific, but it should be a focus of your care every day. *DO NOT* leave the bedside from your rounds without a discussion of the patient's sedation management.

In summary, what can we say about sedation in the ICU? Simple – *LESS IS MORE.* Try to maintain your ICU patient with the least amount of sedation required to maintain patient safety.

18.5.2 Pain Management

How do we determine if our ICU patients have pain that is not appropriately treated? This can be very difficult when the patient has limited communication (e.g., endotracheal tube $+/-$ encephalopathy). Nurses often interpret tachycardia or hypertension as clinical signs of pain – but are we sure these are sensitive or specific indicators in the complex ICU patient? Despite the lack of objective data to guide pain management in the ICU patient population, we can assume that an endotracheal tube and other ICU procedures are at the very least unpleasant, if not painful. Current guidelines for pain management in the ICU have favored an *analgesic first* approach for ICU patients with agitation or delirium. If pain is suspected or uncertain, initial doses of an analgesic are provided, and the patient response is assessed. Ideally, intermittent dosing can be used.

18.5.3 Delirium

Delirium, in general, refers to an acute waxing and waning confusional state that occurs in ICU patients. We know a few crucial concepts about delirium in the ICU patient. It happens a lot. A patient who experiences delirium has a longer ICU length of stay and higher hospital mortality. We are not sure if delirium causes the bad outcome or is just a marker for a sick patient. Now the prevention and treatment of delirium is another story – we have a long way to go! If you are looking for a magical pill for your patient with delirium, you might want to stop reading.

OK, we know a couple of other things:

- Delirium can occur in a hyperactive or hypoactive form in the ICU patient, and both could contribute to a limitation in successful weaning.
- Bedside clinicians do not recognize delirium very well during their daily patient assessment.
- Specific factors seem to predispose the patient to delirium, including advanced age, underlying neurologic conditions (including dementia), the use of sedative agents (especially benzodiazepines), and severe critical illness.

Hyperactive delirium is characterized by agitation, restlessness, pulling at catheters and tubes, or hitting/striking ICU staff. *Hypoactive delirium* is characterized by flat affect, apathy, lethargy, possibly to the point of being nonresponsive. As a general rule, the hyperactive form is more frequently recognized by ICU clinicians than the hypoactive form.

Two scoring systems have evolved to measure delirium in the ICU population. The logic for using an objective scoring system is simple – if we cannot even recognize delirium in our patients, then we probably will never learn how to treat it. *The Confusion Assessment Method (CAM-ICU)* for delirium assessment is illustrated in **Figure 18.8**. The CAM-ICU uses nonverbal tasks such as picture recognition, vigilance task, simple yes/no logic questions and simple commands to assess the patient for delirium. The delirium criteria and algorithm used to determine the presence of delirium include (a) acute mental status change, (b) inattention, (c) disorganized thinking, and (d) altered level of consciousness. Delirium is considered to be present if criteria a and b and either criteria c or d are present.

When using the CAM-ICU, the patient must meet criteria for LEVEL I and LEVEL II – and then have features of either LEVEL III or LEVEL IV. You can learn a great deal about the CAM-ICU and ICU delirium in general by checking the following website: http://www.icudelirium.org/delirium/monitoring.html.

An alternative approach to the CAM-ICU, with relatively comparable sensitivity, is the *Intensive Care Delirium Screening Checklist (ICDSC)*.[138] The ICDSC is shown in **Figure 18-9.** The ICDSC includes eight features of delirium, including: inattention; disorientation; hallucination-delusion psychosis; psychomotor agitation or retardation; inappropriate speech or mood; sleep/wake cycle disturbances; and symptom fluctuation. The ICDSC uses a 0 to 8 scoring system and a score more than 4 is defined as delirium positive.

While current guidelines advocate for the routine use of these scales in your ICU patients, the goal is primarily to recognize delirium. The routine use of the delirium scales has not yet been demonstrated to change the patient outcome.

Confusion Assessment Method (CAM) - ICU
Patients can only be assessed for delirium if the RASS is −3 to −5 or the RSAS > 3.
If true, proceed to Level I
LEVEL I: ACUTE CHANGE OR FLUCTUATING COURSE OF MENTAL STATUS Does the patient have a change in mental status from baseline? Does the patient have a fluctuating mental status over the past 24 hours? If the answer to either question is yes – proceed with the CAM-ICU assessment. If the answer to both questions is no – the patient is CAM-ICU negative and the patient does not have delirium. Proceed to Level II.
LEVEL II: INATTENTION Say, "Squeeze my hand when I say the letter 'A,' and then say the phrase 'S-A-V-E-A-H-A-A-R-T.'" An error is defined if the patient fails to squeeze on "A" and squeezes on another letter than "A." If the rate of error is 0-2, the patient is CAM-ICU negative. If errors > 2, patient is positive at Level II, and then proceed to Level III.
LEVEL III: ALTERED LEVEL OF CONSCIOUSNESS If RSAS = other than 4 or RASS other than 0, the patient is CAM-ICU positive. If RSAS = 4 or RASS = 0 proceed to LEVEL IV

LEVEL IV: DISORGANIZED THINKING
 	
The patient is asked the following questions
    1. Will a stone float on water?
    2. Are there fish in the sea?
    3. Does one pound weigh more than 2?
    4. Can you use a hammer to pound a nail?
 	
Errors are counted when the patient incorrectly answers a question.
 	
Command: "Hold up this many fingers." (Hold up two fingers.)
 	
"Now do the same thing with the other hand."
 	
OR "Add one more finger" if patient unable to move both arms.
 	
An error is counted if the patient is unable to follow the command.
 	
If the patient has > 1 total combined errors – CAM ICU POSITIVE

Figure 18-8 The CAM-ICU.

Intensive Care Delirium Screening Checklist (ICDSC)	
Score 8 items based upon DSM criteria with a 0 = absent and 1= present scale	
Altered level of consciousness	
Inattention	
Disorientation	
Hallucinations	
Psychomotor agitation or retardation	
Inappropriate speech	
Sleep/wake cycle disturbance	
Symptom fluctuation	
TOTAL SCORE	Normal =0 Subsyndromal delirium 1-3 Delirium ⩾ 4

Figure 18-9 Intensive Care Delirium Screening Checklist (ICDSC).

When identified, a multi-faceted approach to delirium in the ICU patient population is advocated. The components of that approach might include:

- Remove all nonessential medications that can cause delirium.
  - o Minimize sedation exposure, especially benzodiazepines.
  - o Stop nonessential anticholinergic medications.
- Use non-pharmacologic interventions.
  - o Provide open visitation for family members.
  - o Focus on noise reduction.
  - o Provide availability of glasses or hearing aids if appropriate.
  - o Provide orientation items, including a clock and calendar.
  - o Promote a sleep/wake cycle.
  - o Advocate for patient mobility (see below).
- Use pharmacologic interventions when appropriate.
  - o Currently, no data exist to support the routine use of prophylactic antipsychotic medication.
  - o Antipsychotic medications should be used cautiously in the ICU population and avoided in patients with a prolonged QT syndrome.

In summary, what can we say about delirium in the ICU?

- Delirium is a frequent clinical problem for mechanically ventilated patients, and when present, contributes to an adverse outcome and prolonged time on mechanical ventilation.
- Clinicians must be alert for signs/symptoms of delirium during their daily patient assessment, using either an objective scoring assessment or *gestalt* diagnosis.
- Treatment currently consists of a multi-faceted patient review focused on both non-pharmacologic and pharmacologic measures. Antipsychotic medications are not effective in the treatment of ICU delirium.[139]

18.5.4 Early Mobility in the ICU

For many years, the typical sequence for an ICU ventilator dependent patient was

- Fix the problem.
- Wake up from sedation.
- Wean to complete spontaneous breathing with extubation.
- Start to mobilize the patient.

More recently, investigators have started to question this sequence and move the goal of patient mobility to the top of the list – often called *early mobility in the ICU*. Two early studies were conducted in this area and showed favorable outcomes.[140,141] The early mobility patients showed a higher functional status at discharge with reduced ICU delirium, a reduction in overall sedative use, greater functional status, and reduced ICU and hospital length of stay. The results are not uniformly positive; however, other investigators have not found an impact on LOS.[142,143]

In summary, what can we say about early mobility in the ICU?

- The practice of early mobility initiatives in the ICU requires significant care coordination among physicians, nurses, and physical/occupational therapy staff.
- Early mobility appears to have favorable effects on delirium and patient functional status.
- Early mobility initiatives currently investigated have not had a consistent impact on length of stay parameters in the ICU or hospital.

18.6 Coordination of Ventilator Care – Know Your Alphabet?

Wow!! That was a lot of information. How can we bring this all together? To simplify, the Society of Critical Care Medicine has advocated a bundle approach to organize this during your daily rounds. The more recent version is the *ABCDEF* bundle for daily management of the patient on mechanical ventilation (http://www.icudelirium.org/medicalprofessionals.html) summarized in **Figure 18-10**.

You may find the bundle serves as a useful checklist for your ICU rounds. After you have amazed the rounding team with your complicated discussion of ventilator physiology and cardiovascular hemodynamics – do not leave that bedside until the whole team has reviewed Pain-Sedation-Delirium-Mobility.

18.7 When Is a Tracheotomy Indicated?

Tracheotomy is one of the most common procedures performed in the patient with acute respiratory failure and ventilator dependence. The procedure is most commonly performed electively in patients who require prolonged mechanical ventilation to facilitate weaning from the ventilator. Less frequently, tracheotomy is performed on an emergent basis due to a "difficult airway" to address upper airway obstruction. The potential advantages of tracheotomy when performed to assist weaning are outlined in **Figure 18-11**.

In contrast, the potential disadvantages of a tracheotomy are outlined in **Figure 18-12**.

BUNDLE	PARAMETER	COMMENTS
A	Assess, Prevent, and Manage Pain	Guidelines favor an objective pain scale monitoring tool. "Treat first" approach to pain in the setting of agitation and delirium
B	Both Spontaneous Awakening Trials and Spontaneous Breathing Trials	Follow the *Wake Up and Breathe* protocols for SI and SBT.
C	Choice of Analgesia and Sedation	Minimal effective dosing to provide for patient pain relief and safety. Use a goal-directed approach with a standardized measurement tool such as RSAS or RASS.
D	Delirium: Assess, Prevent, and Manage	Guided by an objective assessment tool (CAM-ICU or ICDSC), with attention to pharmacologic and non-pharmacologic measures to reduce delirium
E	Early Mobility and Exercise	Consider interventions early after intubation.
F	Family Engagement and Empowerment	Engage the family in all aspects of the patient's ICU care.

Figure 18-10 ABCDEF Ventilator weaning bundle.

Mechanism of Improvement	Clinical Manifestation
Improved respiratory mechanics	Reduction of upper airway anatomic dead space
Reduced laryngeal ulceration	
Improved patient comfort	Reduced sedation requirement Improved patient mobility
Improved secretion clearance	
Improved speech and swallowing	

Figure 18-11 Potential advantages of a tracheotomy.

Complications	Comment
Immediate surgical complications	Bleeding (5%), tracheal wound infection, subcutaneous emphysema
Tracheal tube occlusion	Mucous or soft tissue of tracheal wall
Fistula formation	Tracheoinnominate artery (<0.7%) or Tracheoesophageal (<1%)
False passage	During procedure or during early tube displacement
Tracheal stenosis	1-2% of procedures and more frequent with high pressure cuffs
Persistent stoma	Seen post decannulation

Figure 18-12 Potential disadvantages of a tracheotomy.

18.7.1 Timing and Technique of Tracheotomy

Significant debate exists regarding the optimal timing and technique for tracheotomy in the patient with prolonged mechanical ventilation. A meta-analysis of the published trials has suggested that early (< 10 days post-intubation) compared to late (> 10 days post intubation) tracheotomy did not show an effect on ICU length of stay, mortality, or ventilator-associated pneumonia.[144]

In the absence of strong data favoring early tracheotomy, physician judgment regarding the risk:benefit ratio generally guides the decision to proceed. The decision to perform an elective tracheotomy in the patient with ventilator dependence balances two problems: 1) the likelihood of significant laryngeal injury with the continued use of an endotracheal tube vs. 2) the frequency of surgical and stoma-related complications following tracheotomy. Additional consideration is given to the role of tracheotomy in facilitating the weaning process. Factors other than absolute time should play the major role in the decision to perform a tracheotomy. The timing of tracheotomy should be individualized.

Absolute contraindications to tracheotomy include

- Skin infection at the surgical site
- Prior neck surgery that obscures the normal anatomy
- Coagulopathy

Relative contraindications to tracheotomy include

- High inspired oxygen concentration ($FiO_2 > 0.50$)
- High end-expiratory pressure (PEEP > 10 cm H20)
- Hemodynamic instability

The tracheotomy is performed as an "open" surgical tracheotomy either in the operating room or at the patient's bedside. In an "open" procedure, blunt dissection is used to accomplish a transverse or vertical incision in the trachea. Alternatively, the procedure can be done percutaneously. Percutaneous tracheotomy is performed by progressive blunt dilation of a small tracheal opening produced by passing a wire through a needle in the trachea (*Seldinger technique*). Bronchoscopic visualization confirms the needle and subsequent guide wire are positioned in the trachea. In either trach procedure, the endotracheal tube is slowly withdrawn to a position just above the tracheotomy insertion point. The endotracheal tube is not removed until the tracheotomy tube is placed, and the position confirmed. Currently available data suggest the percutaneous approach has at least an equivalent risk-benefit profile to the open tracheotomy procedure and may reduce the incidence of post-procedure bleeding and peristomal infection.

18.7.2 Type and Size of the Tracheotomy Tube

Tracheotomy tubes are available in graded lengths and diameters. The tubes may contain a single cannula (no removable internal cannula) or a dual cannula (removable internal cannula). The advantage of an internal cannula is related to secretion management as the internal cannula can be changed daily or more frequently when necessary. There is usually no need to change the outer tracheotomy tube. Changing of the tracheotomy should be avoided for at least 1 week after the creation of the stoma. If a difficult tracheotomy tube change is anticipated, a clinician experienced in endotracheal intubation should be present. Tracheotomy tubes may come with or without a cuff for inflation. The cuff is intended to seal the trachea during positive pressure ventilation and may minimize (but not eliminate) a tendency to aspiration. Tracheotomy

tubes with foam cuffs conform to the patient's trachea and maintain a low-pressure seal. The tracheotomy tube may have a small opening in the superior wall of the tube called a *fenestration*. This opening is expected to facilitate speech in the patient who is liberated from mechanical ventilation for specific intervals.

Tracheotomy tube changes are indicated for malfunction, inspissated secretions, or when a different tracheotomy tube design is necessary. Routine changes of tracheotomy tubes are not advised.

Both the initial selection of a tracheotomy tube and subsequent tube changes should involve a careful analysis of tube dimensions. The standard tracheotomy tube has three important dimensions to consider:

1. *Length*. This parameter refers to the distance from the trach tube face plate to the tip of the tube. This distance changes when tracheal tube size changes or sometimes when the manufacturer of the trach tube changes. Adequate length must exist to set the tracheal tube securely within the tracheal airway.
2. *Outer diameter*. An important parameter to compare with tube changes to be sure the stoma is wide enough to accept a replacement tube
3. *Inner diameter*. An important parameter that influences the resistive work of breathing and secretion clearance

All tracheotomy tube manufacturers have numbering systems that identify their tubes. However, *the numbering systems do not necessarily imply equivalent tube dimensions*. Careful comparison of the listed dimensions is essential, especially when changing the brand of the tracheotomy tube.

18.7.3 Care of the Tracheotomy Tube

The tracheotomy cannula should be secured in place and the tracheotomy left to heal for 5-7 days, to allow for the development of a stable and patent cutaneous-endotracheal tract. The tracheotomy wound should remain clean and dry to prevent post-incisional wound infection. When a dual cannula is used, the inner cannula can be changed daily or more frequently if necessary. Changing the outer cannula within 5-7 days after placement is dangerous due to the risk of collapse of the cutaneous-endotracheal tract and subsequent loss of the airway. Tube replacement can be associated with a false passage of the tube into the anterior tracheal space, leading to subcutaneous emphysema. The only indication to change the outer cannula is when the cuff has been damaged or when a tracheotomy tube of different size or shape is necessary. The early change of the outer tracheotomy tube, especially when a percutaneous technique has been performed, should be performed by a practitioner who is trained in the method.

Tracheotomy tube cuffs require monitoring to maintain pressures in a range of 20-25 mmHg. High cuff pressures (> 25-35 mmHg) exceed the capillary perfusion pressure and can result in compression of mucosal capillaries, which promotes mucosal ischemia and tracheal stenosis. The tracheostomy tube should be maintained in a central position in the trachea to minimize damage to the tracheal wall. The goal is to avoid traction as well as unnecessary movement of the tube.

The tracheotomy tube bypasses the functions of the upper airway to filter, heat, and humidify the inspired gas. This function must be replaced by providing appropriately treated inspired air, even if the patient is breathing room air oxygen. The lack of humidification in an early tracheostomy is associated with mucosal damage, loss of mucociliary transport, and thickening of airway secretions. These changes may, in turn, increase the risk for lower respiratory tract infection and provoke airway obstruction by endoluminal mucous impaction.

18.7.4 Swallowing

The replacement of the endotracheal tube by the tracheotomy tube allows the patient to begin consideration of oral dietary intake but may initially interfere with the normal swallowing mechanism, especially with larger tracheotomy tubes. A tracheotomy tube inhibits the physiologic upward movement of the larynx during deglutition, hinders glottic closure, and produces dysphagia due to mechanical compression of the esophagus. Candidates for possible dietary intake include patients with a normal mental status who have adequate oxygenation with low inspired oxygen concentrations and possess sufficient ventilatory reserve such that they can physiologically tolerate an episode of aspiration during the introduction of oral feeding. Ideally, a speech therapist should assess aspiration risk before the institution of an oral diet.

18.7.5 Decannulation

Patients who are successfully liberated from mechanical ventilation and managing their respiratory secretions may be candidates for decannulation. Occlusion of the trach tube can test the patient's tolerance for decannulation. Patients who can breathe around their current tube most likely have an adequate respiratory reserve and a sufficiently preserved native airway to tolerate decannulation. Alternatively, patients unable to accomplish these goals may need to undergo a progressive downsize of their tracheotomy tube. Patients who continue to fail trials of tracheotomy occlusion should undergo laryngoscopic evaluation to exclude the presence of tracheal stenosis or other pathology above the trach tube. Tracheotomy tubes with foam cuffs should not be used for decannulation trials because these cuffs can spontaneously reinflate, providing a risk of airway occlusion if the trachea cannula remains capped.

Suggested Reading

- Devlin JW, Skrobik Y, Gélinas C, et al. Clinical practice guidelines for the prevention and management of pain, agitation/sedation, delirium, immobility, and sleep disruption in adult patients in the ICU. Crit Care Med 2018;46(9):e825–73.
- Neufeld KJ, Yue J, Robinson TN, Inouye SK, Needham DM. Antipsychotic medication for prevention and treatment of delirium in hospitalized adults: A systematic review and meta-analysis. J Am Geriatr Soc 2016;64(4):705–14.
- Rochwerg B, Brochard L, Elliott MW, et al. Official ERS/ATS clinical practice guidelines: noninvasive ventilation for acute respiratory failure. Eur Respir J [Internet] 2017;50(2):1602426.
- Pun BT, Balas MC, Barnes-Daly MA, et al. Caring for Critically Ill Patients with the ABCDEF Bundle. Crit Care Med [Internet] 2019;47(1):3–14.

19

Bleeding, Clotting and Hematological Emergencies

This chapter covers bleeding, clotting and the available drugs that modulate bleeding and clotting. It also summarizes the top four hematology emergencies you will face in the hospital: HIT, DIC, TTP, and CAPS – letter salad now, but it will all be clear to you later! All of these conditions represent medical emergencies and have an impact on multiple organ systems. Let's start with a review of the clotting cascade and relate this to diseases you will see and drugs you will use.

19.1 Clotting Cascade: Help Me Memorize!!!

The clotting cascade involves an extrinsic pathway, and intrinsic pathway, and a common pathway. The extrinsic or tissue factor pathway is activated by external trauma to the vascular system. The instrinsic or contact activation pathway is activated by trauma inside the vascular system. Both the extrinsic and instrinsic pathway meet at the common pathway leading to clot formation.

It is helpful to draw out the clotting cascade yourself as we go (**Figure 19-1**). Let's build this together with some memory tools and integrate this with the diseases and drugs you will face in the intensive care unit. The blue boxes in the figure include mnemonics summarized below.

For memorization it is usually easier to remember in numbers rather than Roman numerals; your modern neurons are programmed to "see" these symbols better. Let's start on the right side, which is the extrinsic pathway and activated by tissue factor, for example during trauma or obstetrical complications.

19.1.1 Extrinsic or Tissue Factor Pathway

Lucky (VII) for you this side is EXtra (extrinsic) simple, with only one factor, lucky 7 (VII). The Extrinsic pathway is the War side, as the drug Warfarin inhibits it. In war, you have to go to basic training and get lots of EXercise (more extrinsic) and Physical Training (PT), which you will have to do 7 days a week. There will be trauma (unlucky 7) and tissue (factor) injury that sets off this pathway. Following damage to the blood vessel, factor 7 leaves the circulation and comes into contact with tissue factor (TF), forming an activated complex (TF-FVIIa). Note that women are now allowed to fight in wars in the U.S., so obstetrical emergencies can also release tissue factor. So your mnemonic for the extrinsic pathway is in italics below.

Lucky 7 Extra simple; War exercise-PT; trauma and tissue (factor) injury

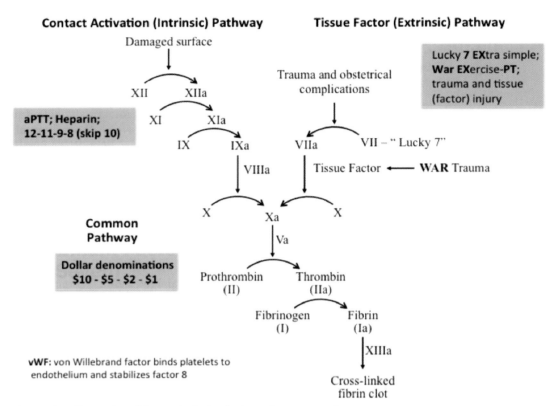

Contact Activation (Intrinsic) Pathway

Damaged surface

XII → XIIa

XI → XIa

IX → IXa

VIIIa

aPTT; Heparin;
12-11-9-8 (skip 10)

Tissue Factor (Extrinsic) Pathway

Trauma and obstetrical complications

VIIa   VII – " Lucky 7"

Tissue Factor ← WAR Trauma

Lucky **7 EX**tra simple;
War EXercise-**PT**;
trauma and tissue
(factor) injury

Common Pathway

Dollar denominations
$10 - $5 - $2 - $1

X   Xa   X

Va

Prothrombin (II)   Thrombin (IIa)

Fibrinogen (I)   Fibrin (Ia)

XIIIa

Cross-linked fibrin clot

vWF: von Willebrand factor binds platelets to endothelium and stabilizes factor 8

Figure 19-1 *Ilustration of the extrinsic, intrinsic, and common pathways.*

19.1.2 Intrinsic or Contact (collagen) Activation Pathway

Once you have that right side memorized, the left side is easier. The Intrinsic pathway is just the other one, so it is monitored by PTT and inhibited by heparin. To remember the factors, they go down in descending order and just skip 10. So:

The left side is aPTT; Heparin; 12-11-9-8 (skip 10)

From a mechanistic standpoint, this intrinsic pathway is the contact activation pathway and begins with a damaged surface of a blood vessel, exposing the underlying collagen. This leads to formation of the primary complex on collagen of high-molecular-weight kininogen (HMWK), prekallikrein, and factor 12 (XII or Hageman factor). Prekallikrein is converted to kallikrein, and XII becomes XIIa to set it all off.

Activation of the intrinsic contact factor pathway or the extrinsic tissue factor pathways both converge at 10, which also helps you remember which one is skipped in the intrinsic pathway. Now just think of dollar denominations, which are the available bills from 10 down:

$10 / $5 / $2 (Prothrombin to thrombin) / $1 (Fibrinogen to fibrin)

Thrombin's primary role is the conversion of fibrinogen to fibrin, which forms the building block of a hemostatic plug.

19.1.3 Anti-Clotting Pathways

Four significant enzymes keep the coagulation cascade in check. These are shown in gray circles added in **Figure 19-2** with the targets that they inhibit. Drugs activate or inhibit these pathways to prevent clotting. Abnormalities in these enzymes can lead to an increased tendency toward thrombosis:

1. *Protein C* is a primary physiologic anticoagulant. Protein C is activated by thrombin into activated Protein C (APC). Activated Protein C, along with Protein S and a cofactor phospholipid, degrades activated factor 7 and 8 (VIIa and VIIIa). Any deficiency of Protein C or S can lead to a risk for thrombosis (thrombophilia). Activated protein C had been developed as a therapy for sepsis that did not work for sepsis, but one of the side effects was that it could promote bleeding.

2. *Antithrombin III* is a serine protease inhibitor that degrades almost *ALL* of the serine proteases: the activated factors XIIa, XIa, IXa, Xa and thrombin (IIa). Note that it targets all the proteases in the light gray circle in **Figure 19-2**. Antithrombin III is continuously active, but its adhesion to these factors is increased by the presence of heparan sulfate (a glycosaminoglycan) or the administration of heparins. The low molecular weight heparins

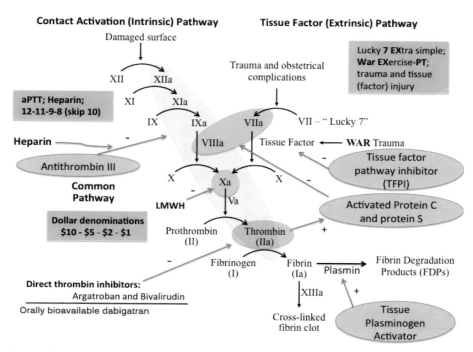

Figure 19-2 *Anti-clotting pathways aligned with the clotting pathways.*

specifically target the sequence of antithrombin to factor Xa.

3. *Tissue factor pathway inhibitor (TFPI)* limits the action of tissue factor (TF). It also inhibits excessive TF-mediated activation of factor 7 (VII). New inhibitors of tissue factor pathway inhibitor are being developed to promote clotting and stop bleeding in hemophilia patients.

4. *Plasmin* is generated by cleavage of plasminogen, a plasma protein synthesized in the liver. This cleavage is catalyzed by tissue plasminogen activator (t-PA), which is synthesized and secreted by endothelium and is given as a drug (alteplase for heart attacks or massive pulmonary embolism). Plasmin proteolytically cleaves fibrin into fibrin degradation products that inhibit excessive fibrin formation.

Here's a silly mnemonic to remember the four inhibitory factors: *Politically Correct People are Anti Tissue Paper and Plastics* (**P**rotein C, **Anti**-thrombin III, **Tissue** factor pathway inhibitor and **Plas**min).

19.2 Overview of Bleeding and Clotting disorders

You have to know what your drugs do and what diseases knock out what factors to diagnose patients

accurately in the hospital. The terminology for the drugs continues to involve but currently we talk about four main categories of medications related to the clotting process:

1. Antithrombotic agents – include anticoagulants and antiplatelet agents.
2. Anticoagulants – includes medications that inhibit steps in the coagulation cascade with a wide variety of mechanisms.
3. Direct factor Xa inhibitors – includes medications that prevent factor Xa from converting prothrombin to thrombin. These medications bind directly to factor Xa, in contrast to heparin which enhances the activity of antithrombin III. These include the oral medications rivaroxaban, apixaban, edoxaban, and betrixaban.
4. Direct thrombin (IIa) inhibitors – prevent thrombin from cleaving fibrinogen to fibrin. The intravenous medications include bivalirudin, argatroban, and desirudin. The oral medication available in this class is dabigatran.

So you can remember all those new direct acting oral anticoagulants (DOAC's) by their mechanism of action which is to "ban Xa" because they include Xa-Ban in their name e.g., rivaro*xaban*. Note that the direct thrombin inhibitor dabigatran does not contain Xa-Ban.

Here are a few concepts that you can work into your coagulation cascade knowledge. Some of these will be reinforced in discussions of the top four ICU hematological emergencies.

19.2.1 Things that Elevate the PT-INR

Warfarin overdose or drug interactions that increase warfarin levels are very common. You now know that your War overdose will increase your Ex-PT. Patients can present with PT values (measured now by INR) of 5-12 times normal! Warfarin inhibits the vitamin K epoxide reductase enzyme (VKOR) required to produce reduced Vitamin K. Reduced vitamin K is required for the synthesis of clotting factors II, VII, IX and X, as well as the anti-clotting factors protein C and S. Since warfarin can lower the levels of factor IX, a severe overdose will start to increase the PTT as well. Many rodent poisons are long-acting warfarin analogs called *coumarins*, and patients can present with overdoses of these drugs, with very high PT/INR values. Treatment with vitamin K, fresh frozen plasma, and prothrombin complex concentrate (PCC) to restore the clotting factors will work.

Warfarin can produce a severe massive thrombosis in blood vessels that can cause skin necrosis and gangrene of limbs. While we think of warfarin as an anti-clotting drug by blocking factor 7, it also inhibits vitamin K-dependent synthesis of the anti-clotting proteins C and S. Since they have the shortest half-lives, when you first start warfarin, the levels of C and S drop before 7, so you get a brief period of hypercoagulability. Patients at the highest risk for this are patients with genetic protein C or S deficiency or sick patients (liver disease, with severe infections or malnourished) whom we see in the ICU who start with lower C and S levels. We *ALWAYS USE A BRIDGE* strategy of starting heparin with warfarin in sick patients to limit the risk of clotting and warfarin skin necrosis. *In fighting a WAR, you always need to build bridges, so bridge with heparin.*

Rare factor 7 inhibitors or autoantibodies to 7 (*rare for 7 to be unlucky*) can cause high PT values and bleeding in the ICU. The direct thrombin inhibitors also elevate the INR.

19.2.2 Things that Elevate the PTT

The PTT rises when the intrinsic and common pathways are inhibited. The PTT is longer than PT and the intrinsic and common are long: PTT reflects inhibition of 12, 11, 9, 8, 10, 5, 2, 1. *You can actually remember this using the descending 12 to 8, skip 10, then 10 to 1 in dollars!!!*

Heparin works by binding to and activating plasma antithrombin III (**Figure 19-1**). The heparin-antithrombin III complex inhibits most of the intrinsic and common pathway-activated clotting factors (XIIa, Xa, IXa) and especially thrombin (IIa), thus preventing the fibrin thrombus formation. Heparin specifically increases the PTT. Since it is an inhibitor, it cannot be reversed by giving the clotting factors back as can be done for the hemophilias. Protamine sulfate is a specific antidote for heparin, used in major bleeding emergencies.

But remember that low molecular weight heparins (LMWH) do not increase PTT. There are a number of these drugs, including *enoxaparin*, *dalteparin*, and *tinzaparin*, which are given as subcutaneous injections. They are about 1/3 the size of heparin, have a long half-life so that they can be given once or twice a day subcutaneously, and have more direct anti-factor Xa activity. To remember this, *think that heparin has been cut down in size and refined to create a low molecular weight cruise missile that knocks out the middle of the intrinsic and common pathway: Xa* (see the specific Xa targeting in **Figure 19-2**). A few critical clinical concepts to remember about the LMWHs:

- Most of the elevation in PTT comes from inhibiting thrombin, so the LMWH do not change PTT much. To monitor activity, you have to send a Xa activity test, which is now commonly ordered.
- They are excreted by the kidney, so they are difficult to dose in renal dysfunction and are typically avoided in these cases.
- They can still cause HIT (a disease described later in this chapter) even though they are small! *Remember: A LMWH cruise missile can HIT factor Xa.*
- *Fondaparinux* is a synthetic pentasaccharide that causes antithrombin III-mediated inhibition of factor Xa, so it is monitored in the same way. *Pearl: This anticoagulant does NOT cause HIT.*

Direct thrombin inhibitors including the drugs argatroban and bivalirudin are treatments for HIT as described below. They work by inhibiting thrombin and will increase the PTT. The direct thrombin inhibitors also prolong the INR with argatroban having the greatest effect.

Dabigatran (trade name *Pradaxa*) is an oral bioavailable direct thrombin inhibitor. Dabigatran is now indicated for the treatment of non-valvular atrial fibrillation, venous thromboembolism, and pulmonary embolism. Since it inhibits thrombin, it also raises PTT, but at therapeutic doses has less effect on PT/INR. In case of overdose or severe bleeding complications, a monoclonal antibody inhibitor of dabigatran (*idarucizumab*) has now been shown to reverse its effects rapidly.[145]

Hemophilia A is a genetic deficiency in factor 8 (VIII), and hemophilia B is a genetic deficiency in factor 9 (IX), so both can elevate the PTT. *Remember that A rhymes with 8.* Patients have normal platelets, so they will stop bleeding initially but cannot form the full fibrin mesh and will rebleed later. Bleeding into the joints and post-operative or trauma-related hematomas and significant bleeds are typical. Specific therapy with recombinant factor VIII and IX is the way to go here. Interestingly, a new approach involves the therapeutic delivery of a liver-targeted silencing RNA (siRNA) that binds to and inhibits the mRNA that encodes antithrombin III. Since Antithrombin III is a serine protease inhibitor that degrades almost *ALL* of the serine proteases (activated factors XIIa, XIa, IXa, Xa and IIa), this helps offset the deficiency of factors VIII or IX (8 or 9). Since antithrombin III inhibits activated thrombin (IIa), this inhibitor will increase clotting ability in hemophilia patients.

von Willebrand factor (vWF) is synthesized in endothelial cells and plays a vital role in helping clot formation by binding platelets to the endothelium to initiate the platelet plug in tears or holes that form in the blood vessel. It also stabilizes factor 8. Patients with von Willebrand disease (vWD), a common genetic disease, usually present with normal platelet counts but a prolonged bleeding time (a measure of platelet dysfunction) and are at risk of bleeding during procedures in the ICU. A key to diagnosis is that vWF stabilizes the half-life of factor 8 (VIII) in the intrinsic (PTT) pathway; so when vWF is low, the factor 8 levels are low, and the PTT is often prolonged as if the patient is taking heparin. Treatment can start with desmopressin (DDAVP), which increases factor 8 formation from the endothelium. If more bang for the buck is needed, one can give FFP or cryoprecipitate, which contain vWF (lots in cryoprecipitate).

Auto-antibodies to factors such as a Factor VIII inhibitor can result in severe bleeding problems.

To diagnose the cause of an elevated PTT one can do a mixing study and a protamine sulfate mixing study. Mixing studies use the patient's plasma mixed with plasma that replaces the missing factors to $\geq 50\%$ of their normal levels. Factor deficiencies will be corrected with mixing studies (hemophilia, vWF, liver disease, disseminated intravascular coagulation) while auto-immune factor inhibitors and heparin will not. Heparin will correct with protamine sulfate which binds the heparin and makes it inactive.

19.2.3 Things that Elevate both PT-INR and PTT

Some conditions are such a mess that they mess up everything!! In liver failure, the liver fails to adequately produce factors 2, 7, 9 and 10 (II, VII, IX, X), and both the intrinsic and extrinsic pathways are deranged, so both PTT and PT-INR are prolonged. In very advanced liver disease, factor V and fibrinogen levels drop and are considered dangerous prognostic signs. Because the liver makes proteins C and S, patients can be at risk of

clotting even with clotting factor deficiencies! The other disease that chews up clotting factors and increases PT-INR and PTT is disseminated intravascular coagulation (DIC), which is discussed later.

As mentioned above, the low molecular weight heparins (LMWH) that directly target factor Xa do not elevate INR or PTT. One must monitor the Xa activity.

A number of direct oral anticoagulants that function as Xa inhibitors have now been developed for oral outpatient therapy for the treatment of venous thromboembolism and to prevent stroke in the setting of non-valvular atrial fibrillation. These include rivaroxaban (trade name Xarelto), apixaban (Eliquis), edoxaban (Lixiana), and betrixaban (Bevyxxa). In case of an overdose or severe bleeding complications from these medications, andexanet alfa is a recombinant modified human factor Xa decoy protein that reverses the inhibition of factor Xa.

The direct oral anticoagulants including dabigatran are cleared rapidly from the blood over 24 to 72 hours depending on the patient's renal and hepatic function. The initial approach to a bleeding complication is supportive and withholding the medication. The reversal agents are reserved for patients with severe bleeding complications (e.g., CNS bleeding) due to an associated risk of thrombosis.

19.3 Top four Bad Boys of ICU Hematology

The next section reviews four hematological emergencies in order of most common to least common. These are diseases you *CANNOT* afford to miss. They often develop while the patient is in the hospital, so you have to be vigilant to think about them and diagnose them rapidly.

19.3.1 Public Enemy #1: Heparin-Induced Thrombocytopenia (HIT)

19.3.1.1 How Common and Why Does it Happen?

About 10% of patients on heparin therapy experience a modest reduction in platelet count that is not immune mediated. This drop happens within the first few days of starting heparin, and the platelet levels rarely drop below 100,000 platelets/uL. The severe disease called HIT (for heparin-induced thrombocytopenia) will occur in 1% of patients on heparin, typically after 5 days, and is characterized by a more significant drop in the platelet count.

Heparins, both unfractionated standard heparin and the low molecular weight heparins, have a high affinity for a platelet protein called *platelet factor 4 (PF4)*, located in platelet α-granules and on the platelet cell surface. Once heparin binds to PF4, it undergoes a conformational change that now makes it immunogenic and can lead to the production of IgG antibodies against the heparin-PF4 complex. These form immune complexes that *ACTIVATE* the platelets, leading to platelet consumption and activation with clot formation. The immune complexes can also cause endothelial injury and activate tissue factor, which generates more thrombin and leads to arterial thrombosis.

19.3.1.2 HIT Clinical Manifestations

A fundamental concept here is that even though platelet counts drop (thrombocytopenia), *HIT causes platelet activation and tissue factor activation* that causes platelets to *clot* in both arteries and veins. In fact, if heparin is stopped, and no other anticoagulant is added, there is an approximate 50% chance of thrombosis and up to 30% risk of death. The degree of thrombocytopenia (how low do they go!) is an independent predictor of the composite occurrence of death, limb amputation, or new thrombosis.

Thromboembolic complications include venous, arterial, or both:

- DVT/PE
- MI
- Stroke
- Limb artery occlusion requiring amputation

Heparin-induced thrombocytopenia HITS the patient from both the arterial and venous side of the circulation (**Figure 19-3**). In the figure, we illustrate a blood vessel with arterial circulation on the left, going to capillaries in the middle, to veins on the right. We see clot in both the artery and the vein and a boxing glove *HITTING both the artery and vein*. Below it we see a man being HIT! in the head with stroke, chest with MI, arm with hand infarction, and leg with DVT.

19.3.1.3 Diagnosis of HIT

When rounding in the ICU you have to ask the question: "Is this patient on heparin and are the platelets stable?" You should really ask this question for *EVERY* patient because heparin is often given for IV flushes, coating of catheters or devices, with hemodialysis, etc. Your nurses and team may not even realize a patient is getting heparin. You must track the platelet counts and trends, and if the platelets start to drop, you should start to worry.

The clinical probability of actually having HIT has been described by the 4 *T*'s and summarized in **Figure 19-4**. Essentially the risk is highest with more *T*'s:

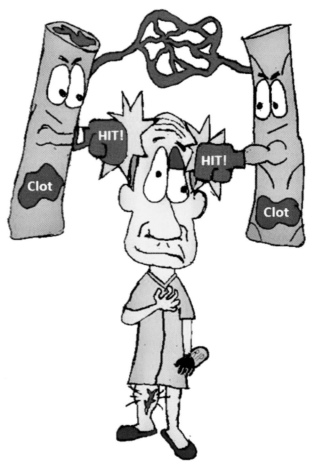

Figure 19-3 A reminder that heparin-induced thrombocytopenia (HIT) hits both the arterial and venous circulation.

1T: *Thrombocytopenia*: The platelets drop more than 50% or drop to a count of 20-100.

2T: *Timing*: The platelets drop 5-10 days after heparin exposure *OR* immediately if the patient has been exposed to heparin in the past (prior anti-PF4 antibody formation).

3T: *Thrombosis*: There is proven arterial or venous thrombosis or skin necrosis.

4T: oTher causes of low platelets are *NOT* present.

Interpretation of score:

- 6-8 points: high probability of HIT
- 4-5 points: intermediate probability of HIT
- 0-3 points: low probability of HIT

A low 4T score indicates a low probability of HIT. For example, in clinical observational studies, 93% of patients with a low 4T score had a negative specific ELISA test for HIT.

If the score is intermediate or high probability, the heparin should be held immediately, and a diagnostic

Category	2 Points	1 Point	0 Points
Thrombocytopenia	>50% fall OR nadir of 20-100 × 10^9/L	30-50% fall OR nadir of 10-19 × 10^9/L	<30% fall OR nadir <10 × 10^9/L
Timing of platelet count fall	5-10 days OR <1 day if prior heparin exposure in past 30 days	> 10 days or unclear OR ≤1 day if heparin exposure in past 30-100 days	≤1 day
Thrombosis or other sequelae	Proven thrombosis, skin necrosis or acute reaction after heparin bolus	Progressive, recurrent, or silent thrombosis or erythematous skin lesions	None
Other causes of thrombocytopenia	None evident	Possible	Definite

Figure 19-4 *Four T score for assessing the risk of heparin-induced thrombocytopenia.*

HIT panel test should be performed. This starts with an ELISA test for the presence of antibodies to PF4. The ELISA test is very sensitive (>95%), so if this test is negative, heparin can be tried again. If ELISA is positive, it can be a false positive (low specificity, ~ 50-80%), so treatment for HIT should be started (non-heparin anticoagulation described below), *BUT* a confirmatory platelet serotonin release test should be performed. This test measures the platelet-activation response (i.e., release of platelet serotonin) to the anti-PF4-heparin complex (rather than just detecting the antibody). This test is reported to have >95% sensitivity and specificity for HIT.

19.3.1.4 Treatment of HIT

Stop the heparin! That is the crucial first step and should be done for all patients at intermediate or high probability of HIT. In patients at a high probability, therapy should be started even before the HIT screening ELISA test is back. Treatment requires anticoagulation to stop the clot from forming or allow the clot to break down. Because we cannot use heparins, the drugs of choice are the direct thrombin inhibitors (**Figure 19-5**). These drugs bind directly to and inhibit thrombin. The drug binding prevents thrombin from converting fibrinogen to fibrin and reduces platelet activation. You can also use fondaparinux to treat HIT because it cannot bind to PF4 to create an antigen. **Figure 19-5** summarizes the available FDA-approved therapies for HIT.

Two concepts about these drugs:

1. Titrate all of the direct thrombin inhibitors to a dose that increases the PTT to 1.5-2.5 times the baseline.
2. Argatroban and bivalirudin are the approved first-line drugs. Use bivalirudin for Liver failure (cleared by the kidney) and argatroban for kidney failure (largely liver-cleared).

19.3.1.4.1 *Argatroban*

Argatroban is your first-line drug for the majority of patients suspected with HIT, as it can be given even with kidney dysfunction, which is very common in the hospital. It is a reversible inhibitor of thrombin. There is no bolus. Start this drug at an infusion dose that depends on the degree of renal impairment. If there is no renal impairment: 0.5 mcg/kg/min. The argatroban is titrated to a goal PTT of 1.5-2.5 times the baseline.

19.3.1.4.2 *Bivalirudin*

This is a synthetic analogue of hirudin. It is reversible and there is no bolus dosing. It is renally cleared, so the starting infusion depends on the degree of renal impairment. No renal impairment: 0.15-0.2 mg/kg/hr; creatinine clearance <30 mL/min: 0.1 mg/kg/hr; critical illness: 0.05 mg/kg/hr. Titrate to a goal PTT of 1.5-2.5 × baseline. The drug can be used in patients with hepatic dysfunction.

19.3.1.4.3 *Fondaparinux*

Fondaparinux is an easy one to use as it is given SQ once a day. Fondaparinux is an inhibitor of factor Xa, like the LMWH, but it is smaller than LMWH; therefore, the drug does not cause a conformational change in PF4 that is required for HIT antibody binding. Base your initial dose on weight:

- < 50 kg: 5 mg SQ daily
- 50-75 kg: 7.5 mg SQ daily
- >100 kg: 10 mg SQ daily

Fondaparinux is cleared by the kidney, so it is contraindicated for use in patients with a creatinine clearance of <30 mL/min. One can monitor the anti-factor Xa levels when attempting to treat patients with renal failure.

So you want a silly mnemonic? OK. In case you need some help, check out **Figure 19-6.** In the next Transformers Movie Sequel, the hero *"Argatron holds a bat (argatroban) and leaps by (bivalirudin) the Fondue Pot (fondaparinux) to HIT the huge, bad salivating leech on the head. Unfortunately, he* accidentally HITS a monster platelet at the same time!"

Drug	Mechanism of Action	Affinity for Thrombin	Metabolism	Half-life	FDA indicated for HIT	ACCP recommendation for treatment of HIT
Argatroban	DTI	+	Hepatic	40-50 min	Yes	Grade 1C
Bivalirudin	DTI	++	20% Renal, 80% Proteolysis	25-40 min	No	Grade 2C
Fondaparinux	Factor Xa inhibitor	n/a	Renal	17-21 hours	No	Grade 2C

Figure 19-5 Treatment options for HIT.

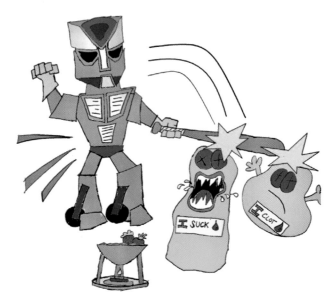

Figure 19-6 Mnemonic for the alternative anticoagulants to use in HIT. See text.

19.3.2 Public Enemy #2: Disseminated Intravascular Coagulation (DIC)

DIC is one of the most frequently encountered bleeding problems in the ICU.[146] DIC can be considered a massive forest fire that is activating and chewing up the coagulation factors along both the intrinsic and extrinsic pathway (**Figure 19-1**). Most commonly, the intrinsic pathway is activated by gram-negative sepsis and other severe infections and shock states, caused, for example, by massive trauma, burns, or drug overdose. The fire lights up and runs down the serine proteases like dominoes: 12 11 9 8 10 5 2: prothrombin (II) to thrombin (IIa) 1: fibrinogen to fibrin. Paradoxically, while this is a clotting process, the massive burn consumes all the factors and results in systemic anticoagulation and a bleeding diathesis *(burns them*

up and bleed!). DIC can also be set off by activation of the extrinsic pathway. DIC occurs through the extrinsic pathway activation, typically with a massive release of tissue factor, for example during massive trauma or obstetrical complications like abruption of the placenta.

The diagnosis of DIC requires an analysis of laboratory evidence showing:

1. Consumption of clotting proteins and platelets, which can be measured by elevation in the PT and drop in platelets
2. Evidence of microvascular fibrin clot formation and degradation, which includes consumption of fibrinogen, with the production of fibrin degradation products and D-dimers

For example, in DIC, the mean values from lab changes include: PT increases from 11-14 seconds to 18 seconds; platelets drop from 150-400,000/microL to 52; fibrinogen falls from 150-400 mg/dL to 137; fibrin degradation products and D-dimers rise to a high titer.

Therapy of DIC requires first and foremost an identification of the primary cause of the forest fire and immediate efforts at putting it out. The source of sepsis must be identified and treated, toxic drugs cleared, and traumatic or surgical or obstetrical injury addressed. If the patient is bleeding, the consumed products can be repleted, with platelet transfusion, cryoprecipitate to restore fibrinogen levels (especially if less than 100 mg/dL), and FFP for prolongation of PT and PTT values.

19.3.3 Public Enemy #3: Thrombotic Thrombocytopenic Purpura (and HELLP! and HUS!)

Thrombotic thrombocytopenic purpura (TTP) is a fascinating disease that requires prompt recognition and emergent plasmapheresis to reduce the mortality dramatically from 90% to 20%.[147] TTP is a member of a family of diseases called the *microangiopathic hemolytic anemias (MAH)*, and includes the *HELLP (hemolysis, elevated liver enzymes, low platelets) syndrome* of pregnancy and *HUS (hemolytic uremic syndrome)* of childhood. HELLP and HUS are named better as they emphasize the importance of hemolysis and organ injury, in addition to low platelets.

What is microangiopathic hemolytic anemia (MAH), and what causes this to happen?

As described earlier, endothelial cells that are injured or subjected to shear-stress will dump von Willebrand factor (vWF) outside of the cell. In fact, vWF can form long chain polymers that stream along endothelial cells. vWF binds to platelets and platelet thrombospondin-1 and activates clotting (both platelets and factor 8). vWF activity is normally checked by a metalloproteinase enzyme called *ADAMTS13* that chews up vWF and prevents it from forming these unusually large multimers of vWF. In TTP and other MAH diseases, there is a hereditary or acquired deficiency or inhibition of ADAMTS13. This deficiency results in accumulation of vWF and platelet thrombosis in the microvasculature where vWF is produced. *TTP is primarily a disease caused by platelet aggregation* with clumping and subsequent vascular obstruction in the vital organs. This process consumes the platelets and causes thrombocytopenia (low platelets).

As the red cells flow through the microvasculature, they are shredded by the strings of vWF and platelet microthrombi that fill the lumen. This process has been likened to the effect of a cheese wire or garrote across the vessel lumen. Think of red cells streaming through a paper-shredding machine in the microvasculature. The result is intravascular hemolysis, which produces torn, damaged red cells, called *schistocytes*. Since this happens in the small vessels, it is called *microangiopathic hemolytic anemia*. **Figure 19-7** illustrates a high-powered

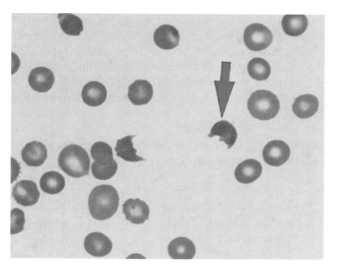

Figure 19-7 Peripheral blood smear with a schistocyte (red arrow).

image of a thin smear of peripheral blood, showing a characteristic schistocyte.

19.3.3.1 Diagnosis and Clinical Presentation

The central features required to diagnose all three diseases (TTP, HELLP, and HUS) are low platelets and microangiopathic hemolytic anemia (MAH). MAH is defined by the presence of schistocytes (torn red cell fragments) (**Figure 19-7**), which are easy to see on microscopy, and by evidence of intravascular hemolysis. Intravascular hemolysis can be diagnosed by

- *High levels of red cell enzymes in plasma (lactate dehydrogenase or LDH, aspartate aminotransferase or AST).* Note that both LDH and AST are also made in the liver and skeletal muscle, so you should measure CPK, which is made in the muscle but *NOT* red cells and measure ALT, which is made in the liver but *NOT* in red cells. So, high LDH and AST but normal CPK and ALT suggests intravascular hemolysis. Note that the LDH levels are *VERY* high in MAH, usually approaching or over 1000 units/Liter.
- *Low hemoglobin and high reticulocytes.* The hemoglobin must drop, as red cells are destroyed and new cells are made, increasing the reticulocyte count. The latter can stay low if there is renal failure.
- *Undetectable haptoglobin.* Hemoglobin released into plasma binds to haptoglobin, and both are cleared and degraded. New synthesis of haptoglobin takes time, so levels should drop to undetectable amounts.
- *High plasma hemoglobin.* Plasma hemoglobin levels are usually not detectable, but these will rise.
- *Schistocytes and Helmit cells.* **Figure 19-7** shows these torn-shaped red cells. These are nonspecific and can also be seen in DIC. But note that TTP and MAH are *NOT* generally associated with elevated PT-INR or PTT, which is characteristic of DIC.

TTP is caused by microangiopathy and microthrombosis that affect the blood vessels to many organs. If fact, most organs in the body can be changed, but especially the central nervous system.

Classically, TTP is diagnosed by the following five clinical features *(The TTP Pentad)*; however, in many cases one or more of these are absent:

1. Thrombocytopenia (low platelet count with petechiae and nosebleeds)
2. Microangiopathic hemolytic anemia (defined above)
3. Neurologic symptoms (fluctuating), such as hallucinations, bizarre behavior, altered mental status, headaches, seizures, and stroke

4. Renal failure
5. Fever

Microangiopathic clots within the circulation can block local blood supply to any organ. While TTP preferentially affects the blood vessels of the brain and kidneys, it can affect any organ, and patients can even develop acute lung injury and pancreatitis.

Idiopathic or auto-immune TTP. Antibodies to ADAMTS13 cause this condition. ADAMTS13 enzyme activity assay can be run by the laboratory and is <5% of normal activity in 80% of patients.

Hereditary TTP. A hereditary form of TTP occurs in less than 1% of all cases and is called the *Upshaw-Schülman syndrome*, caused by frameshift and point mutations in the ADAMTS13 enzyme. Patients with this inherited ADAMTS13 deficiency have a surprisingly mild phenotype but develop TTP in clinical situations with increased von Willebrand factor levels, such as infection. Patients with Upshaw-Schülman syndrome have 5-10% of normal ADAMTS-13 activity.

Secondary TTP. The mechanism of secondary TTP is poorly understood, because the ADAMTS13 activity is generally not as depressed as in idiopathic TTP, and no inhibitors are detected. Probable etiologies may involve, at least in some cases, endothelial damage that increases vWF levels beyond the ability of ADAMTS13 to properly degrade it. This occurs secondary to many diseases commonly seen in the ICU:

- Cancer
- Bone marrow transplantation
- Pregnancy
- Medication use including:
  o Platelet aggregation inhibitors (ticlopidine, clopidogrel, and prasugrel)
  o Immunosuppressants (cyclosporine, mitomycin, tacrolimus/FK506, interferon-α)
- HIV-1 infection

Hemolytic uremic syndrome (HUS) is really a form of TTP that mainly involves the kidneys. It is also a MAH but it tends to occur in children and affects the kidney more than the central nervous system. HUS is classically caused by infection with *E. coli* O157:H7 from infected foods. This shiga-toxigenic group of *E. coli* produces a shiga-like toxin. The shiga-toxin binds to proteins on the surface of glomerular blood vessel endothelium, and there it appears to inactivate ADAMTS13 locally. Once the ADAMTS13 is disabled, multimers of von Willebrand factor (vWF) form, initiate platelet activation, and cause microthrombi formation, just like TTP and all MAH diseases. The arterioles become obstructed by the resulting complexes of activated platelets, and large multimeric vWF shred the red blood cells as they squeeze through the narrowed blood vessels filled with vWF polymer "garrote wire," causing MAH.

HELLP syndrome, another MAH, is associated with pre-eclampsia and eclampsia, and it can occur after delivery. HELLP is just like TTP, but there is liver injury associated with this, so that the ALT can rise as well as the AST.

19.3.3.2 Treatment of TTP, HUS, and HELLP

Plasmapheresis. TTP, HUS, and HELLP are considered medical emergencies and require immediate plasmapheresis. Call your on-call blood bank person and say, *"HELLP, HUSsle!! We have an emergent case of TTP!!!"* Plasmapheresis requires insertion of a hemodialysis catheter into a central vein and a full exchange of plasma for FFP with a pheresis machine. Plasmapheresis removes inhibitors of ADAMTS13 and repletes the enzyme level. This therapy has dramatically improved outcomes. Mortality rates of up to 90% are now well below 20%. If this therapy is not immediately available, you should transfuse FFP while preparing for full plasmapheresis.

Remove inciting agents. For drug-induced TTP (cyclosporine, FK506, for example), the drugs should be discontinued. With HUS, the *E. coli* should be killed with antibiotics. For HELLP, the baby should be safely delivered.

Supportive care. Provide intensive care support for organ failure as required. Examples include anti-seizure agents as needed, mechanical ventilation for acute lung injury, and hemodialysis for renal failure complicating TTP or HUS.

19.3.4 Public Enemy #4: Catastrophic Antiphospholipid Antibody Syndrome (CAPS)

Our last hematological emergency is *catastrophic antiphospholipid antibody syndrome (CAPS)* and, like HIT, it is one of the causes of serious arterial thromboses.[148]

Antiphospholipid antibody syndrome (APS) is an autoimmune, hypercoagulable state caused by antibodies against cell membrane phospholipids, causing blood clots (thrombosis) in both arteries and veins. APS classically causes pregnancy-related complications, such as miscarriage, preterm delivery, and severe pre-eclampsia.

The specific phospholipids that become antibody targets are cardiolipin (anti-cardiolipin antibodies) and β2 glycoprotein I. APS can be a primary condition or can occur in the context of other autoimmune diseases, such as systemic lupus erythematosus.

In rare cases, antiphospholipid antibody syndrome leads to rapid organ failure due to diffuse and severe thrombosis; this is termed *catastrophic antiphospholipid syndrome (CAPS)* and is associated with a high risk of multi-organ injury and death. The most common venous thrombosis is deep vein thrombosis of the lower extremities, which can lead to pulmonary embolism; the most common arterial event is stroke. Many other arterial sites can be thrombosed in CAPS, including the kidney, heart, skin, mesenteric arteries, and extremities.

Laboratory testing in CAPS reveals a prolonged PTT; three additional tests can be performed:

1. High titer anti-cardiolipin IgG and/or IgM measured by ELISA
2. High titer anti-β2 glycoprotein I IgG and/or IgM measured by ELISA on 2 or more occasions
3. Lupus anticoagulant

Therapy for CAPS requires anticoagulation and plasmapheresis.

*You are doing your routine ICU physical examination, which involves running your hand across the arms and legs to feel for edema, temperature and pulses. During your exam you are looking for edema and swelling to identify venous thrombosis, which is common, but you are also feeling the skin temperature and feeling the pulses to look for arterial occlusions. On this particular day you notice that Mr. Jones, a 60you admitted with respiratory failure and pneumonia has a left hand and right foot which are cold. You notice that his right radial pulse and left leg dorsalis pedis pulses are absent. You confirm with Doppler ultrasound, and the nurse indicates that this is new. What is going on? This could be peripheral vascular disease, but that would not affect two vessels at the same time and would not affect the arm. It could be an embolic event from infectious endocarditis. But what types of diseases cause arterial blood clots? There are not many. **One is HIT and the other is CAPS.** You quickly evaluate the platelet count, which is stable, and the patient is not on heparin; a HIT screen was sent the prior week and was normal. You see that the PTT is long, and he has a positive ANA; you begin to suspect this could be APL syndrome. You send a workup and start emergent therapy with plasmapheresis while waiting for definitive lab tests.*

Suggested Reading

- Jaax ME, Greinacher A. Management of heparin-induced thrombocytopenia. Expert Opin Pharmacother 2012;13(7):987–1006.

20

Transfusion Medicine

You will often find yourself in situations where you have to massively transfuse a patient to keep the patient alive. The definition of a massive transfusion is giving 1-2 times the total blood volume. Since we have $> 5L$ of blood in us and a unit of whole blood is 500 mL, we have > 10 units of whole blood in our bodies. There are a few examples where massive transfusion is common: the massive GI bleeds from esophageal varices, an acute surgical bleed in the operating room or post-operatively in the ICU, a surgical complication such as a laceration of a major blood vessel, or during massive trauma (blunt motor-vehicle accident or gunshot wound).

20.1 Quick-Thinking Rapid Transfusion

If the blood pressure is bottoming out and you see red in the room, you probably do not have time to think. In this case, there are three things to do:

1. *Say, "Oh F—"!!! No, no, not that. Say, "O—negative"!* Ask for 4-6 units of O negative blood. Type O is the universal donor blood, which has no A or B antigens and is Rh negative. You save some time not having to match the blood. Ordinarily this is not necessary as the patient has been hospitalized and you have cross-matched blood available.
2. *A bag of white, a bag of red, a bag of yellow.* Run the crystalloid (lactated ringers or normal saline) wide open (a bag of white), run in the packed red blood cells (a bag of red), run in the fresh frozen plasma (a bag of yellow).
3. *Give platelets.* If using random donor platelet units (RDU), give one for every unit of packed red blood cells (RBC) and 1 unit of fresh frozen plasma (FFP) for each unit of packed RBCs. If using single donor phereses units, give one unit for every six units of red cells and FFP.

Massive transfusion blood component ratio: 1 RBC : 1 FFP : 1 RDU

During a massive transfusion, you may develop complications that you have to address as you stabilize the patient and have more time to think. You will need to send labs including a complete blood cell count, electrolytes, blood gas analysis, PT and PTT, and fibrinogen levels. A few of the most common complications are:

1. *Hypothermia.* If you work in a large trauma hospital, you may be able to order blood delivered via a rapid infuser device. This device will infuse the blood very fast (30-1500 ml/min) and warm the blood. Otherwise, you will have to warm the patient during and after the resuscitation to prevent the development of disseminated intravascular coagulopathy (DIC) and other complications of hypothermia.
2. *Electrolyte abnormalities: hypocalcemia and hypokalemia.* Blood contains citrate as an anti-coagulant, and this will chelate calcium in the

body. Hypocalcemia can produce tetany (muscle spasms). Hypokalemia occurs from dilution and can lead to cardiac dysrhythmias.

3. *Dilutional coagulopathy.* If you do not stay on top of one bag of FFP and one bag of platelets (RDU) for every bag of RBC, you will dilute out the clotting factors and platelets, worsening the bleeding situation. With massive transfusion you should send labs to check your fibrinogen, and if less than 100 g/dL, give cryoprecipitate (see below for details on why). If platelets less than 50,000/microL, provide more platelets.

Now that you have saved the patient, let's review the types of transfusion products, indications for transfusion, and complications associated with transfusion.

20.2 Red Blood Cell Transfusions

The blood bank will collect about 500 mL of whole blood and then remove most of the plasma to process for fresh frozen plasma, platelets and sometimes cryoprecipitate, leaving behind about 250-300 mL of packed red blood cells. The packed red blood cell unit has a hematocrit of approximately 70% red cells, with 30% plasma mixed with a storage solution, such as CPD-Adsol (citrate, phosphate, dextrose, adenosine solution) to chelate calcium (inhibit clotting) and provide phosphate, adenosine, and dextrose to maintain cellular ATP production.

Transfusion of red blood cells is very common in the hospitalized patient. Approximately 1/3 of critically ill patients will receive at least one unit, and the mean number transfused is 3-5 units![149]

20.2.1 When to Transfuse?

Transfusion is associated with a number of risks, albeit small, so evidence-based and rational approaches to transfusion should be followed. A consensus has emerged that a more restrictive approach should be followed with no transfusion for hemoglobin values more than 10 g/dL, and with definite transfusion for values less than or equal to 6 g/dL. When should one transfuse for values between 7-10 g/dL? This decision should be tailored to the precise clinical situation and the patient's co-morbidities. For example, if a patient is actively bleeding or has compromised cardiopulmonary function, a higher target may be appropriate. In the relatively stable ICU patient, a more restrictive "transfusion trigger" of 7 g/dL is recommended.[150]

For patients with GI bleeding, similar data exist. A restrictive transfusion group (transfused only if the Hgb < 7 gms/dL) had lower 6-week mortality, lower bleeding recurrence rate, and lower portal pressures in those patients with cirrhosis.[151] Investigators have also studied the septic population with very similar findings.[152]

At the last count, there are 8 published guidelines from various medical and surgical societies related to transfusion. Let's try and summarize:

1. No transfusion for Hgb > 10 gms / dL
2. Pull the transfusion trigger for all patients < 7 g/dL in stable ICU conditions and patients with subacute gastrointestinal bleeding.
3. Consider a higher threshold for patients with an acute coronary syndrome, active symptoms of anemia, or active ongoing bleeding.

20.2.2 Complications of Red Blood Cell Transfusion

To remember the many complications of blood product transfusion, think of the tourist ALI, who was visiting San Francisco and riding on the TRALI eating an OLD, AGED TACO that caused a major REACTION, with fevers, chills, shakes, hemolysis, and lung injury (**Figure 20-1**).

The many complications of blood product transfusion include:

- Multiple organ dysfunction with aged blood transfusion
- Acute and chronic hemolytic transfusion reactions
- Febrile non-hemolytic transfusion reactions
- **A**cute **l**ung **i**njury (ALI) and ARDS
- **T**ransfusion-**a**ssociated acute **l**ung **i**njury (TRALI)
- **T**ransfusion-**a**ssociated **c**irculatory **o**verload (TACO)

20.2.2.1 The Storage Lesion

Red blood cells can be stored for up to 6 weeks (42 days) and then must be discarded. While blood sits in storage, many physiological and biochemical changes occur in the red cells. The level of ATP and DPG are depleted; the membrane ages, forms microparticles, expresses surface phosphatidylserine; and a fraction of the red cells hemolyze. These combined abnormalities have been termed the *storage lesion*. A study in cardiovascular disease patients suggested that transfusion of blood greater than 2 weeks old increased the risk of developing multiple organ system failure and death.[153] The findings remain controversial because people who get older blood tend to get more blood, and if they need ten units, they have a 10-fold increased risk of getting at least one old unit than a person who gets one unit (so in studies you are classified as receiving old blood). Older blood also has less O blood type, as these universal donor units are depleted early, which may have less of an effect on immune activation. While

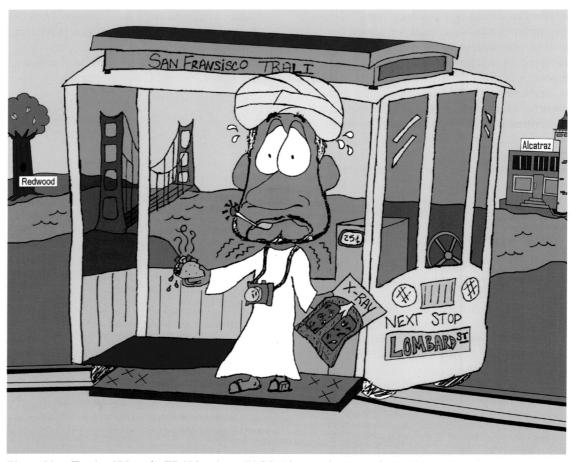

Figure 20-1 *Tourist ALI on the TRALI eating a TACO. The complications of red cell transfusion!*

there is little controversy that receiving lots of blood can cause complications, such as volume overload, ALI, ARDS and TRALI (discussed below), the major debate surrounds whether the problem is with blood in general or with older blood or both.

Two large multicenter randomized clinical trials evaluating the effect of the age of red cells have now been published without confirming an adverse effect of "old" blood.[154,155]

20.2.2.2 Transfusion Reactions

There are three significant types of transfusion reactions:

1. *Acute hemolytic transfusion reactions.* An acute hemolytic transfusion reaction is a severe complication but fortunately very, very rare. It is caused by a major clerical error with the infusion of A, B, or O incompatible blood, which is the reason two readers must match the blood to the patient's correct ID. Infusion of A blood into a B person, or B into A, or A or B into O results in the activation of complement on the red cell and acute and severe intravascular hemolysis. The patient will develop fever; rigors; chest, back and abdominal pain; dyspnea; a sense of doom; nausea and vomiting; hypotension; hemorrhage, and hemoglobinuria. Very, very bad things happen. Fortunately, neither of us has ever seen this in a combined 50 years of ICU work, and hopefully neither will you.

2. *Delayed transfusion reactions.* Now this one is more common, especially if you take care of patients with sickle cell disease or other conditions requiring frequent transfusions, especially in African Americans. A delayed transfusion reaction occurs about three days to two weeks after receiving blood with minor red cell surface antigens (like Rh, Duffy, Kell, etc.) to which the patient has previously developed antibodies. There is an anamnestic immune response, as the patient recognizes the antigen and activates a memory

response to produce new alloantibodies. The signs and symptoms are less severe, as complement is usually not activated. A delayed transfusion reaction can sometimes manifest as a failure to increase hemoglobin levels with transfusions, accompanied by evidence of intravascular hemolysis (increasing lactate dehydrogenase—LDH, bilirubin, aspartate aminotransferase—AST, and dropping haptoglobin). In severe cases, hemoglobin levels plummet, and patients can even develop "bystander hemolysis," where complement is activated and knocks out neighboring host red cells. Since more than 50% of the alloantigens are in the Kell (antigen-K) or Rh group (D, E, C, little e and little c), it is now standard practice in most hospitals to match for these antigens in patients with sickle cell disease (see **Figure 20-2**). In patients with sickle cell disease, transfuse with blood *matched for DECK— or else! A chair is on the DECK of the Titanic, which is listing to one side in the water and sinking. On the chair is a sickle red blood cell. On the upside (out of water) are red blood cells that are negative for DECK (blood negative for Rh group antigens: DECK) and on*

In patients at risk of developing alloantibodies, as in sickle cell disease, the development of alloantibodies is like being vaccinated in that antibodies can develop and then go away with time. So you can have a patient with a past history of antibodies but not detect a positive Coombs antibody test, but then about 3 days after transfusion, the patient develops a severe hemolytic anemia (LDH rises, hemoglobin drops below 5 g/dL). To avoid this, you should call blood banks from hospitals that transfused the patient in the past to check for prior allo-antibodies. Use of medical alert bracelets and routine testing for allo-antibodies is critical.

the water side are red cells positive for DECK. Now you know what happens if you mess this choice up!

3. *Febrile non-hemolytic transfusion reactions.* These are the most common and least severe reactions. During the infusion of any product (red cells, FFP, platelets or cryoprecipitate), the patient develops a fever, chills, or rigors. Anti-leukocyte antibodies

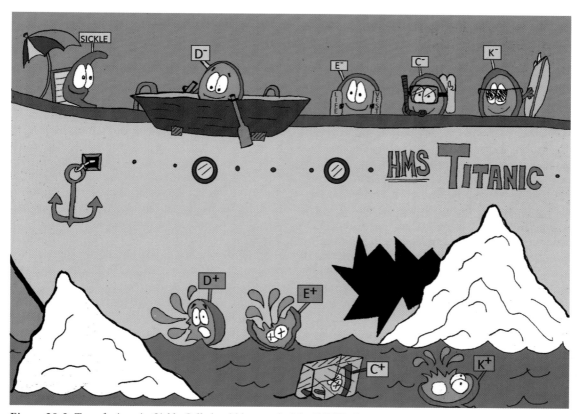

Figure 20-2 *Transfusions in Sickle Cell should be matched for DECK. See text.*

directed against donor white blood cells in the infused product cause this. Pre-treatment with acetaminophen and diphenhydramine and use of leukoreduced products can help prevent or reduce the severity of this reaction.

20.2.2.3 Acute Lung Injury and ARDS

The transfusion of a large number of units of blood or older stored blood has been statistically associated with a significant risk of ALI/ARDS. Many large retrospective studies in trauma patients have shown that transfusion of red blood cells is an independent risk factor for developing ARDS, and this risk increases with the number of units transfused. An intrinsic problem in these studies is that red cell transfusions are given to "sicker" patients, with higher severity of illness and organ dysfunction. However, most studies have adjusted for measurable co-morbidities and seem to show an increased risk that is dose (unit) dependent.[156,157]

20.2.2.4 Transfusion-Associated Lung Injury (TRALI)

TRALI is a unique syndrome of acute lung injury similar in definition to ALI/ARDS, but that occurs during or within 6 hours of a transfusion. Most cases occur within 2 hours of a transfusion. Like ARDS, TRALI is defined by a PaO_2/FiO_2 ratio < 300 mm Hg, diffuse bilateral infiltrates on chest radiograph, and no evidence of cardiogenic pulmonary edema (a low central venous or pulmonary artery occlusion pressure, normal brain natriuretic peptide level, or no evidence of cardiac dysfunction on echocardiogram). For a diagnosis of TRALI, there must be no pre-transfusion ALI or ARDS present. In cases where there are other risk factors for ALI or ARDS (such as sepsis, aspiration, trauma, recent surgery, or massive transfusions), one should refer to a patient with this condition as *possible TRALI*.

TRALI is now considered one of the most common causes of transfusion-associated mortality, based on the number of reports to the FDA. However, many of the suspected cases of TRALI may, in fact, be ALI/ARDS and volume overload. Specific antibodies in the donor's blood are recognized in a confirmed case of TRALI against leukocyte (anti-HLA) and neutrophil (anti-HNA) antigens. Soluble CD40 ligand from platelets, bioactive lipids, and pre-formed cytokines have also been implicated. All blood products with plasma can cause TRALI, including packed red blood cells, FFP, platelets, and cryoprecipitate.

TRALI is also categorized as *immune-mediated* if caused by anti-HLA or anti-HNA antibodies in the donor plasma. Interestingly, immune-mediated TRALI is most commonly associated with donor plasma in blood products from multiparous women. Based on these findings many countries now reduce or exclude women from donating high-volume plasma products, which has decreased the incidence of TRALI. *Non-immune mediated TRALI* is caused by bioreactive lipids, CD40 ligand from platelets, pre-formed cytokines, and other biologic response modifiers that accumulate during storage of blood products.

If acute lung injury develops during or immediately after a transfusion, then TRALI should be suspected, and the transfusion stopped, and the blood bank contacted. The donor product and the recipient blood can be sent to evaluate donor-recipient antibody-antigen HLA and HNA status. Donors with anti-HLA or anti-HNA antibodies should not be allowed to donate in the future.

20.2.2.5 Transfusion-Associated Circulatory Overload (TACO)

TACO is a diagnosis that can be mistaken for TRALI, but is cardiogenic pulmonary edema caused by giving a large fluid volume. TACO is often observed in patients with renal or heart dysfunction and can be diagnosed by a high brain natriuretic peptide level, high filling pressures (central venous pressure or pulmonary artery occlusion pressure), or an abnormal echocardiogram. The treatment is diuresis or dialysis if no urine output.

20.2.2.6 Risk of Infection

Current screening of blood donors and antigen/antibody testing has significantly reduced the risk for transmission of infectious diseases. However, the risk is not zero, and informed consent is needed before transfusion of blood products. You will need to know the mathematical risk to educate patients regarding the risks and benefits of receiving a transfusion. This is easy

Irradiation and leukodepletion can reduce the risk of CMV transmission. This also reduces the number of leukocytes, which can cause the rare complication of transfusion-associated graft-versus-host disease (TA-GVHD). This occurs when blood products are infused into an immunocompromised host, and the contaminating T cells engraft in the donor's bone marrow and start to attack the host, similar to what happens after a bone marrow transplant. Fevers, rash, diarrhea and liver dysfunction can develop with GVHD. So to reduce risk of CMV and TA-GVHD, always use CMV matched and irradiated blood products for immuno-compromised patients.

to remember as almost all the viruses have a risk of less than 1 out of 2 million (for HIV 1 and 2, hepatitis C, and HTLV I and II). While the risk is more for hepatitis B (less than 1 out of 200,000), most people are now vaccinated for hepatitis B. Blood banks now routinely screen for West Nile virus as well.

Cytomegalovirus (CMV) is very common in the donor population and can present a risk if transfused into CMV-negative immunocompromised recipients. Patients in the ICU with bone marrow or solid organ transplant should receive CMV negative units as well as leukoreduced and irradiated units.

Platelets are commonly infected with bacteria, coming from the skin plug in the pheresis catheter. For this reason, platelets are only stored for 5 days (see below).

Other infections are reported but rare, including variant Creutzfeldt-Jakob disease, dengue, babesiosis, Chagas disease and malaria.

20.3 Platelets

There are two types of platelet products, which can be very confusing. The first type comes from the isolation of platelets from the whole blood 500 mL unit. As mentioned, the unit is collected, spun down, red cells removed, and then the plasma is centrifuged faster and the platelet-rich plasma removed, leaving behind the rest of the plasma for fresh frozen plasma or cryoprecipitate (see below). The platelets collected from a whole blood unit are called *random donor units (RDU),* and each unit has about 5×10^6 platelets. Platelets cannot be frozen, or they activate, so they are stored for only five days at room temperature to limit bacterial growth (bacterial contamination occurs in blood collected from small skin plugs in needle puncture sites). A typical transfusion of platelets would be 5-6 random donor units.

Connecting the donor to an apheresis machine and collecting many circulating platelets obtains the second type of platelet product. This device can collect about 4.2×10^{11} platelets from a single donor! These are called *single donor platelets.* A typical transfusion would be a single donor platelet unit, which is more than six units of RDUs.

All platelet products are in plasma, so the risks of febrile transfusion reactions, TRALI, and even ABO incompatibility hemolytic reactions are possible. The use of single donor apheresis units can help reduce this risk, as the plasma can be obtained from one individual rather than 5-6. Patients can also develop *platelet refractoriness,* where infusions of platelets do not result in an increase in the levels in the blood after the transfusion. This is defined by a failure to increase the platelet count by more than approximately 5,000 per microL within 1 hour of a platelet transfusion.

There are two causes of platelet refractoriness:

1. *Immune-mediated.* This is caused by the development of antibodies to class I human leukocyte antigens that exist on platelets, often caused by prior platelet transfusions or pregnancies. The immune response consumes all the platelets that are infused. Specific single donor pheresis units that are HLA matched to the patient can be used to improve platelet transfusion success in these cases.
2. *Non-immune mediated.* Non-immune mediated platelet refractoriness is caused by accelerated platelet activation and consumption and is seen during active infection; disseminated intravascular coagulation (DIC); hypersplenism (liver cirrhosis); and medications, such as heparin, which causes heparin-induced thrombocytopenia (HIT).

20.4 Fresh Frozen Plasma (FFP)

FFP is the plasma that is collected and separated from the red cells in the whole blood unit. Unlike platelets, it can be frozen for one year (at less than $-18°C$). FFP contains all of the clotting factors and is used during a massive transfusion *(remember a bag of red and a bag of yellow!)* to keep the PT and PTT at least 1.5 times normal. It can also be used to reverse warfarin overdose while waiting for the vitamin K to kick in. A typical dose to normalize the levels of clotting factors is 2-4 units of FFP. Patients with severe coagulopathy from liver failure may need a constant infusion of FFP of 2 units every 2-4 hours to help stop bleeding.

FFP also contains the protease ADAMTS13, which is required to cleave von Willebrand factor (vWF). Genetic deficiency or auto-antibodies against ADAMTS13 lead to hereditary or acquired thrombotic thrombocytopenic purpura (TTP). FFP infusions and plasma exchange transfusion can provide much-needed ADAMTS13 to treat the TTP patient. Complications of FFP therapy are discussed above.

20.5 Cryoprecipitate

This product is named based on how it is made. Cryoprecipitate is the cold-insoluble fraction of plasma when FFP is thawed slowly at 1-6°C. Cryoprecipitate contains a highly concentrated amount of Factor VIII, vWF, Factor XIII, and fibrinogen. Cryoprecipitate previously was used for Factor VIII (hemophilia A – *remember, A rhymes with 8*) and vWF deficiency (von Willebrand disease), but there are now concentrated preparations available with no risk of infection. So cryoprecipitate is now mostly used as a source of fibrinogen in patients bleeding with DIC or liver failure, and rarely for Factor XIII deficiency.

Ultimate pimp attack on ICU rounds. Your attending may pimp you, asking, "What blood components are in cryoprecipitate but not in FFP?" If you want to be a smart-ass and counter-attack, tell him,"None, cryo comes from FFP, stupid." *OK, really not the best move.* Instead, let him know that you understand the question, and what implied is what factors are concentrated from FFP during a freeze and slow thaw. This would be factors 8 (VIII), 13 (XIII), vWF, and fibrinogen. We don't have a good way to remember this, so we can only point out that with the first approach, *you ATE (8) his lunch but in turn became unlucky 13 for the rest of the rotation* (vWF and fibrinogen seem easier to remember, sorry!).

20.6 Recombinant Factor VIIa (Novo-Seven)

Recombinant Factor VIIIA product was developed and approved for the treatment of hemophilia patients who have developed inhibitors to their factor replacements. This requires a downstream activation of the clotting cascade by VIIa. It directly boosts thrombin generation and can stop bleeding fast, so it has been used heavily "off label." *Off label* is use that has not been directly approved by the FDA, for example, for central nervous system bleeds, massive hemorrhage, pulmonary hemorrhage, surgery, trauma and many other indications. For these indications, it is often used at doses less than half that used for hemophilia patients. While it clearly stops bleeding, it can cause clotting problems, such as pulmonary embolism and myocardial infarction (venous and arterial thrombosis!). A meta-analysis of the published data has suggested that the risks of this therapy may be worse than the benefits, so this should be used with extreme caution and based on clear risk/benefit analysis.[158]

20.7 Four-Factor Prothrombin Complex Concentrate

Prothrombin complex concentrate (PCC) products are available in a variety of formulations including 3- and 4-factor concentrates. You need to be familiar with your local product to use these effectively in the patient with emergent bleeding in the setting of warfarin administration. These products are favored for the reversal of warfarin-associated bleeding to rapidly replete factors II, VII, IX, and X. The concentrate products are favored over FFP because they offer a more rapid reversal with a smaller volume of product delivery.[159] PCC products have a lower risk profile in comparison to FFP, including volume overload and TRALI. The PCC carries a small but real prothrombotic risk and should be restricted to patients who require rapid reversal of warfarin coagulation.

For the direct oral anticoagulants (DOACs), specific antidotes exist for dabigatran (idarucizumab) and apixaban or rivaroxaban (andexanet alfa). These anticoagulant agents must be treated with supportive care. There is no available evidence to suggest efficacy of the PCC products for the reversal of these medications.

Suggested Reading

- Levi M, Scully M. How I treat disseminated intravascular coagulation. Blood 2018 131:845–854.
- Tobian, A. A., Heddle, N. M., Wiegmann, T. L. & Carson, J. L. Red blood cell transfusion: 2016 clinical practice guidelines from AABB. Transfusion 56, 2627–2630 (2016).
- Carson, J. L., Triulzi, D. J. & Ness, P. M. Indications for and adverse effects of red-cell transfusion. NEJM. 377,1261–1272 (2017).

21

Acute Kidney Injury

A decline in renal function in the hospitalized patient can range from mild impairment to renal failure. To establish a standard definition for Acute Kidney Injury (AKI), the Kidney Disease: Improving Global Outcomes (KDIGO) Group built on the work of prior groups to provide both a definition and staging system.[160] The term *Acute Kidney Injury* is favored over the former name of *Acute Renal Failure,* recognizing that even a small acute decline in renal function in the hospital setting carries an adverse prognosis, independent of whether the patient requires dialysis.

The KDIGO definition requires an acute reduction in kidney function, defined as

- Increase in serum creatinine by $\geq$ 0.3 mg/dL ($\geq$ 26.5 micromol/L) within 48 hours; *OR*
- Increase in serum creatinine to $\geq$ 1.5 times baseline, which is known or presumed to have occurred within the prior seven days; *OR*
- Urine volume < 0.5 mL/kg/h for six hours.

The diagnosis generally requires at least two creatinine values to assess for change or accurate measurement of urine output. It is assumed that a diagnosis of AKI based on the urine output criterion alone will include the exclusion of urinary tract obstruction that reduces urine output or any other readily reversible causes of reduced urine output.

The KDIGO severity stage groups AKI into three stages, as summarized in **Figure 21-1.**

The development of AKI in the hospital setting is a reliable predictive variable of a negative hospital outcome. A creatinine change equivalent to Stage 1 has been associated with a relative risk of hospital death of 2.2. AKI requiring the institution of dialysis therapy is associated with a threefold risk of hospital mortality. Prevention of AKI in the hospital setting is an essential goal for a successful patient outcome.

The clinical value of the KDIGO criteria for the diagnosis of acute kidney injury is debatable. The primary utility is for clinical trials in AKI or efforts to study the epidemiology of AKI. Key summary points for the clinician would include:

- Any decline in renal function is a bad prognostic variable for a hospitalized patient. An early warning sign is an *increase in creatinine of 1.5 × the admission or baseline value.*
- AKI can be recognized as a decline in traditional serum markers of creatinine and blood urea nitrogen (BUN) or in its earliest form by a decline in urine output. *The target urine output is > 0.5 ml/ kg/hr, or for a 60kg person ~ 350 ml per 12-hour shift.*
- AKI can be grouped into stages of severity with a progressive increase in hospital mortality

21.1 Classification of Acute Kidney Injury

The classic approach to AKI in the hospitalized patient generally focuses on the classification of the patient into one of three groups:

Stage	Creatinine	Urine Output
Stage 1	Increase in serum creatinine to 1.5 to 1.9 times baseline, OR increase in serum creatinine by $\geq$ 0.3 mg/dL ($\geq$26.5 micromol/L)	Reduction in urine output to <0.5 mL/kg per hour for 6 to 12 hours
Stage 2	Increase in serum creatinine to 2.0 to 2.9 times baseline	Reduction in urine output to < 0.5 mL/kg per hour for $\geq$12 hours
Stage 3	Increase in serum creatinine to 3.0 times baseline, OR increase in serum creatinine to $\geq$ 4.0 mg/dL ($\geq$353.6 micromol/L), OR the initiation of renal replacement therapy, OR in patients <18 years, decrease in eGFR to <35 mL/min per 1.73 M^2.	Reduction in urine output to <0.3 mL/kg per hour for $\geq$24 hours, OR anuria for $\geq$12 hours

Figure 21-1 *KDIGO classification for acute kidney injury.*

1. *Pre-renal* – an etiology based upon impaired renal perfusion. The kidney is functionally normal.

Clinical examples include volume depletion, hemorrhage, congestive heart failure, abdominal compartment syndrome, hepatorenal syndrome, and drugs altering renal hemodynamics.

2. *Intrinsic renal* – disorders of the renal microvasculature, glomerulus, interstitium, or tubules

Clinical examples include acute tubular necrosis, acute interstitial nephritis, acute glomerulonephritis, HUS/TTP, vasculitis, and atheroembolic disease.

3. Post-renal – also termed obstructive uropathy

Clinical examples include bladder outlet obstruction (blocked Foley is most common), benign prostatic hypertrophy, and bilateral ureteral obstruction.

Pre-renal insufficiency is subclassfied into disorders of

1. Pre-renal insufficiency due to global hypoperfusion

    a. *Hypovolemia* – examples here include diarrhea or hemorrhage
    b. *Hypervolemia* with decreased renal perfusion – examples here include CHF or hepatorenal syndrome

2. Pre-renal insufficiency due to local hypoperfusion

Examples here include renovascular occlusion or specific drug therapies that modify glomerular afferent and efferent vascular tone, including the use of non-steroidal anti-inflammatory agents, calcineurin inhibitors, or ACE inhibitors.

In hospitalized patients, acute tubular necrosis (renal) and pre-renal etiologies make up almost 2/3 of patients presenting with acute renal insufficiency.[161]

We can generally resolve post-obstructive etiologies for AKI the easiest. Although post-renal represents a small fraction of AKI cases, they are reversible with prompt recognition and intervention – *so don't miss the obstructed Foley or distended bladder!* A bedside or formal ultrasound can rapidly assess for bladder enlargement or hydronephrosis and *renal ultrasound is included in any assessment of AKI* when an etiology is not easily determined. Patients with two kidneys usually require a lesion that causes bilateral obstruction to develop AKI.

Once post-renal etiologies are ruled out, focus on distinguishing pre-renal azotemia from intrinsic renal disease. *No single parameter* will make the distinction easy between renal and pre-renal causes, but a comprehensive assessment of the patient with acute kidney injury will be most helpful, including history, physical examination, imaging, urine chemistries, and urine sediment. An additional parameter, bladder pressure, may be indicated in patients with large volume resuscitation or suspected elevation in intra-abdominal pressures.

A significant component of your history will focus on drug exposure, infection (meaning sepsis), or episodes of hypotension. These are the BIG THREE for etiologies of AKI in the hospitalized patient. A patient may have been on ACE inhibitors long-term without AKI, but in the hospital setting with an episode of hypotension, that combination can lead to AKI.

Your physical exam will focus on assessment of your patient's volume status. Both hypovolemia from fluid losses and hypervolemia associated with CHF or cirrhosis can be associated with AKI. Other physical findings such as a drug rash might suggest acute interstitial nephritis.

Urinalysis will assess for evidence of proteinuria. The urine dipstick detects albuminuria primarily with a lower limit of detection of approximately 10-20 mg/dL. The urine dipstick can be falsely positive in highly concentrated urine, in the presence of hematuria, with recent iodinated contrast exposure, or with a markedly alkaline pH. The presence of proteinuria strengthens your suspicion of intrinsic renal disease. Hematuria may suggest the presence of glomerulonephritis or vasculitis. Pyuria may suggest the presence of interstitial nephritis. Multiple granular or epithelial cell casts suggest acute tubular necrosis. Simply stated, *an active urine sediment DOES NOT suggest pre-renal azotemia* as the cause of the intrinsic renal dysfunction.

The most commonly employed urine measure to distinguish pre-renal AKI from acute tubular necrosis is the fractional excretion of sodium (FENa). A normal kidney, in the face of a perceived reduction in perfusion (prerenal), will conserve sodium – meaning the fractional excretion of sodium will be low. The FENa is a more specific measure for pre-renal causes of AKI than the urine sodium. The FENa calculation requires simultaneous measurements of both serum and urine sodium and creatinine.

$$FENa, \% = \frac{UrNa \times SCr}{SNa \times UCr} \times 100$$

where UrNa = urine sodium, SCr=serum creatinine, SNa=serum sodium, and UCr=urine creatinine

A value of $< 1\%$ suggests pre-renal disease. A value $> 2\%$ suggests intrinsic renal disease. Values between 1-2 % are indeterminate. But the FENa is not perfect. A number of intrinsic renal conditions have been reported with a FENa $< 1\%$, including contrast-induced renal failure and severe pre-renal states that transition to ATN. So, a FENa $< 1\%$ is consistent with a pre-renal etiology but is not diagnostic. In addition, the FENa is falsely elevated in the setting of diuretic therapy, which promotes a natriuresis. A similar effect is seen with hyperglycemia and the associated osmotic diuresis.

As an alternative to FENa, the fractional excretion of urea (FEUrea) has been used to assess pre-renal vs. renal etiologies – particularly in patients on diuretic therapy. The FEUrea is calculated using a similar methodology to the FENa calculation. A value $< 35\%$ is consistent with a pre-renal etiology, whereas a value of 50-65% suggests intrinsic renal disease.

$$FEUrea, \% = \frac{UUN \times SCr}{BUN \times UCr} \times 100$$

where UUN = urinary nitrogen, BUN=blood urea nitrogen, SCr=serum creatinine, and UCr=urine creatinine

By the time you complete your detailed history, exam, imaging studies, and urinalysis, you should have a pretty good assessment whether your AKI is pre-renal or renal in origin.

21.2 Drug-induced Acute Kidney Injury

A component of assessing your patient with AKI is a *detailed drug history*. Recognize that <u>any</u> medication exposure within the past 5-7 days will still count as a cause for AKI. Drug-induced renal disease has a myriad of mechanisms – so a very careful drug history is essential to the assessment of your patient with AKI. A broad outline of drug-induced AKI by location of the injury is outlined below:

- *Prerenal azotemia*

Clinical examples include IL-2 induced capillary leak.

- *Alteration in vascular hemodynamics of the glomerulus*

Clinical examples include ACE inhibitors, ARBs, NSAIDs, calcineurin inhibitors, vasopressor agents, contrast agents.

- *Glomerular injury*

Clinical examples include microangiopathic hemolytic anemia (TTP syndrome) caused by calcineurin inhibitors, ticlopidine, clopidogrel, gemcitabine, oral contraceptives, mitomycin C
Glomerulonephritis secondary to NSAIDs, gold, penicillamine, captopril, bisphosphonates

- *Tubulointerstitial injury*

ATN secondary to contrast, aminoglycosides, vancomycin, amphotericin, pentamidine, foscarnet, cisplatin, acetaminophen, tenofovir, cidofovir, ritonavir, bisphosphonates
Acute interstitial nephritis (AIN) secondary to beta-lactams, quinolones, sulfonamides, vancomycin, PPI, phenytoin, allopurinol, diuretics

- *Crystal deposition*

Clinical examples include acyclovir, sulfadiazine, sulfamethoxazole, methotrexate, indinavir.

- *Retroperitoneal fibrosis*

Clinical examples include methyldopa, methysergide, gadolinium.

21.3 Prevention of Acute Kidney Injury

The focus of management in AKI is on prevention. Strategies have been suggested for the prevention of

Etiology of Acute Renal Failure	Prevention steps
Hypoperfusion	• Rapid reversal of MAP < 65 mm Hg with fluids and vasopressors as clinically appropriate • Avoidance of large volume hyperchloremic fluid resuscitation • Avoidance of hetastarch colloid solutions • Avoidance of over-resuscitation and significant interstitial edema
Contrast Nephropathy	• Avoidance of volume depletion with the administration of normal saline. No definite evidence favors bicarbonate solutions over the standard isotonic saline administration. • Stop medications which alter renovascular hemodynamics, including non-steroidal anti-inflammatory agents. The need to discontinue ACE inhibitors before contrast exposure remains controversial. • Minimize the dose of contrast, if feasible, and avoid short-term repetitive exposure (< 48 hours) • Administer the antioxidant N-acetylcysteine • Use low or iso-osmolar nonionic contrast agents
Aminoglycoside Nephropathy	• Single daily dosing • Careful monitoring of drug levels
Amphotericin Nephrotoxicity	• Use liposomal preparations • Use azole antifungal agents and/or the echinocandins rather than conventional amphotericin B, if equal therapeutic efficacy can be assumed • If standard amphotericin is required, discontinue diuretics and employ fluid loading protocols • Correct hypokalemia and hypomagnesemia
Tumor Lysis Syndrome	• Hydration accompanying allopurinol (moderate risk) or rasburicase (high risk)
Cirrhosis	• Albumin for patients with spontaneous bacterial peritonitis or for large volume paracentesis

Figure 21-2 *Prevention strategies for common hospital conditions causing acute renal failure.*

specific causes of AKI in the hospitalized patient. The prevention strategies are outlined in **Figure 21-2.** We will review the more common conditions.

21.3.1 Hypoperfusion

Very commonly, you will be managing the patient with sepsis and hypotension. While your focus will be on the initial resuscitation of the cardiopulmonary system, you should also be considering those interventions that will serve to prevent the delayed development of acute renal injury.

Patients with sepsis present with complex hemodynamics that involves vascular dilation (both arterial and venous), decreased cardiac output (septic cardiomyopathy), and reduced preload secondary to vascular leak. Initial resuscitation often focuses on volume administration to address preload but may have a delay in the administration of vasopressors. Vasopressor agents may be needed to address the additional hemodynamic manifestations of sepsis. A MAP < 65mm Hg is very predictive of mortality in the patient population presenting with septic shock. Early restoration of effective perfusion pressure (mean arterial pressure ≥ 65 mm Hg) is needed to

minimize organ injury. Often restoration of perfusion pressure requires a combination of fluid resuscitation and vasopressor (norepinephrine) administration. Remember, norepinephrine acts quickly to cause venoconstriction to correct preload deficits and can facilitate a prompt return of organ perfusion. Timely restoration of normal perfusion pressure is believed critical to renal protection.

Recent data has suggested the *type of resuscitation fluid* may influence renal function in the patient presenting with hypoperfusion. A reduction in renal perfusion has been demonstrated in healthy volunteers after the administration of 2L of normal saline in comparison to a buffered solution.[162]

Clinical trials have suggested the composition of crystalloid resuscitation fluids in ICU patient populations may influence metabolic function. All internists have recognized that large volume saline resuscitation is associated with a non-anion gap metabolic acidosis. Beyond this identified metabolic abnormality, are there additional adverse effects produced by the composition of resuscitation fluids on renal function?

Hyperchloremic solutions (normal saline) have been associated with a higher degree of renal injury in comparison to more balanced solutions (Ringer's lactate or Plasmalyte) in post-operative and general ICU patient clinical studies.[16,17,18,19] Whether a beneficial effect is restricted to larger volume administration, or only in sicker patients, remains undetermined.

A logical approach, given the existent clinical trials, might be to *target normochloremia*. This approach favors limiting saline solutions by volume (~ 1 liter) or by laboratory monitoring of serum chloride.[163] This approach restricts the administration of high volume saline administration to specific conditions that warrant this therapy, based upon electrolyte monitoring or tonicity, including metabolic alkalosis, hyponatremia, or brain injury.

In contrast to the controversy with crystalloid solutions, the adverse impact of hydroxyethyl starch solutions on renal failure is well recognized.[22] These fluids should be avoided in the resuscitation of patients with hypoperfusion to protect renal function.

The use of albumin is controversial in the resuscitation of the patient with sepsis, but this fluid, in comparison to crystalloid solutions, has not particularly been linked to an adverse impact on renal function. The exception is patients with liver disease, including patients with spontaneous bacterial peritonitis and those undergoing large-volume paracentesis. In these settings, intravenous albumin appears to be beneficial in preserving renal function.[164]

Finally, the *volume of fluid administered* may be significant in preserving renal function. The data here are again controversial and perhaps counterintuitive. As outlined by Prowle and colleagues, from a broad range of clinical studies in ICU patients with sepsis, we have "association" data that a markedly positive fluid balance has been associated with a higher risk of AKI.[165] Marked interstitial edema could contribute to abdominal compartment syndrome, which compromises renal blood flow. Marked positive fluid balance could also contribute to interstitial and renal subcapsular edema, compromising renal function. In this hypothesis, fluid overload in ICU septic patients is associated with adverse clinical outcomes and might contribute to the persistence of AKI. Obviously, these associations are not confirmatory of pathogenesis, but they do suggest that optimal fluid management in critical illness and AKI might involve early, targeted resuscitation to correct preload, but then is followed by active management to maintain an appropriate fluid balance. *Not too little, not too much, just right!! Easy to say, but hard to do.*

Neither diuretics nor dopamine (low dose at 3 mcg/kg/min) is helpful in preventing AKI. Diuretics are only indicated to manage volume overload in the setting of progressive AKI.

At the current time, no specific resuscitation strategy has been defined to limit the risk of AKI. Currently structured protocols for sepsis resuscitation do not appear to lower the risk of AKI in hospitalized patients with sepsis.

21.3.2 Contrast-Induced AKI

The best treatment for contrast-induced AKI (CI-AKI) is prevention, and the best prevention is avoidance! Think carefully before you expose your ICU patient with unstable hemodynamics to contrast. But even with significant caution, you will have situations that require contrast administration. What to do?

Is your patient at risk? Risk factors for CI-AKI have been variably defined in the literature but include[166]

- Presence of underlying renal insufficiency – target creatinine clearance of < 60 ml/min/1.73 M^2
- Diabetes
- Dehydration
- Malignancy
- Advanced age
- NSAIF agent use
- Biguanide use (metformin)
- Chemotherapy

The presence of these risk factors, especially underlying renal insufficiency, should trigger you to consider preventive measures to limit the risk of CI-AKI. This area has been extensively investigated without definitive solutions. The available clinical trials are limited by inadequately powered clinical trials with variable methodology. Numerous meta-analyses have been published, but they are limited by the inadequate clinical trials upon which they are based.

Intravenous saline (in contrast to more hypotonic saline) would be the preferred saline crystalloid to achieve volume expansion before and following contrast exposure. Comparison to bicarbonate administration has not clearly shown a benefit to the latter.[167] No difference in renal protection could be identified between these two regimens. There are no commercially available isotonic bicarbonate formulations, and that limitation could lead to compounding errors with the use of these solutions. Given their equivalency, we favor the use of normal saline. The use of mannitol is not favored for renal protection and may be harmful.

N-acetylcysteine (NAC) is a thiol compound with both antioxidant and vasodilating properties. This compound has been extensively investigated for possible renal protection effects in patients at high risk for CI-AKI. Both oral low dose (600 mg) and high dose (1200 mg) studies exist, with the dose given bid on the day prior and day of the procedure. The effectiveness of acetylcysteine is widely debated. Even the meta-analyses cannot agree on the efficacy of this regimen. Comparison of existing studies is limited by variable patient characteristics, variable dosing, and variable outcome measures. Given the excellent safety profile of oral NAC administration, in contrast to IV, this method of prevention alone may be of sufficiently low risk to justify its use in high-risk patients.

Statins have also been investigated as preventive measures for CI-AKI. Statins may improve endothelial function and reduce inflammation and oxidative stress. Some data, primarily from cardiac angiography patients, suggest that administration of statins in high-risk patients who also receive pre-intervention saline hydration and NAC benefit from statin administration. Given that patients with CAD have strong indications for statin therapy, it makes sense to initiate this therapy before contrast angiography if possible.

Finally, the selection of the contrast agent may also influence the risk of CI-AKI. Non-ionic, low osmolarity agents appear to provide lower risk and should be used whenever possible.

In summary

- Identify high-risk candidates for CI-AKI. No precautions other than avoidance of dehydration are needed for low-risk patients.
- Avoid contrast agents if other imaging modalities will provide clinically equivalent information.
- Pre-hydrate with normal saline at 1 mL/kg/hour for 6 hours before the procedure, intra-procedure, and 6-12 hours post procedure. The rate of fluid administration can be modified, based upon a patient's risk factors for fluid overload.
- Consider the additional administration of oral NAC at a dose of 600-1200 mg PO q12 hrs the day prior and day of the procedure. The current efficacy data are conflicting, but the oral medication is associated with a low-risk profile. The use of intravenous NAC is not favored. The administration of NAC *does not* preclude the need for isotonic fluid hydration.

21.3.3 Aminoglycoside Nephropathy

AKI, in addition to ototoxicity, represents the major risk factor to the use of aminoglycosides in the treatment of life-threatening infections. AKI may occur in up to 20% of patients receiving aminoglycosides in the hospital setting, and the toxicity can occur even with appropriate monitoring of serum levels. Current strategies to minimize the risk of aminoglycoside nephrotoxicity include

- Avoid using aminoglycosides for the treatment of infections unless no suitable, less nephrotoxic alternatives are available.
- Carefully monitor serum drug levels if therapy extends beyond 24 hours for multiple daily dosing

regimens and at 48 hours and beyond for single-daily dosing.
- Aminoglycoside selection should be based upon their perceived rate of AKI, which would favor selection in the following order: tobramycin > amikacin > streptomycin > gentamycin.
- Correct volume depletion and avoid simultaneous administration of additional potentially nephrotoxic agents.
- Use single-dose aminoglycoside dosing, if feasible.
- Correct low serum magnesium and potassium prior to administration of aminoglycosides, if possible.
- Use topical or local applications of aminoglycosides (e.g., respiratory aerosols, instilled antibiotic beads) rather than IV application, when feasible.

21.4 Management of Acute Kidney Injury

At the first sign of AKI, you want to walk through a series of steps in your patient management algorithm. The management of AKI is primarily supportive. The five key management items for you to consider each day are

1. Have all identified etiologies for AKI been removed or modified?
2. Have all necessary medication dosages been adjusted?
3. Are acid-base and electrolyte disorders corrected?
4. Are diuretics needed for volume overload only?
5. Is dialysis appropriate for *A-E-I-O-U* indications? (see mnemonic below)

21.4.1 Diuretic Use in AKI

Loop diuretics do not alter the course of AKI but can increase the volume of urine output. Simply put, they do not prevent or "cure" AKI. They may allow easier management of AKI because of their ability to control volume. Loop diuretics have a high risk of temporary deafness if used at high dosing in this patient population and should be dosed cautiously.

21.4.2 Dialysis Therapy

The primary indications for acute dialysis therapy can be remembered with the mnemonic *A-E-I-O-U*.

- *Acid-base disturbance* – significant metabolic acidosis (pH < 7.2) especially if resistant to bicarbonate replacement therapy or unable to replace due to volume overload
- *Electrolytes* – especially hyperkalemia associated with any ECG changes

- *Ingestions* – indicated for specific intoxications with marked clearance by dialysis intervention, including lithium, toxic alcohols, and salicylates
- *Overload* – fluid overload, especially in the setting of pulmonary edema resistant to diuretic therapy
- *Uremic symptoms*—including pericarditis, encephalopathy or seizures, platelet dysfunction with bleeding, intractable nausea with vomiting

The goals of hemodialysis are really twofold:

1. Remove kidney-failure-related small molecules, based upon a gradient of concentration = dialysis
2. Remove excess salt and water, based upon a gradient of pressure = ultrafiltration

Existing clinical data do not define an optimal time to initiate hemodialysis. However, a more delayed approach to initiating hemodialysis (based upon the presence of hyperkalemia or metabolic acidosis resistant to medical therapy, pulmonary edema, a blood urea nitrogen level > 112 mg/dL, or oliguria for > 72 hours in the AKIKI trial) was not associated with a greater mortality at 60 days compared to an earlier intervention.[168] Further, a delayed approach allowed several patients to avoid dialysis.

21.4.3 Dialysis Methods

Intermittent hemodialysis (IHD) involves solute clearance by diffusion across a semipermeable membrane, driven by a concentration gradient between the blood and a dialysate solution. In **Figure 21-3**, a basic hemodialysis circuit is illustrated. Blood is drawn from the arterial side of the patient's vascular access and pumped through tubing to the dialysis machine. Within the dialyzer, the membrane tubing is bathed by dialysate fluid running in opposite direction to the blood flow. Smaller molecules and metabolic waste products diffuse across the semipermeable membrane and into the dialysate fluid. Large molecules and blood cells remain in the tubing and are returned to the patient on the venous limb of their vascular access. Pressure monitors are present on both the arterial and venous side of the dialysis circuit. Heparin can be added to the circuit before the dialyzer to limit the risk of clotting. An air detector and filter are located on the venous limb to protect the patient from the introduction of air bubbles.

A number of variables interact to determine the *rate of solute clearance*, including the membrane characteristics, the rate of dialysate and blood flow, and the solute

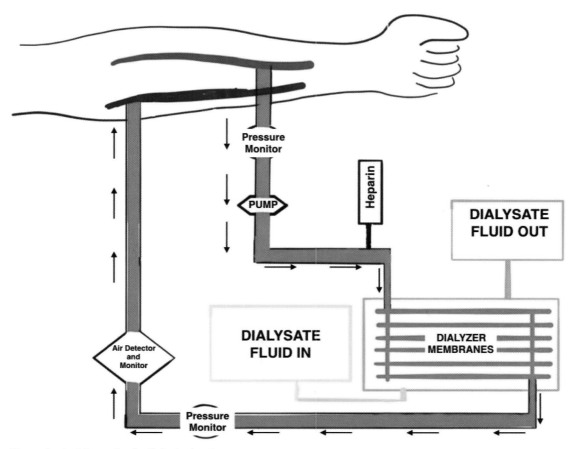

Figure 21-3 Schematic of a dialysis circuit.

characteristics (molecular weight). For IHD, typical pump speed is in the range of 200-500 mL/min with a dialysis flow rate of 500-750 mL/min. No replacement fluid is provided. Fluid removal rates are 500-1000 mL/hr. A typical IHD treatment will last ~ 4 hours and be provided on a three day per week schedule (M-W-F or T-Th-S). In the ICU, a modification of IHD is called *slow efficiency daily dialysis (SLEDD)*, which is provided at a reduced blood flow over a longer time interval (8 to 12 hours). This allows a more gradual fluid and solute removal over an extended period.

Continuous renal replacement therapy (CRRT) refers to a form of dialysis that is provided continuously over a 24-hour interval. There are a number of different modifications in the CRRT modality that lead to variable terms, including continuous venovenous hemofiltration (CVVH), continuous venovenous hemodialysis (CVVHD), and continuous venovenous hemodiafiltration (CVVHDF). A typical pump speed for CRRT is in the range of 100-180 mL/min with a dialysis flow rate of 0-2 L/hr. Replacement fluid is provided at a rate of 1-3 L/hr. Fluid removal rates are 100 mL/hr to 500 mL/hr. Although solute clearance is reduced per unit time, the 24-hour duration of this therapy allows CRRT to provide greater solute clearance over a 48-hour interval than IHD.

The forms of acute dialysis therapy are summarized in **Figure 21-4**. Currently, data do not suggest one form is advantageous in terms of mortality. The selection of dialysis modality is traditionally based upon the hemodynamic status of the patient. Slower or more continuous types of dialysis are favored in patients with hemodynamic instability. CRRT is generally considered a more costly form of dialysis treatment for the hospitalized patient with AKI.

Peritoneal dialysis is a fourth method of dialysis that uses the peritoneum as a natural semi-permeable membrane for solute removal. Although considered of equal efficacy to hemodialysis in the patient with chronic kidney failure, this form of dialysis is very rarely initiated in the acute care setting.

Anticoagulation is commonly employed for both IHD and CRRT if there is no contraindication. Passage of blood through the dialyzer membrane is associated with platelet activation and prothrombotic mediators that place the dialyzer membrane at risk for clotting and fibrin deposition on the filter membranes. This process can compromise the efficiency of the dialyzer membrane with time. Unfractionated heparin is the traditional agent employed for anticoagulation on dialysis, as the kidney clears low molecular weight heparins. A dose of heparin is given at the start of dialysis and repeated mid-dialysis to maintain a target clotting time. In high-risk patients, heparin may be avoided, especially if the patient is coagulopathic. A number of protocols exist for no-heparin hemodialysis, minimum dose heparin, and regional anticoagulation for the patient with a high bleeding risk.

For the patient who develops heparin-induced thrombocytopenia, the options for anticoagulation are limited. The options include no heparin dialysis, regional citrate hemodialysis, or the use of an alternative anticoagulant. Protocols exist for the use of argatroban, danaparoid, and lepirudin as alternative anticoagulants.

21.4.4 Dialysis Dose

In contrast to many other areas of AKI management, the dose of dialysis for patients with AKI has been carefully investigated. The adequacy of intermittent hemodialysis is most commonly assessed by a measurement that reflects the adequacy of urea clearance called the *Kt/V*. The measurement requires a blood sample for urea at the beginning and end of dialysis.

The *Kt/V* abbreviation includes the following:

- *K* stands for the dialyzer clearance or the rate at which blood passes through the dialyzer, expressed in milliliters per minute (mL/min).
- *t* stands for time measured as the duration of the dialysis treatment, measured in minutes.
- *Kt*, the top part of the fraction, is clearance multiplied by time, representing the volume of fluid completely cleared of urea during a single treatment.
- *V*, the bottom part of the fraction, is the volume of water a patient's body contains, which is estimated as 60% of the body weight.

So, if we assume a dialysis treatment with a clearance of 300 mL/min for 3 hours in a 70kg male, we would calculate

- Kt = 300 mL/min × 180 min = 54,000 mL or 54 liters

Dialysis method	Advantage	Disadvantage
Intermittent HD (IHD)	Easy to perform Solute control	Hemodynamic instability Anticoagulation
Slow efficiency daily dialysis (SLEDD)	Solute control Hemodynamic stability	Anticoagulation
Continuous renal replacement therapy (CRRT)	Solute removal Volume management Hemodynamic stability	Labor intensive Anticoagulation

Figure 21-4 Comparison of different dialysis methods.

- $V = 70 \text{ kg} \times 0.60 = 42$ liters
- $Kt/V = 54/42 = 1.3$

A common standard for the measure of dialysis adequacy per treatment session is a $Kt/V > 1.2$.

In studies involving CRRT, the dose has been prescribed as a weight-based hourly effluent rate, and the delivered dose of dialysis is considered to be the measured effluent volume.

Two clinical trials have compared dialysis regimens of varying intensity.[169,170] In both studies, no recognized benefit was seen to the more intensive dialysis strategy.

The orders for hemodialysis will generally require a discussion of multiple factors by the nephrologist:

1. Hemodialyzer membrane
2. Dialysate composition
3. Blood flow rate
4. Ultrafiltration goal
5. Anticoagulation method and dose
6. Dialysis dose

The good news is that unless you are a nephrologist, you will not have to set most of these parameters. But you don't get a free pass either! You need to work daily with your nephrologist, and two parameters are key for you to understand: 1) dialysate composition and 2) ultrafiltration goal.

The *dialysate composition* consists of the common electrolytes potassium, sodium, calcium, magnesium, bicarbonate, and glucose. The composition of the dialysate fluid will influence your post-dialysis electrolyte values. In the AKI patient on dialysis, you may need to alter the dialysate composition on a daily basis to maintain normal serum levels of these electrolytes. ***TALK TO YOUR NEPHROLOGIST!*** If your nephrologist writes orders and does not talk to you, find a new nephrologist. In a similar fashion, you need to agree on the daily ultrafiltration requirements based upon the patient's volume status and hemodynamic indices.

Suggested Reading

- Kellum JA, Chawla LS, Keener C, et al. The effects of alternative resuscitation strategies on acute kidney injury in patients with septic shock. Am J Respir Crit Care Med 2016;193(3):281–7.
- Weisbord SD, Palevsky PM. Prevention of contrast-associated acute kidney injury: What should we do? Am J Kidney Dis 2016.
- Pannu N, Manns B, Lee H, Tonelli M. Systematic review of the impact of N-acetylcysteine on contrast nephropathy. Kidney Int 2004;65(4): 1366–74.
- Husain-Syed, F., Slutsky, A. S. & Ronco, C. Lung-Kidney Cross-Talk in the critically ill patient. Am. J. Respir. Crit. Care Med. 194,402–14 (2016).
- Darmon, M. et al. Diagnostic work-up and specific causes of acute kidney injury. Intensive Care Med 43, 829–840 (2017).
- Joannes-Boyau O, Velly L, Ichai C. Optimizing continuous renal replacement therapy in the ICU. Curr Opin Crit Care [Internet] 2018;24(6):476–82.

22

Gastrointestinal Bleeding

Gastrointestinal bleeding is one of the most common conditions admitted to the intensive care unit. The clinical symptoms can range from frank hematemesis (vomiting blood) or hematochezia (bright red blood in the stool) to more occult signs with an isolated decline in the blood hematocrit and hemoglobin levels. The intensivist is focused on issues of fluid and transfusion resuscitation and medical management to diagnose and stop the bleeding—*fill up the tank and plug the holes!* Control of bleeding usually requires a multidisciplinary effort, which may involve the gastroenterologist, surgeon, and interventional radiologist.

The clinical manifestations of gastrointestinal bleeding are a history of hematemesis, melena, or hematochezia. Additional historical items include a history of ulcer disease, reflux symptoms, a prior history of abdominal aortic aneurysm, diverticulitis, or liver disease. A past use of alcohol, aspirin or corticosteroids suggests a potential etiology for bleeding (upper GI source), while a history of anticoagulant medications introduces a particular issue to address in the patient management. While the patient with hematemesis confirms an upper GI source, the patient presenting with melena or hematochezia is more difficult to assign a specific bleeding location. Bright red blood passed per rectum with stable hemodynamic indices suggests a source in the left colon. A hemodynamically stable patient with darker blood may be bleeding from the right colon or small bowel. Mild-moderate bleeding from the upper GI tract is characterized by loose, black bowel movements (melena).

These clinical parameters provide only a rough guide to the potential source of a GI bleed. An early assessment for possible upper GI bleeding in these patients can be made using nasogastric lavage. A positive aspirate from the stomach including blood or coffee ground material confirms the source as an upper tract bleed. However, the value of a nasogastric lavage is debated. An aspirate may be negative with an upper tract source if bleeding has stopped or the bleeding is post pylorus. Importantly, approximately 16% of upper GI bleeds from duodenal ulcer disease are reported to have a negative nasogastric (NG) aspirate.

An overall assessment of hemodynamics and tissue perfusion is a critical component of management for the hospital physician. The majority of patients present with intravascular volume contraction leading to tachycardia, hypotension, and a reduction in urine output. The reduced preload leads to a fall in stroke volume and cardiac output with compensatory increases in sympathetic output, renin/angiotensin production, and vasopressin release. These compensatory mechanisms promote salt and water retention and lead to systemic vasoconstriction, compromising organ perfusion. Depending on the magnitude of the compensatory response, the patient with GI bleeding may present hypo or normotensive with intravascular volume contraction.

22.1 ABC's (and D) of GI Bleeding

The management of the GI bleeding patient is focused on four components using your *ABC...D*'s:

1. **A**ccess for aggressive volume resuscitation to reverse organ hypoperfusion

2. **Blood** products for correction of hematocrit and reversal of defects in systemic coagulation
3. **Call** for additional expertise to control bleeding
4. **Determine** and treat the source of bleeding

56 yo woman presents with no recognized medical history other than being told of an enlarged liver in the past on routine exam. She suffers from modest obesity. She has a 12-hour history of recurrent hematemesis and hypotension. On presentation to the emergency department, she is having frequent emesis of bright red blood. Her heart rate is 115 bpm, RR 22, BP 80/70. She is cold and clammy on exam. Her lungs are clear, and her cardiac exam shows the tachycardia with no gallop. Her abdomen is non-tender. She has limited communication but responds to name appropriately. She has mild asterixis on examination. Her admission laboratories include a HCT of 32%, a (PT) INR of 1.9, and a platelet count of 90K. Note that the patient is in shock with visible bleeding, which represent the best markers of active bleeding. The hematocrit is not a reliable marker of active hemorrhage; it does not decrease immediately with acute bleeding, since you lose whole blood (equal plasma and red cells, so hematocrit is unchanged).

Our patient is unstable with evidence for active bleeding and hemodynamic instability. Immediate access with a peripheral 16-gauge catheter is appropriate, but early preparation for the placement of a central 8.5 French introducer is indicated with active bleeding and hemodynamic instability. The placement of a triple lumen central venous catheter in this situation is less than optimal for large volume resuscitation.

22.1.1 Access

Adequate resuscitation is always the first step in the management of gastrointestinal bleeding, and this requires appropriate intravascular access. Because resistance is proportional to length times radius to the 4th power, the bigger the diameter (lower the gauge) and shorter the catheter, the faster the flow. For this reason, a larger bore (~16 gauge) peripheral venous angiocatheter or central venous catheter is immediately indicated to begin resuscitation. Note that a simple 16 gauge IV (angiocatheter) can give close to one 400-450 mL unit of blood in two minutes (220 mL per minute)! A summary of intravenous catheters and their associated maximal flow rates are outlined in **Figure 22-1**.

22.1.2 Blood and Blood Products

The primary focus of resuscitation is to administer volume as quickly as possible to reverse the decline in preload, improve stroke volume, and achieve better overall systemic perfusion. Debate has existed over the appropriate target for transfusion in patients with GI bleeding. Current evidence supports a more restrictive transfusion target in the range of ~ 7-8 gms/dL

Catheter	Diameter (mm)	Length (mm)	Maximum flow ml/min
20-gauge angiocath	0.8	30	60
18-gauge angiocath	1.0	30	105
16-gauge angiocath	1.3	30	220
3-lumen catheter 16-gauge angiocath	1.3	200	52
8F introducer catheter	2.8	100	126

Figure 22-1 *Comparison of different venous access catheters by dimensions and maximum flow rates.*

hemoglobin.[151] The more restrictive strategy in this trial was associated with a 45% relative-risk reduction in 45-day mortality due to fewer deaths from bleeding that could not be successfully controlled. Also reduced were rates of further bleeding, transfusion reactions, cardiac events, and length of hospital stay. Animal studies have suggested a restrictive transfusion strategy might benefit the patient with portal hypertension to prevent transfusion-associated increases in portal pressure.

Exceptions to this threshold for transfusion may exist. Patients with hypotension (shock) in the setting of GI bleeding may have significant intravascular volume depletion prior to a fall in their hematocrit. Patients with cardiac disease remain controversial with respect to transfusion targets. The available data suggest we can safely also use a restricted transfusion target in these patients without risk. However, many of the trials enrolled patients with exclusion of varying degrees of cardiac dysfunction, especially acute coronary syndrome. In the absence of clinical symptoms, our available data suggest that a transfusion target of 7-8 gms/dL is appropriate, even for patients with cardiac disease.

Complications are recognized in the patient who receives transfusion with multiple units of packed RBCs. Hypothermia is associated with the transfusion of multiple units of chilled blood and can be related to arrhythmias. A blood warmer can be used to minimize this complication any time > 3 units of blood are transfused, as hypothermia can also be associated with coagulation complications. Each transfused unit of blood can increase the blood potassium concentration, which is usually inconsequential except in the patient with impaired excretion (renal disease). Blood is anticoagulated with sodium citrate, and citric acid can potentially lead to a metabolic alkalosis and a decline in the plasma free calcium level. This complication is most frequent in the setting of advanced liver disease.

You will often find yourself in situations where you have to massively transfuse a patient with GI bleeding in order to keep the patient alive. In these cases, you will be at risk for a number of complications from giving so much blood products. For massive transfusion guidelines, review our *Chapter 20, Transfusion Medicine.*

Keep three basic targets in mind:

- Hemoglobin 7-8 gms / dL
- Platelet count > 50,000 /mm^3
- INR ≤ 1.5

And our simple rule:

- Massive transfusion blood component ratio: 1 RBC : 1 FFP : 1 RDU

22.1.3 Call for Help

Patients with active bleeding need urgent consultation with other specialists, often including a gastroenterologist, interventional radiologist, and a surgeon. It's better to call early and figure out they may not be needed.

The management of GI bleeding is broken into three management algorithms based upon the location of the bleeding site:

1. *Upper GI bleeding* – considered to be an origin proximal to the ligament of Treitz

   a. Non-variceal upper GI bleeding
   b. Variceal upper GI bleeding

2. Lower GI bleeding

Our patient needs aggressive resuscitation with blood products. Using a rapid infuser, she receives 5 units of packed red blood cells and 4 units of fresh frozen plasma. Because of the large volume infused, the blood is warmed, and a schedule of ongoing monitoring for HCT and coagulation parameters is established. After venous access is achieved, she undergoes elective intubation because of ongoing hematemesis and the need for urgent endoscopy with sedation.

For the patient with an upper GI bleeding source, the intensivist can assist with the prep for endoscopy by managing the patient's airway. Intubation and airway protection may be needed to protect the patient from blood aspiration. The complexity of airway management is significantly increased in the presence of active upper GI bleeding, and a rapid sequence approach is preferred to avoid gastric distention from insufflation during bag-mask ventilation. NG lavage can be used to clear the stomach of retained clots and improve the effectiveness of endoscopy to achieve an accurate diagnosis and intervention.

22.1.4 Diagnose the Bleeding Source

22.1.4.1 Non-Variceal Upper GI Bleeding

The most common etiology of upper GI bleeding is non-variceal bleeding (80-90% of cases). The most common

etiology of non-variceal bleeding is related to peptic ulcer disease (30%). *Heliobacter pylori,* non-steroidal anti-inflammatory agents, and aspirin are major risk factors for upper GI bleeding. Early endoscopy (within 24 hours of admission) is advocated to reduce the risk of recurrent bleeding and the need for surgical intervention. For the patient with non-variceal GI bleeding, a number of risk-stratification models have been developed to promote efficient use of resources for this very common type of GI bleeding. Current models rely on both clinical and endoscopic parameters. Prior to endoscopy, the *Blatchford scoring system* can be used to define high risk for patients with upper GI bleeding (**Figure 22-2**).[171]

Using this scoring system, a score of 0-1 is associated with a low-risk patient, and the endoscopy can be delayed. The Blatchford scoring system has a high sensitivity for identifying patients with a severe bleeding risk. The advantage of this scoring system is that it does not incorporate endoscopy data and can be used at the time of the patient's initial clinical presentation.

Once endoscopy has been performed, the *Rockall model* is used to predict the risk of recurrent bleeding, as outlined in **Figure 22-3**.[172]

The score is obtained for each individual parameter in the far-left column and totaled. For patients with a score of < 2, rebleeding occurs in less than 5% of

Admission Risk Marker	Value	Score Component Based Upon Value
BUN	< 18.2 mg/dL	0
	≥ 18.2 but < 22.4 mg/dL	2
	≥ 22.4 but < 28 mg/dL	3
	≥ 28 but < 70 mg/dL	4
	≥ 70 but < 22.4 mg/dL	6
Hemoglobin	Male > 13 g/dL	0
	Male ≥ 12 but < 13 g/dL	1
	Male ≥ 10 but < 12 g/dL	3
	Female ≥ 12 g/dL	0
	Female ≥ 10 but < 12 g/dL	1
	Male or Female < 10 g/dL	6
Systolic blood pressure	≥ 110 mmHg	0
	100 to 109 mm Hg	1
	90 to 99 mm Hg	2
	< 90 mm Hg	3
Other markers	Heart rate ≥ 100 per minute	1
	Melena at presentation	1
	Syncope at presentation	2
	Hepatic disease present	2
	Cardiac failure present	2

Figure 22-2 Blatchford scoring systems for high risk upper gastrointestinal bleeding.

Score	0	1	2	3
Age	< 60yo	60-79yo	> 80yo	
Shock	Shock absent Systolic BP > 100 mm Hg and HR < 100 bpm	Tachycardia HR > 100 with systolic BP > 100	Hypotension Systolic BP < 100	
Comorbidity	None		Cardiac failure Ischemic heart disease Malignancy of the upper tract	Renal failure Liver failure Disseminated malignancy
Diagnosis	Mallory-Weiss tear No lesion identified	All other	Malignancy of the upper tract	
Stigmata of recent Hemorrhage	None or dark spot only	All other diagnoses	Blood in upper GI tract Adherent clot Visible or spurting vessel	

Figure 22-3 Rockall model for recurrent bleeding risk post endoscopy in upper gastrointestinal bleeding.

patients, and mortality was very low in a validation series. This represents a very low-risk group, and the variables can be incorporated into triage decisions for hospital location (ICU vs. floor) or discharge.

The value of these scoring systems is debated, and clinicians do not use them on a regular basis. But the modeling does highlight clinical variables that predict patients with a very high risk of rebleeding. Rebleeding is one of the strongest predictors of mortality. These risk factors include

- Age > 60
- Comorbid illness
- Hemodynamic instability
- Active arterial bleeding at endoscopy
- Nonbleeding visible vessel at endoscopy
- Ulcer > 2 cm
- Adherent clot

The primary medical therapy for upper GI non-variceal bleeding is the administration of proton pump inhibitors (PPI), which reduce the rate of rebleeding and the need for surgical intervention after endoscopic therapy.[173] The high dose continuous infusion (80 mg omeprazole followed by 8 mg per hour for 72 hours) is a standard regimen that is advised for patients with suspected upper GI non-variceal bleeding. However, equally effective may be the use of intermittent dosing.[174]

Octreotide, a long acting analogue of somatostatin, could have theoretical benefit in non-variceal upper GI bleeding. The drug reduces splanchnic blood flow and inhibits gastric acid secretion. Although some studies suggest octreotide is beneficial in non-variceal upper GI bleeding, the findings are inconsistent. The use of octreotide for non-variceal bleeding remains controversial.

Your friendly gastroenterologist may ask you to administer a medication that promotes gastric motility (erythromycin or metoclopramide) 20 to 120 minutes prior to endoscopy. The administration of these agents in patients with a high likelihood of having fresh blood or a clot in the stomach may help increase the yield of diagnostic endoscopy.[175]

Endoscopy is favored within 24 hours of admission for any patient in higher risk categories. Endoscopic treatment modalities include injection, cauterization, and mechanical therapy. In the case of peptic ulcer disease, the appearance of lesions at endoscopy can be used to define the risk of recurrent bleeding and the need for a specific endoscopic intervention beyond diagnosis, such as a mechanical method (i.e., clips), thermal coagulation, or fibrin/thrombin treatment with epinephrine.[176]

Endoscopic intervention is indicated for peptic ulcer disease lesions considered at high risk for failing medical therapy alone. These conditions include

- Ulcers with signs of active spurting or oozing blood
- Ulcers with a nonbleeding visible vessel (~ 50% rebleeding rate)

In these high-risk lesions, epinephrine injection treatment should not be used alone but rather combined with a second endoscopic treatment modality. In contrast, lower-risk lesions can be approached without the need for endoscopic intervention and with more conservative medical therapy. These lesions include

- Flat pigmented spots in the ulcer bed (< 8 % rebleeding rate)
- Clean-based ulcers (< 3 % rebleeding rate)

Intermediate risk lesions show signs of adherent clots (8-35% rebleeding rate) with the prognosis influenced by the underlying lesion.

Patients with rebleeding after PPI administration and initial endoscopy should undergo a repeat endoscopy. Patient who recurrently bleed after endoscopy interventions should be offered interventional radiology procedures. Patients with a bleeding peptic ulcer should be tested for H. pylori and treated if present. Empiric treatment is not advised.

22.1.4.2 Variceal Upper GI Bleeding

Gastroesophageal varices are present in a significant fraction of patients with cirrhosis, and variceal bleeding accounts for approximately 1/3 of all deaths in patients with cirrhosis. Although prevention is a major component of variceal management, this discussion will focus on the acute management of an active bleed. Although patients with cirrhosis can bleed from other causes (e.g., Mallory-Weiss tear, peptic ulcer disease), the presumed etiology is gastroesophageal varices, pending endoscopic confirmation. Patients with non-variceal bleeding stop spontaneously in 90% of cases, in contrast to the $\leq$ 50% rate of spontaneous resolution in patients with variceal bleeding. The high risk of rebleeding and mortality risk seen in patients with variceal bleeding mandates that they be managed in an intensive care unit until bleeding is controlled.

Similar to non-variceal bleeding, there are three principles in the management of variceal upper GI bleeding, remembered by the parameter you are always chasing in the bleeding patient, the *HCT*:

1. *Hemodynamic resuscitation*
2. *Complication management*
3. *Treatment of bleeding*

Fluid and blood product replacement are the key components of early management. Vascular access to allow rapid blood product administration is essential. Target parameters for resuscitation are similar for the non-variceal population. The overall goal is a target hemoglobin of 7-8 gms/dL and hemodynamic stability. Avoid over-resuscitation, which can lead to elevated portal venous pressures.

The initial treatment of patients with esophageal varices is also focused on efforts to control portal hypertension. In an effort to lower portal venous pressures, patients with suspected variceal bleeding are initially treated with continuous infusions of one of two agents associated with reduced portal blood flow:

- *Octreotide.* This is your best first-line agent. It is a long-acting analog of somatostatin, which inhibits the release of vasodilator hormones in the GI tract, indirectly leading to vasoconstriction.

The medication may also have some direct vasoconstrictor properties. The primary advantage of octreotide is a very favorable safety profile, and it can be used continuously for 5 days or even longer. Following a 50 mcg bolus of somatostatin, portal venous inflow, portal pressures, and intravariceal pressures decrease almost immediately. The formulation is administered as a 50 mcg bolus followed by an infusion of 50 mcg/hr for five (5) days. Reduction of portal venous pressures to < 12 mm Hg or a 20% reduction from baseline measurements are associated with control of active bleeding and a reduced rebleeding rate. This therapy can be initiated as soon as variceal bleeding is suspected.

- *Vasopressin.* Alternatively, intravenous vasopressin (0.4 unit bolus followed by a continuous infusion of 0.4 – 0.8 unit/min) is a potent vasoconstrictor of mesenteric arterioles, reducing portal venous inflow and therefore portal venous pressures. The major risk of vasopressin administration is the nonspecific vasoconstrictive effect on non-mesenteric blood vessels, including the coronary circulation. Administration of nitroglycerin (10 to 50 mcg /min) with vasopressin can attenuate some of the adverse hemodynamic effects. Comparative studies suggest that somatostatin has a greater rate of bleeding cessation in the setting of variceal bleeds and a lower risk of adverse effects. For these reasons, octreotide is generally the preferred agent.

Although Beta-blockers are frequently used to reduce the rate of recurrent variceal bleeding, they would not be used in the acute setting. These medications could complicate hemodynamic resuscitation by lowering blood pressure and blocking the necessary heart rate response.

22.1.4.2.1 Complications of Variceal Bleeding

Complications that arise in association with esophageal hemorrhage are a significant mortality risk for patients. They include aspiration pneumonia, spontaneous bacterial peritonitis, hepatic encephalopathy, hepatorenal syndrome, and sepsis.

The *risk of aspiration* for patients with variceal bleeding, prior to and in association with endoscopy can be significant. Endotracheal intubation is used to protect the airway in high-risk esophageal bleeding cases prior to endoscopy, especially if the patient has altered mental status (e.g., intoxication or hepatic encephalopathy). Use precautions to avoid over-distending the stomach during the intubation (i.e., limit bag-mask ventilation) in order to prevent emesis and minimize this risk.

The risk of *infection* complicating the course of patients presenting with variceal bleeding is very high, both spontaneous bacterial peritonitis and other infections. This has led to a large number of trials using antibiotic prophylaxis to minimize this risk.[177] Antibiotic prophylaxis in these patients has been associated with significantly reduced bacterial infections, rebleeding events, hospitalization length, and mortality. These findings have led to the recommendation that any patient with cirrhosis and GI hemorrhage receive short-term ($\leq$ 7 days) antibiotic prophylaxis, which might include ciprofloxacin, trimethoprim-sulfamethoxazole, or ceftriaxone.

Patients with advanced cirrhosis and GI bleeding will be at significant risk for *hepatic encephalopathy*. Patients should receive lactulose to promote clearance of blood from the GI tract soon after resuscitation and stabilization of the active GI bleeding.

Bleeding and the associated hemodynamic complications will place the patient at risk for *acute renal injury*, including acute tubular necrosis. This risk can be minimized with adequate intravascular volume resuscitation.

22.1.4.2.2 Treatment of Variceal Bleeding

Esophagogastroduodenoscopy (EGD) should be performed promptly after the patient admission as soon as the patient can be hemodynamically stabilized. In general, EGD should be completed within 12 hours of presentation. The majority of bleeding from esophageal varices can be controlled by endoscopic therapy. Endoscopic variceal ligation (EVL) is the preferred method of endoscopic therapy for acute esophageal variceal bleeding, although sclerotherapy is advised in patients when EVL is not technically feasible.[178] The combination of pharmacologic and endoscopic therapy is the favored treatment option for patients presenting with variceal bleeding.[179] Pharmacologic treatment is

extended over a 5-day interval when the risk of rebleeding remains significantly elevated. Approximately 10-20% of patients with variceal bleeding will fail initial therapy. These patients are then addressed with balloon tamponade and/or creation of a portosystemic shunt.

22.1.4.2.2.1.1 Balloon Tamponade

Balloon tamponade can be used in patients with variceal bleeding who fail to respond to initial endoscopic therapy. Although highly effective, balloon tamponade is associated with several potentially lethal complications, including aspiration, balloon migration, and necrosis/perforation of the esophagus. The use of balloon tamponade should be restricted to a temporizing procedure to control bleeding until a more definitive procedure (see TIPS below) can be accomplished. Because of the high association with complications, balloon tamponade should be attempted only by experienced individuals who place the tubes with precautions.

A number of specialized tubes exist to accomplish balloon tamponade including the following:

1. *Sengstaken-Blakemore tube* – consists of a 250cc gastric balloon, an esophageal balloon, and a single gastric suction port
2. *Minnesota tube* – consists of a 250cc gastric balloon, an esophageal balloon, and gastric suction port, and a suction port above the esophageal balloon
3. *Linton-Nachlas tube* – consists of a single 600cc gastric balloon

A sample balloon tamponade tube is illustrated in Figure 22-4.

Prior to placement of the tube for balloon tamponade, all patients should undergo elective intubation for definitive airway control to prevent aspiration and accidental airway occlusion if the balloon tamponade were to slip.

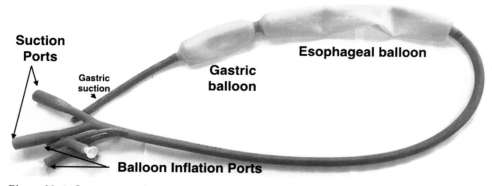

Figure 22-4 *Components of a sample Minnesota tube used for balloon tamponade.*

First check the balloons to confirm their integrity, and then the tube is passed into the stomach. Initial positioning can be verified with auscultation. The gastric tube is partially inflated (~50cc) with air, *followed by a radiograph obtained to confirm a subdiaphragmatic location* of the gastric balloon. The importance of radiographic confirmation of the tube position prior to full inflation of the gastric balloon cannot be understated. Inflation of the gastric balloon to full volume in the esophagus can produce an esophageal perforation, a potentially lethal complication. Once the correct position is confirmed, the gastric balloon can be inflated to the full volume (~450-500ml). At this point, the tube is pulled until tension is appreciated, at which point the balloon is compressing the GE junction. The tube can then be taped to a football helmet or connected to 1-2 lb traction to maintain tension. In many cases, inflation of the gastric balloon alone will stop active variceal bleeding.

If bleeding continues after inflation of the gastric balloon, the esophageal balloon is inflated. Rather than a specific volume, the inflation of the esophageal balloon occurs to a pressure target. Initially the balloon is inflated to 30 to 45 mmHg, and the pressure is checked frequently (~q1 hour). Overinflating the esophageal balloon to accomplish higher pressures can create excessive ischemia of the esophagus mucosa, leading to esophageal necrosis or rupture. Once the bleeding is controlled, the pressure in the esophageal balloon is reduced by 5 mmHg to a goal pressure of 25 mmHg for 12 to 24 hours.

The gastric and esophageal balloons can be periodically deflated to examine for recurrent bleeding. The use of balloon tamponade is typically combined with a more definitive procedure to control bleeding, due to a high recurrence rate with balloon deflation.

22.1.4.2.2.1.2 Portosystemic Shunt Therapy

Transjugular intrahepatic portosystemic shunt (TIPS) or transjugular intrahepatic portosystemic stent shunting (TIPPS) is used acutely to lower portal hypertension in the patient with active bleeding. The TIPS procedure, most commonly performed by an interventional radiologist, establishes a communication between the inflow portal vein and the outflow hepatic vein of the liver, decreasing the vascular resistance of the liver. By creating a "shunt" from the portal to systemic circulation, portal venous pressures are acutely lowered, and vascular pressures in the intestinal circulation fall. As a result, bleeding risk is controlled. This procedure is now the most common approach to the treatment of portal hypertension and the associated complications. TIPS has replaced the past use of surgical portocaval shunting procedures.

Access to the circulation is typically achieved through the internal jugular vein. The hepatic vein is cannulated from this route, and a needle is passed from the hepatic vein to the portal vein. An angioplasty balloon is used to create a tract from the two veins, followed by placement of a stent in the tract. Pressure measurements can be made to confirm a lowering of portal vein pressures with the established shunt. The risks of the procedures include bleeding or hepatic injury, but this risk is low in the hands of an experienced operator (~ 1%). The primary complication of the TIPS procedure is hepatic encephalopathy, which can occur in up to 25% of patients due to the bypass of the hepatic circulation.

The patient's active bleeding was controlled with placement of a Minnesota tube and inflation of the gastric balloon only. She was taken for urgent TIPS, and 24 hours following this procedure her gastric balloon was deflated without recurrence of her bleeding.

Frequently, variceal bleeding can be controlled with balloon compression at the level of the GE junction. This provides a temporary measure until a permanent solution can be achieved by performance of either a transjugular intrahepatic portal-systemic shunt (TIPS) or surgical shunt. TIPS placement is successful in 90-95% of cases, with the primary adverse effect being a relatively high rate of post-TIPS encephalopathy (15-30%).

22.1.4.2.3 Gastric Varices

There is much less data on specific therapy for gastric varices. These varices, when they occur in isolation, can be difficult to treat. EVL is a therapeutic option for gastroesophageal varices that arise as an extension of esophageal varices along the lesser curvature of the stomach (GOV1). Although fundal varices might be approached with injection therapy or banding by experienced endoscopists, the incidence of rebleeding is very high. Emergency TIPS appears to be the procedure of choice for these patients.

22.1.4.3 Lower GI Bleeding

Lower gastrointestinal (LGI) bleeding has traditionally been defined as bleeding beyond the ligament of Treitz. However, a more recent definition, which recognizes mid-gut bleeding (small bowel), now classifies LGI bleeding as beyond the ileocecal valve. Classically, lower GI bleeding presents with hematochezia or clots per rectum, in contrast to melena, which suggests upper GI bleeding. However, right colon bleeding from the cecum can present with melena, and brisk upper GI bleeding can present with hematochezia, so the distinction is not absolute. The majority of patients with lower GI bleeding have a self-limited bleed with an uncomplicated hospitalization. In comparison to upper GI bleeding, patients generally require fewer packed red blood cell transfusions and have greater hemodynamic stability.

The most common cause of acute LGI bleeding is *diverticular bleeding* (30%), yet only a small fraction of patients with diverticuli actually develop bleeding (~3%). The patient most frequently presents with painless hematochezia. Bleeding resolves spontaneously in the majority of patients. Bleeding from *ischemic colitis* typically results from a sudden episodic reduction in blood flow. The most commonly affected areas are the watershed zones located in the splenic flexure and the rectosigmoid junction. Mesenteric occlusion may result from cardiac thromboembolic disease. The majority of patients with ischemic colitis improve with conservative management that includes hydration. Additional etiologies for LGI bleeding include angioectasias, hemorrhoids, colorectal neoplasia, and post-polypectomy bleeding.

The principles for the initial resuscitation for LGI bleeding are similar to those for UGI bleeding. Of all patients with bright red blood per rectum, those who require multiple unit transfusions or have hemodynamic instability and/or significant comorbidity should be hospitalized with monitoring in the ICU.

The role of nasogastric tube placement in the evaluation of patients with LGI bleeding is controversial. The procedure may be most valuable in a patient presenting with hematochezia and hemodynamic instability. An algorithm for the evaluation of the patient with suspected lower GI bleeding based upon the NG aspirate is outlined in **Figure 22-5**.

In hemodynamically stable patients with significant hematochezia, *colonoscopy is considered the initial step* in the evaluation, when an upper GI source has been excluded by NG lavage or EGD. Colonoscopy has a higher diagnostic yield and allows possible therapeutic control of bleeding in comparison to radionucleotide scanning or angiography. Gastroenterologists favor a variety of techniques for colon preparation, which continues until the effluent is free of fecal material. Radiographic studies are indicated prior to the procedure if perforation or obstruction is suspected. For patients with diverticular bleeding, epinephrine injection combined with thermal coagulation or endoscopic clip are utilized to control bleeding,

If colonoscopy is unable to achieve visualization, due to an accelerated bleeding rate, then radionuclide imaging is indicated. Radionuclide imaging is more sensitive to bleeding (bleeding rate of ~ 0.5ml/min), compared to arteriography (bleeding rate of ~ 1.0ml/min), providing a potential role for nuclear imaging to screen patients prior to arteriography for active bleeding.

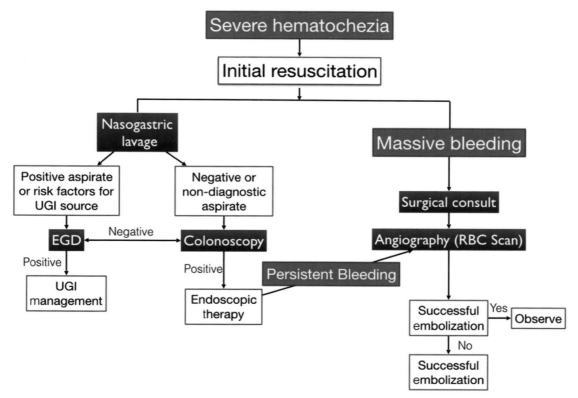

Figure 22-5* *Approach to the patient with lower gastrointestinal bleeding.*

*Adapted from180 ASGE Standards of Practice Committee, Pasha SF, Shergill A, et al. The role of endoscopy in the patient with lower GI bleeding. Gastrointestinal Endoscopy 2014;79(6):875–85.

The two standard nuclear scans include technetium sulfur colloid (99mTc) and 99mTc pertechnetate-labeled autologous red blood cells. The primary advantage of 99mTc pertechnetate-labeled autologous red blood cells is a longer half-life in the circulation, allowing the scans to be obtained repeatedly up to 24 hours post injection. The major limitation of radionuclide imaging is a wide range in reported accuracy from 25-90%. This wide variability and the nonspecific nature of positive findings from radionuclide imaging has led to *colonoscopy being the initial procedure of choice.*

Arteriography requires a rate of bleeding between 1-1.5 mL/minute for detection of active bleeding. The procedure is 100% specific but has widely reported sensitivity. The superior mesenteric artery is the most common source for LGI bleeds and is typically examined first if a particular location is not suspected, followed by the inferior mesenteric and celiac arteries. The procedure does not require bowel preparation, and therapeutic intervention with either embolization or local vasopressin administration will often control active bleeding. The primary risks of arteriography with embolization include arterial thrombosis with intestinal infarction and acute renal failure (post contrast). As a result, colonoscopy is again favored over this procedure in patients if satisfactory visualization can be achieved.

Suggested Reading

- D'Hondt A, Haentjens L, Brassart N, Flamme F, Preiser J-C. Uncontrolled bleeding of the gastrointestinal tract. Current Opinion in Critical Care 2017;23(6):549.

23

Acid-Base Disorders

Arterial blood gases (ABG) are one of the most frequently ordered tests in the hospital. With the widespread availability of non-invasive methods to measure oxygenation (pulse oximetry), the need for ABGs may be less frequent. But ABGs remain a critical tool for the assessment of gas exchange efficiency, ventilation, and acid-base disturbances.

An arterial blood gas is obtained from a small (1ml) sample of blood obtained from puncture of the radial artery or from an indwelling arterial catheter. ABG analysis includes the direct measurement of PaO_2, $PaCO_2$, and pH. The SaO_2 can be calculated based upon the standard oxygen-hemoglobin dissociation curve or alternatively measured if the blood gas analyzer includes a co-oximeter. The co-oximeter actually measures the ligand-binding (oxygen, carbon monoxide, deoxyhemoglobin, methemoglobin) saturations of hemoglobin using absorbance spectrophotometry, and is the most accurate way of assessing these different hemoglobin species.

Acidemia is defined as a pH < 7.36 and alkalemia as a pH > 7.44. Alternatively, an acid-base disorder can be suspected when the $PaCO_2$ is outside the normal range of 35-45 mm Hg, the plasma bicarbonate concentration is outside the normal range of 22-26 mEq/L, or the arterial base excess is > 3 or < -3 mEq/L. However, any analysis of the patient's acid-base status *always requires an assessment of the blood pH* before an analysis of the acid-base condition of the patient can begin.

Because arterial blood sampling can be painful for patients, often there is a desire to use venous blood

sampling for pCO_2 and acid-base assessment. Venous blood sampling is considered more convenient, less painful, and generally easier to perform. Most studies suggest that venous pH, bicarbonate, and base excess provide an acceptable alternative to arterial parameters in clinical practice. However, the reliability of venous parameters in more advanced shock states is poorly studied and favors the continued use of arterial measurements for these patients. Central venous pH is usually 0.03 to 0.05 pH units lower than arterial blood. The serum HCO_3^- will show minimal variation between venous and arterial blood. The gradient between arterial pCO_2 and central venous pCO_2 is traditionally reported as 4-5 mm Hg, but the differences can vary widely. For shock states and complex acid-base disorders, arterial blood specimens are preferred. For more stable patients, we often follow the trends of the venous CO_2 values for patients on the ventilator or on BiPAP therapy, rather than stick the artery or place A-lines. The following analysis of acid-base applies to either origin for the blood gas samples.

23.1 Simple Acid-Base

An excellent resource on acid-base disorders and the logic and illogic behind how we teach them is covered on http://www.acid-base.com/index.php, Acid-Base Tutorial, by "Grog" (Alan W. Grogono). He points out a few critical paradoxes in terminology that are all based on historical nomenclature, e.g., hydrogen missing an electron is called H^+, a decrease in pH represents more

H+ and more acidity, and metabolic acidosis is defined by a negative base excess *(that one can give you a headache!)*. Furthermore, the Henderson-Hasselbalch equation has been used to teach acid-base disorders to legions of medical students, yet it is intrinsically counterintuitive as it describes a negative log relationship:

$$pH = pK_A + \log \{[\,HCO_3^-]/[CO_2]\}$$

For OUR approach let's start by throwing Hasselbalch in the trash!

Let's scrape this Hasselbalch part and start over with simple chemistry and physiology that we can use to build a clinical acid-base analysis. To do this we will think about proton (H^+), bicarbonate (HCO_3^-), and carbon dioxide (CO_2). Since you know that more proton means more acid and lower pH, then you can just avoid the Hassel (balch)!

Let's start with the primary buffer systems in blood, bicarbonate (HCO_3^-), and its major protonation product: carbonic acid (H_2CO_3). This amazing system maintains a tight pH control in the body, between 7.35 and 7.45. This system's entire job is to regulate *hydrogen ion balance.*

This is simply described as the concentration of ionization products on the left (proton and bicarbonate) and dissociation products on the right (water and carbon dioxide), catalyzed by carbonic anhydrase:

$$[H+] + [HCO_3^-] \leftrightarrow [H_2CO_3] \leftrightarrow [H_2O] + [CO_2]$$

If you think of this relationship and the fact that it is balanced in the body, then everything is easy. This can also be conceptualized as:

$$[H+] = [CO_2]/\,[HCO_3^-]$$

This simple relationship describes the mass action of the PCO_2 and HCO_3^- buffering system. This system maintains the proton concentration in just the right place. The hydrogen ion concentration is therefore set by the ratio of these two components. A normal proton concentration is maintained by a PCO_2 of about 40 mm Hg and by a HCO_3^- of 24-26 mEq/L.

As illustrated in **Figure 23-1**, imagine a balance that maintains hydrogen ion concentration. If $PaCO_2$ goes up, then HCO_3^- must be added (retained by kidney) to keep the hydrogen ion balanced. If $PaCO_2$ goes down, then HCO_3^- must be wasted by kidney to balance. Vice versa for changes in HCO_3^- relative to $PaCO_2$.

For acidosis. Increasing CO_2 increases hydrogen ion, and decreasing bicarbonate likewise increases hydrogen ion.

For alkalosis. Decreasing CO_2 decreases hydrogen ion, and increasing bicarbonate likewise decreases hydrogen ion.

Easy.

23.2 Primary Disturbance and Secondary Compensation

When you have a primary disturbance or disease that changes the hydrogen ion concentration, the body will attempt to compensate to keep the hydrogen ion in the right place and maintain a normal pH. The lung defends (compensates) the hydrogen ion concentration (and pH) by changing PCO_2, and the kidney defends (compensates) the hydrogen ion concentration by changing HCO_3^-. The lung can do this by hyperventilating or hypoventilating. The kidney can do this by retaining HCO_3^- at the proximal tubule or by increasing fixed acid excretion at the distal tubule. The proximal tubule reabsorption of bicarbonate is massive, with up to 4,500 mEq per day reabsorbed! This prevents

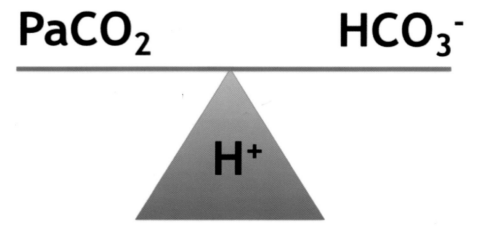

Figure 23-1 *The balance of arterial hydrogen ion concentration is achieved by the relationship of PaCO₂ and HCO₃⁻.*

For those of you math nerds who DO want to know how to derive the HH equation you start with the dissociation constant for carbonic acid, our bodies major buffer system

$$Ka = \{[H^+] + [HCO_3^-]\}/[H_2CO_3]$$

Or

$$Ka = \{[H^+] + [HCO_3^-]\}/[H_2O + CO_2] \text{ with } H_2O \text{ dropped}$$

And then take the negative log (-log) of both sides and solve for the negative log of $[H^+]$, which is pH. A nice summary of the algebraic steps for this task can be found on:
    http://blog.science-matters.org/2012/03/01/deriving-the-henderson-hasselbach-equation/

the loss of bicarbonate. However, other tricks are needed to clear the acid being generated from metabolism. The kidney has two tricks to do this: The first is a high-capacity ATP-dependent proton pump that pumps out a proton and recovers a bicarbonate. One proton removed, *AND* one bicarbonate saved! The second trick is to hydrolyze glutamine and generate NH_4^+ ions, which are excreted in the urine. This removes H^+ and saves a HCO_3^-. This is a major way of eliminating hydrogen ion and saving bicarbonate.

Let's consider a few examples, keeping **Figure 23-1** in our brains...

Respiratory acidosis. The patient is not ventilating well and does not blow off enough CO_2. This increases the CO_2, which reacts with water to increase carbonic acid, which increases protons, causing an acidosis. Note that bicarbonate will also increase as the full balanced equation drives to the left, and the patient's kidneys begin to compensate by excreting protons and retaining bicarbonate.

Respiratory alkalosis. The patient is hyperventilating (from pain, sepsis, liver failure), and is removing too much CO_2. This "pulls" the equation to the right, so the proton is removed, bicarbonate is removed, carbonic acid is down, and the patient develops an alkalosis. The patient's kidney responds by reducing proton/bicarbonate exchange and letting go of the bicarbonate.

Metabolic acidosis. In this case, the patient is adding protons $[H+]$ from some source, like lactic acid or diabetic ketoacids, or you are losing bicarbonate, such as with renal dysfunction (type II RTA). The proton reacts with bicarbonate to form carbonic acid, so the bicarbonate is consumed as it buffers this reaction. The lungs will compensate, and hyperventilate to clear the CO_2 (respiratory alkalosis compensation, so CO_2 drops).

Metabolic alkalosis. In this case, the bicarbonate goes up and it sucks up the proton, or the hydrogen ion is lost (gastric suction removing HCL), causing the alkalosis. The patient's lungs want to hold on to the PCO_2 to try to compensate.

So, in the case of a respiratory acidosis or alkalosis, a change in ventilation changes the levels of PCO_2 to cause the disturbance; while in the case of metabolic acidosis or alkalosis, a change in hydrogen ion or bicarbonate drives the disturbance. The compensation works in the opposite way to try and maintain hydrogen ion levels. So, if $PaCO_2$ rises, so does the HCO_3^-, and vice versa to try to keep $H+$ the same.

23.3 The Four Steps of Acid-Base Analysis

The analysis of an arterial blood gas involves four steps:

1. *Define the primary disorder.* Measurement of blood pH, $PaCO_2$, and HCO_3 defines the primary acid-base disorder and determines whether it is respiratory or metabolic.
2. *Assess the compensation.* Calculations of compensation have to be memorized and applied. If the compensation is inadequate or excessive, then the patient has a mixed acid-base disorder.
3. Calculate the anion gap.
4. Rule out associated second or third disorders, using the delta AG / delta HCO_3.

23.3.1 STEP 1: Define the Primary Disorder

In order to interpret an acid base disturbance, you first have to diagnose the primary problem. This starts off easy. If the pH is less than 7.36, it is an acidosis; and if more than 7.44, it is an alkalosis.

Now you have to figure out if it is metabolic or respiratory. This requires you to evaluate the PCO_2 and HCO_3^- as the major buffering systems maintaining the hydrogen ion balance.

$$[H+] = [CO_2] \text{ Respiratory}/[HCO_3^-] \text{ Metabolic}$$

If you have an acidosis—high $[H+]$-→ with high PCO_2 = respiratory; or with low HCO_3^- = metabolic.

If you have an alkalosis—low $[H+]$→ with low PCO_2 = respiratory; or with high HCO_3^- = metabolic.

In the unusual case that the pH is normal *BUT* the PCO_2 and the HCO_3^- are very abnormal, then pick the worst one to start with. For example, in the case of a blood gas analysis of pH 7.42, PCO_2 of 61 mm Hg, and

Acid-base disorder	pH	PaCO$_2$	HCO$_3^-$
Respiratory acidosis	↓	↑	Normal or ↑
Respiratory alkalosis	↑	↓	Normal or ↓
Metabolic acidosis	↓	↓	↓
Metabolic alkalosis	↑	↑	↑

Figure 23-2 *Directional change in pH, PaCO$_2$, and HCO$_3^-$ associated with acid-base disorders.*

HCO$_3^-$ of 34 mEq/L, you have a respiratory acidosis and a metabolic alkalosis. To understand this, you have to understand compensation, which will come next.

A summary of Step 1 is outlined in Figure 23-2.

23.3.2 STEP 2: Assess the Compensation

In this case, compensation is not talking about money! We are talking about the body's response to the initial pH disorder. As described above, the body responds to an acid-base disorder by making compensatory changes in either the PaCO$_2$ (respiratory compensation) or HCO$_3^-$ (renal compensation) to protect the proton concentration. The compensation serves to protect the PCO$_2$ and the HCO$_3^-$ ratio, and therefore the compensatory response should occur in the same direction as the primary disorder (low PCO$_2$ leads to low bicarbonate, high to high, etc.). For simple acid base disorders, there will be a primary derangement and a secondary compensation. To know if an acid base disturbance follows this simple situation, you have to calculate how much the PCO$_2$ or the HCO$_3^-$ has changed. The compensatory response can be predicted from known equations in order to answer the question, "Is the compensatory response of an expected magnitude?" If the compensation is expected, that is consistent with your calculation, then there is a simple disorder with a simple correction.

Note that corrections move towards a normal pH but are *NEVER* entirely correct! It is not normal to overcorrect, since the goal is to maintain the hydrogen ion concentration in a narrow range. If the compensation is more or less than the calculated compensation, then you have more than one primary disorder!!! Some of these compensatory calculations are easy to memorize, and some are not. You will have to pick a compensation formula for each disorder and commit it to lifelong memory. You do not have to use the ones we use, but we have selected the ones that we find the easiest to memorize and apply.

Keep it simple—remember that the relationship between CO$_2$ (Respiratory) and HCO$_3^-$ changes in a predictable way. How much they change relative to each other depends on whether the change is respiratory or metabolic, and whether it is acute (less time to change) or chronic (more time to change the bicarbonate).

23.3.2.1 Respiratory Compensation

For respiratory compensations, you can use the PaCO$_2$ 10's Rule as outlined in **Figure 23-3**:

It takes ATP and energy to pump out protons and hold onto bicarbonate. So, it is much easier for the kidney to dump bicarbonate than to hold on to it. (Decreases in bicarbonate are always bigger than increases.)

As shown in **Figure 23-4**, think of acid-base compensation like a hot air balloon floating in the air with the balloon filled with PaCO$_2$ and the basket with a ballast of HCO$_3^-$. If the CO$_2$ falls, the person in the balloon is throwing off ballast to maintain altitude. Remember, with the rule of 10's it is easier to throw the HCO$_3^-$ off the balloon than to make more, so change in HCO$_3^-$ is always more for a respiratory alkalosis (*dump it overboard!*) than a respiratory acidosis.

For an acute respiratory acidosis with a PCO$_2$ of 60, the bicarbonate should change by 1 × 2 = 2, from 24 to 26. For chronic respiratory acidosis, the bicarbonate should change by 3.5 × 2 = 7, from 24 to 31. If the value is lower than the expected value, then you have a second metabolic acidosis! If the value is higher than the expected value, then you have a second metabolic alkalosis. *Easy!*

For acute and chronic respiratory alkalosis with a PCO$_2$ of 20, the compensation of bicarbonate is also down by either 2 x 2 or 5 x 2 (20 or 14 meq bicarbonate), as you dump bicarbonate to compensate.

Another method is to calculate compensatory changes in pH. For every change of PCO$_2$, the pH should change by 0.8 or 0.8 × (40 - new PCO$_2$). Another way of thinking of this is for every change of PaCO$_2$ of 10, the pH should change by 0.08 units.

So, for a respiratory acidosis with a PCO$_2$ of 60, the pH should be about 7.24, based on 0.8 × (40−60) = −0.16; so 7.4 − 0.16 = 7.24. If the value is lower than this, then you have a second metabolic acidosis! If the value is higher than this, you have a second metabolic alkalosis. *Easy!*

For an acute respiratory alkalosis with PCO$_2$ of 20, the pH would be 7.4 + 0.16, or 7.56. If the value is higher

Acid-base disorder	Change in PaCO$_2$	Change in HCO$_3^-$
Acute respiratory acidosis	↑10	↑1
Acute respiratory alkalosis	↓10	↓2
Chronic respiratory acidosis	↑10	↑3.5
Chronic respiratory alkalosis	↓10	↓5

Figure 23-3 Compensation in HCO$_3^-$ in respiratory acid-base disorders for every 10 change in PaCO$_2$.

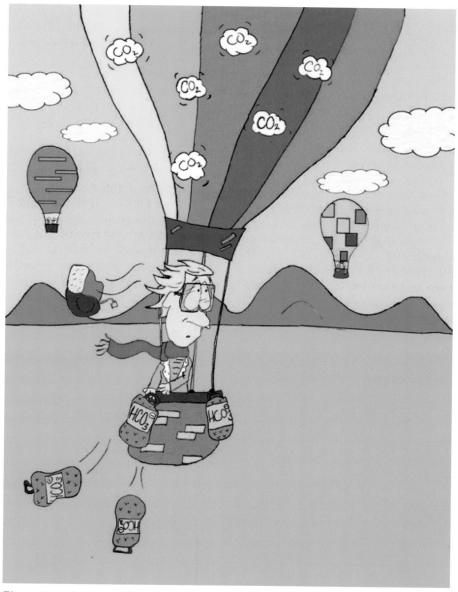

Figure 23-4 *Consider pH compensation like the balloonist that needs to maintain a constant altitude, keeping a balance of PaCO$_2$ and HCO$_3^-$.*

than this, you have a second metabolic alkalosis. If the value is lower than this, you have a second metabolic acidosis. *Easy!*

For chronic conditions, the change in pH is less for every change in PCO_2 because the kidneys have time to compensate and regulate proton and bicarbonate levels. In this case, the change in pH is 0.3 times the change in PCO_2, rather than 0.8.

23.3.2.2 Metabolic Compensation

For a primary metabolic disorder, you start with changes in bicarbonate and have to assess compensatory changes in $PaCO_2$.

Metabolic acidosis. Acidemia with a low HCO_3^- and a normal or reduced $PaCO_2$ suggests that the primary acid-base disorder is a metabolic acidosis. For a metabolic acidosis, the respiratory compensation is rapid, and the distinction between an acute and chronic acidosis is often difficult. The *Winters formula* is most commonly used to analyze the compensation by using the bicarbonate value:

$$PaCO_2 = 1.5\ (HCO_3^-) + 8$$

A measured $PaCO_2$ above or below the calculated value suggests a superimposed secondary respiratory acid-base disorder. For a bicarbonate value of 17, the PCO_2 should be 33 mm Hg, as the patient compensates for the acidosis by breathing down the PCO_2. If the value is higher, then you have a second respiratory acidosis. If the value is lower, you have a second respiratory alkalosis. *Another simple rule to consider is that an appropriately compensated metabolic acidosis leads to* a $PaCO_2$, *which is equivalent in value to the last two numbers in the pH.*

Metabolic alkalosis. Alkalemia with a high HCO_3^- and normal or elevated $PaCO_2$ suggests that the primary acid-base disorder is a metabolic alkalosis. Respiratory compensation for a metabolic alkalosis is achieved through a reduction in tidal volume to increase PCO_2, but is limited by the development of hypoxemia, with progressive hypoventilation making this compensation limited in magnitude. You analyze the compensation for metabolic alkalosis by using the bicarbonate value:

$$PaCO_2 = 0.9\ [HCO_3] + 15$$

A measured $PaCO_2$ above or below the calculated value suggests a superimposed second respiratory acid-base disorder.

Remember that corrections move towards a normal pH but *NEVER fully correct. It is not normal to overcorrect in biology!* If the compensation is more or less than the calculated compensation, then you have more than one primary disorder!!!

A summary of the compensation rules for acid-base disorders is outlined in **Figure 23-5**.

23.3.3 STEP 3: Calculate the Anion Gap

Assessment of the anion gap is an important tool in the analysis of acid-base disorders. The plasma in the body is normally electro-neutral, so all anions must equal all cations. This balance can be summarized as the balance of the unmeasured cations (UC) and measured cations (sodium) and the unmeasured anions (AU) and measured anions (chloride and bicarbonate):

Disorder		Primary Disturbance	Compensatory Response	Expected Compensation
RESPIRATORY				
Acute Acidosis	↑↑↑ $PaCO_2$		↑HCO_3^-	$\Delta pH = 0.8\ \Delta pCO_2$ or $10\Delta[HCO_3^-] = \Delta pCO_2$ Limits - HCO_3^- not > 30
Chronic Acidosis	↑↑↑ $PaCO_2$		↑↑HCO_3^-	$\Delta pH = 0.3\ \Delta pCO_2$ or $10\Delta[HCO_3^-] = 3.5\ \Delta pCO_2$ Limits - HCO_3^- not > 45
Acute Alkalosis	↓↓↓ $PaCO_2$		↓HCO_3^-	$\Delta pH = 0.8\ \Delta pCO_2$ or $10\Delta[HCO_3^-] = 2\ \Delta pCO_2$ Limits - HCO_3^- not < 20
Chronic Alkalosis	↓↓↓ $PaCO_2$		↓↓ HCO_3^-	$\Delta pH = 0.7\ \Delta pCO_2$ or $10\Delta[HCO_3^-] = 5\ \Delta pCO_2$ Limits - HCO_3^- not < 15
METABOLIC				
Acidosis	↓↓ HCO_3^-		↓ $PaCO_2$	$PaCO_2 = 1.5\ (HCO_3^-) + 8$ (Winter's Formula) Limits $PaCO_2$ not < 16-20
Alkalosis	↑↑ HCO_3^-		↑ $PaCO_2$	$PaCO_2 = 0.9\ [HCO_3^-] + 15$ Limits $PaCO_2$ not > 55

Figure 23-5 *A summary of compensation rules for acid-base disorders.*

$$UC + Na^+ = UA + Cl^- + HCO_3^-$$

The unmeasured cations include potassium, calcium, magnesium, and gamma globulins. The unmeasured anions are albumin, sulfate, phosphate, and organic anions. The anion gap (AG) is calculated as the difference between measured cations and measured anions; it is defined as

$$AG = Na^+ - (Cl^- + HCO_3^-)$$

The normal AG is 9-16 mEq/L; just remember 12. An increasing anion gap is caused by the accumulation of hydrogen ion $[H^+]$ that is sucking up the bicarbonate.

If the AG is normal, you are finished and have a primary acid-base disturbance with a compensatory response. Normal anion gap acidosis is caused by the accumulation of HCl, so that the drop in bicarbonate that buffers the H^+ is offset by an increase in chloride anion.

In clinical practice, we separate metabolic acidosis into two categories: 1) anion gap positive or 2) anion gap negative metabolic acidosis (also referred to as non-gap).

23.3.4 STEP 4: Calculate the Delta Gap

The $\Delta AG / \Delta HCO_3^-$ (sometimes called *the delta/delta*) compares the measured change in AG (from a normal of 12 to the new value) to the measured change in HCO_3^- (from the normal baseline value of 24 mEq/L to the new value). Under normal conditions, these values should be relatively equal in amount or within + 6 mmol. The reason for this is that as you titrate the hydrogen ion, the bicarbonate should drop 1:1. In fact, it is not always this perfect. In the case of lactic acidosis, it can drop 1.5:1 because of bone buffering of hydrogen ion; while in the case of ketoacidosis, it remains 1:1. But if the relationship is not close, it suggests there is another thing modulating the HCO_3^-. The +6 mmol fudge rule lets you deal with the loose connection between $\Delta AG / \Delta HCO_3^-$.

- *A HCO_3^- value that is higher than the value predicted by the rise in the AG suggests a hidden metabolic alkalosis.*
- *A HCO_3^- value that is lower than the value predicted by the rise in the AG suggests a hidden non-gap metabolic acidosis.*

For example, a normal patient should have an AG of 12 and a HCO_3^- value of 24 mEq/L. Let's say the patient develops a lactic acidosis with an AG of 25. What should the HCO_3^- be? The answer: Change in AG is 25-12 = 13. So, the HCO_3^- should change by 24-13 = 11 ± 6. If the measured HCO_3^- is > 17, then you have an additional metabolic alkalosis. If the value is less than 5, then you have an additional non-gap acidosis.

If your patient has a primary disorder and secondary compensation, with an anion gap plus a delta-delta gap, then there are three processes going on!

Now let's move from the basic physiology of acid-base homeostasis and interpretation to the differential diagnosis and management of the major acid-base disorders. We will briefly review respiratory acid-base disorders and then spend more time on metabolic acidosis and alkalosis.

23.4 Respiratory Acid-Base Disorders

23.4.1 Respiratory Acidosis

Respiratory acidosis is caused by low alveolar ventilation and can be caused by expiratory airflow obstruction (as in asthma and COPD); by severe parenchymal lung disease with increased physiologic dead space (high V/Q) (as seen in severe ARDS); or from severe weakness and hypoventilation (as in neuromuscular disorders). The causes of respiratory acidosis can be organized as outlined in **Figure 23-6**.

Because CO_2 has a central nervous system narcotizing effect and causes a severe acidosis as it rises, the patient's

Etiology of respiratory acidosis	Examples
Upper airway obstruction	Laryngospasm, tracheal tumor
Lower airway obstruction	COPD, status asthmaticus
Parenchymal lung disease	ARDS, pneumonia, pulmonary edema
Central drive disorders	Drug overdose
Neuromuscular disorders	Guillain-Barre, myasthenia gravis, critical illness neuropathy
Chest wall disorders	Kyphoscoliosis, morbid obesity
Iatrogenic disorders	Permissive hypercapnia
Disorders of CO_2 production	Hyperthermia, hypermetabolism

Figure 23-6 Etiology for respiratory acidosis and clinical examples.

clinical symptoms may range from confusion, lethargy, and agitation to more advanced phases, including seizures, coma, cardiac arrhythmias, and pulmonary hypertension. The patient may also be asymptomatic. Permissive hypercapnia is used in the setting of advanced ARDS or status asthmaticus as a form of therapy, allowing us to ventilate with low tidal volumes to avoid lung injury. Current data suggest that this produces little adverse effect and that hypercapnia and respiratory acidosis may actually be protective in these settings. Permissive hypercapnia is contraindicated in the setting of disordered cerebral blood flow (e.g., cerebral edema) due to the cerebral vasodilating effects of hypercapnia.

23.4.2 Respiratory Alkalosis

Respiratory alkalosis is caused by either an iatrogenic increase in the ventilator settings or with spontaneous hyperventilation. This can occur in the hospital patient secondary to a broad range of disorders, as outlined in **Figure 23-7**.

Alkalemia is usually associated with an adverse outcome when the pH > 7.60. This level of pH change is associated with electrolyte abnormalities (e.g., hypokalemia), pulmonary vasoconstriction, decreased cardiac contractility, and seizures.

A 33 yo woman with a newborn baby of 2 months of age is brought into the emergency room by ambulance, having been found down at home. She is breathing spontaneously but is not responsive. The team reports that she was found in her bed with a number of empty open bottles of non-prescription over-the-counter medications. They note only that no narcotics or anti-depressant medications are identified. Her alcohol metabolite, narcotic, and benzodiazepene tox screens are negative. Acetaminophen levels are undetectable. Her CXR is clear, and her ABG shows pH 7.45; $PaCO_2$ 22; PaO_2 118; HCO_3^- 14; Na^+ 135; Cl^- 92.

What is your diagnosis?

It sounds like an overdose, but screens are negative. Let's start with an evaluation of her acid-base status.

Step 1: Define the primary disorder. Respiratory alkalosis. The pH is high, but the bicarbonate is low, so it cannot be metabolic. The $PaCO_2$ is low, so it must be a respiratory alkalosis.

Step 2: Calculate the compensation. Use our respiratory rule of 10's. For an acute respiratory alkalosis, for every drop of 10, the HCO_3^- drops by 2, and for chronic by 5. Remember it is easier to dump bicarb so we can dump more with a respiratory alkalosis. The $PaCO_2$ dropped (40-22 = 18), so the HCO_3^- would drop by about 4 for acute. It has in fact dropped from 24 to 14 or by 10! We see a bigger drop than in an acute compensation. This suggests that we have a second disorder: a metabolic acidosis.

Step 3: Calculate the anion gap. Your calculated gap is 135-(92+14)= 29. So, we have an anion gap acidosis.

Step 4: Calculate the delta gap. Assuming your AG started at 14 and your bicarb started at 24, then your delta-delta is (29-14) and (24-14), or 15-10= 5. Even for a lactic acidosis, the AG/1.5 would be 10, so the delta-delta would be zero. This means we have an expected drop in bicarbonate for the AG, so there is no other disorder. The final answer is a respiratory alkalosis with an anion gap metabolic acidosis. This is unusual with poisonings, which usually slow down the brain and the breathing. *What could this be? The answer is aspirin overdose!* This interesting "classic" can cause a primary central respiratory alkalosis and a lactic acidosis.

23.5 Metabolic Acid-Base Disorders

Metabolic acidosis is the most interesting and complicated type of the acid-base disorders that you will face *DAILY* in the busy ICU. In general, this is a process that decreases HCO_3^- and is caused by either a gain of acid, which sucks up HCO_3^-, or a loss of HCO_3^-.

Gain of acid:

1. Increased production by the body of hydrogen ion in the form of a number of endogenous acids, including lactic acid (from tissue hypoxia or drugs) and ketoacids (from diabetes or starvation or alcoholism)
2. Metabolism of drugs or poisons to form acids, including methanol (metabolized to formic acid) and ethylene glycol (metabolized to oxalic acid)
3. Decreased renal excretion of hydrogen (renal failure and distal type I renal tubular acidosis)

Etiology of respiratory alkalosis	Examples
Central disorders of ventilation	Intracranial hemorrhage, cerebrovascular accident, fever, anxiety
Peripheral disorders of ventilation	Hypoxemia, pain, sepsis
Non-respiratory disorders	Advanced liver disease, pregnancy
Drug-related disorders	Salicylate (aspirin) overdose
Iatrogenic disorders	Ventilator-induced hypercapnia

Figure 23-7 *Etiology for respiratory alkalosis and clinical examples.*

Loss of HCO_3^-:

1. GI loss from diarrhea
2. Renal loss from proximal tubule

23.5.1 Metabolic Acidosis and the Anion Gap

As described in the last section, a metabolic acidosis is defined by acidemia and a low bicarbonate. We then determine the compensation and the anion gap. The anion gap helps us differentiate between the major kinds of metabolic acidosis.

This anion gap examines the balance between unmeasured cations (UC) and measured cations (sodium) and the unmeasured anions (UA) and measured anions (chloride and bicarbonate) as defined by

$$UC + Na^+ = UA + Cl^- + HCO_3^-$$

A high anion gap is caused by the production of endogenous acids that have a hydrogen ion and that are partnered with an unmeasured anion. For example, lactic acidosis is H^+ and lactate. Typical acids are natural L-lactic acids, rare D-lactic acids, ketoacids, and uremic acids from severe renal failure. A very high anion gap (i.e., > 25) suggests the presence of an organic acid from a poison, like formic acid (methanol poisoning) or oxaloacid (ethylene glycol poisoning).

To help remember the important causes of anion gap acidosis, you can focus on the major concept that this is caused by toxic alcohols and things that increase lactic or keto acids. If you need a silly mnemonic, you can try our Aunt Grandma Ethyl Anion Gap story. *(We apologize ahead of time to all Proper Methodists.)* (See **Figure 23-8** and **Figure 23-9**.) *Remember: Aunt Grandma Ethyl Met a Proper Lactating Methodist Urinating and Singing out of Key.*

A normal anion gap typically is caused by a primary loss of HCO_3^- that is balanced with an increase in

Because albumin is an unmeasured anion, when it is low the anion gap will decrease. This happens because the levels of the measured anions (Cl^- and HCO_3^-) increase, as they are retained to maintain electroneutrality. Since we use these to calculate the anion gap, the gap is less. A general rule of thumb is to add 3 mmol/L to your anion gap for every decrease of 1 g/dL of albumin below 3 g/dL. So for an albumin of 1.5, you would add 4.5 to your anion gap estimate.

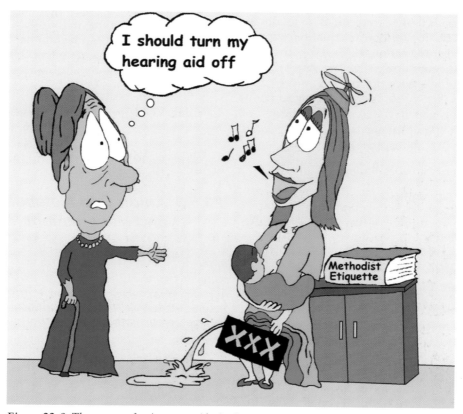

Figure 23-8 The causes of anion gap acidosis. See text.

Anion Gap (AG) Acidosis	Aunt Grandma	Comments
Ethylene Glycol	Ethyl	Toxic ingestion
Metformin	Met	Often seen in association with renal insufficiency
Propylene Glycol	Proper	Toxic ingestion
Lactic Acidosis	Lactating	
Methanol	Methodist	Toxic ingestion
Uremia (ESRD)	Urinates	Mild renal insufficiency is non-anion gap. Advanced is AG
Salicylate Overdose	Sings Out	Toxic ingestion. Often a mixed disorder with respiratory alkalosis
Ketoacidosis	Key	Diabetic or alcoholic

Figure 23-9 *Causes of an anion gap acidosis by the Aunt Grandma mnemonic.*

chloride to maintain the normal AG. Alternatively, a failure to excrete hydrogen ion can causes a normal anion gap acidosis (in kidney for example, which also increases chloride).

Other things that will lower your anion gap are high levels of immunoglobulin light chain paraproteins in multiple myeloma. This increase in unmeasured cations will lower the measured cation (Na^+) resulting in a lower calculated anion gap. Similarly, increases in the other unmeasured anion (phosphate) or an increase in the other unmeasured cations (calcium, potassium and magnesium) will lower the gap. The opposite direction does the opposite thing to the anion gap!

To remember these concepts, consider that the body (kidney) retains charged molecules to maintain electroneutrality. Each side of the AG equation remains balanced, so if unmeasured cations (UC) go up, the $Na+$ goes down. If the UC goes down, the $Na+$ goes up. On the other side, if the UA goes up, the Cl^- and HCO_3^- must go down, and vice versa. Now it is easy to know what happens to the gap if you remember the list of unmeasured cations (paraproteins, K^+, Ca^+, Mg^+) and unmeasured anions (Cl^-, phosphate).

$$\uparrow up\ UC + then \downarrow Na^+ = up \uparrow UA + then \downarrow CL^- + \downarrow HCO_3^-$$

OR

$$\downarrow up\ UC + then \uparrow Na^+ = up \downarrow UA + then \uparrow CL^- + \uparrow HCO_3^-$$

23.5.2 Metabolic Acidosis and the Osmolar Gap

The calculation of an osmolality gap can help you in cases of anion gap metabolic acidosis, because certain diseases or toxic drugs can lead to increases in both, the classic being the toxic alcohols, ethylene glycol, methanol, and propylene glycol.

This is mainly used to diagnose toxic alcohols!

The osmolality gap is simply calculated as the serum osmolality, measured using a laboratory test, and the calculated osmolality from the molecules in blood plasma that contribute the most to the osmolality: sodium, glucose, and blood urea nitrogen (BUN).

Measured OSM = lab test and normally 290-300 mOsm/L

Calculated OSM = $2 \times Na^+$ + Glucose/18 + BUN/2.8

The calculated OSM is typically about (2×140) + 100/18 + 20/2.8 = 288. A normal OSM gap is < 10 mOsm/L.

Alcohol overdose is very common and will cause a large OSM gap. However, if there is no starvation or alcoholic ketoacidosis, there will be no anion gap acidosis. To determine if the OSM gap is caused by alcohol or if there might be another toxic alcohol in the blood, one should calculate the OSM gap and include alcohol. This is done by adding alcohol (ETOH in mg/dL) to the Calculated OSM

Calculated OSM = $2 \times Na^+$ + Glucose/18 + BUN/2.8 + ETOH/4.6

Things that cause a high OSM gap are shown in Figure 23-10.

23.5.3 Anion Gap Metabolic Acidosis and Management

A 44 yo man is admitted from the emergency room intubated, mechanically ventilated on assist-control mode, on norepinephrine (0.15 mcs/kg/min) with a mean arterial blood pressure of 55 mm Hg and heart rate of 112, sinus rhythm, respiratory rate of 35. He was febrile to 39.5 C and his chest radiograph showed bilateral patchy consolidations at the bases. His laboratory studies revealed a leukocytosis of 35K with a bandemia. His ABG revealed a pH 7.28; $PaCO_2$ 26; PaO_2 of 67 on 0.8 FiO_2 and PEEP 10 cm H_2O. His Na^+ 142; K^+ 3.6; Cl^- 96; HCO_3^- 12.

What is going on?

High osmolality gap with anion gap metabolic acidosis	High osmolality gap with non-anion gap metabolic acidosis
Ethylene glycol Methanol Propylene glycol Alcoholic or diabetic ketoacidosis	Mannitol Ethanol Isopropyl alcohol

Figure 23-10 *Causes of a high osmolality gap grouped by effect on anion gap.*

Step 1: Define the primary disorder. This is a metabolic acidosis. The pH is low and the bicarbonate is low.

Step 2: Calculate the compensation. For an acute metabolic acidosis, your $PaCO_2$ should be $= 1.5(12) + 8$, which equals 26. Your patient's value is 26, so the respiratory compensation is appropriate.

Step 3: Calculate the anion gap. Your calculated gap is $142 - (96 + 12) = 34$. There is a significant anion gap.

Step 4: Calculate the delta-delta. $(32-14) - (24-12)$, so 18-12 is 6, so within 6. Note: For lactic acidosis, the anion gap/1.5 is a better estimate (bone buffering in addition to bicarb), so that would be $12 - 12 = 0$. There is no significant delta-delta to suggest a second metabolic disorder. You have a major anion gap acidosis with appropriate respiratory compensation. Now you need more clinical and laboratory information, while reviewing your differential diagnosis for anion gap acidosis.

Your patient does not have a history of alcoholism or alcohol binge drinking, including drinking anti-freeze or other alcohols. There is no history of insulin-dependent diabetes, renal failure, or excessive aspirin use or overdose. There is certainly clear evidence of hypoxemia and shock (hypoperfusion).

Clinically the case is consistent with shock, since your patient is on norepinephrine (0.1-0.5 mcgm/kg/min is a "stiff dose"). You send glucose and urine and serum ketones, which are normal. A blood toxic alcohol screen is negative, and a plasma lactic acid level returns at 17 mmoles/L, consistent with your diagnosis of lactic acidosis from septic shock secondary to possible pneumonia. It is now critical that you continue goal-directed resuscitation therapy and maintain a mean arterial blood pressure > 65 mm Hg.

This classic case is a high anion gap acidosis > 30 and a high osmolality gap > 30. This suggests the presence of a toxic alcohol and you have to send tests for this rapidly or treat empirically to avoid renal failure (ethylene glycol) or blindness (methanol). For more details of these conditions, read on! If the osmolality gap is very large but there is no anion gap, this could be isopropyl alcohol or regular ethanol overdose, which is not such a bad toxin.

23.5.3.1 Lactic Acidosis

Lactic acidosis is the most common cause of a high anion gap metabolic acidosis. Lactic acidosis is common in shock states (septic shock, heart failure, cardiac arrest, massive GI bleeding, ischemic intestines, etc.), which are characterized by altered cellular metabolism. Lactate can also increase after a significant seizure due to cellular ischemia. Other causes of lactic acidosis include genetic deficiencies in glycolytic pathway enzymes or in mitochondria, drugs such as metformin, HIV nucleoside reverse transcriptase inhibitors, and cyanide poisoning.

Lactic acidosis is classified as groups A and B:

- *Group A* – hypoxic lactic acidosis with shock states or abnormal tissue oxygenation
- *Group B* – normoxic lactic acidosis with normal perfusion and oxygenation
  - Genetic diseases (oxygen is normal but cannot be utilized well by the mitochondria to form ATP via oxidative phosphorylation)
  - Medication or poisoning, such as metformin or cyanide
  - Underlying disease, like diabetic ketoacidosis, liver failure, and large cancers that produce lactate (non-Hodgkin's and Burkitt lymphomas)

The management of lactic acidosis does *NOT* merely involve the repletion of HCO_3^-. The primary treatment is to *reverse the cause!* The role of HCO_3^- replacement in the ICU patient with lactic acidosis is controversial. In fact, this is considered risky because the HCO_3^- will react with hydrogen ion to form H_2CO_3, which can dissociate via carbonic anhydrase to H_2O and CO_2. The CO_2 can diffuse into tissues like the heart and react again to form H_2CO_3 and release hydrogen ion to paradoxically lower the intracellular pH!!! For this reason, bicarbonate is not recommended for lactic acidosis unless the pH is very low (ph<7.0) and the patient is not responsive to vasopressors, such as during prolonged cardiopulmonary arrest. Even in this case, bicarbonate is a controversial recommendation.

The primary therapy of lactic acidosis is adequate resuscitation and treatment of the underlying condition.

23.5.3.2 D-Lactic Acidosis

D-lactic acidosis is an uncommon complication of short bowel syndrome from surgical jejunal-ileal bypass or small bowel resection. This results in higher delivery of carbohydrates to the colon, where gram-positive anaerobes, such as Lactobacilli, are able to metabolize carbohydrates and form the D-lactate stereo-isomer of lactate. D-lactate is then absorbed, causing lactic acidosis and mental status changes, presenting as "drunkenness." It is tough to diagnose as it is so rare, and standard laboratory assay for lactic acid only measures the L-lactate form. Treatment is with antibiotics to kill the offending bacteria.

23.5.3.3 Ethylene Glycol Intoxication

A 31 yo alcoholic is admitted from the emergency, confused and somnolent, breathing spontaneously on 40% oxygen delivered by face mask, with a mean arterial blood pressure of 55 mm Hg and heart rate of 105, sinus rhythm, respiratory rate of 35. He was afebrile and his chest radiograph showed only small areas of atelectasis at the bases. His laboratory studies revealed a normal complete blood count. His ABG revealed a pH 7.26; $PaCO_2$ 23; PaO_2 of 67 on 0.8 FiO_2 and PEEP 10 cm H_2O. His Na+ 140; K+ 4.0; Cl^- 102; HCO_3^- 10; glucose 192 mg/dL and BUN of 32.

What is going on? Similar to the case above, you have an anion gap metabolic acidosis with appropriate respiratory compensation. The delta gap is also normal. Because of the decreased mental status and history of alcoholism, you need to send a serum osmolality lab test and calculate the osmolality gap. The lab result comes back at 364, and your calculated osmolality is 2 x 142 + 192/18 + 32/2.8 = 306 and the OSM gap is therefore 364 – 306 = 58. So, you are now very anxious about a differential diagnosis of high anion gap and high osmolar gap. This could be ketoacidosis, so you send the ketones, but it could also be a toxic alcohol. You send a toxic alcohol screen. The urine shows calcium oxalate crystals, which form from the metabolism of ethylene glycol by alcohol dehydrogenase to form glycolic acid, then glyoxylic acid, and, finally, oxalic acid. Oxalic acid binds with calcium to form calcium oxalate crystals, which may deposit and cause damage to many areas of the body, including the kidneys, brain, heart, and lungs. Your toxic alcohol blood screen returns with a positive result for ethylene glycol. You send a stat order for fomepizole antidote therapy, to block the metabolism of the ethylene glycol to glyoxylic acid, and hemodialysis to remove the ethylene glycol!

Ethylene glycol is a component of anti-freeze and is a major cause of poisoning worldwide. Because of its sweet taste, children and animals may also drink it. Interestingly, the use of bittering additives like Bitrex has not significantly reduced the high rate of poisoning.

The major organ damaging complications with this toxic alcohol are due to its metabolites, glyoxylic acid and oxalic acid, which take about 12-36 hours to form, giving you time to intervene and save the patient! With this poison, you are working on a time-bomb. There are

three phases to the poisoning:

- *Stage 1 (30 minutes to 12 hours). Drunk as a skunk.* The ethylene glycol directly causes neurological impairment with slurred speech, confusion, gait instability, nystagmus, and headache. GI symptoms like nausea, vomiting and diarrhea can occur. Similar to ingestion of any major alcohol, it causes an osmolar gap.
- *Stage 2 (12-36 hours). Acids start to burn the body!* The ethylene glycol is metabolized by alcohol dehydrogenase to glycolaldehyde, which is then oxidized to glycolic acid → glyoxylic acid → oxalic acid. These metabolites can cause heart dysfunction, hypotension, and cerebral edema, as well as shut off mitochondria, to increase lactic acid. This all causes the anion gap metabolic acidosis, which is due mainly to accumulated glycolic acid.
- *Stage 3 (24-72 hours).* Acute tubular necrosis and renal failure are caused by the accumulation and deposition of calcium oxalate crystals.

As illustrated in **Figure 23-11**, alcohol, ethylene glycol and methanol are all metabolized by alcohol dehydrogenase (ADH). We can block the enzyme by giving excess alcohol or fomepizole. Either compound can inhibit the metabolism of methanol → formaldehyde → formic acid, and prevent the metabolism of ethylene glycol → glycoaldehyde → glycolic acid → glyoxylic acid → oxalic acid.

23.5.3.3.1 Treatment of Ethylene Glycol Intoxication

Stop the metabolism and dialyze it off! Fomepizole is an FDA-approved specific antidote that potently blocks the enzyme alcohol dehydrogenase to prevent the metabolism to toxic acids. Alternatively, good old 100% ethanol can be given as an IV infusion. Because ethanol has a 100 times greater affinity for alcohol dehydrogenase, it successfully blocks the breakdown of ethylene glycol into glycoaldehyde. At the same time, hemodialysis should be initiated, and the patient clinically stabilized with mechanical ventilation and hemodynamic support.

23.5.3.4 Methanol Intoxication

This smallest, most simple, and sweet-tasting alcohol (CH_3OH) is also used as an antifreeze, solvent, and fuel. Like ethylene glycol and alcohol, it causes early central nervous system effects and is metabolized by alcohol dehydrogenase. It is converted to formaldehyde and then by aldehyde dehydrogenase to formic acid (also called *methanoic acid*, by the way!)

To remember the key features of methanol poisoning, use **Figure 23-12**. Visualize a drunk pouring

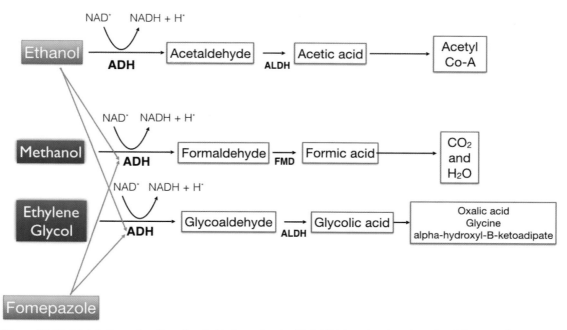

Figure 23-11 *Metabolism of methanol and ethylene glycol with inhibition sites for ethanol and fomepazole.*

METHANOL over his EYES. The methanol contains ANTS and FORMIC acid (formica is "ant" in Latin) that are now biting his eyes and causing blindness. This will remind you of the three critical features in this intoxication: methanol, anti-freeze, and blindness.

Formic acid inhibits the mitochondrial cytochrome C oxidase (complex IV). This stops mitochondrial oxidative phosphorylation and causes an anion gap lactic acidosis. While the patient presenting with methanol intoxication starts out drunk as a skunk, this progresses within 10-30 hours to blurred vision, retinal edema, and blindness, caused by the formic acid. Like ethylene glycol, the use of fomepizole or ethanol will block the first-step conversion of methanol by alcohol dehydrogenase to formaldehyde. Interestingly, formic acid occurs naturally in the venom of bees and ants. This is what hurts with their bite! In fact, the name *formic acid* comes from the Latin word for ant, *formica*, referring to its early isolation by the distillation of ant bodies.

23.5.3.5 Diabetic Ketoacidosis (DKA)

A 23 yo insulin-dependent diabetic woman is admitted from the emergency room. About 3 days ago she developed a fever with lower back pain over her left flank. Over the last 24 hours she developed some nausea, polyuria, and polydipsia. On arrival to the ICU, she has stable blood pressure, heart rate of 115, temperature of 38.1°C, is breathing at a respiratory rate of 35 per minute with deep almost gasping breaths (Kussmaul respiration) and is somnolent. Her mucous membranes appear dry, and her skin has low turgor. Her chest radiograph is clear, and her urinalysis has +bacteria, +leukocyte esterase, with leukocytes too-numerous-to-count, +ketones, and +glucose. Her laboratory studies reveals a leukocytosis of 15 with a bandemia. Her glucose is 350, BUN is 34, and creatinine is 1.4 on her chemistry examination. Her ABG reveals a pH 7.16; PaCO$_2$ 14; PaO$_2$ of 134. His Na$^+$ 142; K$^+$ 4.1; Cl$^-$ 103; HCO$_3^-$ 6.

DKA and lactic acidosis are the two most common forms of anion gap acidosis you will see in the ICU. On most admission days, you will get a DKA case. It is good to really understand this condition clinically and how to manage it correctly.

Diabetic ketoacidosis (DKA) most commonly affects patients with Type 1 diabetes, but it can occur in those with type 2 diabetes, more commonly in African-American and Hispanic populations; this is called "ketosis-prone type 2 diabetes." DKA results from high glucose, which causes an osmotic diuresis, polyuria, polydipsia, volume depletion, and potassium and magnesium depletion. A shortage of insulin results in a metabolic shift for the body to burn fatty acids and to produce acidic ketoacids, resulting in the anion gap acidosis and significant compensatory respiratory alkalosis.

Presenting symptoms include vomiting, dehydration, polyurea, polydipsia (thirst), deep breathing (compensatory respiratory alkalosis to clear CO$_2$ and remove hydrogen ion), confusion, and occasionally coma (caused by severe DKA, leading to cerebral edema).

DKA is often triggered by intercurrent illness (pneumonia, influenza, gastroenteritis, a urinary tract

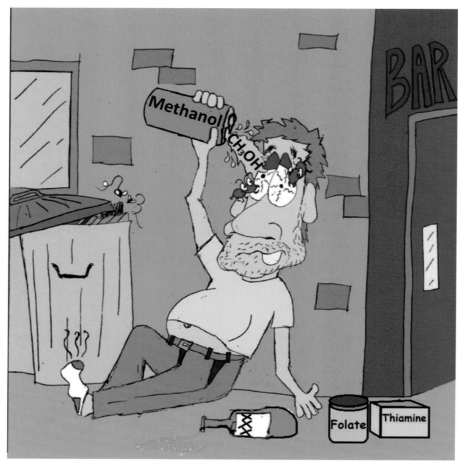

Figure 23-12 *Methanol poisoning. See text.*

infection), pregnancy, stroke, myocardial infarction, inadequate insulin therapy, or the use of illicit drugs, such as cocaine. This magnifies the underlying problem of low insulin production and insulin resistance. Since insulin's normal job is to store glucose away in the liver, a lack of insulin and unopposed increased glucagon cause an increased release of glucose from glycogen and increased gluconeogenesis. There are *two major consequences* of this:

1. *High glucose induces osmotic diuresis.* Glucose levels usually exceed 13.8 mmol/L or 250 mg/dL. The increase in osmotically active glucose causes an osmotic diuresis (polyurea), volume depletion (dehydration, thirst), and loss of electrolytes, such as potassium. A DKA patient has a total body water shortage of around 6 liters and loses sodium, potassium, chloride, phosphate, magnesium, and calcium.
2. *Ketoacidosis causes anion gap acidosis.* The absence of insulin leads to a shift to other forms of energy, since the glucose cannot be used. There is a release

from adipose tissue of free fatty acids, which are converted in the liver into the ketoacids acetoacetate and β-hydroxybutyrate. It is these acids that cause the metabolic acidosis.

DKA is diagnosed with blood and urine tests, including the assessments of ketones in the blood and urine, high glucose level (to distinguish from alcoholic or starvation ketoacidosis), and assessment of the anion gap and arterial blood gas.

Remember that DKA can be distinguished from other forms of ketoacidosis (such as alcoholic or starvation) by the presence of high blood glucose levels.

23.5.3.5.1 Treatment of DKA

The big picture is that treatment of DKA involves intravenous fluids to correct dehydration, insulin to suppress the production of ketoacids, treatment for any underlying triggers (such as infections), repletion of potassium and electrolytes, and close observation in the intensive care unit to prevent and identify complications. The detailed management can be complex, but many hospitals have treatment protocols to help prevent major complications.

There are a number of DKA "booby traps" that can get you and your patient into trouble.

Hydration. Normal saline should be administered to replete the volume. Fluids can be started at 150-300 mL per hour. One liter should be given immediately, and the fluid deficits calculated. The average patient is 6 liters negative on presentation. This hydration will rapidly bring the glucose down.

Insulin. This is typically started at 0.1 units per kg per hour as long as the glucose level is >300 mg/dL and the potassium levels are not low. If the presentation glucose is low, it can be added to the saline (D5 or D10 normal saline) to allow you to safely keep the insulin dose high in order to suppress the ketosis and correct the anion gap. A typical patient would start with 7 units per hour of insulin and then add dextrose to ½ normal saline when glucose is less than 300 mg/dL. The addition of dextrose will allow you to maintain the insulin infusion with a blood glucose at 100-200 mg/dL. *This is your first booby trap: You elect to stop the insulin too early when the glucose is controlled, but the anion gap is not normal.* While things look OK, the anion gap has not corrected and will spiral out of control. This is a major reason a patient stays too long in the ICU. *The trick is to keep the insulin going by adding glucose to your intravenous fluids.*

The second booby trap is potassium. While the plasma K^+ level may look normal, it is actually very low systemically. Why is this? You lose a lot of K^+ with the osmotic diuresis, as it is washed out in the urine. Also, the acidosis and increasing hydrogen ion levels in blood increase the H^+/K^+ exchange pump activity in organs, so that the H+ goes into the organs and what little K^+ is there comes out. But this hides the actual low levels in the body. As you correct the acidosis, this reverses and insulin also causes H^+/K^+ exchange, so the K^+ levels will plummet with therapy. *So, the rule you must follow is to start repleting K+ in your saline for a plasma K^+ level of <5.3 mmol/L.* In fact, all IV fluids should have 20-40 mEq/L potassium after your first bolus. If the level drops below 3.3, you should stop insulin until you replete the levels.

The third boopy trap relates to bicarbonate and mechanical ventilation. While you will be tempted to give bicarbonate, the data suggest that this can actually worsen cardiac arrhythmias by increasing intracellular CO_2 and hydrogen ion (see mechanism in lactic acidosis section above). *Just treat with saline and insulin and your acidosis will correct.* You will also be tempted to want to intubate the patient who has agonal deep Kussmaul breathing with a $PaCO_2$ as low as 6 mm Hg. However, it turns out that a young, strong patient can do a better job of ventilating than you can with the machine, so just treat and watch carefully.

23.5.3.5.2 DKA Management Summary

- *Look for a trigger!* Usually an infection is lurking. Turn over every stone (Hx and physical exam, UA, CXR, ECG and rule out MI, blood cultures, tox screen, etc.).
- *Fill the tank!* Give lots of fluids. Average deficit is 6L!
- *Close the anion gap, kill the ketones!* Start glucose in saline for glucose < 300 mg/dL.
- *Don't let a potassium deficiency blow you up!* Add KCL to saline for K <5.3 mmol/L; hold insulin and more aggressive repletion for levels <3.3.
- You do not need to intubate or give bicarbonate, even if things look pretty bad!

A sample order set for DKA management is outlined in **Figure 23-13.**

23.5.3.6 Alcoholic Ketoacidosis

Severe chronic alcohol use with low caloric intake (starvation) can lead to ketogenesis. This occurs because of low glucose intake and an effect of alcohol on inhibiting gluconeogenesis. These patients can present in a very complicated way with nausea, vomiting, and abdominal pain, GI bleeding, pancreatitis, a second metabolic alkalosis from vomiting and dehydration, and electrolyte depletion (especially phosphorus and Mg+).

Patients with alcoholic ketoacidosis have a high β-hydroxybutyrate/acetoacetate ratio. The ketones in the dipstick may not be as high as DKA, since this test does not measure the β-hydroxybutyrate.

23.5.3.7 Renal Failure and Uremic Acidosis

In early mild-to-moderate renal failure, an acidosis develops, since the failing kidney is not able to pump out hydrogen ion by the normal pathway of production and excretion of NH_4^+. This causes a non-anion gap acidosis, because the kidney can still retain chloride to maintain electroneutrality. When renal failure advances (uremia), then the kidney cannot retain chloride. This lowers both the chloride and bicarbonate and the AG increases.

23.5.4 Non-Anion Gap Acidosis

A normal anion gap typically is caused by a primary loss of HCO_3^- that is balanced with an increase in chloride, to maintain a normal AG. The causes of a non-anion gap acidosis are outlined in **Figure 23-14.**

DKA order set	
Notify MD for blood work	Blood sugar < 100, Blood sugar > 300, K+< 3.5, K > 5.0, HCO3 < 16
Notify MD for vital signs	T > 101, HR > 100, SBP < 90. DBP > 50, UOP < 30
Notify MD	Anion Gap > 20
Vital signs	q 2hours
I/O	Routine, q 2hours
Glucose level, capillary	q 1hour
IVF	NS + 20 meq KCL IV at _____ Suggested rate 500-1000 ml/hour for 1-4 hours. Hold any continuous infusion containing KCL if urine output < 30 ml/hr or serum potassium (K+) > 5 meq/L and call MD.
Insulin	Bolus 0.1 units/kg and initiate insulin infusion with suggested rate 0.1 units/kg/hour OR 5 units/hour. If blood glucose > 250 and decreasing by < 50 mg/dL, call MD for adjustment of insulin infusion.
Electrolytes	q2 hours x 4, then q 4 hours
Sodium bicarbonate	50 mEq IV in 1000 nL 1/2NS to infuse over 30-60 minutes Indicated only for life-threatening hyperkalemia
Potassium phosphate	15 mMol IV over 4 hours. Give only when serum phosphate level < 1.5 mg/dL with adequate urine output (provides 22 mEq of K+).
Transition	When anion gap is closed, transition to subcutaneous insulin. Stop IV insulin 60 minutes after injection of subcutaneous short or rapid acting insulin. Stop IV insulin 90 minutes AFTER NPH or Insulin glargine (Lantus) if no short or rapid acting insulin is also given.

Figure 23-13 Sample order set for diabetic keto acidosis.

Non-anion gap (AG) acidosis	Comments
Mild to Moderate Renal Insufficiency	In contrast to AG acidosis in End-Stage Renal Disease
Diarrhea (GI Loss of Bicarbonate)	Loss of bicarbonate in the stool can lead to an acidosis. Chloride is retained to maintain electrical neutrality, and there is no increase in anion gap.
Dilutional Acidosis	Large volume resuscitation using saline solutions will dilute out the 24mmol/L bicarbonate, which is replaced by the chloride in the saline, causing a mild non-anion gap acidosis.
Renal Tubular Acidosis	Types I, II, and IV

Figure 23-14 Causes of a non-anion gap metabolic acidosis.

The first three conditions are commonly related to problems that result in hospital admissions, such as acute renal failure, severe infectious diarrhea, and large volume saline resuscitation. The final class (called the *renal tubular acidosis*) is not typically an ICU problem, but your patient may commonly have this in the context of a baseline problem or renal insufficiency.

Let's start with the proximal tubule and move through the kidney:

23.5.4.1 Renal Tubular Acidosis

Type I (distal) RTA. This is caused by failure of the distal tubular cells apical H+/K+ antiporter, a distal tubular acidosis where the kidney cannot excrete hydrogen ion, cannot acidify the urine, and cannot reabsorb potassium.

This leads to a hypokalemic non-anion gap acidosis. The urine pH *CANNOT* drop below 5.3 with an acid load. Calcium stones often form with this disease, because they require a high urine pH to crystallize. Type I RTA can be caused by acquired chronic tubulointerstitial disease, injury from drugs like amphotericin B, and hereditary conditions.

Type II (proximal)I RTA. This is a problem with the proximal tubule's ability to work well. Remember that most of the system's bicarbonate is absorbed here, so if the proximal tubule is on the blink, then bicarbonate is wasted. This can be a generalized failure to function, called *Fanconi's syndrome*, caused by injury from multiple myeloma, mercury, lead, or copper poisoning. It can also be hereditary, such as the case of cystinosis. Acetazolamide inhibits carbonic anhydrase and also prevents bicarbonate reabsorption from the proximal tubules, so it can present as a type II RTA. Because the distal tubule that excretes hydrogen ion works fine, if you give an acid load, the urine will acidify normally to pH <5.3, allowing you to tell a type II RTA from types I and IV.

Type III is rarely used as a classification for RTA and most commonly represents a combination of Type I and Type II.

Type IV RTA. This is not really a tubular disorder, but a normal physiological reduction in proximal tubular ammonium and, therefore, hydrogen ion excretion (impaired ammoniagenesis). Type IV RTA is caused by hypoaldosteronism or tubular resistance to aldosterone. Its cardinal feature is hyperkalemia, and measured urinary acidification is normal; hence, it is often called *hyperkalemic RTA* or *tubular hyperkalemia.* Aldosterone increases ammonium excretion, opens the sodium–K^+ exchange channels, and activates the sodium–K^+ ATPase, to increase sodium absorption and waste K^+. So, with adrenal insufficiency, the sodium drops (hyponatremia), K^+ rises, and there is a mild non-anion gap acidosis.

The causes of Type IV RTA are outlined in **Figure 23-15**:

23.6 Metabolic Alkalosis

Metabolic alkalosis is caused by either a loss of hydrogen ion or a gain of bicarbonate. Usually this has to be compounded by a problem with the kidney holding on to too much bicarbonate, since the kidney has the ability to retain a massive amount of bicarbonate.

23.6.1 Contraction Alkalosis

Most commonly a contraction alkalosis relates to extracellular volume depletion, called a *contraction*

alkalosis. The response from the kidney is to retain sodium at the proximal tubule, and bicarbonate follows the sodium to maintain electrical neutrality (since the chloride concentration is lower than sodium). Etiologies for this disorder include vomiting or NG suction, diuretic therapy, and chronic diarrhea (if not acute bicarb wasting).

This is also called *chloride-* or *saline-responsive alkalosis.* If you give normal saline, it has high chloride (150 mEq/L) in it with no bicarbonate, so the kidney can resorb sodium with chloride and let more of the bicarbonate go.

A patient can also lose fluids that have hydrogen ion, as in the case with vomiting or nasogastric suction of HCL containing stomach juice. The volume contraction from fluid loss is coupled with proximal tubule retention of sodium and bicarbonate to try to restore fluid status.

23.6.2 Post-Hypercapnic Metabolic Alkalosis

A patient with severe COPD has the following ABG: pH 7.35; $PaCO_2$ 60 mm Hg; PaO_2 56 mm Hg; and CO_2 on chemistry (HCO_3^-) value of 32 mEq/L. Note that this is a respiratory acidosis, with a chronic compensation: A change in 10 of $PaCO_2$ should change the HCO_3^- by 3.5 for chronic compensation. So, in this case the HCO_3^- should increase by 7, from 24 to 31, close to the measured value. You intubate the patient and tell the therapist to set the vent at a respiratory rate of 15 and a tidal volume of 600 mL. Your gas comes back: pH 7.51; PaCO2 40; HCO_3^- 28.

This looks like a metabolic alkalosis with a second primary respiratory alkalosis (there is no expected increase in $PaCO_2$ above 40). Since you know the clinical scenario and the prior ABG, you can make the correct diagnosis! Note that the HCO_3^- value dropped acutely from 32 to 28 because of the acute change in CO_2 from

Aldosterone deficiency
Primary adrenal insufficiency
Hyporeninemic hypoaldosteronism associated with diabetes mellitus
Aldosterone resistance
Chronic interstitial nephritis (analgesic nephropathy, obstructive nephropathy, chronic pyelonephritis)
Drugs that cause Type IV RTA
Spironolactone
Amiloride
Heparin therapy
NSAIDS
ACE-inhibitors

Figure 23-15 Causes of Type IV RTA.

60 to 40 (for every 10 drop in CO_2 with acute respiratory alkalosis, the HCO_3^- value drops by 2).

This is an interesting case where you have chronic $PaCO_2$ retention from COPD, sleep apnea, obesity hypoventilation, neuromuscular weakness, etc.; and then the patient is intubated, and ventilated to a normal level of pCO_2 (~ 40 mm Hg). This brings the normally high $PaCO_2$ down to normal quickly, revealing the underlying chronic compensatory increase in HCO_3^-. This is an iatrogenic complication of your ventilator settings, a typical ICU complication worth remembering and understanding!!!

23.6.3 Mineralocorticoid Excess

Mineralocorticoid excess is the opposite of the type IV RTA. High levels of aldosterone can come from

- An adrenal tumor or Cushing's syndrome
- Secondary hyperaldosteronism from activation of the renin-angiotensin-aldosterone axis (e.g., with renovascular hypertension and heart failure)
- Giving too much mineralocorticoid (hydrocortisone or fludrocortisone)

The reason for the metabolic alkalosis is related to aldosterone's effects on the kidney. It increases ammonium excretion (retaining H^+), and it opens the sodium–K^+ exchange channels and activates the sodium–K^+ ATPase, to increase sodium and waste K^+. So, with excess aldosterone, the sodium rises (hypernatratremia), K^+ drops (hypokalemia), and there is a mild metabolic alkalosis.

The key to learning to interpret acid-base disorders is to practice, practice, practice.

Suggested Reading

- Preston RA. Acid-base, Fluids, and Electrolytes Made Ridiculously Simple. Edition 3. Published by MedMaster Inc. Miami FL. 2018.
- http://www.acid-base.com/index.php. Acid-Base Tutorial. by "Grog" (Alan W. Grogono). Tulane University
- Adrogué HJ, Gennari FJ, Galla JH, Madias NE. Assessing acid–base disorders. Kidney International 2009;76(12):1239–47.
- Rastegar A. Clinical utility of stewart's method in diagnosis and management of acid-base disorders. Clinical Journal of the American Society of Nephrology 2009;4(7):1267–74.
- Berend K. Diagnostic use of base excess in acid–base disorders. NEJM 2018;378(15):1419–28.
- Brent J. Fomepizole for ethylene glycol and methanol poisoning. NEJM 2009;360(21):2216–23.
- Kraut JA, Kurtz I. Toxic alcohol ingestions: Clinical features, diagnosis, and management. Clinical Journal of the American Society of Nephrology 2008;3(1):208–25.

24

Drug Overdose

24.1 The Basics

Management of the patient with a drug overdose really focuses on four simple concepts:

1. Resuscitate and stabilize
2. Confirm diagnosis and toxin
3. Use antidotes and toxin elimination if appropriate
4. Avoid the overdose Occult Booby Traps!

24.1.1 Resuscitate and Stabilize

The care of the patient with a drug overdose is focused around the basics of resuscitation, including airway management; ventilation; and cardiovascular stabilization. In addition to the *ABC's*, the overdose management typically incorporates neuroresuscitation for the comatose patient with a cocktail of thiamine, glucose (D_{50}), and naloxone.

24.1.2 Confirm Diagnosis and Toxin

The patient history will focus on the type of overdose and timing. However, the self-reported drug history is notoriously unreliable in the population. The time of ingestion provides some perspective on the time course of expected drug effects. The expected time course is markedly altered if the patient had access to long-acting or sustained-release medication forms. A history of bottles and pills found in the home and medications potentially available for ingestion is also helpful.

The physical exam in the overdose patient is focused on classifying the patient into a toxidrome or clinical exam pattern. This pattern is then used to create a list of likely "suspects" that might have contributed to the patient's presentation. Common toxidromes are based upon vital signs, mental status, and pupillary reflexes. Based upon the assessment of these variables, patients can be grouped into patterns of physiologic excitation or depression. Patterns of *physiologic excitation* are characterized by tachycardia, hypertension, tachypnea, and fever. Physiologic excitation is characteristic of intoxications that are sympathomimetic, anticholinergic, or withdrawal states. Drugs in this grouping might include cocaine, amphetamines, phencyclidine (PCP), central hallucinogens, alcohol and/or narcotic withdrawal. *Physiologic depression* is characterized by mental status depression, with a reduction in heart rate, blood pressure, and respiratory rate. The physiologic depression pattern would be more characteristic of sedative hypnotic agents (including alcohol), cholinergic agents, and sympatholytic compounds.

Common toxidromes are outlined in **Figure 24-1 and Figure 24-2**.[181]

Patients may not demonstrate all features of each syndrome, due to variable time intervals to ingestion and mixed ingestions. But repeated examinations will help to guide initial management, pending confirmation by laboratory testing.

Electrocardiography is an important component in the initial assessment of patients with suspected

Toxidrome	Vital Signs				Physical Exam				
	HR	BP	RR	Temp	Pupils	Mental Status	Bowel Sounds	Reflexes	Mucous Membranes
Physiologic Excitation									
Sympathomimetic	↑	↑	↑	↑	↑	hallucinations, agitation, seizures	→↑	↑	moist/diaphoretic
Anticholinergic	↑↑	→	↑	↑	↑	delirium, hallucinations, mumbling speech, picking at objects	↓		dry
Hallucinogen	↑	↑	↑	↑	↑	hallucinations, depersonalization, agitation		→↑	
Sedative withdrawal	↑↑	↑	↑	↑	↑	agitation	→↑	↑	moist/diaphoretic
Physiologic Depression									
Opioid	→	→	↓	→↓	↓	depressed, coma		→↑	
Sedative hypnotic	→	→	→	→↓	→↓	depressed, coma, stupor	→↓	↓	
Cholinergic	↑↓	↑↓	↑		↓	confusion, coma, fasciculation, seizures	↑↑		moist
Misc syndromes									
Serotonin syndrome	↑	↑	→	→↑	↑	confusion, agitation, coma	→↓	↓	moist/diaphoretic
Neuroleptic Malignant syndrome	↑	↑↓	→	↑		variable		→↓	moist/diaphoretic

Figure 24-1 *Clinical features of toxidromes.*

ingestions. Evidence for QRS or QTc prolongation suggests the ingestion of potentially cardiotoxic agents and might warrant immediate therapy.

Important laboratory clues to the ingested substance can be suggested by the *"gap analysis."* Three gaps are essential to consider in the assessment of the toxicology patient:

1. *Anion gap.* The anion gap reflects the difference between measured cations and anions in the serum. The serum anion gap is most frequently calculated as [serum Na - (serum Cl + serum HCO_3^-)]. Alternatively, some information systems include the cation potassium in the equation. The normal value can vary based upon analyzer performance, but ranges around 12 ± 4 if potassium is excluded.

A high anion gap metabolic acidosis is associated with numerous intoxications identified by the mnemonic *MUDPILES* (**Figure 24-3**).

2. *Osmolar gap.* An osmolar gap is calculated as the difference between the calculated and measured serum osmolarity (Sosm).

Sosm = (2 x serum [sodium, in mmol/L]) + [glucose, in mg/dL]/18 + [blood urea nitrogen, in mg/dL]/2.8)

A difference greater than 10 mosmol/L is considered significant. An elevated osmolar gap raises the suspicion of a toxic alcohol ingestion (ethanol, methanol, propylene glycol, isopropyl alcohol).

Toxidrome	Key Features	Examples
Physiologic Excitation		
Sympathomimetic	agitation	cocaine, amphetamine, methamphetamine, theophylline, ephedrine, cathinones
Anticholinergic	urinary retention myoclonus, picking behavior	tricyclic antidepressants, antihistamines, scopolamine, cyclobenzaprine, antiparkinson medications
Hallucinogen		phencyclidine (PCP), LSD, mescaline,
Sedative withdrawal		
Physiologic Depression		
Opioid		opioids (morphine, fentanyl, dilaudid, methadone, oxycodone)
Sedative hypnotic		benzodiazepines, barbituates, alcohols, zolipidem, baclofen
Cholinergic	salivation, bronchorrhea, urinary and fecal incontinence	organophosphates and carbamate insecticides, nicotine, bethanechol, urecholine
Misc syndromes		
Serotonin syndrome	myoclonus, lead-pipe rigidity, flushing	SSRIs, MAO inhibitors, meperidine, TCAs, dextromethorphan
Neuroleptic malignant syndrome	lead pipe rigidity	typical or atypical antipsychotic medication, withdrawal from pro-dopaminergic medications

Figure 24-2 Key features and examples of toxidromes.

M	Methanol, metformin	**P**	Propylene glycol, paraldehyde, propofol
U	Uremia	**I**	Iron, isoniazid, ibuprofen
D	Diabetic ketoacidosis	**L**	Lactate
		E	Ethylene glycol, etoh ketoacidosis
		S	salicylates

Figure 24-3 Mnemonic for anion gap acidosis.

3. *Oxygenation gap.* An oxygenation gap refers to the difference between the oxygen saturation measured by pulse oximetry and the value from a blood gas analyzer with a co-oximeter. Commercial pulse oximeters fail to distinguish saturated hemoglobin from carboxyhemoglobin and methemoglobin. In contrast, hospital blood gas machines that use multiple wavelength co-oximeters can distinguish these forms of hemoglobin. A gap in arterial oxygen saturation > 5% between these two analyzers suggests the presence of significant carboxyhemoglobin, methemoglobin, or sulfhemoglobin.

Screening for intoxication can be helpful in patients where limited history is available. Toxicology screening often begins with "drugs of abuse" immunoassays. These tests are readily available in most emergency departments with a rapid turnaround time. These urine assays commonly assess for cocaine, opioids, benzodiazepines, tricyclic antidepressants, phencyclidine, and tetrahydrocannabinols. These immunoassays rely upon an antibody recognizing a specific chemical structure. Due to the variable clinical structures of drugs within a class (e.g., opioids), these screens have a risk of both false positives and false negatives. Therefore, the screen results should always be considered within the clinical context of the patient.

Assays for acetaminophen and salicylates are commonly available with a rapid turnaround time and should be included in any undefined or suspected possible ingestion, due to the emergent need to institute recognized therapy. Additional blood assays are generally obtained, based upon clinical suspicion (i.e., lithium, neuroleptics, digoxin, theophylline).

More comprehensive qualitative toxic screens can be used for difficult cases but are expensive, delayed in return, and infrequently change patient management. Urine assays are generally preferred for toxicology screening, as the detection interval for most drugs is prolonged for blood assays.

24.1.3 Antidotes and Toxin Elimination

Drug elimination from the GI tract historically has focused on ipecac, activated charcoal, gastric lavage, and whole bowel irrigation. Due to limited effectiveness and risk of the other modalities, only activated charcoal remains in use. Activated charcoal is most effective if administered within 1-2 hours of ingestion at a dose of 1mg/kg. Repeated dosing of activated charcoal is generally not indicated except for rare overdoses of barbiturates, theophylline, and carbamazepine.

Alkaline diuresis (target urine pH > 7) is favored for barbiturates and salicylate intoxications only. The target is to achieve a urine pH ≥ 7.5.

Toxins may also be eliminated using extracorporeal elimination techniques, the most common of which is hemodialysis. Ideal toxins for the use of hemodialysis are characterized by a low volume of distribution, high intravascular concentration, low protein binding, and high water solubility. A list of toxins effectively removed by hemodialysis is shown in **Figure 24-4**.

Antidote administration can be life-saving for those limited overdoses where an antidote exists. The decision to give an antidote is based upon the severity (real or expected) of the poisoning, and the risk:benefit profile associated with the antidote administration. A summary of the more common antidotes is listed in **Figure 24-5**.

When an antidote is administered, the pharmacology of both the antidote and the poisoning must be considered. If the toxin (i.e., opioid) has a longer elimination half-life compared to the antidote (i.e., naloxone), signs of toxicity may be recurrent and require repeat administration of the antidote.

Alternatively, the risk of antidote administration can limit its use. Flumazenil, an effective antidote for

Medications cleared by dialysis	
Ethylene glycol	Lithium
Methanol	Theophylline
Isopropyl alcohol	Phenobarbital
Salicylates	Carbamazepine
Valproic acid	

Figure 24-4 *Medications that are cleared by dialysis in a patient with a drug overdose.*

Drug	Antidote
Narcotic	Naloxone
Benzodiazepine	Flumazenil
Methanol and Ethylene Glycol	Fomepizole
Acetaminophen	Acetylcysteine
Iron	Deferoxamine
Digoxin	Digibind
Calcium channel blocker	Glucagon
Cyanide	Hydroxocobalamin

Figure 24-5 *Common antidotes for selected drug intoxications.*

a suspected benzodiazepine overdose, can precipitate seizures; therefore, the routine use of this antidote is not advised.

A number of newer strategies have been described to antagonize the effects of specific toxic ingestions of medications. These strategies include *hyperinsulinemic euglycemia (HIE)* and *lipid emulsions.*

HIE is a form of treatment that involves high-dose insulin and glucose administration. HIE has been reported to be effective in calcium channel blocker and Beta-blocker overdoses. The specific mechanism of action for this therapy is not established. Calcium channel blockers appear to disrupt fatty acid metabolism and create relative insulin resistance in the myocardium, an effect that could be reversed with HIE. No randomized trials exist to confirm the benefits of this therapy, but case reports suggest a benefit primarily to reverse the negative inotropic and vasopressor effects of calcium channel blockade. HIE does not reverse the cardiac conduction abnormalities. Continuous monitoring to maintain a normal serum potassium concentration is required with HIE.

Intravenous *lipid emulsions (ILE)* have been employed for intoxications that involve lipophilic medications, including local anesthetics. Lipid emulsions are a commonly used caloric source in patients receiving total parenteral nutrition. Case reports have suggested that this treatment may be effective for some tricyclic antidepressants, Beta-blockers, verapamil, chlorpromazine, and flecainide intoxications. Again, the specific mechanism of action is not clear, although altering the drug volume of distribution to target organs is suspected.

Both HIE and ILE can create significant risks during administration and should be considered only after consultation with an experienced toxicologist.

24.1.4 The Overdose Booby Traps

Avoid the overdose Occult Booby Traps! There are a number of key occult booby traps that you should memorize and run through like a checklist or by visualizing your poor overdosed patient in **Figure 24-6:**

1. *Tylenol, Tylenol, Tylenol (OK, acetaminophen).* You should always suspect this and send blood levels since if you miss this, the liver is shot. As you see below, an antidote, N-acetyl-cysteine or NAC, is readily available for IV dosing.
2. *Consider the risk of co-ingestions.* Acetaminophen again! And send a salicylate level while you are thinking about co-ingestions.
3. *Toxic alcohols.* Always measure the anion gap and osmolar gap to search for toxic alcohol ingestion. This is the primary reason why you do an OSM gap. If you miss this, you can kill the eyes (methanol) or the kidneys (ethylene glycol).
4. *Occult infection.* Expect and look for aspiration pneumonia. This can jump up and bite you on day 1-3 after overdose.
5. *Occult trauma.* Always CT the head and look for a subdural bleed. Physical examination can identify an occult fracture from a fall.

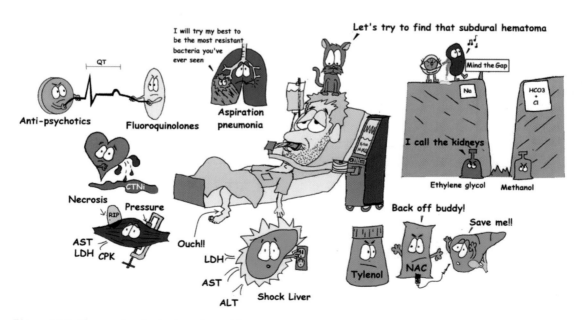

Figure 24-6 *The overdose booby traps to avoid.*

6. *Occult rhabdomyolysis and myocardial infarction.* Shock after overdose is common, and you can see infarction of multiple organs. Hypo-perfusion of the heart will increase troponin levels; shock liver increases the AST, ALT, and LDH; shock or pressure necrosis of the muscle will increase the AST, LDH and CPK (not ALT, which is liver specific).
7. *Occult Q-T prolongation.* Always check the ECG, as many drugs can prolong this QT and increase risk of ventricular tachycardia and cardiac arrest (*Torsades De Pointes*)
8. *Occult alcohol and narcotic withdrawal.* Many patients will have co-dependencies and will suffer withdrawal. You will have to try to evaluate severe delirium and determine if you are seeing withdrawal, brain injury from shock, or delirium related to SIRS (from a new infection, like aspiration pneumonia or multi-organ injury from shock).

24.2 Specific Overdoses

24.2.1 Acetaminophen

Acetaminophen is one of the most frequent ingestions that, not infrequently, presents as a co-ingestion with some other toxic agent, like a sedative hypnotic or pain reliever. Acetaminophen toxicity may occur from a single acute ingestion or from repeated ingestions of the medication at supra therapeutic levels. The primary toxicity is hepatic due to accumulation of a toxic metabolite, N-acetyl-para-benzoquinoneimine (NAPQI), leading to depletion of glutathione stores and subsequent hepatotoxicity. Peak hepatic injury occurs approximately 4 days post an acute ingestion. Patients also may develop renal injury, which can occur in isolation.

For single acute ingestions only, a drug level is obtained initially at least 4 hours post ingestion to ensure a peak level post absorption. Patients who ingest an extended-release preparation should have a second level obtained 4 hours following the initial level. The level is assessed using the *Rumack-Matthew nomogram* (**Figure 24-7**). This nomogram does not apply to ingestions more than 24 hours prior to assessment, chronic iatrogenic intravenous ingestions, or recurrent ingestions. For these chronic ingestions you should assess transaminases. The level is plotted against the time of the ingestion with levels above the line being an indication for therapy.

The treatment antidote is oral or IV N-acetylcysteine (NAC), which restores glutathione levels. The drug is most effective if administered within the first 8 hours of ingestion, when the antidote is highly effective in eliminating the risk of hepatic necrosis. In addition to guidance from the nomogram, the clinician should appreciate that any of the following are considered indications for the administration of NAC:

- A serum acetaminophen concentration > 4 hours post-acute ingestion of an immediate release preparation that is above the treatment line
- A patient with a history of ingestion and any evidence for hepatic injury
- A suspected ingestion ≥ 150 mg/kg, where the drug level results will be delayed beyond 8 hours
- Patients with an unknown time of ingestion with a drug level > 10 mcg/mL

A 20-hour intravenous and a 72-hour oral protocol for the administration of NAC are both recognized. These two methods of treatment are considered equivalent. The intravenous route is generally favored for any patient with GI intolerance (i.e., nausea and/or vomiting) or actual hepatic injury.

24.2.2 Alcohols

The frequency of alcohol (ethyl, methanol, ethylene glycol, and isopropyl) ingestions in clinical medicine pales in comparison to their appearance on internal medicine, critical care, and emergency medicine board exams. *They are a favorite of question writers across the U.S., so you better know this one!* A detailed description of diagnosis, pathogenesis, and treatment is covered in *Chapter 23 Acid-Base Disorders.*

All of these alcohols create an osmolar gap and begin their metabolism via alcohol dehydrogenase. The

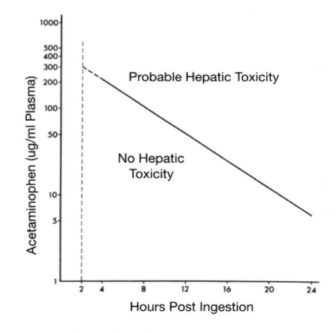

Figure 24-7 *Rumack-Matthew nomogram for analysis of acute acetaminophin toxicity.*

presence of any alcohol can be suspected if an osmolar gap is present while the actual level of the specific substance is being measured. Toxic alcohol ingestions with ethylene glycol and methanol are characterized by both an osmolar gap and an anion gap. The osmolar gap reflects the toxic alcohol, and the anion gap reflects the acid metabolite, the latter of which can poison the eye (methanol to formic acid) or the kidney (ethylene glycol to oxalic acid crystals). All metabolism for these substrates occurs through alcohol dehydrogenase, which has the greatest affinity for the metabolism of ethyl alcohol. An osmolar gap can be absent in known toxic alcohol ingestions if the alcohol has been metabolized to the acid metabolite. But an anion gap will be present to indicate the unmeasured anion, which is the base partner of the acid. If the osmolar gap is absent in a toxic ingestion, then the substrate has been fully metabolized. Visual disturbances suggest methanol ingestion, while the presence of oxalate crystals indicates ethylene glycol intoxication.

Isopropyl alcohol is metabolized directly via alcohol dehydrogenase to acetone. For isopropyl alcohol, an osmolar gap without an anion gap is characteristic. Clinical features will include CNS depression or GI manifestations. Treatment is supportive only.

The primary therapy for a *methanol or ethylene glycol ingestion* is focused on slowing the metabolism to the toxic product, using competitive inhibition of the alcohol dehydrogenase. This can be accomplished by giving ethyl alcohol or fomepizole, both of which tie up the enzyme. Dialysis removes both the acid metabolites and the alcohol and should be initiated early. Generally, dialysis is indicated in the presence of an acidosis or end-organ damage. Thiamine and pyridoxine should also be administered.

A unique form of toxic alcohol ingestion occurs with *propylene glycol intoxication*. This type of ingestion typically occurs when the drug is used as a diluent for another medication. The classic ICU overdose occurs during prolonged and or higher dose (>0.1mg/kg/hr) lorazepam infusions. The overdose is recognized by the presence of both an osmolar and anion gap. Propylene glycol is also used as the diluent for diazepam but not midazolam.

24.2.3 Benzodiazepines

The benzodiazepine (BZD) category of medications is frequently prescribed and not surprisingly is a frequent cause of intoxications. BZDs mediate their pharmacologic effect via modulation of the gamma-aminobutyric acid A (GABA-A) receptor, increasing the affinity for the GABA neurotransmitter. GABA is a primary inhibitory neurotransmitter in the central nervous system.

Isolated oral benzodiazepine ingestions rarely cause respiratory depression, but mixed overdoses that involve medications with varied mechanisms can cause profound respiratory depression. The most common co-ingestion is with alcohol. Although an antidote (flumazenil) is readily available, concerns regarding the short half-life of the antidote, the risk of withdrawal symptoms, and the risk of seizures make flumazenil infrequently used. Care is primarily supportive for this intoxication.

24.2.4 Slow it Down: Beta Blockers and Calcium Channel Blockers

The presence of bradycardia with hypotension on initial assessment should suggest the possibility of a Beta-blocker or calcium channel blocker overdose. The hypotension is attributable to the negative inotropic effects of these medications more than the frequently associated bradycardia. Obviously, structural heart disease must also be considered in the differential diagnosis.

Calcium channel blockers can produce cardiac (negative inotropy and chronotropy) and peripheral vasodilator effects. The diagnosis depends primarily on the patient history, as assays for the various calcium channel blockers are not routinely available. The clinical manifestations are determined by the interaction of the drug's pharmacology and the patient's underlying cardiac condition. Bradycardia would be more common with diltiazem or verapamil, whereas peripheral vasodilation might be more dominant with amlodipine or nifedipine. Verapamil is considered the most lethal of the calcium channel blocker overdoses.

The physical exam of the patient with a calcium channel blocker overdose can be deceptive, as the peripheral vasodilation can produce a "warm" shock state, inappropriately suggesting adequate tissue perfusion. The time course for a calcium channel blocker overdose can be challenging to predict due to the existence of sustained-release preparations and delayed gastric motility. Rapid clinical deterioration is often seen. Treatment is generally supportive, initially with volume resuscitation for hypotension and atropine for bradycardia. In more advanced cases, vasopressors and/or temporary pacing may be required. For very advanced cases, extracorporeal support might be needed. In patients with resistant hypotension, very high dosing of vasopressor infusion has been successfully employed.

Intravenous calcium (intermittent or by continuous infusion) can be attempted, but the effects are variable, and monitoring for hypercalcemia is required. Intravenous glucagon increases intracellular cyclic AMP and has been shown to be effective for the bradycardia in calcium channel blocker overdoses. Hyperinsulinemic-euglycemia and lipid emulsions have also been described as an "antidote" for this intoxication, but, as previously noted, no clear benefit from randomized trials has been confirmed.

Beta-blocker overdoses present with similar findings of bradycardia and hypotension. Again, the clinical manifestations will be variable, based upon the specific pharmacology of the Beta-blocker and the patient's background cardiovascular physiology. The time course will again be variable due to both short-acting and extended preparations. In addition to changes in cardiovascular hemodynamics, propranolol, which crosses the blood-brain barrier, can cause central nervous system findings of seizures and coma.

The initial antidote of choice for Beta-blocker overdose is glucagon, which has an inotropic effect independent of acting at the *B* receptors. Initial doses can be given by IV push followed by continuous infusion.

The challenge for both overdoses is that the traditional medications used to treat these hemodynamic abnormalities (i.e., atropine, dopamine, epinephrine) are frequently ineffective.

24.2.5 Speed it Up: Cocaine and Cathinones

Patients who present with fever, tachycardia, and hypertension should suggest an acute sympathomimetic syndrome and a likely stimulant overdose. A young patient with a coronary event in this setting would raise suspicion for cocaine intoxication, which is second to only alcohol as the most common cause of emergency department intoxications. In addition to coronary events, these patients can present with intracranial complications, including ischemic stroke and hemorrhages. Cocaine blocks the presynaptic reuptake of biogenic amines, including catecholamines and serotonin, leading to stimulation of both alpha and beta receptors. The vascular pathophysiology includes vasoconstriction in cardiac and peripheral vascular beds, leading to organ ischemia. Cocaine also increases the risk of intra-arterial thrombosis.

Patients present with clinical manifestations of tachycardia and hypertension. At high doses, cocaine may adversely impact Na channel activity, leading to QRS prolongation and negative inotropy. Central nervous system manifestations can include headaches, psychomotor agitation, seizures, and even coma. Pulmonary complications can include direct airway injury from inhalation (i.e., crack cocaine) and pulmonary infarction. GI manifestations include ischemic colitis and infarction. In essence, any organ can suffer from the vascular pathology that characterizes cocaine abuse.

The cocaine metabolite benzoylecgonine is assessed in traditional drugs of abuse screens in emergency departments. Unlike cocaine, which is rapidly cleared form the blood, benzoylecgonine can be detected in urine specimens for several days. False positives and negatives may occur. The assay is also limited by the prolonged positivity, so that a positive test today does not necessarily correlate with an acute intoxication but may reflect past exposure.

Aspirin is appropriate therapy in these conditions, as the intoxication is associated with platelet aggregation. No specific antidote exists. Treatment usually involves higher doses of benzodiazepines to offset the centrally mediated adrenergic stimulation. For more severe cases with hypertension, bolus IV phentolamine to achieve peripheral alpha blockade is the preferred agent. Beta-blockers, including labetalol, are generally to be avoided because they can lead to imbalanced alpha stimulation.

Amphetamines, methamphetamines, and synthetic cathinones can have a similar clinical presentation to cocaine intoxication. Fever, hypertension, tachycardia, mydriasis, diaphoresis, and hyperagitation are features of the sympathomimetic toxidrome. The combination of adrenergic stimulation with an agitated delirium suggests this category of intoxicants. The synthetic cathinones (i.e., bath salts) in particular are recognized for their prominent neuropsychiatric manifestations, including hallucinations, combativeness, paranoia, myoclonus, and confusion. In contrast to cocaine, which is generally short-acting, the synthetic cathinones can have prolonged clinical manifestations for days. Patients can also develop significant hyponatremia, which can also adversely affect mental status.

Many of the synthetic cathinones are not detected by traditional urine drug screens. The clinical diagnosis is based upon patient history and recognition of the key clinical features. This intoxication is included in the differential diagnosis of the acutely agitated patient. Important considerations in the differential diagnosis for sympathomimetic intoxication include the withdrawal syndromes.

Patients with amphetamine, methamphetamine, and synthetic cathinone intoxications are similarly treated to cocaine intoxication with IV benzodiazepines. Airway control may be necessary, as high doses of benzodiazepine are often required. Serum electrolytes and glucose should be monitored, and adequate hydration maintained. Patients may be at risk for rhabdomyolysis, which mandates ongoing monitoring of electrolytes, renal function, muscle biomarkers, and checking for compartment syndromes.

In addition, patients can develop a cardiomyopathy and valvular heart disease from the more chronic stimulation of these medications.

24.2.6 Hypoglycemia Secondary to Insulin and Oral Hypoglycemic Agents

Hypoglycemia can be a manifestation of an overdose of insulin or oral hypoglycemic agents. These overdoses may be intentional or accidental, the latter in association with polypharmacy or changing renal function. The differential diagnosis will include endocrine disorders (hypocortisolism, hypoglucagon), alcohol abuse, or critical illness (sepsis, hepatic failure).

The initial treatment is supplemental glucose (i.e., 25 gms of D_{50} [50ml] in an adult, followed by a 20% dextrose infusion), recognizing that the drug effect (particularly in the case of oral hypoglycemic agents) can be prolonged. Parenteral thiamine (100 mg IV) is also provided if deficiency is expected. Glucagon (5 mg IM) will support the mobilization of liver glycogen and can also be supportive initially but is not a substitute for dextrose administration. Because both dextrose and glucagon promote the release of insulin from the pancreas, their use can be self-defeating in these overdoses. Octreotide reduces insulin secretion from the pancreas and can be very effective for this problem. The dose is 50 to 100 mcg q 6 hours subq or IV.

24.2.7 Antidepressants and the Abnormal ECG

A presentation with an abnormal ECG, including wide complex tachycardia and prolonged QT, can be highly suggestive of an antidepressant overdose. Although classically associated with the older tricyclic antidepressants, this syndrome can occur with any of the medications in the antidepressant class. The tricyclic antidepressants (TCAs) are considered more toxic than the selective serotonin reuptake inhibitors (SSRIs).

TCA overdoses may present with shock secondary to peripheral alpha blockade or shock from a myocardial depressant effect due to sodium channel blockade. Cardiac arrhythmias in association with intraventricular conduction delays are also recognized. Central nervous system manifestations may include anticholinergic toxicity or seizures.

Treatment for TCA intoxication includes intravenous sodium bicarbonate, fluid resuscitation, and vasopressor medications. Intravenous sodium bicarbonate attenuates the sodium channel blockade and is indicated in all patients with intraventricular conduction delay and/or hypotension. The medications affect the Na-K channel of the myocardium; therapy with sodium bicarbonate involves sodium's impact at these channels as much as the alkalization. For refractory cases, hypertonic saline can be used when maximum alkalization (pH > 7.55) has not been successful.

The clinical features of *overdose for the SSRIs and serotonin-norepinphrine reuptake inhibitors (SNRIs)* are generally milder in severity and managed with supportive care only. The clinical features include sedation and gastrointestinal upset. Venlafaxine and citalopram have been associated with conduction abnormalities and ventricular arrhythmias. Bupropion has been associated with delayed onset of seizures.

24.2.8 Salicylates and the Pseudosepsis Syndrome

Patients with acute salicylate intoxication can present with abdominal pain and vomiting, tinnitus, and vertigo, which can progress to more advanced symptoms of altered mentation, noncardiogenic pulmonary edema, and coma. Clinical features include tachycardia, tachypnea (hyperventilation), delirium, and seizures. Drug absorption will usually manifest symptoms within 2 hours of ingestion, but may be delayed, especially with enteric coated preparations. The complete manifestations may not be seen for up to 24 hours. Symptoms do not perfectly correlate with blood levels but, generally, patients are symptomatic above a salicylate serum concentration of > 40 mg/dL. Monitoring the time trend of salicylate levels (q 2 hours) can help assess the response to therapy and guide specific interventions. Patients frequently present with a lactic acidosis in more severe intoxications. This lactic acidosis is due to the effect of salicylates on oxidative phosphorylation.

An elderly patient with altered mental status, fever, respiratory alkalosis, and metabolic acidosis may be suffering from chronic salicylate ingestion but suspected erroneously of having sepsis syndrome. This salicylate ingestion is more characteristic of chronic rather than acute ingestion.

Salicylate intoxication is a common co-ingestion and should be screened for routinely to allow early appropriate intervention.

The treatment is hydration and urine alkalization. The target urine pH is 7.5 to 8.0. Even patients with a respiratory alkalosis should receive bicarbonate therapy to achieve the urine pH target, as long as the blood pH is not severely alkalemic. These modalities serve to minimize central nervous system penetration and enhance elimination. Careful electrolyte monitoring is needed to maintain normal potassium levels. Respiratory alkalemia is protective and serves to trap salicylate anions in the blood. Respiratory alkalosis should be maintained even if the patient requires ventilator support. Hemodialysis is effective in removing salicylate and is indicated for severe cases with metabolic acidosis, encephalopathy, or cardiovascular compromise.

24.2.9 Serotonin Syndrome

Serotonin toxicity, often called the *serotonin syndrome,* occurs due to excess activity of the neurotransmitter serotonin in the central nervous syndrome. The diagnosis is based upon clinical findings that can range from mild to life-threatening. Serotonin syndrome manifests with variable components, from a classic triad of altered mental status, autonomic dysfunction, and neuroexcitability (seizures, rigidity, and tremors). This syndrome can be seen with an excess of antidepressants (SSRI medications and MAO inhibitors) and other medications, including linezolid, and tramadol. The syndrome occurs with intentional and non-intentional drug overdose, or from unappreciated drug interactions. The syndrome may result from any combination of events that increases serotonergic neurotransmission. Patients may manifest the signs of serotonin syndrome after a simple dose change in their chronic medications.

Patients present with altered mentation, ranging from mild agitation to frank delirium (**Figure 24-8**). Autonomic dysfunction includes temperature dysregulation (hyperthermia), as well as cardiovascular (tachycardia, hypertension), respiratory (tachypnea), and GI manifestations (vomiting and/or diarrhea). Neuroexcitability may range from tremors to hyperreflexia and clonus, to rigidity, or seizures. The neuromuscular findings are typically greatest in the lower extremities.

Because the diagnosis is clinical in origin, consideration of disorders that fit in the differential diagnosis is important. Neuroleptic malignant syndrome (NMS), withdrawal states, malignant hyperthermia, as well as adrenergic and anticholinergic toxicity states must be considered in the patient presenting with some of the clinical features. Sepsis syndrome, encephalitis, and meningitis are often considered as alternative infectious causes of the mental status changes. NMS can be the most challenging in patients with neuropsychiatric disease. NMS is caused by dopaminergic excess and tends to be more delayed in onset and resolution. Hyporeflexia is more common in NMS, while myoclonus is rare. Lead pipe rigidity is characteristic of NMS (**Figure 24-9**). Likewise, hyperreflexia and myoclonus are rare in the infectious syndromes.

The treatment for the serotonin syndrome is primarily supportive. Patients with significant clinical findings require monitoring in an ICU. All serotonergic medications must be discontinued. Benzodiazepines may help to address agitation or manifestations of neuroexcitability. A specific antidote, cyproheptadine, is available for more severe intoxications. Use of this antidote should be conducted in consultation with an experienced toxicologist.

24.2.10 Opioids

Opioid intoxications include a large group of compounds that occur naturally, are synthetic, or are semi-synthetic. Opioids, a common cause of acute intoxication, characteristically present with depressed mentation, miosis, hypoventilation, and decreased to absent bowel sounds. Although miosis is often considered the key feature of opioid intoxication, hypoventilation is the most characteristic finding. Secondary complications

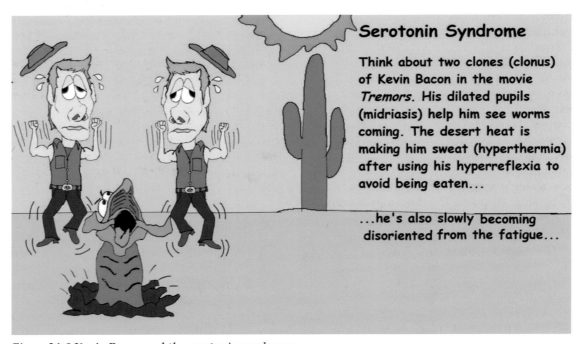

Serotonin Syndrome

Think about two clones (clonus) of Kevin Bacon in the movie *Tremors.* His dilated pupils (midriasis) help him see worms coming. The desert heat is making him sweat (hyperthermia) after using his hyperreflexia to avoid being eaten...

...he's also slowly becoming disoriented from the fatigue...

Figure 24-8 Kevin Bacon and the serotonin syndrome.

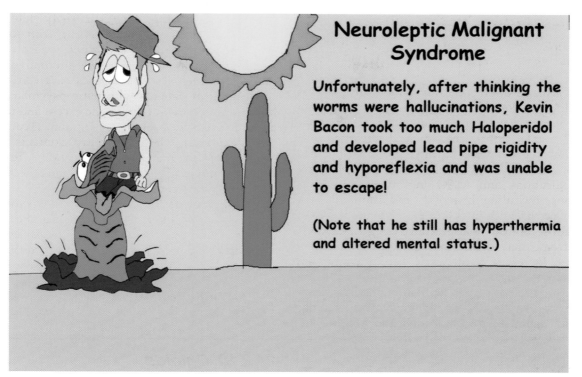

Figure 24-9 *Kevin Bacon and neuroleptic malignant syndrome (NMS).*

of co-ingestion (think acetaminophen) or trauma can complicate the presenting clinical features. Both tramadol and meperidine can present with seizures. Both oxycodone and methadone can be complicated by QT prolongation.

Treatment is initially focused on support of the respiratory system. Pulse oximetry may be deceptively normal in the hypoventilating patient if he is receiving supplemental oxygen. Monitoring of arterial blood gases (preferred) and/or ETCO2 is needed to assist your assessment of alveolar ventilation.

Naloxone is a specific opioid antagonist that is administered to any patient with a suspected opioid intoxication. The dosing is adjusted between 0.2 and 2.0 mg, based upon the patient's clinical status. Naloxone is generally available as a 0.4 mg/ mL solution (1 ampule) or the equivalent of 4 mg/10 ml.

For patients with suppressed but spontaneous respirations, a single ampule can be administered over 30 seconds by slow IV push. The dose may be repeated q 5-10 minutes to achieve a respiratory rate > 12 breaths per min. If a total dose of 5 to 10 mg is not effective, an alternative etiology should be considered.

Patients with long-term opioid dependence will experience withdrawal with the administration of naloxone. To minimize withdrawal symptoms, one ampule of naloxone (0.4mg / mL) can be mixed with 9 ml of normal saline to achieve a concentration of 0.04 mg/ ml. This dose can be administered in 1-2 ml increments. The target is to achieve a respiratory rate > 12 bpm – not a normal mental status.

The half-life of naloxone is generally shorter than most opioid intoxications. Repeated administration or a continuous infusion may be required to maintain the effect of the antidote.

Because opioids, in general, have a large volume of distribution in the body, they cannot be removed by dialysis.

Patients with opioid intoxication risk development of non-cardiogenic pulmonary edema. Originally termed *heroin lung*, this clinical picture of ARDS will manifest when the patient is recovering from the initial opioid effects on respiratory depression. The clinical syndrome has also been attributed to the combined opioid-reversal effects of naloxone. Naloxone is associated with prompt reversal of the opioid and a potential catecholamine surge. This catecholamine surge has been theorized as a potential cause of the non-cardiogenic edema. Positive pressure therapy (BVM ventilation) might be protective of this complication, but remains to be determined.

Suggested Reading

- Brooks DE, Levine M, O'Connor AD, French RNE, Curry SC. Toxicology in the ICU Part 2: Specific toxins. Chest 2011;140(4):1072–85.
- Levine M, Ruha A-M, Graeme K, Brooks DE, Canning J, Curry SC. Toxicology in the ICU Part 3: Natural toxins. Chest 2011;140(5):1357–70.

25

Neurologic Emergencies

A complete summary of neurologic emergencies is beyond the scope of this book and frequently requires advanced training in neurocritical care. However, we will discuss the acute care management of four common emergencies seen on hospital floors and general intensive care units including:

1. Acute Ischemic Stroke
2. Acute Intracerebral Hemorrhage
3. Generalized Convulsive Status Epilepticus
4. Acute Myasthenic Crisis

25.1 Acute Ischemic Stroke

The sudden loss of cerebral function is the primary clinical manifestation of an acute stroke. All patients presenting with an acute change in neurologic status should be evaluated for an acute stroke, although the differential diagnosis for this clinical presentation includes many conditions which can *mimic a stroke* such as seizures, hypoglycemia, and drug toxicity. The initial focus is similar to all critically ill patients, and that is to manage the basics of airway, breathing, and circulation. Patients with an acute change in neurologic status may require airway control for patency and to support secretion clearance due to acute bulbar dysfunction. Supplemental oxygen is only provided if necessary to maintain the oxygen saturation > 92%.

Patients may also require support of the circulation to maintain a target cerebral perfusion. The *optimal blood pressure* for management of the patient with acute stroke

is not known. Hypotension and hypovolemia should be corrected to maintain systemic perfusion and support organ function. Patients with an elevated blood pressure that are otherwise eligible for treatment with fibrinolytic therapy should have their BP cautiously lowered into the range of < 185 mm Hg systolic and < 110 mm Hg diastolic before administration of IV fibrinolytic therapy. For specific therapeutic options, please see Chapter 10 on *High Systemic Arterial Blood Pressure.* More intensive blood pressure control is initiated after the acute stroke phase has stabilized. Patients that are not candidates for fibrinolytic therapy are allowed permissive hypertension (treatment only for a blood pressure greater than 220/110 mm Hg) to maintain adequate perfusion in brain areas at risk of injury.

A key requirement of the patient history is to establish the *timing of the stroke onset.* The stroke onset is based upon timing from when the patient was last *known to be "normal."* As an example, a patient that lives alone and is not seen for 12 hours is assumed to have a stroke which is 12 hours in duration. The optimal time window for lytic therapy in acute stroke is < 3 hours from symptom onset, although evidence exists that a subset of patients between 3 and 4.5 hours also benefit.[182]

Although a few clinical features (e.g., headache and sudden loss of consciousness) can favor the diagnosis of intracerebral or subarachnoid hemorrhage over an acute stroke, all patients must undergo *urgent CNS imaging with a brain CT* scan to evaluate for intracerebral hemorrhage vs. stroke. The brain imaging studies should be performed within 20 minutes of arrival to the

ED or floor notification. The benefit of intravenous lytic therapy is recognized to be time-dependent with earlier treatment having more favorable results. Acute brain ischemia may not be evident on this initial CT scan, but we treat the patient with a persistent neurologic defect as an acute ischemic stroke.

The assessment of the patient's neurologic function is accomplished using the National Institute of Health Stroke Scale (NIHSS) (https://www.ninds.nih.gov/sites/default/files/NIH_Stroke_Scale_Booklet.pdf). The *NIHSS provides an 11-item assessment of neurologic function*. Training of the examiner in the performance of the scale improves reliability. This scale provides a reliable assessment tool that can even be assessed remotely (using telemedicine). The scores range from 0 (best) to 42 (worst). The score is a valid predictor of long-term outcome following an acute stroke. A higher NIHSS core (> 10) predicts occlusion of a main intracerebral artery. The tool has limited discriminating power between carotid and vertebrobasilar vascular involvement.

Laboratory studies are needed to exclude alternative etiologies for the acute neuro status change and support the diagnosis of acute stroke, with a *blood glucose* mandatory to r/o hypoglycemia as the etiology for a patient's change in neurologic status. Additional studies should include coagulation parameters, complete blood count, and a metabolic profile.

Once stabilized from a cardiovascular perspective and the initial assessment completed, a decision regarding the need for *reperfusion therapy* in acute stroke must be considered. In the current era, most hospitals will have consultation available with a stroke expert, either on-site or via telemedicine. Specialized stroke units with defined care protocols improve patient outcomes. The timing of stroke onset, objective assessment via the NIHSS, and initial brain imaging is rapidly obtained to support the stroke service consultation.

Consultation with stroke expertise will also be essential to define patients that may be eligible for mechanical thrombectomy. Mechanical thrombectomy can be provided for patients with large vessel occlusion in the proximal anterior circulation up to 24 hours post stroke onset, independent of whether they receive IV fibrinolytic therapy for the same event.

Based primarily upon the NINDS study group evaluation and the ECCAS 3 trial, the inclusion and exclusion criteria for intravenous alteplase therapy are summarized in **Figure 25-1**.[182,183] Consultation with a stroke expert is advised. The primary risk of lytic therapy is symptomatic intracranial hemorrhage (sICH) as a complication of reperfusion therapy (~ 6 %).

The dose for IV alteplase is 0.9 mg/kg (maximum dose 90 mg) over 60 min, with 10% of the treatment given as an initial bolus over 1 min. *Admit the patient to an intensive care unit* for frequent monitoring of the NIHSS and blood pressure. *Delay any invasive procedures* such as nasogastric tubes, foley, or intravascular catheters if possible. If the patient develops a severe headache, hypertension, nausea or vomiting, or a change in the neurologic exam a STAT head CT is needed, and any remaining alteplase infusion is held. The blood pressure is closely monitored to maintain systolic blood pressure <180 mm Hg and diastolic blood pressure < 105 mm Hg throughout the infusion. A *routine head CT or MRI is obtained at 24 hours* to evaluate for hemorrhage prior to the provision of anticoagulants or antiplatelet agents. If the patient has evidence for an intracranial bleed, stop any residual alteplase infusion. Urgent hematology and neurosurgical consultation is obtained. If bleeding occurs within 24 hours of alteplase administration, the patient can be treated with cryoprecipitate (includes factor VIII) with 10 U infused over 10–30 min (onset in 1 h, peaks in 12 h); administer an additional dose for fibrinogen level of <200 mg/dL. Further treatment includes tranexamic acid 1000 mg IV infused over 10 min OR ε-aminocaproic acid 4–5 g over 1 h, followed by 1 g IV until bleeding is controlled (peak onset in 3 hours).[184]

Clinical trials have suggested some patients may benefit from intra-arterial thrombolysis or mechanical thrombectomy. These procedures continue to be evaluated for outcomes, and the patients should be considered in consultation with a stroke neurologist.

Fluid replacement therapy is indicated in acute stroke management if the patient has evidence for intravascular volume contraction. Fluid management is individualized to the patient, but as a general rule, *isotonic fluid* without dextrose (e.g., normal saline) is favored over hypotonic fluid (e.g., ½ normal saline) to minimize the risk for exacerbating cerebral edema.

Close monitoring of blood glucose is indicated in acute stroke as both hypoglycemia and hyperglycemia are problematic. Hypoglycemia can mimic an acute stroke, while hyperglycemia is associated with a poor outcome. Current guidelines target treatment to maintain glucose in the range of 140-180 ng/dL.[183]

Patients begin *aspirin within 48 hours* of stroke onset and *statin therapy* is favored to reduce recurrent events. Urgent anticoagulation with the goal of preventing recurrent stroke is not favored.

Anticoagulation is indicated in patients with ischemic stroke due to atrial fibrillation based upon the CHA_2DS_2-VASC score. Anticoagulation is frequently withheld during the initial stroke treatment interval due to the risk of hemorrhagic transformation of the ischemic stroke.

Patients with immobility due to ischemic stroke benefit from *prophylaxis for deep venous thrombosis*. Intermittent pneumatic compression (with aspirin therapy) is recommended over routine care to reduce the risk of deep vein thrombosis. The benefit of prophylactic subcutaneous heparin in these patients is less clear.

Criteria for Intravenous Thrombolysis for Acute Ischemic Stroke
Inclusion Criteria
Clinical diagnosis of ischemic stroke with the sudden onset of neurological functional deficit (NIHSS $\geq$ 4 points or a functionally significant deficit)
Onset of the symptoms < 4.5 hours before treatment, with the exception of an acute occlusion of the basilar artery (in this case, a longer therapeutic window may be accepted)
Age > 18 years
Exclusion Criteria
Ischemic stroke or severe head trauma within the last 3 months
Suspicion of subarachnoid hemorrhage
Arterial puncture in non-compressible locations in the last 7 days
Previous history of intracranial hemorrhage
Patients with a history of intra-axial intracranial neoplasm
Arterio-venous malformation or aneurysm of the cerebral arteries
Cerebral or spinal operation within the past 3 months
Persistent arterial hypertension (systolic BP > 185 and/or diastolic BP > 110 mmHg)
Presentation consistent with infectious endocarditis
Stroke associated with aortic arch dissection
Serious bleeding event within the last 3 weeks or hemorrhagic diathesis
Childbirth in the last 10 days or the third trimester of the pregnancy
Platelet count < 100,000
Administration of heparin in the last 48 h and APTT over the normal range
Therapy by anti-vitamin K and INR > 1.7
Therapy by thrombin direct inhibitors or activated factor X inhibitors with a significant alteration of the monitoring laboratory tests (APTT, INR, thrombocytopenia, and relevant tests of activated factor X activity)
Hypoglycemia < 50 mg/dL
Evidence of intracranial hemorrhage by CT scan
Relative Contraindications
Minor neurological deficit (NIHSS < 4 points) or rapidly resolving symptoms
Structural GI malignancy
Myocardial infarction in the past 3 months
Major surgery in the past 14 days
History of GI or GU bleeding within 21 days of stroke onset
Serious trauma in the past 14 days
Premorbid severe neurological deficit (mRS>4 points)
Pregnancy
Epileptic seizure with the postictal neurological deficit

Figure 25-1 *Inclusion and exclusion criteria for fibrinolytic therapy in acute stroke.*

Fever is not uncommon in stroke patients and is associated with an adverse outcome. The source of fever should be promptly identified and treated, and antipyretic medications provided to lower body temperature

Patients with acute stroke are at risk for *swallowing dysfunction* due to the associated neurologic complications. Swallowing dysfunction places the patient at high risk for the complication of aspiration pneumonia. This risk must be carefully considered when administering oral medications and food. Specialized assistance from speech therapy can assist with accurate patient assessment.

25.2 Acute Intracerebral Hemorrhage

Acute intracerebral hemorrhage (ICH) is a medical emergency that demands prompt diagnosis and management. Hematoma expansion and early neurologic deterioration are a significant risk in ICH after onset. A severe headache, vomiting, decreased level of consciousness, and more rapid neurologic decline all favor the diagnosis of ICH over acute stroke, but none of the clinical findings are specific. Non-contrast head CT is therefore mandatory, and highly sensitive in distinguishing acute ischemic stroke from acute intracerebral hemorrhage (ICH).

Patients with evidence for ICH are closely monitored in the ICU due to a higher risk for neurologic instability, increased intracranial pressure, and poorly controlled blood pressure. In general, these patients have a greater need for neurocritical care, neuroradiology, and neurosurgical intervention. Common management principles apply to both acute ischemic stroke and acute intracerebral hemorrhage including fever control, glucose management, DVT prophylaxis (intermittent pneumatic compression), isotonic fluid administration, and monitoring for aspiration risk. Clinical seizures should be treated with anticonvulsant medication, but prophylactic treatment is not advised.

The three pillars of patient management for acute intracerebral hemorrhage include:

1. Blood pressure control
2. Reversal of coagulopathy
3. Possible management of elevated intracranial pressure

25.2.1 Blood Pressure Control

BP is elevated in patients with acute intracerebral hemorrhage (ICH), often to a greater degree than in ischemic stroke. Severe blood pressure elevation could worsen ICH by creating a continued force for bleeding. Higher arterial pressure may, alternatively, be required to maintain cerebral perfusion in ICH complicated by intracranial hypertension. For patients suspected to have elevated intracranial pressure (ICP), ICP monitoring may be used to guide treatment based on the measurement of cerebral perfusion pressure.

American Heart Association guidelines, admittedly arbitrary and not evidence-based, suggest *a target MAP of less than 110 mm Hg or a blood pressure of less than 160/90 mm Hg* while maintaining a reasonable cerebral perfusion pressure in patients with suspected elevations of intracranial pressure.[185] Based upon the results of INTERACT 1 and 2, showing a trend toward a reduction in the primary outcome of death or severe disability, significant improvements in secondary functional outcomes, and reassuring safety data, many investigators advocate acute blood-pressure reduction to a target systolic blood pressure of 140 mm Hg for patients with spontaneous ICH.[186] Short-acting titratable therapeutic agents are used for blood pressure control in the setting of ICH. See *Chapter 10 High Systemic Arterial Pressure* for review and suggested treatment options.

25.2.2 Reversal of Coagulopathy

Patients taking anticoagulants present a particular problem in the management of intracerebral hemorrhage. For all patients taking anticoagulants or antiplatelet medications, these should be immediately discontinued. As reviewed in *Chapter 20 Transfusion Medicine*, the traditional agents for the rapid reversal of warfarin-induced coagulopathy have been vitamin K and fresh frozen plasma. More recently, *prothrombin complex concentrate (PCC) products* are available in a variety of formulations including 3 and 4 factor concentrates. PCC's contain Factor II, IX, X and small amounts of VII. The concentrate products are favored over FFP for high-risk bleeding such as intracerebral hemorrhage because they offer a more rapid reversal with a smaller volume of product delivery.[159] Recombinant Factor VIIa is not routinely recommended for reversal of oral anticoagulants.

For the direct oral anticoagulants (DOACs), a specific antidote exists for dabigatran (idarucizumab). Adexanet alfa is available for the direct factor Xa inhibitors (apixaban, betrixaban, edoxaban, and rivaroxaban). Additional unproven strategies include administration of an antifibrinolytic agent and drug removal from the gastrointestinal tract (activated charcoal). Non-specific agents including the prothrombin complex concentrates may be tried in severe cases of ICH but remain unproven. Consultation with hematology expertise is strongly advised.

Protamine sulfate should be administered to patients on therapeutic heparin complicated by ICH. Patients on antiplatelet medications without thrombocytopenia complicated by ICH do not benefit from platelet transfusions.[187]

Patients with a coagulation factor deficiency or thrombocytopenia should undergo appropriate factor replacement or platelet transfusion.

Despite the recognized bleeding risk, patients with ICH remain at risk for thromboembolic complications. Intermittent pneumatic compression with elastic stockings is advised for prevention of deep venous thrombosis. Low dose subcutaneous heparin may be considered after cessation of bleeding.

25.2.3 Elevated Intracranial Pressure

Patients with ICH are at risk for intracranial hypertension either from hydrocephalus or mass effect from the hematoma. The decision to introduce intracranial pressure monitoring is complicated by limited outcome data that defines the specific indications and benefits from this intervention. This intervention requires neurosurgical expertise. Basic measures to address elevated intracranial pressure (ICP) include:

- Head of bed elevation > 30 degrees
- Avoid any obstruction of cervical veins
- Use only isotonic fluids
- Mild sedation as required to limit agitation, coughing, gagging
- Control fever

Guidelines suggest patients with a GCS score < 8, with evidence for transtentorial herniation, significant intraventricular hemorrhage, or hydrocephalus are candidates for invasive monitoring.[185] A target cerebral perfusion pressure of 50 to 70 mm Hg may be an appropriate target to maintain. The role of surgical resection for expanding hematoma with mass effect remains uncertain. The exception may be patients with cerebellar hemorrhage with brainstem compression or hydrocephalus where surgical resection is favored.

Elevated ICP can be treated medically with either mannitol or hypertonic saline. Hyperosmotic therapy reduces brain volume by moving water from the brain parenchyma to the circulation and excreting it through the kidney. Mannitol has been the traditional agent for osmotic therapy in acute conditions. The medication is administered as a bolus of 0.25 to 1 g/kg. The dose may be repeated every 6 to 8 hours. The effects of mannitol are rapid in onset (i.e., minutes). The risks associated with mannitol administration include hypernatremia and renal dysfunction. In addition, the administration may be associated with hypotension and careful hemodynamic monitoring is needed to avoid a reduction in cerebral perfusion pressure during mannitol administration. A rebound adverse effect on cerebral edema following mannitol administration in cerebral edema is recognized.

Hypertonic saline is an alternative agent to mannitol for use as osmotic therapy. A variety of regimens have been proposed. Comparative clinical trials are reported but a concensus on the treatment duration and best agent to use for medical therapy of elevated intracranial pressure is not resolved.

25.3 Status Epilepticus

Generalized convulsive status epilepticus (GCSE) is a common neurologic emergency that warrants prompt recognition and treatment. GCSE is currently defined based upon two specific criteria:

1. ≥ 5 minutes of continuous seizures or
2. ≥ 2 discrete seizures between which there is an incomplete recovery of consciousness

The narrow time frame in this definition of GCSE provides focus on the need for emergent therapy to limit patient morbidity and mortality.

GCSE is characterized by generalized tonic-clonic movements of the extremities, mental status impairment, and possibly focal neurologic deficits. Additional "motor" forms of status epilepticus include focal motor status epilepticus, myoclonic status epilepticus, and tonic status epilepticus. Neurologic expertise will be required to assist with this differential which has prognostic significance. Of note, patients with focal status epilepticus may retain consciousness during periods of focal motor activity.

Other categories of sustained seizure activity include:

- Non-convulsive status epilepticus (NCSE) – refers to seizure activity on the EEG without the associated clinical findings that characterize GCSE.
- Refractory status epilepticus (RSE) – refers to patients that do not respond to standard treatment with continued clinical or electroencelphalographic seizures despite initial treatment.

The etiologies for seizure disorder can be grouped into major categories as outlined in **Figure 25-2.**

The diagnostic workup includes EEG monitoring even if GCSE is no longer evident. The EEG is necessary when the clinical features of GCSE have resolved to exclude nonconvulsive status epilepticus, and can include "spot" EEG or continuous EEG for patients that fail to awaken or show signs of ongoing seizure activity. Additional clinical workup attempts to address the underlying etiologies as outlined in **Figure 25-2.** A careful history of prior blood pressure treatment, past seizures, and medication or toxin exposure is required. In addition, CNS imaging and a comprehensive metabolic profile is warranted in all patients. Drug levels should be obtained urgently if the patient is taking anticonvulsant medication. Based upon the initial assessment a lumbar puncture with analysis of the cerebral spinal fluid indices can be diagnostic but will not be necessary in all patients.

The initial management of the patient with GCSE is focused on both diagnosis and treatment. The urgency to terminate seizure activity mandates that diagnostic testing not delay initial therapy. The initial resuscitation should focus on management issues common to all critically ill patients including airway control, ventilation, and hemodynamic resuscitation.

Acute Conditions	
	Acute structural brain injury – stroke, ischemia, or tumor CNS infection – meningoencephalitis, brain abscess, Lyme disease Drug toxicity or withdrawal – including alcohol, opioid, benzodiazepine Hypertensive encephalopathy Immune encephalitis – SLE, vasculitis Metabolic disturbances – hypoglycemia, low Na, low calcium Post-cardiac arrest, hypoxemia, hypoglycemia Stroke and neurovascular injury Traumatic brain injury
Chronic Conditions	
	Chronic alcohol use Remote structure brain injury – prior head trauma, benign brain tumors Pre-existing epilepsy – exacerbated by low blood concentrations of antiepileptic medications

Figure 25-2 Etiologies for GCSE.

The treatment of GCSE has been divided into three phases by the Neurocritical Care Society guidelines including emergent initial therapy, urgent control, and treatment of refractory disease.[188] For initial emergent therapy, benzodiazepines are the agent of choice. If IV access is available, lorazepam is the preferred agent. Alternative agents are based on the route of administration and include midazolam (intramuscular or nasal) or diazepam (rectal). The initial dose of IV lorazepam is 0.1 mg/kg up to a maximum of 4mg per dose. The treatment may be repeated every 5-10 min.

Following initial emergent therapy, urgent control of seizures in indicated with the most common regimens including phenytoin/fosphenytoin, valproate sodium, and levetiracetam. Few comparative studies exist to guide agent selection. Fosphenytoin/ phenytoin or levetiracetam may be considered the initial agent of choice in the majority of patients. The medicine is administered by IV infusion and a bolus is provided to rapidly achieve a therapeutic blood level. Generally speaking, fosphenytoin is favored over phenytoin due to a lower risk of adverse hemodynamics. Frequent cardiac and hemodynamic monitoring is indicated during the infusion of phenytoin/fosphenytoin.

For refractory status epilepticus, the key decision will be to increase dosing of the same anticonvulsant therapy or move to continuous intravenous infusion. The urgent control agents are most effective at seizure prevention rather than termination. For this reason, many neurologists turn to continuous infusion of midazolam, propofol, or pentobarbital in the setting of refractory status epilepticus.

A treatment algorithm for GCSE is outlined in **Figure 25-3**.

25.4 Acute Myasthenic Crisis

Acute myasthenic crisis refers to weakness from myasthenia gravis leading to respiratory failure with intubation or the requirement for non-invasive ventilation. Respiratory failure can manifest as a new requirement for mechanical ventilation or persistent ventilator dependence following surgery. Oropharyngeal (bulbar) muscle weakness often occurs in association with the respiratory muscle weakness leading to swallowing dysfunction and aspiration risk. The primary differential diagnosis for conditions leading to neuromuscular respiratory failure includes Guillain-Barre syndrome and amyotrophic lateral sclerosis (ALS).

The most common precipitant of myasthenic crisis is a concurrent infection. Other factors include surgical interventions, pregnancy, or tapering of immunosuppressive medications. A key element to consider as contributing to a myasthenic crisis are medications. **Figure 25-4** provides a list of medications that contribute to muscle weakness in patients with myasthenia gravis that should be avoided.

Patients with acute myasthenic crisis are admitted to an intensive care unit environment for close monitoring of respiratory and bulbar muscle function. Clinical signs of respiratory distress such as reduced respiratory effort, weak cough, swallowing dysfunction, or difficulty in speech can warn of impending respiratory failure. Dyspnea in this patient population is aggravated by the supine condition as the diaphragm is depending on gravity for optimal function.

Measurement of the vital capacity with a portable bedside spirometer provides an objective measure of respiratory muscle capacity independent of the clinical signs and symptoms. A vital capacity value < 30 ml/kg

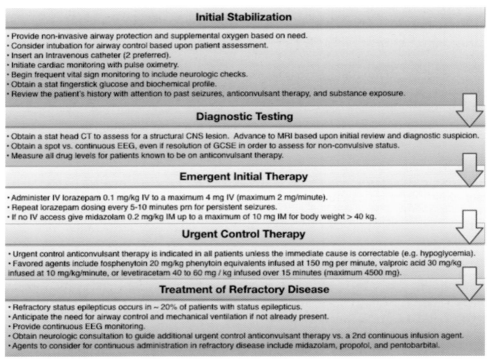

Initial Stabilization

- Provide non-invasive airway protection and supplemental oxygen based on need.
- Consider intubation for airway control based upon patient assessment.
- Insert an intravenous catheter (2 preferred).
- Initiate cardiac monitoring with pulse oximetry.
- Begin frequent vital sign monitoring to include neurologic checks.
- Obtain a stat fingerstick glucose and biochemical profile.
- Review the patient's history with attention to past seizures, anticonvulsant therapy, and substance exposure.

Diagnostic Testing

- Obtain a stat head CT to assess for a structural CNS lesion. Advance to MRI based upon initial review and diagnostic suspicion.
- Obtain a spot vs. continuous EEG, even if resolution of GCSE in order to assess for non-convulsive status.
- Measure all drug levels for patients known to be on anticonvulsant therapy.

Emergent Initial Therapy

- Administer IV lorazepam 0.1 mg/kg IV to a maximum 4 mg IV (maximum 2 mg/minute).
- Repeat lorazepam dosing every 5-10 minutes prn for persistent seizures.
- If no IV access give midazolam 0.2 mg/kg IM up to a maximum of 10 mg IM for body weight > 40 kg.

Urgent Control Therapy

- Urgent control anticonvulsant therapy is indicated in all patients unless the immediate cause is correctable (e.g. hypoglycemia).
- Favored agents include fosphenytoin 20 mg/kg phenytoin equivalents infused at 150 mg per minute, valproic acid 30 mg/kg infused at 10 mg/kg/minute, or levetiracetam 40 to 60 mg / kg infused over 15 minutes (maximum 4500 mg).

Treatment of Refractory Disease

- Refractory status epilepticus occurs in ~ 20% of patients with status epilepticus.
- Anticipate the need for airway control and mechanical ventilation if not already present.
- Provide continuous EEG monitoring.
- Obtain neurologic consultation to guide additional urgent control anticonvulsant therapy vs. a 2nd continuous infusion agent.
- Agents to consider for continuous administration in refractory disease include midazolam, propofol, and pentobarbital.

Figure 25-3 Treatment algorithm for generalized convulsive status epilepticus.

Anesthetic agents	Neuromuscular blocking agents
Antibiotics	Aminoglycosides, clindamycin,fluoroquinalones, ketolides, vancomycin
Cardiovascular medications	Beta-blockers, procainamide, quinidine
Misc medications	Botulinum toxin, chloroquine, hydroxychloroquine, magnesium, penicillamine, quinine, anti-PD-1 monoclonal antibodies

Figure 25-4 Medications associated with compromise of neuromuscular function in patients with myasthenia gravis.

measured in the sitting position suggests compromised respiratory function. Repeated measurements (i.e., every 2 hours) provide an objective trend in respiratory muscle capacity during treatment. This parameter, combined with clinical signs and symptoms, can suggest the need for elective endotracheal intubation.

Attention to airway hygiene is paramount and support with bronchodilators, chest physiotherapy, and "cough-assist" positive pressure therapy can help to limit the need for mechanical ventilation. Non-invasive ventilation can be considered for short-term use in myasthenia gravis patients that retain upper airway secretion control and can achieve a satisfactory interface with the mask. Prolonged use of non-invasive ventilation may further impair secretion clearance and should be avoided.

The treatment of myasthenic crisis is focused on two interventions:

1. Short-term – plasma exchange (PLEX) and intravenous immunoglobulin (IVIG) are effective therapies within days of institution. Plasma exchange removes acetylcholine receptor antibodies from the circulation. The beneficial effect is usually limited to a few weeks. Plasma exchange is typically provided as five exchanges on an alternate day interval over 10 days.

Alternatively, intravenous immunoglobulin is administered in the acute setting to treat myasthenic crisis. The mechanism of action for IVIG is believed to be a competitive inhibition of the myasthenia autoantibodies, but this is not confirmed.

Comparative trials between plasma exchange and IVIG do not favor one particular therapy, although consensus opinion suggests PLEX may achieve a faster therapeutic effect. The treatment decision is based on individual patient factors (e.g., PLEX is not used in patients with sepsis, IVIG is contraindicated in renal failure). PLEX requires a vascular access which introduces additional risk which can be minimized by using peripheral catheters if possible.

2. Long-term – sustained treatment in myasthenic crisis requires immunomodulatory therapy to limit the autoantibody production which sustains the disorder. High dose glucocorticoid therapy (e.g., prednisone 60-80 mg daily) is provided with an expected effect delayed for 2-3 weeks. This delayed onset of definitive treatment explains the need for a dual intervention (i.e., plasma exchange and corticosteroids). A transient worsening of neuromuscular function can occur with corticosteroid administration in these patients at day 5-10 in the treatment course but this effect is minimized with the short-term interventions. The initiation of corticosteroid therapy may be delayed initially to allow the short-term intervention to be effective.

Alternative immunosuppressive agents may be considered for long-term therapy including azathioprine, mycophenolate, and calcineurin inhibitors.

During any period of mechanical ventilation, cholinesterase inhibitor therapy used for the treatment of myasthenia gravis is discontinued to minimize excess respiratory secretions.

Suggested Reading

- Steiner T, Weitz JI, Veltkamp R. Anticoagulant-associated intracranial hemorrhage in the era of reversal agents. Stroke [Internet] 2018;48(5): 1432–7.
- Sanders, D. B. et al. International consensus guidance for management of myasthenia gravis: Executive summary. Neurology 87,419–25 (2016).

References

1. Seif D, Perera P, Mailhot T, et al. Bedside ultrasound in resuscitation and the rapid ultrasound in shock Protocol. Critical Care Res Pract Vol 2012:1-14

2. Levy MM, Fink MP, Marshall JC, et al. 2001 SCCM/ESICM/ACCP/ATS/SIS International sepsis definitions conference. Intensive Care Medicine 29(4):530–8.

3. Singer M, Deutschman CS, Seymour CW, et al. The Third International Consensus Definitions for Sepsis and Septic Shock (Sepsis-3). JAMA 2016;315(8):801–10

4. Ferreira FL, Bota DP, Bross A, et al. Serial evaluation of the SOFA score to predict outcome in critically ill patients. JAMA 2001;286(14):1754–8.

5. Cecconi M, Backer DD, Antonelli M, et al. Consensus on circulatory shock and hemodynamic monitoring. Task force of the European Society of Intensive Care Medicine. Intensive Care Medicine 2014;40(12):1795–815.

6. Robin ED. Dysoxia: Abnormal tissue oxygen utilization. Archives of Internal Medicine 1977;137(7):905–10.

7. Seymour CW, Gesten F, Prescott HC, et al. Time to treatment and mortality during mandated emergency care for sepsis. NEJM 2017; 376:2235–44.

8. Asfar P, Meziani F, Hamel J-F, et al. High versus low blood-pressure target in patients with septic shock. NEJM 2014;370(17):1583–93.

9. Mouncey PR, Osborn TM, Power SG, et al. Trial of early, goal-directed resuscitation for septic shock. NEUJM2015;372(14):1301–11.

10. The ProCESS Investigators. A randomized trial of protocol-based care for early septic shock. NEJM 2014;370(18):1683–93.

11. The ARISE Investigators and the ANZICS Clinical Trials Group. Goal-directed resuscitation for patients with early septic shock. NEJM 2014;371(16):1496-1506.

12. Marik PE, Linde-Zwirble WT, Bittner EA, et al. Fluid administration in severe sepsis and septic shock, patterns and outcomes: an analysis of a large national database. Intensive Care Med 2017;43(5):625–32.

13. Sadaka F, Juarez M, Naydenov S, et al. Fluid resuscitation in septic shock: the effect of increasing fluid balance on mortality. J Intensive Care Med 2014;29(4):213–7.

14. Leisman DE, Doerfler ME, Schneider SM, et al. Predictors, prevalence, and outcomes of early crystalloid responsiveness among initially hypotensive patients with sepsis and septic shock. Critical Care Medicine 2018;46(2):189–98.

15. Atkinson PR, Milne J, Diegelmann L, et al. Does point-of-care ultrasonography improve clinical outcomes in emergency department patients with undifferentiated hypotension? An international randomized controlled trial from the SHoC-ED Investigators. Ann Emerg Med. 2018; 72:478-489

16. Semler MW, Self WH, Wanderer JP, et al. Balanced crystalloids versus saline in critically ill adults. NEJM 2018;378(9):829–39.

17. Self WH, Semler MW, Wanderer JP, et al. Balanced crystalloids versus saline in noncritically ill adults. NEJM 2018;378(9):819–28.

18. Young P, Bailey M, Beasley R, et al. Effect of a buffered crystalloid solution vs saline on acute kidney injury among patients in the intensive care unit: The SPLIT randomized clinical trial. JAMA 2015;314(16):1701–10.

19. Yunos NM, Bellomo R, Hegarty C, et al. Association between a chloride-liberal vs chloride-restrictive intravenous fluid administration strategy and kidney injury in critically ill adults. JAMA 2012;308(15):1566–72.

20. The Safe Study Investigators. A comparison of albumin and saline for fluid resuscitation in the intensive care unit. NEJM;350(22):2247–56.

21. Caironi P, Tognoni G, Masson S, et al. Albumin replacement in patients with severe sepsis or septic shock. NEJM;370(15):1412–21.

22. Myburgh JA, Finfer S, Bellomo R, et al. Hydroxyethyl starch or saline for fluid resuscitation in intensive care. NEJM 2012;367(20):1901–11.

23. Backer D, Biston P, Devriendt J, et al. Comparison of dopamine and norepinephrine in the treatment of shock. NEJM;362(9):779–89.

24. Russell J, Walley K, Singer J, et al. Vasopressin versus norepinephrine infusion in patients with septic shock. NEJM 2008;358(9):877–887.

25. Vallée F, Vallet B, Mathe O, et al. Central venous-to-arterial carbon dioxide difference: an additional target for goal-directed therapy in septic shock? Intensive Care Medicine 2008;34(12):2218–25.

26. Marik PE, Bellomo R. Lactate clearance as a target of therapy in sepsis: a flawed paradigm. Critical Care 2103;01(1):1–6.

27. Kiyatkin ME, Bakker J. Lactate and microcirculation as suitable targets for hemodynamic optimization in resuscitation of circulatory shock. Current Opinion in Critical Care 2017;23(4):348.

28. Jones AE. Lactate clearance for assessing response to resuscitation in severe sepsis. Academic Emergency Medicine 2013;20:1-4.

29. Venkatesh B, Finfer S, Cohen J, et al. Adjunctive glucocorticoid therapy in patients with septic shock. NEJM 2018;378(9):797–808.

30. Annane D, Renault A, Brun-Buisson C, et al. Hydrocortisone plus fludrocortisone for adults with septic Shock. NEJM 2018;378(9):809–18.

31. Keh D, Trips E, Marx G, et al. Effect of hydrocortisone on development of shock among patients with severe sepsis: The HYPRESS Randomized Clinical Trial. JAMA 2016;316(17):1775–85.

32. Ferrer R, Martin-Loeches I, Phillips G, et al. Empiric antibiotic treatment reduces mortality in severe sepsis and septic shock from the first hour: results from a guideline-based performance improvement program. Crit Care Med 2014;42(8):1749–55.

33. Kalil AC, Metersky ML, Klompas M, et al. Management of adults with hospital-acquired and ventilator-associated pneumonia: 2016 clinical practice guidelines by the Infectious Diseases Society of America and the American Thoracic Society. Clin Infect Dis 2016;63(5):e61–e111.

34. Klompas M. Monotherapy Is adequate for septic shock due to gram-negative organisms. Crit Care Med 2017;45(11):1930-32.

35. Paul M, Lador A, Grozinsky-Glasberg S, et al. Beta lactam antibiotic monotherapy versus beta lactam-aminoglycoside antibiotic combination therapy for sepsis. Cochrane Database of Systematic Reviews (Online) 0AD;(1):CD003344.

36. Blomström-Lundqvist C, Scheinman MM, Aliot EM, et al. ACC/AHA/ESC guidelines for the management of patients with supraventricular arrhythmias — executive summary. Journal of the American College of Cardiology 2003;42(8):1493–531.

37. Olesen JB, Torp-Pedersen C, Hansen ML, et al. The value of the CHA2DS2-VASc score for refining stroke risk stratification in patients with atrial fibrillation with a CHADS2 score 0-1: a nationwide cohort study. Thromb Haemost 2012;107(6):1172–9.

38. Neumar RW, Shuster M, Callaway CW, et al. Part 1: Executive Summary 2015 American Heart Association guidelines update for cardiopulmonary resuscitation and emergency cardiovascular care. Circulation 2015;132(18 suppl 2):S315–67.

39. Andersen LW, Kurth T, Chase M, et al. Early administration of epinephrine (adrenaline) in patients with cardiac arrest with initial shockable rhythm in hospital: propensity score matched analysis. Brit Med J 2016;353:i1577

40. Dick WF, Eberle B, Wisser G, et al. The carotid pulse check revisited: what if there is no pulse? Critical Care Medicine ;28(11 Suppl):N183–5.

41. Littmann L, Bustin DJ, Haley MW. A simplified and structured teaching tool for the evaluation and management of pulseless electrical activity. Med Princ Pract 2013;23(1):1–6

42. Breitkreutz R, Walcher F, Seeger FH. Focused echocardiographic evaluation in resuscitation management: Concept of an advanced life support–conformed algorithm. Crit Care Medicine 2007;35(5):S150.

43. Jabre P, Penaloza A, Pinero D, et al. Effect of bag-mask ventilation vs endotracheal intubation during cardiopulmonary resuscitation on neurological outcome after out-of-hospital cardiorespiratory arrest: A randomized clinical trial. JAMA 2018;319(8):779–87.

44. Arrich J, Holzer M, Havel C, et al. Hypothermia for neuroprotection in adults after cardiopulmonary resuscitation. Cochrane Database of Systematic Reviews (Online) 2012;9:CD004128.

45. Nielsen N, Wetterslev J, Cronberg T, et al. Targeted temperature management at 33°C versus 36°C after cardiac arrest. NEJM 2013;369:2197-2206.

46. Coppler PJ, Elmer J, Calderon L, et al. Validation of the Pittsburgh cardiac arrest category illness severity score. Resuscitation 2015;89:86–92.

47. Bentzer P, Griesdale DE, Boyd J, et al. Will this hemodynamically unstable patient respond to a bolus of intravenous fluids? JAMA 2016;316(12):1298–309.

48. Connors AF, McCaffree DR, Gray BA. Evaluation of right-heart catheterization in the critically ill patient without acute myocardial infarction. NEJM 1983;308(5):263–7.

49. Rajaram SS, Desai NK, Kalra A, et al. Pulmonary artery catheters for adult patients in intensive care. Cochrane Database Syst Rev 2013;2(2):CD003408.

50. Wiener R, Welch GH. Trends in the use of the pulmonary artery catheter in the United States, 1993-2004. JAMA 2007;298(4):423–9.

51. Backer D De, Vincent J-L. Should we measure the central venous pressure to guide fluid management? Ten answers to 10 questions. Crit Care [Internet] 2018;22(1):43.

52. Jabot J, Teboul J-L, Richard C, Monnet X. Passive leg raising for predicting fluid responsiveness: importance of the postural change. Intensive Care Medicine 2009;35(1):85–90.

53. Monnet, X., Rienzo, M., Osman, D., et al. Passive leg raising predicts fluid responsiveness in the critically ill*. Critical Care Medicine, 2006;34: 1402.

54. Monnet, X., Osman, D., Ridel, C., et al. Predicting volume responsiveness by using the end-expiratory occlusion in mechanically ventilated intensive care unit patients. Critical Care Medicine 2009;37: 951–956.

55. Michard F, Boussat S, Chemla D, et al. Relation between respiratory changes in arterial pulse pressure and fluid responsiveness in septic patients with acute circulatory failure. AJRCCM 2000;162(1):134–8.

56. Hadian M, Kim HK, Severyn DA, Pinksy MR. Cross-comparison of cardiac output trending accuracy of LiDCO, PiCCO, FloTrac and pulmonary artery catheters. Critical Care 2010;14(6):1–10.

57. Marik PE, Cavallazzi R, Vasu T, et al. Dynamic changes in arterial waveform derived variables and fluid responsiveness in mechanically ventilated patients: A systematic review of the literature. Crit Care Medicine 2009;37(9):2642–7.

58. Ibarra-Estrada M, López-Pulgarín JA, et al. Respiratory variation in carotid peak systolic velocity predicts volume responsiveness in mechanically ventilated patients with septic shock: a prospective cohort study. Critical Ultrasound Journal 2015;7(1):29.

59. Vistisen ST, Juhl-Olsen P. Where are we heading with fluid responsiveness research? Current Opinion in Critical Care 2017;23(4):318–2

60. Hofmann R, James SK, Jernberg T, et al. Oxygen therapy in suspected acute myocardial infarction. NEJM, 2017;377:1240–1249.

61. O'Gara PT, Kushner FG, Ascheim DD, et al. 2013 ACCF/AHA guideline for the management of ST-elevation myocardial infarction. Circulation [Internet] 2013;127:e364-e425

62. Wiviott SD, Antman EM, Braunwald E. Prasugrel. Circulation 2010;122(4):394–403.

63. Bavry AA, Kumbhani DJ, Rassi AN, et al. Benefit of early invasive therapy in acute coronary syndromes: a meta-analysis of contemporary randomized clinical trials. JACC 2018;48(7):1319–25.

64. Antman EM, Cohen M, Bernink PJLM, et al. The TIMI risk score for unstable angina/non–ST eevation MI: A method for prognostication and therapeutic decision making. JAMA 2000;284(7):8

65. Lichtenstein DA. BLUE-Protocol and FALLS-Protocol Two Applications of lung ultrasound in the citically ill. Chest 2015;147(6):1659

66. Yancy CW, Jessup M, Bozkurt B, et al. 2013 ACCF/AHA Guideline for the management of heart failure: Executive Summary: A Report of the American College of Cardiology Foundation/American Heart Association Task Force on Practice Guidelines. Journal of the American College of Cardiology 2013;62(16):1495–539.

67. Pinsky MR. Cardiopulmonary interactions: physiologic basis and clinical applications. Annals of the American Thoracic Society 2018;15 (Supplement): S45-47

68. Ellison DH, Felker MG. Diuretic Treatment in heart failure. NEJM 2017;377(20):1964–75.

69. Felker MG, Lee KL, Bull DA, et al. Diuretic strategies in patients with acute decompensated heart failure. NEJM 2018;364(9):797–805.

70. Felker MG, Benza RL, Chandler BA, et al. Heart failure etiology and response to milrinone in decompensated heart failure: results from the OPTIME-CHF study. JACC 2018;41(6):997–1003.

71. Stamm JA, McVerry BJ, Mathier MA, et al. Doppler-defined pulmonary hypertension in medical intensive care unit patients: Retrospective investigation of risk factors and impact on mortality. Pulmonary Circulation 1(1):95–102.

72. Bull TM, Clark B, McFann K, et al. Pulmonary vascular dysfunction is associated with poor outcomes in patients with acute lung injury. Am J Resp Crit Care 2018;182(9):1123–8.

73. Khan AM, Cheng S, Magnusson M, et al. Cardiac natriuretic peptides, obesity, and insulin resistance: evidence from two community-based studies. Journal of Clinical Endocrinology and Metabolism 2011;96(10):3242–9.

74. Hrymak C, Strumpher J, Jacobsohn E. Acute right ventricle failure in the intensive care unit: assessment and management. Can J Cardiol [Internet] 2017;33(1):61–71

75. Lenfant C, Chobanian AV, Jones DW, et al. Seventh report of the Joint National Committee on the Prevention, Detection, Evaluation, and Treatment of High Blood Pressure (JNC 7): resetting the hypertension sails. Hypertension 2018;41(6):1178–9.

76. Sobrinho S, Correia L, Cruz C, et al. Occurrence rate and clinical predictors of hypertensive pseudocrisis in emergency room care. Arq Bras Cardiol 2007;88(5):579–84.

77. Czosnyka M, Miller C. Monitoring of cerebral autoregulation. Neurocritical Care 2014;21(S2):95–102.

78. Katz JN, Gore JM, Amin A, et al. Practice patterns, outcomes, and end-organ dysfunction for patients with acute severe hypertension: The Studying the Treatment of Acute HyperTension (STAT) Registry. American Heart Journal 2009;158(4):599–606.

79. Schwartz RB. Hyperperfusion encephalopathies: hypertensive encephalopathy and related conditions. Neurologist 2002;8(1):22–34

80. Jauch EC, Saver JL, Adams HP, et al. Guidelines for the early management of patients with acute ischemic stroke. Stroke 2013;44(3):870–947.

81. Anderson CS, Heeley E, Huang Y, et al. Rapid blood-pressure lowering in patients with acute intracerebral hemorrhage. NEJM 2013;368(25):2355–65.

82. Committee on Obstetric Practice. Emergent therapy for acute-onset, severe hypertension during pregnancy and the postpartum period. Obstetric Anesthesia Digest 2015;35(4):184.

83. Aronson S, Dyke CM, Levy JH, et al. Does perioperative systolic blood pressure variability predict mortality after cardiac surgery? An exploratory analysis of the ECLIPSE trials. Anesthesia and Analgesia 2011;113(1)

84. Goldhaber SZ, Visani L, Rosa MD, ICOPER F. Acute pulmonary embolism: clinical outcomes in the International Cooperative Pulmonary Embolism Registry (ICOPER). The Lancet 1999;353(9162):1386–9.

85. Kasper W, Konstantinides S, Geibel A, et al. Management strategies and determinants of outcome in acute major pulmonary embolism: Results of a multicenter registry. Journal of the American College of Cardiology 1997;30(5):1165–71.

86. Giusti G, Coerezza A, Cernuschi G. Clinical decision rules for excluding pulmonary embolism. Annals of Internal Medicine 2012;156(2):168.

87. Freund Y, Cachanado M, Aubry A, et al. Effect of the pulmonary embolism rule-out criteria on subsequent thromboembolic events among low-risk emergency department patients: The PROPER randomized clinical trial. JAMA 2018;319(6):559–66.

88. Donzé J, Gal G, Fine MJ, et al. Prospective validation of the Pulmonary Embolism Severity Index. Thrombosis and Haemostasis 2008;100(05):943–8.

89. Konstantinides SV. 2014 ESC Guidelines on the diagnosis and management of acute pulmonary embolism. Eur Heart J 2018;35(45):3145–6.

90. Jaff MR, McMurtry MS, Archer SL, et al. Management of massive and submassive pulmonary embolism, iliofemoral deep vein thrombosis, and chronic thromboembolic pulmonary hypertension. A scientific statement from the American Heart Association. Circulation 2011;123(16):1788–830.

91. Ikesaka R, Carrier M. Clinical significance and management of subsegmental pulmonary embolism. Journal of Thrombosis and Thrombolysis 2015;39(3):311–4.

92. Wan S, Quinlan DJ, Agnelli G, Eikelboom JW. Thrombolysis compared with heparin for the initial treatment of pulmonary embolism: A meta-analysis of the randomized controlled trials. Circulation 2004;110(6):744–9.

93. Skaf E, Beemath A, Siddiqui T, et al. Catheter-tip embolectomy in the management of acute massive pulmonary embolism. The American Journal of Cardiology 2007;99(3):415–20.

94. Kline JA, Steuerwald MT, Marchick MR, et al. Prospective evaluation of right ventricular function and functional status 6 months after acute submassive pulmonary embolism frequency of persistent or subsequent elevation in estimated pulmonary artery pressure. Chest 2009;136(5):1202–10.

95. Meyer G, Vicaut E, Danays T, et al. Fibrinolysis for patients with intermediate-risk pulmonary embolism. NEJM 2014;370(15):14

96. Weingart SD, Trueger NS, Wong N, et al. Delayed sequence intubation: A prospective observational study. Annals of Emergency Medicine 2015;65(4):349–355

97. Braude D, Richards M. Rapid Sequence Airway (RSA)—A novel approach to prehospital airway management. Prehospital Emergency Care 2009;11(2):250–2.

98. Rosenstock CV, Thøgersen B, Afshari A, et al. Awake fiberoptic or awake video laryngoscopic tracheal intubation in patients with anticipated difficult airway management: A randomized clinical trial. Anesthesiology 2012;116(6):1210.

99. Miguel-Montanes R, Hajage D, Messika J, et al. Use of high-flow nasal cannula oxygen therapy to prevent desaturation during tracheal intubation of intensive care patients with mild-to-moderate hypoxemia*. Critical Care Medicine 2015;43(3):574.

100. Vourc'h M, Asfar P, Volteau C, et al. High-flow nasal cannula oxygen during endotracheal intubation in hypoxemic patients: a randomized controlled clinical trial. Intensive Care Medicine 2015;41(9):1538–48.

101. Frat J-P, Thille AW, Mercat A, et al. High-flow oxygen through nasal cannula in acute hypoxemic respiratory failure. NEJM 2015;372:2185–96.

102. Force A, Ranieri MV, Rubenfeld GD, et al. Acute Respiratory Distress Syndrome: The Berlin Definition. JAMA 2012;307(23):2526–33.

103. ARDS Network. Ventilation with lower tidal volumes as compared with traditional tidal volumes for acute lung injury and the acute respiratory distress syndrome. NEJM 2000;342(18):1301–8.

104. Brower, R. G., Lanken, P. N., MacIntyre, N., et al. Higher versus lower positive end-expiratory pressures in patients with the acute respiratory distress syndrome. NEJM, 2004;351(4), 327–336.

105. Briel, M., Meade, M., Brower, R. G., et al. Higher vs lower positive end-expiratory pressure in patients with acute lung injury and acute respiratory distress syndrome: systematic review and meta-analysis. JAMA 2010;303(9), 865–873.

106. Calfee, C. S., Delucchi, K., Parsons, P. E., et al. Subphenotypes in acute respiratory distress syndrome: latent class analysis of data from two randomized controlled trials. The Lancet Respiratory Medicine, 2014:2(8), 611–620.

107. Talmor, D., Sarge, T., Malhotra, A., et al. Mechanical ventilation guided by esophageal pressure in acute lung Injury. NEJM 2008:359(20), 2095–2104.

108. Grasso S, Terragni P, Mascia L, et al. Airway pressure-time curve profile (stress index) detects tidal recruitment/hyperinflation in experimental acute lung injury. Critical Care Medicine 2004;32(4):1018.

109. Gattinoni L, Cressoni M. Quantitative CT in ARDS: towards a clinical tool? Intensive Care Medicine 2010;36(11):1803–4.

110. Amato MBP, Meade MO, Slutsky AS, et al. Driving pressure and survival in the acute respiratory distress syndrome. NEJM 2015;372(8):747–55.

111. Chiumello D, Cressoni M, Carlesso E, et al. Bedside selection of positive end-expiratory pressure in mild, moderate, and severe acute respiratory distress syndrome. Crit Care Med 2014:42(2):252–64.

112. ARDSNet. Wiedemann HP, Wheeler AP, et al. Comparison of two fluid-management strategies in acute lung injury. NEJM; 2006;354(24):2564–75.

113. NHLBI PETAL Clinical Trials Network. Early Neuromuscular Blockade in the Acute Respiratory Distress Syndrome. N Engl J Med 2019;380:1997–2008.

114. Guérin C, Reignier J, Richard J-C, et al. Prone positioning in severe acute respiratory distress syndrome. NEJM 2013;368(23):2159–68.

115. Sud S, Friedrich JO, Adhikari NKJ, et al. Effect of prone positioning during mechanical ventilation on mortality among patients with acute respiratory distress syndrome: a systematic review and meta-analysis. Canadian Medical Association Journal 2014;186(10):E381–90.

116. Pham T, Combes A, Rozé H, et al. Extracorporeal membrane oxygenation for pandemic influenza A(H1N1)–induced acute respiratory distress syndrome. American Journal of Respiratory and Critical Care Medicine 2013;187(3):276–85.

117. Cooke CR, Shah CV, Gallop R, et al. A simple clinical predictive index for objective estimates of mortality in acute lung injury*. Critical Care Medicine 2009;37(6):1913.

118. Herridge MS, Tansey CM, Matté A, et al. Functional disability 5 Years after acute respiratory distress syndrome. NEJM 2011;364(14):1293–304.

119. Ambrosino N, Vagheggini G. Non-invasive ventilation in exacerbations of COPD. International Journal of Chronic obstructive pulmonary disease 2007;2(4):471–6

120. Hill NS, Brennan J, Garpestad E, et al. Noninvasive ventilation in acute respiratory failure. Critical Care Medicine 2007;35(10):2402

121. Vogelmeier CF, Criner GJ, Martinez FJ, et al. Global strategy for the diagnosis, management, and prevention of chronic obstructive lung disease 2017 report. GOLD Executive Summary. American Journal of Respiratory and Critical Care Medicine 2017;195(5):557–82.

122. Jong YP de, Uil SM, Grotjohan HP, et al. Oral or IV prednisolone in the treatment of COPD exacerbations. Chest 2007;132(6):1741–7.

123. Niewoehner DE, Erbland ML, Deupree RH, et al. Effect of systemic glucocorticoids on exacerbations of chronic obstructive pulmonary disease. NEJM 1999;340(25):1941–7.

124. Leuppi JD, Schuetz P, Bingisser R, et al. Short-term vs conventional glucocorticoid T\therapy in acute exacerbations of chronic bbstructive pulmonary disease: The REDUCE randomized clinical trial. JAMA 2013;309(21):2223–31.

125. Rodrigo G, Pollack C, Rodrigo C, et al. Heliox for nonintubated acute asthma patients. The Cochrane Library 2003;(1). 2003, Issue 2. Art. No.: CD00288

126. Wildman MJ, Sanderson C, Groves J, et al. Implications of prognostic pessimism in patients with chronic obstructive pulmonary disease (COPD) or asthma admitted to intensive care in the UK within the COPD and asthma outcome study (CAOS): multicentre observational cohort study. BMJ 2007;335(7630):1132.

127. Girard TD, Kress JP, Fuchs BD, et al. Efficacy and safety of a paired sedation and ventilator weaning protocol for mechanically ventilated patients in intensive care (Awakening and Breathing Controlled trial): a randomised controlled trial. The Lancet 2008;371(9607):126–34.

128. Esteban A, Frutos F, Tobin MJ, et al. A comparison of four methods of weaning patients from mechanical ventilation. NEJM 1995;332(6):345–50.

129. Ely EW, Bennett PA, Bowton DL, et al. Large scale implementation of a respiratory therapist– driven protocol for ventilator weaning. American Journal of Respiratory and Critical Care Medicine 1999;159(2):439–46.

130. Yang KL, Tobin MJ. A prospective study of indexes predicting the outcome of trials of weaning from mechanical ventilation. NEJM 1991;324(21):1445–50.

131. Epstein S. Decision to extubate. Intensive Care Medicine 2002;28(5):535–46

132. Esteban A, Frutos-Vivar F, Ferguson ND, et al. Noninvasive positive-pressure ventilation for respiratory failure after extubation. NEJM 2004;350(24):2452–60.

133. Burns KE, Meade MO, Premji A, et al. Noninvasive positive pressure ventilation as a weaning strategy for intubated adults with respiratory failure. The Cochrane Database of Systematic Reviews 2013;12:CD004127.

134. Thille AW, Boissier F, Ben-Ghezala H, et al. Easily identified at-risk patients for extubation failure may benefit from noninvasive ventilation: a prospective before-after study. Critical Care 2016;20(1):48.

135. Kress JP, Pohlman AS, O'Connor MF, Hall JB. Daily interruption of sedative infusions in critically ill patients undergoing mechanical ventilation. NEJM 2000;342(20):1471–7.

136. Mehta S, Burry L, Cook D, et al. Daily sedation interruption in mechanically ventilated critically ill patients cared for with a sedation protocol: a randomized controlled trial. JAMA 2012;308(19):1985–92.

137. Strøm T, Martinussen T, Toft P. A protocol of no sedation for critically ill patients receiving mechanical ventilation: a randomized trial. Lancet 2018;375(9713):475–80

138. Plaschke K, Haken RV, Scholz M, et al. Comparison of the confusion assessment method for the intensive care unit (CAM-ICU) with the Intensive Care Delirium Screening Checklist (ICDSC) for delirium in critical care patients gives high agreement rate(s). Intensive Care Medicine 2008;34(3):431

139. Girard TD, Exline MC, Carson SS, et al. Haloperidol and ziprasidone for treatment of delirium in critical illness. NEJM 2018;379: 2506-2516.

140. Schweickert WD, Pohlman MC, Pohlman AS, et al. Early physical and occupational therapy in mechanically ventilated, critically ill patients: a randomised controlled trial. The Lancet 2005;373(9678):1874–82.

141. Needham DM, Korupolu R, Zanni JM, et al. Early physical medicine and rehabilitation for patients with acute respiratory failure: A quality improvement project. Archives of Physical Medicine and Rehabilitation 2010;91(4):536–42.

142. Morris PE, Berry MJ, Files DC, et al. Standardized rehabilitation and hospital length of stay among patients With acute respiratory railure: A randomized clinical trial. JAMA 2016;315(24):2694–702.

143. Wright SE, Thomas K, Watson G, et al. Intensive versus standard physical rehabilitation therapy in the critically ill (EPICC): a multicentre, parallel-group, randomised controlled trial. Thorax 2018;73(3):213–21.

144. Huang H, Li Y, Ariani F, Chen X, Lin J. Timing of tracheostomy in critically ill patients: A meta-analysis. PLoS ONE 2014;9(3):e92981.

145. Pollack CV, Reilly PA, Eikelboom J, et al. Idarucizumab for dabigatran reversal. NEJM 2015;373(6):511–20.

146. Hook KM, Abrams CS. The loss of homeostasis in hemostasis: New approaches in treating and understanding acute disseminated intravascular coagulation in critically ill patients. Clinical and Translational Science 2012;5(1):85–92.

147. Koyfman A, Brém E, Chiang VW. Thrombotic thrombocytopenic purpura. Pediatric Emergency Care 2011;27(11):1085.

148. Erkan D, Espinosa G, Cervera R. Catastrophic antiphospholipid syndrome: Updated diagnostic algorithms. Autoimmunity Reviews 2010;10(2):74–9.

149. Lelubre C, Vincent J-L. Red blood cell transfusion in the critically ill patient. Annals of Intensive Care 2011;1(1):1–9.

150. Hebert P, Wells G, Blachman M, Marshall J. Transfusion requirements in critical care: A multicentre randomized controlled clinical trial Hebert PC, Wells G, Blajchman MA, et al. N Engl J Med 340:409–417, 1999. New England Journal of Medicine 1999;340(3):409–17.

151. Villanueva C, Colomo A, Bosch A, et al. Transfusion strategies for acute upper gastrointestinal bleeding. NEJM 2013;368(1):11–21.

152. Holst LB, Haase N, Wetterslev J, et al. Lower versus higher hemoglobin threshold for transfusion in septic shock. NEJM 2014;371(15):1381–91.

153. Koch CG, Li L, Sessler DI, et al. Duration of red-cell storage and complications after cardiac surgery. NEJM 2008;358(12):1229–39.

154. Cooper DJ, McQuilten ZK, Nichol A, et al. Age of red cells for transfusion and outcomes in critically ill adults. NEJM 2017;377(19):1858–67.

155. Lacroix J, Hébert PC, Fergusson DA, et al. Age of transfused blood in critically ill adults. NEJM 2015;372(15):1410–8.

156. Zilberberg MD, Carter C, Lefebvre P, et al. Red blood cell transfusions and the risk of acute respiratory distress syndrome among the critically ill: a cohort study. Critical Care 2007;11(3):1–9.

157. Chaiwat O, Lang JD, Vavilala MS, et al. Early packed red blood cell transfusion and acute respiratory distress syndrome after trauma. Anesthesiology 2009;110(2):351.

158. Simpson E, Lin Y, Stanworth S, et al. Recombinant factor VIIa for the prevention and treatment of bleeding in patients without haemophilia. The Cochrane Database of Systematic Reviews 2012;3:CD005011.

159. Sarode R, Milling TJ, Refaai MA, et al. Efficacy and safety of a 4-Factor prothrombin complex concentrate in patients on vitamin K antagonists presenting with major bleeding. A randomized, plasma-controlled, Phase IIIb study. Circulation 2013;128(11):1234–43.

160. Khwaja A. KDIGO clinical practice guidelines for acute kidney injury. Nephron Clinical Practice 2012;120(4):c179–84.

161. Liaño F, Pascual J, et al. Epidemiology of acute renal failure: A prospective, multicenter, community-based study. Kidney International 1996;50(3):811–8.

162. Chowdhury AH, Cox EF, Francis ST, et al. A randomized, controlled, double-blind crossover study on the effects of 2-L infusions of 0.9% saline and plasma-lyte® 148 on renal blood flow velocity and renal cortical tissue perfusion in healthy volunteers. Annals of Surgery 2012;256(1):18.

163. Vincent J-L, Backer DD. Saline versus balanced solutions: are clinical trials comparing two crystalloid solutions really needed? Critical Care 2016;20(1):250.

164. Garcia Martinez R, Caraceni P, Bernardi M, et al. Albumin: Pathophysiologic basis of its role in the treatment of cirrhosis and its complications. Hepatology 2013;58(5):1836–46.

165. Prowle JR, Kirwan CJ, Bellomo R. Fluid management for the prevention and attenuation of acute kidney injury. Nature Reviews Nephrology 2013;10(1):232.

166. Tao SM, Wichmann JL, Schoepf UJ, et al. Contrast-induced nephropathy in CT: incidence, risk factors and strategies for prevention. European Radiology 2016;26(9):3310–8.

167. Solomon R, Gordon P, Manoukian SV, et al. Randomized trial of bicarbonate or saline study for the prevention of contrast-induced nephropathy in patients with CKD. Clinical Journal of the American Society of Nephrology 2015;10(9):1519–24.

168. Gaudry S, Hajage D, Schortgen F, et al. Initiation strategies for renal-replacement therapy in the intensive care unit. NEJM 2016;375(2):122–33.

169. Renal Replacement Study Investigators, Bellomo R, Cass A, et al. Intensity of continuous renal-replacement therapy in critically ill patients. NEJM 2009;361(17):1627–38.

170. Palevsky PM, Zhang JH, et al. Intensity of renal support in critically ill patients with acute kidney injury. NEJM 2008;359(1):7–20.

171. Stanley AJ, Laine L, Dalton HR, et al. Comparison of risk scoring systems for patients presenting with upper gastrointestinal bleeding: international multicentre prospective study. BMJ 2017;356:i6432

172. Rockall TA, Logan RF, Devlin HB, et al. Risk assessment after acute upper gastrointestinal haemorrhage. Gut 1996;38(3):316–21.

173. Leontiadis GI, Sharma VK, Howden CW. Proton pump inhibitor therapy for peptic ulcer bleeding: Cochrane Collaboration Meta-analysis of Randomized Controlled Trials. Mayo Clinic Proceedings 2007;82(3):286–96.

174. Sachar H, Vaidya K, Laine L. Intermittent vs continuous proton pump inhibitor therapy for high-risk bleeding ulcers: A systematic review and meta-analysis. JAMA Internal Medicine 2014;174(11):1755–62

175. Barkun AN, Bardou M, Martel M, Gralnek IM, Sung JJY. Prokinetics in acute upper GI bleeding: a meta-analysis. Gastrointestinal Endoscopy 2010;72(6):1138–45.

176. Szura M, Pasternak A. Upper non-variceal gastrointestinal bleeding - review the effectiveness of endoscopic hemostasis methods. World Journal of Gastrointestinal Endoscopy 2015;7(13):1088–95.

177. Chavez Tapia NC, Barrientos Gutierrez T, Tellez Avila F, et al. Meta analysis: antibiotic prophylaxis for cirrhotic patients with upper gastrointestinal bleeding – an updated Cochrane review. Alimentary Pharmacology & Therapeutics 2011;34(5):509–18.

178. Garcia-Tsao G, Sanyal AJ, Grace ND, et al. Prevention and management of gastroesophageal varices and variceal hemorrhage in cirrhosis. The American Journal of Gastroenterology 2007;102:2086–2102

179. Bañares R, Albillos A, Rincón D, et al. Endoscopic treatment versus endoscopic plus pharmacologic treatment for acute variceal bleeding: A meta analysis. Hepatology 2002;35(3):609–15.

180. ASGE Standards of Practice Committee, Pasha SF, Shergill A, et al. The role of endoscopy in the patient with lower GI bleeding. Gastrointestinal Endoscopy 2014;79(6):875–85.

181. Levine M, Brooks DE, Truitt CA, Wolk BJ, Boyer EW, Ruha A-M. Toxicology in the ICU part 1: General overview and approach to treatment. Chest 2011;140(3):795–806.

182. Hacke W, Kaste M, Bluhmki E, et al. Thrombolysis with alteplase 3 to 4.5 hours after acute ischemic stroke. NEJM 2008;359(13):1317–29.

183. Tissue plasminogen activator for acute ischemic stroke. NEJM 1995;333(24):1581–8.

184. Powers WJ, Rabinstein AA, Ackerson T, et al. Guidelines for the early management of patients with acute ischemic stroke. Stroke 2018;49(3): e46-e256

185. Hemphill JC, Greenberg SM, Anderson CS, et al. Guidelines for the management of spontaneous intracerebral hemorrhage. Stroke 2015;46:2032-2060

186. Anderson CS, Heeley E, Huang Y, et al. Rapid blood-pressure lowering in patients with acute intracerebral hemorrhage. NEJM 2013; 368(25):2355–65

187. Baharoglu IM, Cordonnier C, Salman R, et al. Platelet transfusion versus standard care after acute stroke due to spontaneous cerebral hemorrhage associated with antiplatelet therapy (PATCH): a randomized, open-label, phase 3 trial. The Lancet 2016; 387(10038):2605–13.

188. Brophy GM, Bell R, Classen J. et al. Guidelines for the evaluation and management of status epilepticus. Neurocrit Care 17, 3–23 (2012).

Index

chylothorax 16
cisatracurium 230-1, 244, 263
clevidipine 127, 143-6, 150
clonidine 145, 149
clopidogrel 104, 127-8, 112, 114, 292, 203
clotting cascade 283, 300
coagulopathy 249, 281, 294-5, 299, 351
cocaine 104, 125, 141, 149, 332, 337,
    339, 344
colloids 45
colonoscopy 317-8
comet tails 31, 118
compliance/elastance 199
computed tomographic pulmonary
    angiogram 157
congestive heart failure 2, 10, 16, 19-20,
    23, 61, 67, 106, 121, 224, 269, 302
constrictive pericarditis 16, 80, 86, 91
continuous positive airway pressure
    120-2, 179, 221-4, 241, 270-1
continuous renal replacement
    therapy 308
contraction alkalosis 335
contrast nephropathy 304
contrast-induced AKI 305
control breaths 208-227, 237, 248-9, 265
control ventilation 211, 220-4, 237,
    249, 265
coronary artery bypass grafting 112
coronary thrombosis 72, 103, 108-12,
    119, 127, 135, 246, 251, 284-293, 300,
    318, 344, 349-51, 361
corticosteroids in COPD 251, 263-7,
counter-pulsation 124
CPAP 120-3, 159, 171, 179, 221-5, 247-8,
    270-2
CPR 69-78, 192
crash intubation 168
cryoprecipitate 287, 290, 295-300, 349
crystalloids 45, 358
CT angiogram 132, 154, 157-9
CTPA 157
Cushing syndrome 141
CvO2 41, 43, 49-53, 93, 180-1, 226, 243-4
CVP waveform 84
cyanide 122, 144, 329, 340

D
D-dimer 155-7, 161, 290
DAPT 103, 107-113, 122, 214, 264, 274, 317
decannulation 280, 182
decubitus ulcer 3
deep venous thrombosis 36-7, 246,
    349-71
deep Y or X descent 86
defibrillators 56, 62, 70-1
delirium 3, 275-82, 338, 342-46, 364
delta gap 325-6, 330
demand ischemia 119

denitrogenation 171
diabetes mellitus 3, 67, 104-5, 115, 335
diabetic ketoacidosis 329, 331, 339
dialysis therapy 301, 306, 308
diastolic pressure augmentation 124
difficult intubation 168-70
digoxin 61-5, 127, 340
diltiazem 58, 61-2, 104, 127, 343
dilutional coagulopathy 295
direct factor Xa inhibitors 285, 351
direct thrombin (IIa) inhibitors 185
Disseminated Intravascular
    Coagulation (DIC) 272, 290, 299
distended bladder 34-5, 302
distributive shock 80, 94
diverticular bleeding 317
DKA 168, 331-4
DO2 41, 49-53, 92, 96, 182
dobutamine 40, 48-9, 120, 123-4, 135-39,
    160
dopamine 40, 47-9, 78, 145, 272, 305,
    339, 344 -6, 358
Doppler echocardiography 98
driving pressure 201, 213-4, 241, 362
drug overdose 194, 253, 290, 324, 337-46
dual anti-platelet therapy (DAPT) 107
dynamic hyperinflation 72-5, 91, 201-3,
    208-13, 224, 253-73

E
echocardiography 232, 242, 30, 45, 72,
    96, 98, 100, 105, 119, 128, 131, 159
eclampsia 140-2, 149-50, 292
ECMO 136, 139, 162, 249-50
ECMO 136, 139, 162, 249-50
Effient 114
effusions 4-5, 16-9, 23, 116, 200, 232
electrical cardioversion 61-2, 67, 127
elevated intracranial pressure 148, 172-
    3, 272, 351-2
empyema 16-7
enalapril 145
end-expiratory occlusion pressure 258
end-tidal CO2 69-70, 76, 174, 192
endoglin 1 129
endothelin A and B receptor
    blockers 137
endothelin pathway 135
endothelin receptor antagonists 136
endotracheal intubation 3, 65-6, 168-76,
    205, 234, 264, 281, 314, 354, 359, 362
endotracheal tube 5-6, 13, 17-8, 60, 65-6,
    170-6, 192-4, 203, 208, 218, 221, 234,
    245, 258, 262, 266, 269-282
enoxaparin 108-9, 112, 114, 284
EPAP 223-4, 264
epinephrine 3, 47-51, 72-5, 94, 123-4,
    160, 171, 174, 227, 265, 272, 304, 313,
    317, 328-9, 344-5, 358-9

epoprostenol 136-9, 245-6
eptifibatide 107
equation of motion 196-202, 210-11
esmolol 61, 127, 144, 147
esophageal balloon 100, 240, 315-6
esophageal Doppler 98, 101
esophageal perforation 16, 316
ETA blockers 62, 136, 343
ethylene glycol intoxication 330, 343
etomidate 123, 172-3, 176
expiratory airway occlusion 258, 260
extrinsic pathway 283, 287, 290
exudate 16, 147
exudative effusion 16-7

F
Factor Xa inhibitors 67, 108, 285, 251
Fast Flush Test 81-2
fibrin-rich clots 107
FiO2 4, 187, 219
flat line 75
Flolan 137
flow-based triggering 207-8
fondaparinux 108-9, 112-4, 286, 289-10
four-factor prothrombin complex
    concentrate 300
fresh frozen plasma 286, 294-5, 299, 312
furosemide 121-3, 139
fusion beats 60

G
gap analysis 338
gastric varices 316
gastrointestinal bleeding 107, 295, 310-
    18, 364-6
GCS 5, 77, 352-3
Geneva Score 156
giant V waves 86
Glasgow Coma Scale 77
Guillain-Barre syndrome 141, 353

H
head tilt-chin lift maneuver 165-6
heart block 58, 86, 104, 145
heart failure 2-23, 48, 6-8, 61-7, 72, 79,
    82, 88-94, 114-9, 104-9, 115-163, 224-9,
    269, 302, 329, 336, 360
heart failure with reduced ejection
    fraction 115, 119
HELLP syndrome 292
hemodynamic monitoring 3, 34, 45, 79-
    100, 119, 133-4, 141-2, 352-3, 357
hemolytic uremic syndrome 291-2
hemophilia A 286, 299
hemophilia B 286
hemothorax 16
Henderson-Hasselbalch equation 177, 320
heparin-induced thrombocytopenia
    (HIT) 160, 288, 299